THE CLINICAL MANAGEMENT
OF
BASIC MAXILLOFACIAL
ORTHOPEDIC APPLIANCES

VOLUME II: DIAGNOSTICS

Terrance J. Spahl, DDS

in collaboration with
and presenting the case studies of

John W. Witzig, DDS

PSG PUBLISHING COMPANY, INC.
LITTLETON, MASSACHUSETTS

Library of Congress Cataloging-in-Publication Data
(Revised for vol. 2)

Spahl, Terrance J.
    The clinical management of basic maxillofacial
orthopedic appliances.

    Includes bibliographies and indexes.
    Contents: v. 1. Mechanics—v. 2. Diagnostics.
    1. Orthodontic appliances. I. Witzig, John W.
II. Title. [DNLM: 1. Orthodontic Appliances.
WU 400 S733c]
RK527.S63   1987   617.6′43   86-91476
ISBN 0-88416-558-2 (v. 1)
ISBN 0-88416-559-0 (v. 2)

Published by:
PSG PUBLISHING COMPANY, INC.
545 Great Road
Littleton, Massachusetts 01460

International Standard Book Number: 0-88416-559-0

Library of Congress Catalog Card Number: 86-91476

9 8 7 6 5 4 3 2 1

To Hans Peter Bimler

ABOUT THE AUTHORS

Terrance J. Spahl, D.D.S. has been in private practice in St. Paul, Minnesota since 1971. He is a dental products consultant for the 3M Company and Ohlendorf Company Orthodontic Laboratory, and a clinical consultant for Ortho-Diagnostics Ltd.

Dr. Spahl is principal author of *The Clinical Management of Basic Maxillofacial Appliances, Volume I: Mechanics* and has published numerous papers in the field of orthodontics. He has lectured widely to dental and medical groups on the subject of the temporomandibular joint and co-developed the Witzig-Spahl Analysis, the first computerized method for analyzing TMJ x-rays.

A clinician with extensive orthodontic and TMJ experience, Dr. Spahl has studied under noted experts in the United States and abroad. He is a member of the American Equilibration Society, the American Endodontic Society, the American Dental Association, the American Academy of General Dentistry, and the American Association of Functional Orthodontics.

John W. Witzig, D.D.S. maintains a private practice devoted exclusively to orthodontics and TMJ pain patients, in Minneapolis, Minnesota. He is regional editor of *The Journal of Cranio–Mandibular Practice* and contributing editor to *The Functional Orthodontist*.

Dr. Witzig is author of *Orthodontic and Orthopedic Appliances* and co-author of *The Clinical Management of Basic Maxillofacial Orthopedic Appliances, Volume I: Mechanics, Orthodontics and Its Effect on the TMJ*, and *Clinical Management of TMJ Pain*. He developed and patented the Orthopedic Corrector I Appliance and the Orthopedic Corrector II Appliance and is co-holder of the U.S. patent on the Sagittal III Appliance. Dr. Witzig is a member of the American Equilibration Society, the American Association of Functional Orthodontics, the European Orthodontic Society, the International Association of Orthodontics, and the American Dental Association.

An experienced clinician who has studied in the United States and Europe, he was honored as "Man of the Year" in 1984 by the American Association of Functional Orthodontics. Since 1972, Dr. Witzig has conducted dental education courses for more than 20,000 doctors in North America.

CONTENTS

Foreword **vii**

Preface **ix**

Acknowledgments **xii**

Section I Cephalometrics

1 On the Way **1**

2 The Early Architects **26**

3 The Knights of Euclid **117**

4 The Apostles of Charm **168**

5 The New Breed **294**

References Section I **367**

Section II Sequential Treatment

6 Sequential Treatment **381**

7 Appliance Sequencing in Conventional Treatment: Class I Malocclusions **422**

8 Class II Malocclusions **479**

9 Class III Adult Dentition Treatment **585**

10   The Final Steps   **590**

11   Interlude   **599**

References   Section II   **607**

Index   **609**

FOREWORD

In any type of orthodontic treatment, it is extremely important to make the proper diagnosis. But the question always comes up, with so many different concepts of diagnosis and philosophies of treatment out there, where does one start to weed out the sound concepts from the others? A practitioner must never be restricted to one diagnostic process, one therapeutic method, or one appliance system, nor can one expect to be able to apply the limited spectrum of such a singular approach to every patient that presents for treatment. A broad base is now required in both diagnosis and treatment methodologies.

At last there is a book on diagnosis and treatment techniques that *does not preach one diagnostic method or treatment philosophy*! This second book by Drs Spahl and Witzig on diagnosis and treatment planning is truly unique! In one book, it explains practically every commonly used clinically oriented cephalometric diagnostic method in great detail, from those of the original pioneers to several of the most recent methods. Early in the book, the anatomical and cephalometric landmarks of the skull are defined and well illustrated so the reader can understand the "language of cephalometrics."

Section I of this text deals with a clinician's view of cephalometrics. The text's principle author, Dr Spahl, has gone to great lengths to explain each analysis as it was intended to be used by its originator. He then goes on to explain these analyses with respect to their strong points and also their limitations. In many cases, comparisons are made between analyses to help the reader understand the differences. And for the first time the concept of temporomandibular joint protection and facial esthetics has finally been accorded its proper position of prominence in the orthodontic diagnostic and treatment-planning process.

In section II of the book, Sequential Treatment, the application of the previously discussed cephalometric analyses is demonstrated in the diagnosis and treatment of Class I, II-1, II-2, and III malocclusions. Treatment of the basic components of these commonly seen types of malocclusions in the primary, mixed, and adult dentitions is explained in detail.

I have never read any other book that explains such a broad and complex subject so clearly and yet so thoroughly. In the flowing style characteristic of Volume I, Dr Spahl goes into great detail in such a way as to hold the reader's attention, whether he or she is a new graduate or a seasoned practitioner with many years of experience. Not only is it an excellent textbook, but I am convinced it will continue to be an excellent reference book for decades to come.

Grant R. N. Bowbeer, DDS, MS

PREFACE

For those involved in the treatment of malocclusion, there is no excuse for being cephalometrically illiterate. The state of the art of maxillofacial orthodontic and orthopedic therapeutics has evolved to a level at which comprehensive cephalometric analysis of both dental and osseous structures has become critical to the successful resolution of the case. This is especially true now, when the powers of the treating clinician include the ability to effect wholesale orthopedic alterations of the *maxilla*, mandible, and temporomandibular joints. No longer will traditional cephalometric standards suffice that merely concern themselves with alignments of anterior teeth or the angulation of the dental occlusal plane. Although important, these considerations have now been relegated to a role accessory to the more important considerations of the orthopedic demands of the case. The location of the maxilla, its influence on the location and action of the mandible through the medium of the teeth, and the interrelated action of these entities on the all-important functional integrity of the temporomandibular joints are paramount concerns that any responsible clinician must directly address in every treatment plan. Yet pursuit of academic knowledge and clinical skills in the cephalometric component of the diagnostic process has always been looked upon as an endeavor fraught with the problems of wading through and deciphering copious amounts of unmanageable and/or clinically irrelevant information and data. Well, in the words of the great American composer George Gershwin, "It ain't necessarily so!"

At first glance the discipline of cephalometrics appears not only didactic and authoritarian but also conceptually amorphous. However there is a story-line here, and once the general evolutionary plot is deciphered, new meaning and clarity to the subject emerge. Although there are a variety of texts that address this subject, they are, unfortunately, limited in scope, a shortcoming that contributes to the confusion. Cephalometrics is, indeed, a language, and as such, it is governed by its own set of rules, just as any other language is governed by rules of spelling, punctuation, and grammar. What has been lacking until now is an attempt not only to explain the details of the science, but also to place these details in their proper perspective in the overall scheme of things. It must be emphasized that the cephalometric language must not only be read but also properly interpreted. The diagnostician must be able not only to determine what the cephalometric analysis says, but also what it means.

In order for proper interpretation to be possible, consideration must be given to the significance a variety of factors may have on the ultimate meaning of compilations of cephalometric information. By virtue of their geometric designs, a certain mathematical bias may occur with respect to some components of certain analyses. The validity of statistical data bases or sample sizes may be of significance. One must be able to determine whether or not certain cephalometric analysis techniques reveal findings that are, in fact, compatible with Nature and the knowledge we have of how components of the maxillofacial complex actually grow and develop. Additionally, the clinician must determine if the standards and/or norms of a given analysis can serve as a proper treatment goal for a given patient, ie, will the needs of the patient tolerate the dictates of certain so-called ideal normative cephalometric standards.

What we have attempted to achieve in this text is a brief survey of the anatomy and methods of growth of the major bony components of the maxillofacial complex in order to give the reader a feel for what we know to be happening in Nature. We have then surveyed the languid and meandering path that cephalometric analysis has taken from its inception to the present day. Of course, we emphasize the clinical aspects of cephalometrics and have selected commonly known analyses that are representative of a given philosophy or the period of time in which they were developed. This is why the reader will note a difference in the artistic styles of the cephalometric drawings that appear throughout the text. Where a specific analysis is discussed in detail, every effort was made to use the original artwork produced by the doctor or institution responsible for that particular analysis. This was done in the hopes that perhaps a little of the historic flavor of the people and the times surrounding the appearance of that analysis might be captured. No one analysis is all good or all bad. All have some contribution to make if interpreted correctly, but all have certain problems associated with them, also. Such a survey not only gives the clinician greater insight as to the overall meaning of cephalometrics, but also allows him or her to cross-check one system against another in treatment planning. This in turn allows for reasoned deviation from cephalometric normative standards when necessary, as per the superseding dictates of the all-important temporomandibular joints.

A healthy and properly functioning temporomandibular joint should be the first and foremost treatment goal of every orthodontic case. Although no cephalometric analysis system is completely dominated by this concept, some are more compatible with it than others. A careful consideration of cephalometric history and development reveals the appearance of a gradual tendency that is directed more recently toward orthopedic and facial profile considerations, and away from the mere tooth-oriented orthodontic considerations. This is only fitting, as it brings us back full cycle to where clinical cephalometrics conceptually began even before the advent of the roentgenocephalogram itself. A text containing such a survey of cephalometric "recipes" can act as a valuable reference source to give clinicians a wealth of information from a wide variety of sources that will enable them to make better treatment-planning decisions. Such an approach will allow diagnosticians to pick and choose the most appropriate (and correct) observations from a variety of analyses and therefore obtain information and insights that will enable them to more easily untangle the stubborn knot of the malocclusion.

The final portion of the text discusses treatment of some of the more common types of malocclusion. Before and after computerized cephalometric tracings of various analyses are also included with each case. In certain cases, it may be seen that the cephalometrics from a variety of sources generally concur, while in other cases they may not. It must also be noted that "perfect" cases were not selected; rather, more commonly seen types of cases were used, which in turn exhibit commonly seen results. These cases do, however, reveal both orthopedic as well as orthodontic changes. It is felt that more is to be learned about the clinical coordination of removable appliances with fixed appliances in this manner. Once one thoroughly understands what is common, one is more prepared to deal with what is uncommon.

Terrance J. Spahl, DDS
St. Paul, Minnesota

Dictionaries are like watches: the worst is better than
none, and the best cannot be expected to run true.

Dr. Samuel Johnson, English lexicographer
1709−1784

ACKNOWLEDGMENTS

It would be a monumental breach of human courtesy to fail to acknowledge the many individuals who gave so freely of their time and efforts to bring this text into existence. In a time when the sharp controversies and deep divisions among our ranks reveal the less admirable traits of our common human natures, the long list of fine individuals who assisted with this effort bears mute testimony to the truly good heart that lies securely at the foundation of our profession.

Once again I would like to begin with the Germans. One of the key contributors of time and material to this text has been my very good friend and colleague Dr Hans Peter Bimler of Wiesbaden, West Germany. As one of the world's supreme cephalometricians, the many hours of his wise personal counsel and the numerous contributions of his superb artwork are deeply appreciated. We are also grateful to Dr Anna Barbara Bimler for her many supportive contributions to this effort. Those warm fall days in Wiesbaden, the nights in Rudesheim, the grace of the Rhine Valley, and the many wonderful days we've spent together in Germany and here in America, too, will long be remembered and appreciated.

On the American side of what Dr Bimler refers to as the "Atlantic River" we have many friends. The help of Dr Richard "Tubes" Beistle with our work on both the Sassouni Analysis and the Sassouni Plus Analysis is deeply appreciated. The hospitality he and his lovely wife Jill extended to me during my stay in Buchanan, Michigan, is gratefully acknowledged. The work of Dr Jack Lynn of Pittsburgh, Pennsylvania, provided an extremely important link in the chain of our story. And of course, the most generous contributions of Dr Alex Jacobson were of enormous benefit, as were the contributions of two men of true cephalometric genius, Dr D. D. Smith of Painted Post, New York, and his brother Mr Norman K. Smith of St Louis, Missouri.

It would be impossible to imagine the completion of this project with out the further assistance of many other fine individuals, the first and foremost of whom would have to be Mr Mark Ohlendorf of Ohlendorf Company, St Louis. The range of knowledge this kind and patient man commands in this discipline can only be described as phenomenal. His enormous compilation of technical skills never ceases to amaze me. A great debt of gratitude is also owed to Jolene Baker and the staff of the Biomedical Library and the Wilson Library of the University of Minnesota.

Many thanks are also owed to Lacinda Kiester and Jan Lazarus of the National Library of Medicine, Bethesda, Maryland, to Mr Robert Adelsperger of the Special Collections Division of the Library of Health Sciences of the University of Illinois, Chicago, and to Judy Chelerik of the Allen Memorial Library at Case Western Reserve University and the Dittrick Museum of Medical History. Additional thanks are due to Dawn Vohsen and Jerry Freeland of the *American Journal of Orthodontics*, to Dr John Kloehn of the Angle Orthodontist, and to Mrs Ruth Schultz, reference librarian of the Bureau of Library Services of the American Dental Association, Chicago. Thanks are also due to Sigmund Spaeth.

Once again, the close support of Judy Cloutier is deeply appreciated, as are the superb artistic contributions of Amy Remes and Jan Bilek. The constancy of my personal staff of Nancy Elert, Marilyn Wiedell, Louise Stoffel, Jackie Blossom, June Cline, Bonnie Westphal, MaryJo Cichy, Lisa Vono, and Dr Peter Hill is also grately appreciated.

Personal support was also provided at critical points during the production of this second volume by the noted dental author Dr Joe Dunlap of Clearwater, Florida. I would also like to thank Dr Steven P. Kulenkamp and Dr James M. Gayes for their continued support. A special thanks is truly owed to Stan and Nancy Weaver of Big Sandy, Montana. The human concern and idyllic sanctuary that they provided acted as a source of strength and inspiration that can never be measured.

Last, but certainly not least, I would like to thank my friend and colleague Dr John Witzig for being so patient with me and my insistence on writing this particular text and including it in our work. His total commitment to excellence, his kind consideration for myself, in conjunction with the continuing sacrifices of my wife Susan and my three children Emma Lee, Teddy, and Joey, generated the sustaining element no other source could have provided. I sincerely hope this particular effort will prove worthy of their constancy as well as that of the reader.

NOTE

Cephalometric analysis is based on the presumption that the condyles are in their normal position in the TMJs. Approximately 50% of all patients presenting for correction of malocclusion exhibit "TMJ clicking" and abnormal pretreatment joint relationships. The correction of improper TMJ relationships should be the first priority of any orthodontic treatment plan.

Omne ignotum pro magnifico est.
(*Everything unknown is taken as marvelous.*)

Tacitus, Roman historian, 55?—117

"It is my belief that much of the confusion among clinical orthodontists concerning cephalometrics stems from the fact that most of the literature concerning cephalometrics has been written by and for research workers. It is my intention to write an article in the only language I know, 'shop talk.'
Cecil Steiner
1953

CHAPTER 1
On the Way

THE SEARCH FOR STRUCTURE

Cephalometrics is the language in which the poetry of orthodontic diagnosis and treatment planning is written. It is not an end unto itself, but rather a means by which the clinician may not only solidify and ensure the accuracy of his diagnosis, but also clearly and precisely communicate his orthodontic ideas and problems to the complete understanding of his fellow colleagues. Cephalometrics can reveal important anatomical information relative to internal structures of the maxillofacial complex of a given case that is totally inaccessible by any of the other diagnostic procedures available, either two-dimensional (radiological) or three-dimensional (model analysis or clinical examination). Cephalometrics can be used to help determine problems that exist and give insights as to the best treatment methods for correcting them. The cephalometric x-ray can also act as a precautionary source of information, alerting the practitioner to circumstances which may exist that would preclude treatment of a case with certain appliances or techniques the operator may already have in mind.

Cephalometrics has not been solely the exclusive instrument of orthodontics, but was initiated originally in the 1800s by the physical anthropologists who used it as a method of comparing the fossil remains of the skulls of early man. But the use of the cephalometric x-ray for orthodontic diagnosis and treatment planning in modern times owes much to some of the early work laid down by these founders of the science, who so carefully and meticulously studied the osteology of the cranium. Some of their original definitions of anatomical planes still survive as a vital component to cephalometric analysis.

Though the cephalometric x-ray, occasionally in the form of the anteroposterior view, but most often in the form of the lateral view, is as common to orthodontic diagnosis and treatment planning as the periapical x-ray is to endodontics, its interpretations and the systems used to define its meaning vary widely. At first inspection of the average lateral cephalogram, it is obvious that an enormous amount of osteological and dental anatomy is visible to the eye. Over the years experts have defined and elaborated upon all sorts of theoretical relationships between the various anatomical parts. So much information has become available that entire corporations have evolved, which use sophisticated computers to manage it. The vast amount of information can be intimidating to beginners in the study of cephalometrics, but harnessing all of this data into a manageable medium is a simple matter of breaking the science down into its component parts so that it may be approached in an organized and orderly fashion. Looking at a cephalometric x-ray is analogous to looking at a large and detailed road map before taking a long trip. After a clinician gains experience in studying the cephalometric x-ray, all of the extraneous anatomy out of the spectrum of his concern for the moment is ignored by his mind's eye; his attention focuses on one area, invariably revealed via the cephalometric tracing and the particular analysis system used—even as one would follow the route of a particular freeway one plans on taking across the face of the map. The eye is concerned only with the particular highway as it follows it past all the other lines and markings on the map to the destination. Then, standing back, the mind evaluates the general path of the route as a whole, whether it is direct, straight, curved, or meandering; and still all the rest of the maze of roads depicted on the map remain semioblivious to the observer's attention. Once this main route is clear in the observer's mind, he may turn his attention to other routes that may offer shortcuts or side trips, and compare them mentally with the original route. Thus his spectrum of attention is increased to include more data, but still, the main bulk of information available from the map remains untapped. Careful and lengthy study soon reveals all that the observer cares to know about the various means available to effect his transit to his destination. As he embarks on the trip, he may even take the map with him so that he may compare his progress of his ever-changing location. Should trouble arise, as in the form of an unexpected detour or washed out road, he again consults the map for alternative routes, but this time his attention is drawn to different areas of the map, which, though originally not considered important, are now studied in a new light by virtue of the unexpected extenuating circumstances that have arisen.

Such is the reading and interpretation of the cephalogram. One quickly deciphers what is important on it from what is extraneous. As much or as little information may be gleaned from it as the clinician needs. Growth and development research studies have been performed on almost every osteological and dental aspect of the maxillofacial-cranial complex as divulged by the cephalometric x-ray, and the information obtained from these studies is prodigious. But in daily practice, the practitioner may be concerned with only a handful of the more common points of anatomical interest; and as he repeatedly gains skills in interpreting these points, his use of the cephalogram becomes an increasingly valuable tool in his treatment planning. He may use a given analytical system or a series of systems or even parts of various systems to interpret his films. Keep in mind that though the cephalogram is valuable for the otherwise unobtainable anatomical information it may provide, it is not the only standard against which diagnosis and treatment planning are to be judged. The cephalogram is merely another servant to the clinician in his efforts to produce excellent orthodontic care for the patient; it is not his master. The data that the cephalogram can provide serves only as a guide, a reference point toward which the course of the orthodontic treatment may direct itself. It is not a mandate as to what must be done in order to consider the treatment results as acceptable. Salzmann eloquently writes,

> Cephalometrics includes measurements, description and appraisal of the morphologic configuration, and growth changes in the skull by ascertaining the dimensions of lines, angles, and planes between anthropometric landmarks established by physical anthropologists and points selected by orthodontists.

The cephalometric film is indeed all of these things and more: It may be used for a wide variety of diagnostic and comparative procedures, and its potential for research purposes seems limitless. It may be used to assist the clinician in the correct definition and classification of the malocclusion he is dealing with. It may be used to establish the facial type and as a quantitative analysis of craniofacial structures. Some practitioners theorize that the cephalometric film can be used to help predict future growth patterns and help to properly select treatment modalities. The cephalogram may be used to check orthodontic progress during treatment. It can be used to check posttreatment changes and to determine the success of the patient in attaining the pretreatment goals. The cephalogram can tell the practitioner how hard he will have to work on a given case to obtain the most satisfactory results; and once treatment is complete, it can tell him how good a job he did. But these things are all due to arbitrary systems of interpretation imposed on the film by the science itself. In its most reduced and basic form, this radiological repository of the patient's hard and soft tissue diagnostic data, known as the lateral cephalogram, is nothing more than an x-ray of the side of the head.

"But he answered that there was no royal road to geometry." (when King Ptolemy asked if there was not a shorter method)
Proclus
Commentary on Euclid, Prologue

ANATOMICAL LANDMARKS: THE GUIDEPOSTS OF CEPHALOMETRICS

The science of cephalometrics literally means "head measurement" (Greek *cephalo*, "head," and *metros*, "measure"). It must be borne in mind that cephalometrics has its origins in 19th-century anthropometrics and physical anthropology. This was long before the discovery of the x-ray by Wilhelm Roentgen in 1895. Thus the earliest efforts at cephalometrics consisted of the external measurement of human skull specimens with some type of calipers. This was the origin of some of the first planes of description for the human skull, such as Blumenbach's plane and Broca's line.

Once x-rays of the skull became available, the term "roentgenocephalometrics" appeared as a delineation between that form of cephalometrics and the earlier techniques which were concerned with the external physical measurement of the actual specimen. This cumbersome term was used for about a decade throughout the dental literature after the appearance of the x-ray—oriented technique in the early 1930s, but then was gradually replaced by the shorter term "cephalometrics," which now has come to imply the roentgenocephalometric technique, even though the more general term originally had a different meaning.

Once cephalometric x-rays became standardized and widespread, a whole new raft of cephalometric terminology came into vogue. This was a result of the appearance on the scene of (1) the newly defined landmarks of integumental, osseous, and dental anatomy now made visible by the cephalogram, and (2) a newly defined series of planes and lines constructed as a result of linearly connecting the appropriate respective landmark points. At the time of the early embryonic stages of development of this discipline, this seemed to be perfectly appropriate and logical. In all the excitement over the meaning and significance of the newfound diagnostic technique of these early days, not much rebuttal was generated over what initially seemed to be simple, straightforward, and basic components of the system as its own defined anatomical points and planes. But after careful consideration and scrutiny, it was later (surprisingly, quite a bit later) discovered that the heretofore all but unchallenged definitions of landmarks seen on the x-ray might not always coincide with what actually existed in the real specimen, and that the interpretation of these landmarks or points and planes might not be as straightforward as it at first appeared. Things were not always as they seemed.

Any reasonable discourse on cephalometrics is predicated on a mutually accepted and universally clear understanding of the terminology used in its discussion. Therefore, we first thoroughly examine the definitions and significance of some commonly used landmarks along with the definitions of major lines and planes, which are themselves composed of these various landmarks.

Because it is clinically oriented, this book is concerned chiefly with the points and planes found on the lateral view of the skull, since this is the view used almost exclusively by practicing clinicians. In the dental literature the lateral cephalogram provides a view referred to as "norma lateralis." The landmark points observed from this aspect will obviously be discussed first, because the various lines and planes are predicated upon the existence of at least two of these landmark points. These points and planes may be located on hard tissues, soft tissues, or a combination of the two. Some points are not even actual physical anatomical entities, but are points in space—positions that do not even exist on the actual specimen, but are conveniently created figments (albeit well-defined figments) of the diagnostician's interpretive imagination![1,2]

Anatomical Landmarks of Norma Lateralis

Acanthion (Ac). Acanthion represents a true oddity in cephalometric circles, since it is an actual anatomical structure—the tip of the anterior nasal spine—but it is almost never seen, because it is so thin and finely pointed that it is almost invariably "burned out" on the x-ray film. Fortunately, its role in cephalometric discussions is quite limited.

Alveolar Point (Al.P.).   See Prosthion.

Antegonial Notch (No).   This point is one that belongs to the group that requires a limited degree of interpretation, because it is defined as the highest point of the Antegonial Notch on the lower border of the mandible. Sometimes this point is quite sharp and reasonably well demarcated naturally, but at other times the inferior border of the mandible may be so smooth and gracefully concave along the surface of its inferior border that this point is completely nonexistent.

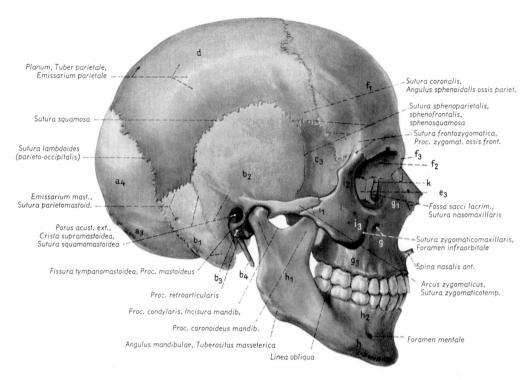

Planum, Tuber parietale,
Emissarium parietale

Sutura squamosa

Sutura lambdoides
(parieto-occipitalis)

Emissarium mast.,
Sutura parietomastoid.

Porus acust. ext.,
Crista supramastoidea,
Sutura squamomastoidea

Fissura tympanomastoidea, Proc. mastoideus

Proc. retroarticularis

Proc. condylaris, Incisura mandib.

Proc. coronoideus mandib.

Angulus mandibulae, Tuberositas masseterica

Linea obliqua

Sutura coronalis,
Angulus sphenoidalis ossis pariet.

Sutura sphenoparietalis,
sphenofrontalis,
sphenosquamosa

Sutura frontozygomatica,
Proc. zygomat. ossis front.

f_3

f_2

k

e_3

Fossa sacci lacrim.,
Sutura nasomaxillaris

Sutura zygomaticomaxillaris,
Foramen infraorbitale

Spina nasalis ant.

Arcus zygomaticus,
Sutura zygomaticotemp.

Foramen mentale

Figure 1–1   Adult skull viewed from right side. The bones of the neurocranium and visceral cranium are shown in different colors, visceral cranium in blue, violet, green. a_3/a_4 = Squama ossis occipit.; b_1 = Pars mastoidea o. tempor.; b_2 = Pars squamosa o. temporalis; b_3 = Pars tympanica o. temporalis; b_4 = Processus styloideus; c_3 = Ala major o. sphenoid.; d = Os parietale; e_3 = Lamina orbitalis o. ethmoid.; f_1 = Squama frontalis; f_2 = Pars orbitalis ossis frontalis; f_3 = Pars nasalis ossis frontalis; g = Maxilla (corpus); g_1 = Maxilla, processus frontalis; g_3 = Maxilla, processus alveolaris; h = Mandibula (corpus); h_1 = Mandibula (ramus); h_2 = Mandibula, processus alveolaris; i = Os zygomaticum; i_1 = Os zygomaticum, processus temporalis; i_2 = Os zygomaticum, processus frontalis; i_3 = Os zygomaticum, processus maxillaris; j = Os nasale; k = Os lacrimale (Reprinted from Pernkopf E: *Atlas der topographischen u. angewandten Anatomie.* Munich, Urban & Schwarzenberg, 1963, p 10 with permission.)

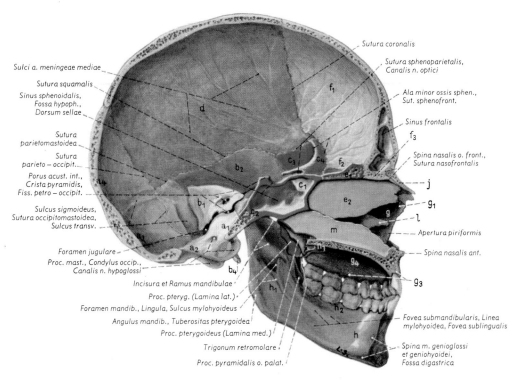

Figure 1−2   Adult skull, midsagittal section. a_1 = Os occipitale, pars basilaris (corpus); a_2 = Os occipitale, pars lat.; a_3/a_4 = Squama o. occipitalis; b_1 = Os temporale, Pars petrosa; b_2 = Squama ossis temporalis; b_4 = Processus styloideus; c_1 = Os sphenoidale (praesphenoid); c_2 = Os sphenoidale (basisphenoid); c_3 = Ala major o. sphenoidalis; c_4 = Ala minor o. sphenoidalis; d = Os parietale; e_1 = Os ethmoidale, lamina cribrosa; e_2 = Os ethmoidale, lamina mediana (perpendicularis); f_1 = Os frontale, squama; f_2 = Os frontale, pars orbitalis; f_3 = Os frontale, pars nasalis; g = Maxilla (corpus); g_1 = Maxilla, processus frontalis; g_3 = Maxilla, processus alveolaris; g_4 = Maxilla, processus palatinus; h = Mandibula, corpus; h_1 = Mandibula, ramus; h_2 = Mandibula, processus alveolaris; j = Os nasale; l = Concha inf.; m = Vomer; n_1 = Os palatinum, lamina horizontalis.

(Reprinted from Pernkopf E: *Atlas der topographischen u. angewandten Anatomie.* Munich, Urban & Schwarzenberg, 1963, p 19 with permission.)

Anterior nasal spine (ANS).   This particular landmark is one that appears both as a point for certain proportional geometric ratio-type linear measurements, such as the juncture between upper and lower facial heights, and as a defined point for certain planes, such as the palatal plane. It is defined as the median sharp bony process that protrudes anteriorly from the superior edge of the maxilla, where it is joined by the anterior floor of the nasal opening and the inferior, almost frenumlike bony midline portion that forms the inferior portion of the spine. This particular point (no pun intended; it is truly a sharp bony point) may be easily felt by placing the tip of the index finger against the base of the nose, where the external midnasal septum meets the filtrum area of the upper lip, and by pressing up and in at an oblique angle.

Conceptually easy to understand, this landmark, ironically, is sometimes difficult to interpret on the cephalogram! It is sometimes mistakenly defined as the tip of the ANS, but this is Ac, the actual finely pointed tip which is always burned out on the film. Therefore, the "tip" of the spine that actually shows up on the film is due to the somewhat stouter osseous structure just distal (by about 1–2 mm) to Ac. Therefore, it may be seen that what actually determines the pinpoint location of this landmark on the film is the degree of penetration of the x-ray beam. Where Ac quits being burned out, ANS begins. It may also be surmised that the two are quite close together, separated usually by only 1 or 2 mm at the most, and the two are always on the same horizontal level of the overall palatal plane. Therefore, the actual delination between the two most often resolves to a moot point! The ANS that actually shows up on the xray image is that area of the bony spinous structure where the bone is laterally about 1 mm thick.

Apicale (Ap).   Apicale is defined as the tip of the root of the maxillary first bicuspid. It is a point used exclusively in the cephalometric analysis system of Hans Peter Bimler, and is one of three points of a line that is also an exclusive of the Bimler, the famous "Stress Axis" or Factor 6.

A-point (subspinale).   This is one of the most famous and widely used of all cephalometric landmarks. It may also often be seen written Point-A or Point-A (Downs), after the first man to adopt its use in an orthodontic context. Its original definition is from an anthropological source and defines it as the deepest or innermost midline point on the anterior profile of the maxilla between ANS and the crest of the alveolar ridge between the maxillary central incisors. But the actual location of this point in a real specimen often lies in a trough between the roots of

---

Figure 1–3   **(A)** Roentgenocephalogram in norma lateralis, dried skull. **(B)** Roentgenocephalogram, living patient.

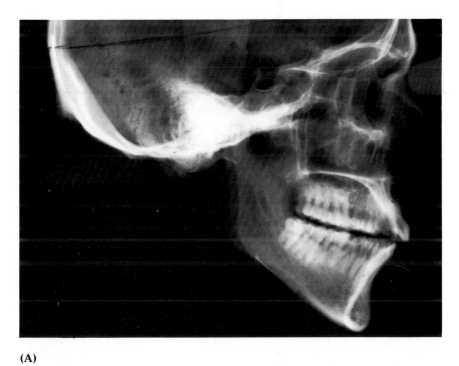

(A)

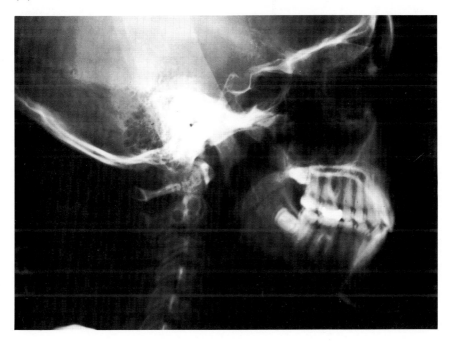

(B)

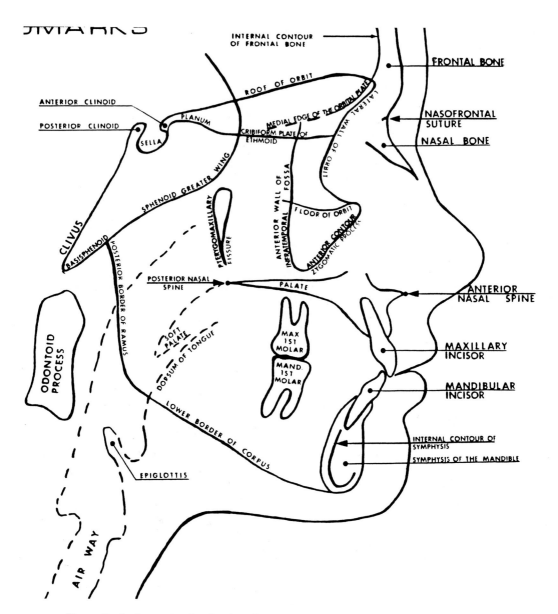

Figure 1–4   Image tracing landmarks.

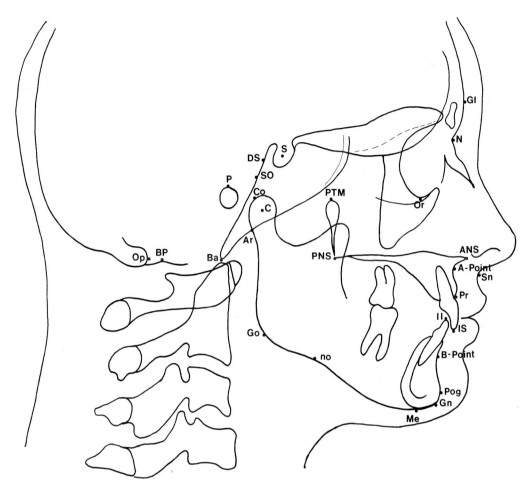

Figure 1–5 Anatomical points   ANS = Anterior nasal spine; A-point (Downs);
Ar = Articulare; Ba = Basion; B-point (Downs); BP = Bolton Point; C = C-point
(Bimler); Co = Condylion; DS = Dorsum sellae; Gl = Glabella; Gn = Gnathion
(anatomic); Go = Gonion; II = Incisor inferius; IS = Incisor superius; Me =
Menton; N = Nasion; No = Antegonial Notch; Op = Opisthion; Or = Orbitale;
P = Porion; PNS = Posterior nasal spine; Pog = Pogonion; Pr = Prosthion;
PTM = Pterygomaxillary fissure; S = Sella; Sn = Subnasion; SO = Spheno-
occipital synchondrosis

the central incisors.[3] This dip in the surface of maxillary alveolar bone
between the roots of the central incisors may easily be palpated with the
fingertip. While gently sliding the fingertip upward over the labial gingivae of the upper central incisors, you can feel the beginning of the base
and the somewhat sharp inferior edge of the ANS. If the bulge of the
roots is great enough, which it usually is, the aforementioned trough is
obliterated on the x-ray in norma lateralis. Thus the point were the labial

surface of bone over the maxillary incisor roots meets the ascending and forward-curving arc of the inferior border of the ANS serves as the innermost or deepest contour of the profile of the maxilla, even though there usually exists an even deeper anatomical location for the point which is obliterated by root structure.

Thus the size and stage of development of the ANS (the inferior border, specifically) has a great bearing on the cephalometrically compromised location of A-point. In the deciduous dentition this trough between the primary maxillary incisors is quite shallow or may not even exist. In such cases the location A-point is often seen to be at least at the level of the root tips of the deciduous teeth, or even higher. However, in the adult dentition stage, A-point is usually found below the level of the apices of the maxillary central incisors.

This apparent "migration" of the landmark is due to several factors. One factor is that in the transition from the deciduous dentition to the full adult dentition, a certain amount of overall skull growth takes place, ANS included. It grows longer and more protrusive, larger and generally more robust. Another factor affecting this area is the eruption of the permanent maxillary incisors. This causes a revamping of the maxillary alveolar process in the area, and the anterior outline of the maxilla becomes more proclined as the permanent incisors tend to be tipped more labially than their more vertically situated deciduous precursors. This change in anterior maxillary profile due to growth can easily change the relative location of A-point by several millimeters. This is an important consideration in the light of interpreting changes in lines or angles that might be concerned with this particular landmark. Growth can change not only the vertical but also the horizontal location of this point, and it is the specific growth of the actual ANS that influences this area most directly.

One remarkable aspect to this whole business of A-point location is in the way its *mis*interpretations manifest themselves. Studies have shown that clinicians tend to err more in the vertical location of the point than in its horizontal placement, no doubt because the operator is asked to interpret the deepest point of a curve. The more gradual and graceful the curve, the more the individual interpretations will be subject to error. Since the arc of the curve is basically in a vertical direction, it is reasonable that most errors in the placement of the landmark will vary in that particular plane. This has little effect on the usefulness of A-point, since most of the measurements in which it is a component are either linearly or angularly along the vertical axis through A-point, where vertical errors in registration of the location of the point are more tolerable.

Articulare (Ar).   This point is nonexistent in nature, it is merely an artifact of the x-ray image due to the fact that it represents the two-dimensional shadow of a three-dimensional object. (Obviously there will be many superimpositions of one structure's x-ray image over another.)

It is defined as the intersection of the image of the edge of the dorsal (distal) contour of the mandibular condyle with the temporal bone.

Basion (Ba). This point is important in the construction of reference planes. It is defined as the midpoint of the anterior border of the foramen magnum. It has also been described as the most inferior posterior point on the occipital bone. Either way, it is a difficult landmark to decipher, due to the superimposition of surrounding osseous structures. However, it is generally quite stable and offers a good opportunity for use as a base reference point.

Bolton Point (BP). This point was named after Charles W. Bolton, a philanthropist who helped fund early studies in cephalometrics during the late 1930s. It is defined as the highest point at the notches of the posterior end of the occipital condyles of the occipital bone in norma lateralis.

B-point (supramentale). This is the mandibular counterpart to A-point in the maxilla. It is defined as the deepest point of contour of the lateral profile of the mandibular alveolar projection, and it represents the anteriormost limits of the mandibular basal arch. This point is also a matter of interpreting the most inward point of a gradual curve and is subject to similar problems of arbitrary placement of the landmark by the clinician. Again, as with its counterpart in the maxilla, errors in placement of the landmark are usually along a vertical axis, which for this landmark's particular use in various analyses is the type of error that is fairly well tolerated.[4]

Broadbent Registration Point (R). This is another nonanatomical point or "space mark" that was devised by B. Holly Broadbent to act as a reference point to permit superimposition of a series of films of the same individual (in what are termed "longitudinal" studies) to analyze changes in bony shape and position due to growth and/or treatment. As such, an extremely stable reference point is desirable.

Registration Point is the midpoint on a perpendicular line drawn from sella (the center of the sella turcica or the hypophyseal fossa) to the Bolton-Nasion line. This was the first in what would become a series of various "stable" reference points or lines devised by various clinicians and researchers over the years to permit serialized superimposition of films to evaluate progress of the individual with respect to growth and/or treatment.

Capitulare (C). This is the arbitrary center of the head of the mandibular or condyle. Though this point may actually be represented on the specimen, its location in norma lateralis is strictly a matter of the individual's own judgment as to just what constitutes the actual center of the condylar head. However, due to the shape of the outline of the condyle, this becomes a fairly easy task with little chance for gross misinterpretation. Again, as with A- and B-points, it is more apt to be misplaced along a vertical plane than along the horizontal.

Clivus. The middle section of this bony line is usually obscured by the superimposed surrounding osseous structure. However, the superior and inferior sections are easily visible. It is defined as the inclined surface of bone arising from the anterior border of the foramen magnum to the dorsum sella (the posterior major bony portion of the sella turcica). It is a composite of the basilar portion of the occipital bone (in the area of the foramen magnum) and a small portion of the sphenoid bone. As previously stated, the middle portion of this landmark is obscured by other structures, but the inferior end of it may be seen as a small fingerlike projection of bone just distal and inferior to the point Ar. The superior portion of the landmark is continuous with the posterior clinoid process of the sella turcica; a plane represented by a line connecting the lower end, clivion inferior, to the upper end, clivion superior, may be seen to take about a 50- to 80-degree angle to the horizontal.

Condylion (Cd or Co). This is defined either as the top or most superior and posterior point on the outline of the mandibular condyle. A seemingly simple enough definition, it is not without its problems of interpretation. First of all, a lot of osseous overlapping of images of the temporal bones obscures much of the condylar head. Second, there is a considerable amount of variation of the location of the right and left condyles with respect to norma lateralis. It is seldom, however, that both condylar heads may be deciphered on the same film.

Dorsum sellae (DS). This quatralateral or square bone forms the posterior boundary of the sella turcica. The posterior clinoid process projects from its superior aspect, and it is continuous inferiorly with the clivus. It is part of the sphenoid bone.

Glabella (Gl). This point represents the crest of the anterior portion of the smooth area of the frontal bone in the midsagittal plane, in the area of the bony prominence joining the supraorbital ridges.

Gnathion (Gn). This again is an arbitrary judgment landmark that is defined as a point halfway between pogonion and menton, each of which is an arbitrary judgment point. Still, this point is reasonably easy to locate due to the curved outline of the mandible and the unobstructed view. Mentally dividing something in half seems to come quite naturally to most people, which is the essence of the selection of the point gnathion, since it is supposed to represent a locus on the outer mandibular border halfway between the most anterior and inferior points of the bony chin. A more modern definition of this point has been derived in order to facilitate its use with computers. It consists of that point at which the facial plane and the mandibular plane intersect, which places the point out in space, albeit in close proximity to the actual surface of the mandible.

Gonion (Go). This point is used to define the general physical location of the angle of the mandible. It is arbitrarily placed at the most outward, lowest, posterior point on the angle of the jaw. There is fairly good symmetry observed in this area, and the unobstructed view should simplify the clinician's choice of where to place the mark. Yet, surprisingly, this is the most misinterpreted point location in all of cephalometrics! This misinterpretation is due to the large and gradual arc the inferior border of the mandible displays in the gonial region. Its wide sweep gives the clinician a relatively broad choice of location for the mark. Yet, it must be kept in mind that though the gonion is to be the most inferior point on the distal border of the ramus, it is also to be the most posterior point on the inferior border of the mandible. Keeping this in mind allows the observer to mentally "rock" the point back and forth along the mandibular gonial outline until the mind "settles it in" to a location that is a fair compromise between the two components.

Incision inferius (II).   The most forward incisal point of the most prominent mandibular central incisor.

Incision superius (IS).   The most forward incisal point of the most prominent maxillary central incisor.

Menton (M, Me).   This is the lowest point on the inferior border of the outline of the symphysis of the mandible.

Nasion (N).   This key landmark, critical to many cephalometric analysis systems, appears as a slight oblique notch at the juncture of the frontal bone with what would be the bones of the bridge of the nose. It was originally defined from an anthropological point of view as the juncture of the internasal suture with the nasofrontal suture. However, since the first of these two sutures is not visible on a lateral cephalogram, a new definition was devised, which describes it as the most anterior point of the suture between the frontal bones and the nasal bones. More specifically, it is the most anterior point of the nasofrontal suture. Due to variation in the direction of the sutures and the size and shape of the nasal bones (and even their number in the case of accessory bones), nasion often reflects a lack of clear definition. In such instances some experts advise placing nasion at the most posterior point on the curve of the juncture of the frontal and nasal bones.[5]

Opisthion (Op).   A logical counterpart to basion, opisthion is the posterior midline point on the posterior margin of the foramen magnum.

Oribitale (Or).   This is the lowest point on the inferior margin of the orbit. In the event two orbital margins are decipherable, the point is placed at the average distance between them.

Pogonion (P, Pg, Po, or Pog).   This landmark is used in many aspects of various cephalometric analysis systems and is defined as the anteriormost point of the profile of the bony chin.

Porion (P).   Three areas have qualified at one time or another for this term. One area is "soft tissue" porion, which is the midpoint on the upper edge of the soft tissue external auditory meatus. This was used as a method of determining the Frankfort plane externally on live individuals. "Machine porion," used briefly during the developmental stages of the science of roentgenocephalometrics, was defined as the center of the image of the metal ear rods inserted in the patient's auditory meatuses in a head-stabilizing device known as a cephalostat. Machine porion has since fallen out of favor and true anatomical porion is used.

Anatomical porion is defined as the most superior point of the upper edge of the external auditory meatus (osseous) and, as such, represents an important and major landmark for base reference line constructions in various cephalometric analysis systems. Due to the density of the petrous portion of the temporal bone and general superimposition of other osseous structures, porion may be difficult to decipher, especially when further obstructed by the image of the metal stabilizing ear rod. Sometimes, if alignment is just right, the image of the ear rod may obliterate the shadow of the edge of true anatomical porion altogether. In such a case the superior point on the machine image may be used. Generally, however, due to the presence and compressibility of soft tissues in the ear canal and the fact that the auditory canal is not perfectly straight, there will be a discrepancy between the outline of the image of machine porion and anatomical porion, with anatomical porion being slightly superior and posterior to machine porion.

Remember that as the ear canal travels inward to the inner ear, it follows a slightly posterior and superior pathway from its original starting place in the external ear. This fact causes much confusion to beginners in cephalometric interpretation. As this pathway travels posteriorly and superiorly, it also makes a slight caudal bend. This bend allows the x-ray beam to pass directly through the superior edge of the canal for a brief portion directly edge on, creating a white circular image that is often mistaken for porion, but is actually the deeper portions of the internal auditory meatus.

The clue that it is the deeper internal meatus is the distance and size of the image from machine porion. The internal auditory meatus is usually about half the size of the external meatus. It is located superiorly and posteriorly to machine porion, and its entire image is usually decipherable, whereas due to the proximity of the external auditory meatus to the ear rods of the cephalostat, in spite of how much variance of alignment there is due to compression of soft tissues, a portion of true anatomical porion is always obliterated by the ear rod.

If plastic ear rods are used and no machine porion is visible, the key to deciphering the difference between internal and external auditory meatuses on the film is size and location. The external auditory meatus will appear larger and more inferior and anterior of the two. This is the reason why physicians pull the pinna of the ear superiorly and posteriorly to facilitate insertion of the otoscope into the ear canal in examinations of the eardrum.

Another clue to the location of true porion is that it generally resides fairly close to a horizontal plane confluent with condylion.

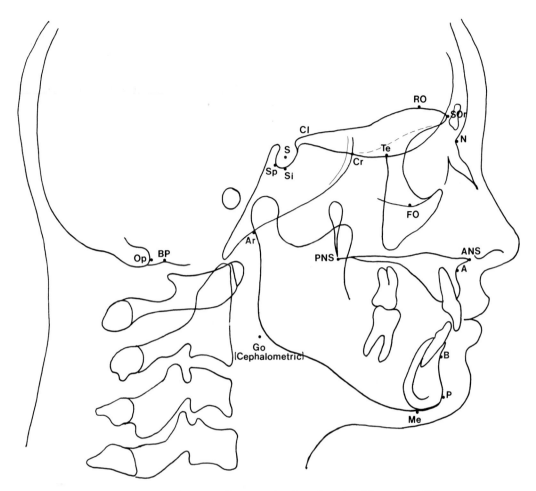

Figure 1–6 Anatomical points (Sassouni) A = A-point (Downs); ANS = Anterior nasal spine; Ar = Articulare; B = B-point (Downs); BP = Bolton Point; CR = Cribriform point; Cl = Anterior clinoid process; FO = Floor of orbit; Go = Cephalometric gonion; Me = Menton; N = Nasion; OP = Opisthion; P = Pogonion (Sassouni) (not to be confused with porion); PNS = Posterior nasal spine; RO = Roof of orbit; S = Sella; Si = Sella inferior; SOr = Supraorbital point; Sp = Sella posterior; Te = Temporale

Posterior nasal spine (PNS). In norma lateralis what may be seen as the palate or roof of the mouth travels posteriorly and tapers off, in what would be the beginning of the soft palate area, to a sharply pointed image called the posterior nasal spine. It represents the process formed by the union of the projecting ends of the posterior borders of the palatal processes of the palatal bones.

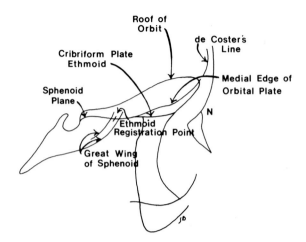

Figure 1−7   Anatomical detail of the cranial base area.

Prosthion (Pr).   Here is yet another example of a landmark that had to have its original anthropological definition altered in order to be compatible with the limitations of roentgenocephalometrics. It was originally defined as the lowest and most forward point on the maxillary alveolar process between the central incisors. Obviously, such a point would be impossible to see in norma lateralis due to the obstruction provided by the labial surfaces of crowns and roots of the upper incisors. Hence, the definition which represents what is really seen on the x-ray is the most anterior inferior crest of the bony lamella over the most prominent maxillary central incisor.

Pterygomaxillary fissure (PTM, T).   This landmark is not a point but an outline. It appears as an upside-down teardrop-shaped area of radiolucency, the tip of which generally points toward the PNS area. It also usually has a slightly forward graceful curve to the tip. It is almost always clearly defined in the cephalogram in spite of being surrounded by considerable amounts of superimposed osseous anatomy. It is especially easy to find in younger patients, the chief concern of most clinicians. In the adult, however, it becomes clouded over, usually by the coronoid process of the mandible, although this is usually only in the inferior region of the landmark. It represents the point where the pterygoid process of the sphenoid bone and the pterygoid process of the maxilla unite to form the characteristic teardrop shape. It is popular for its usefulness in acting as a component of base reference lines.

Sella (S).   This is an example of a point that exists only in norma lateralis and is not an actual anatomical entity but a point in space, that has been called a "space mark." Sella is defined as the arbitrary geometric center of the outline of the sella turcica. It is extremely important as a component in the construction of base reference lines in many cephalometric analyses.

Spheno-occipital synchondrosis (SO).   This represents the cartilaginous union of the forward end of the basal portion of the occipital bone to the posterior surface of the body of the sphenoid. It is very popular with researchers as a component for the construction of reference lines because of its high degree of relative stability. It is also quite difficult to decipher.

Subnasion (Sn).   This is a soft tissue point that represents the point of the angle formed between the inferior external border of the midnasal septum and the upper lip in norma lateralis.

Tuberculum sellae (TS).   This is the anterior boundary of the sella turcica and represents an anatomical area, not a point locus.

Now that some of the major cephalometric landmarks are understood, the next logical progression would be a consideration of lines and planes. A line connects two points, whereas a plane connects three or more points and implies a flat two-dimensional surface area. However, in the dental literature one occasionally sees the terms interchanged. Lines and planes have played such important roles throughout the history of craniometrics and roentgenocephalometrics because of their potential for allowing both description and comparison.

In the earliest days of the science, over a century and a half ago, the first scientists to study physical anthropology were preoccupied with determining types, and describing differences, in human skulls. The age, racial type, and even sex of the skulls studied were of primary interest. Numerous measurements, definitions, tables, and indices were recorded. An endless variety of classification systems were also proposed. Yet despite anthropologists' extensive early attempts to describe skulls anatomically and numerically, there still remained the problems of easily defining and visualizing general skull types. The problem was solved by the formulation of characteristic skull types that were representative of a given group, age, race, or sex. This process entailed the use of normative descriptions and, more importantly, outline drawings, against which a specific specimen's own morphology or outline drawing could be superimposed for comparison. However, this superimposition process was predicated upon the existence of standardized base reference loci for comparative orientation of the respective drawings—hence the development of base reference lines and planes.

Obviously, base references should be as relatively stable and close to that mythological entity known as "the center of growth" as possible. Superimposition of consecutive drawings about such planes would give the anthropologist or craniometrician the opportunity to decipher and interpret variations due to growth, lineage, etc. It also laid the seeds of the methodology of the science of roentgenocephalometrics, which would come over a century later. Over the years a considerable number of such lines and planes have been developed and defined to be used as base references for comparison. Some are extremely important and have proven to be of great value, while others enjoyed only brief popularity and/or faded into obscurity. Some are strictly anthropological in origin, while others have been invented by orthodontists.

Lines and Planes of Norma Lateralis

Blumenbach's plane.   This plane is referred to as a "resting horizontal plane," that is, it is the plane formed as the skull, minus the mandible, rests on a flat horizontal surface. This usually entails the skull resting anteriorly on the maxillary teeth and posteriorly either on the occipital condyles or on the mastoid processes.

Broadbent's line.   This line was devised in the late 1920s by one of the founding fathers of roentgenocephalometrics, B. Holly Broadbent, and has remained as the famous S-N reference base line. It runs of course from sella to nasion.

Broadbent-Bolton line.   Another vintage-level base reference line developed by orthodontists, this line runs from Bolton Point to nasion.

Broca's line.   Sometimes also seen as Broca's plane, it dates back to 1875 and was devised as an attempt to improve on Blumenbach's plane. It extends from the true anatomic prosthion to the lowermost point of the occipital condyle when the skull is resting on a horizontal surface.

Camper's line.   This represents one of the senior members of the family of craniometric lines and planes, as it dates back to 1791. (George Washington was president, and the country only had 14 states!) It is defined as the line extending from Ac (tip of the ANS) to the center of the external auditory meatus. Camper's plane is the triangular plane formed by the two lines from Ac to each external auditory meatus. Camper's triangle represents the triangle formed between Camper's line and a line tangent to the facial profile. This would also form an angle known as "Camper's Facial Angle." This also represents one of the earliest attempts to construct an angle for descriptive and visualization purposes.

DeCoster's line.   This is the only "line" that is not a linear connection of two points. It represents an actual anatomical contour of the planoethmoidal line from the internal plate of the frontal bone down through the roof of the cribriform plate to the anterior portion of sella turcica.

Frankfort Horizontal plane (FH).   This is another one of the oldest and most prestigious planes of cephalometrics. It may be visualized on the living individual, the dried skull, and the lateral roentgenocephalogram of the living patient as well. It has recently "reemerged" as a favorite of modern cephalometricians as the best all-around compromise

Figure 1–8   Anatomical lines and planes. **(A)** Conventional anatomical lines and planes. **(B)** Ricketts' version of mandibular plane. **(C)** Bimler version.

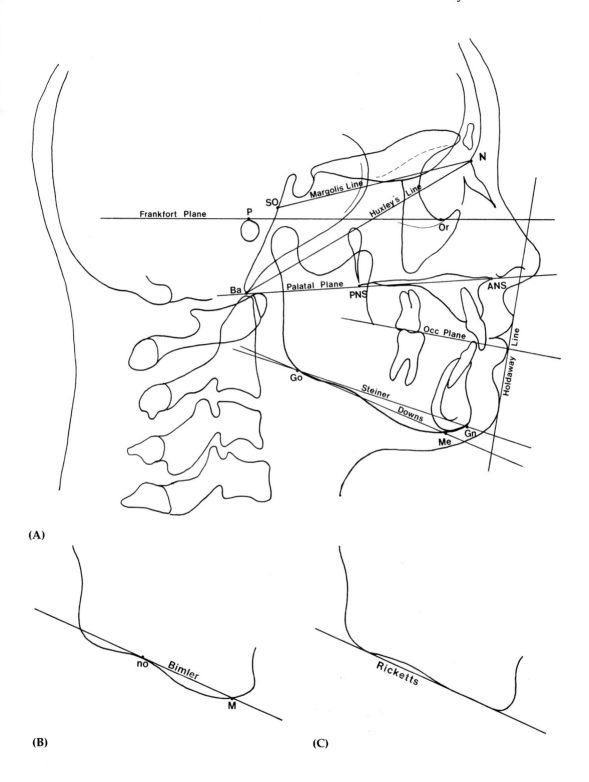

(A)

(B)   (C)

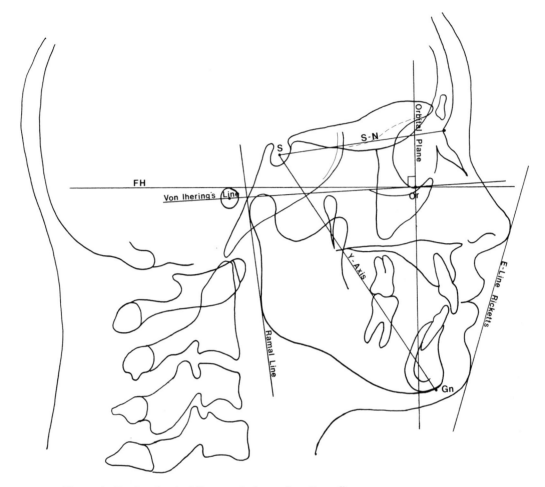

Figure 1–9   Anatomical lines and planes (continued).

for a base reference line against which other points and lines may be measured for interpretation. Its origins date back to the International Congress on Prehistoric Anthropology and Archaeology, held in Frankfort in 1882. The line runs from orbitale to porion. In actual specimens, the left orbitale and left porion are used. It is supposed to represent the ideal horizontal position of the head when the patient stands erect; hence it is usually used as a plane of horizontal orientation of the cephalometric image in norma lateralis.

Palatal plane.   This is the line running from the ANS to the PNS and denotes the general limitations of the hard palate superiorly.

His' plane.   Of the vintage of Broca's plane, the plane of His dates back to 1874 and runs from acanthion to opisthion. This is more practical in the study of skull specimens because it allows for anterior tooth loss and alveolar resorption.

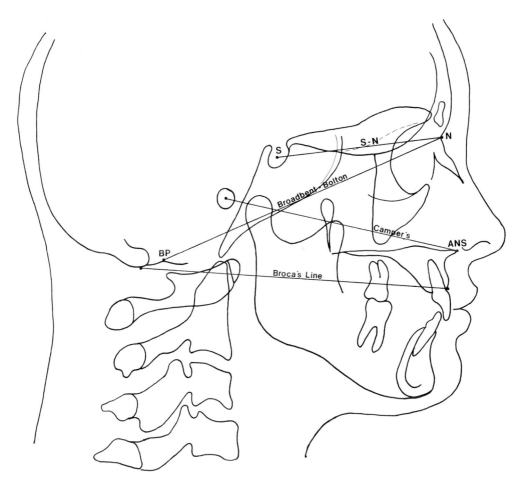

Figure **1−10**   Anatomical lines and planes (continued).

Holdaway line.   This line, also referred to as the harmony line, was developed by R. A. Holdaway at the University of Texas[6] and is strictly a soft tissue profile assessment reference line. It is specific for determination of the balance and harmony of the lower lip. It theorizes that the vermilion border of the lower lip should fall within 1 mm of a line drawn from the unstrained soft tissue chin to the vermilion border of the upper lip. Also soft tissue A-point should be 5 mm (±2) from the harmony line.

Huxley's line.   This is another time-honored member of the cephalometric reference line family. It runs from nasion to basion and is more frequently referred to as the nasion-basion line. It is quite popular in the computerized cephalometrics field as a reference line that exhibits little relative change during growth and development. It also separates the cranial skeleton from the facial skeleton. For this reason it is also referred to as "Huxley's basiocranial axis." As some experts[7] have pointed out, if it were not for the extreme difficulty of locating basion on the cephalogram, it would be the near-perfect base reference line for research purposes on growth and development.

Mandibular plane.   The inferior border of the mandible is easily seen on the x-ray image in norma lateralis; therefore, it is surprising that there are four different mandibular planes used to describe it! Each one is popular with various clinicians and researchers of great renown. Tweed and Ricketts define the mandibular plane as a straight line tangent to the lowermost border of the mandible. Downs, one of the founding fathers of clinical cephalometric analysis, defines this plane as the line joining gonion to menton. A third definition, used by Steiner, is the line joining gonion and gnathion. A fourth is Bimler's line M-No (menton to antegonial notch).

Margolis line.   This line runs from nasion to the spheno-occipital synchondrosis. It is usually used in conjunction with the mandibular plane in the "Margolis Triangle" method of cephalometric assessment. However, it represents similar problems, as does the use of Huxley's line, in that the end point of the line at the spheno-occipital synchondrosis is difficult to decipher on the x-ray image.

Occlusal plane.   There are three occlusal planes.[8] The first plane is the line joining the midpoint of the overlap of the mesiobuccal cusps of the upper and lower first molars with the point bisecting the overbite of the incisors. This appears to be the most popular, and is used by both Downs and Steiner. A second plane, used by Ricketts and in the "Wits" analysis, is called the functional occlusal plane, and is a line joining the midpoint of the overlap of the mesiobuccal cusps of the first molars and the buccal cusps of the premolars or deciduous molars. The third plane is the line joining the midsection of the molar cusps to the tip of the upper incisor.

Orbital plane.   This is a plane perpendicular to the Frankfort Horizontal plane at orbitale.

Ramus line.   This is a line tangent to the posterior border of the ramus of the mandible. It may originate in the posterior border of the condyle, in a point immediately below the condyle, or in articulare (Ar).

Ricketts' esthetic line.   This is the second of the soft tissue profile reference lines. It extends from the soft tissue tip of the nose to the most anterior portion of the profile of the soft tissue chin. At age 8 the lower lip should be 1 mm (±2 mm) behind the esthetic line. The lips will have a tendency to recede compared with the tip of the nose (which actually grows forward, especially in males). In the adult female the lower lip should be 2 mm behind the line; in the adult males, 3 mm.

Von Baer's line.   This line is anthropological in origin and follows the anteroposterior axis of the zygomatic arch tangent to its uppermost conversity.

Von Ihering's line. This too is an old line of anthropological origins. It is similar to the Frankfort Horizontal plane, except that it extends from orbitale to the center of the external auditory meatus instead of porion.

Y-axis. This is a line first devised by Downs, which extends from sella to gnathion. Its angulation with the Frankfort Horizontal is used as an indication of the general direction of growth (either predominantly vertical or predominantly horizontal) of the facial skeleton.

"All the keys hang not at one man's
girdle."
A Dialogue
J. Heywood (ed.), 1546

CHAPTER 2
The Early Architects

HISTORY AND DEVELOPMENT

We have taken the rather unusual course of discussing cephalometric landmarks, points, planes, and lines prior to beginning this discussion of cephalometric history and development. But then, the discipline of cephalometrics is an unusual science. As stated at the outset, cephalometrics is a language. It is only fitting and proper that the individual words of that language are clearly understood prior to discussions of the language. Due to the demands of modern practicality, not every point or plane that has ever been used throughout the history of cephalometrics has been discussed here, merely the ones of major clinical or historical significance. Since the study of cephalometrics is a dynamic science, there is always the potential for developing new points and planes, or for resurrecting old ones and using them in new ways. We can better understand how such processes take place, and will continue to take place, if we study the history of the development of cephalometrics.

Various authorities like to ascribe the introduction of cephalometrics to orthodontics to various individuals; however, considering the position occupied by those who subscribe to the basic tenets of the philosophy of functional jaw orthopedics (FJO), the beginnings of cephalometrics might best be ascribed to J. A. W. Van Loon of Utrecht, Holland. In a paper published in 1915, he described a technique concerned with relating the teeth to the rest of the face and skull.[9] It must be remembered that in those distant times such prestigious members of the orthodontic profession as E. H. Angle were writing things like "...the degree of perfection of the (study) models (the orthodontist) makes is indicative of the knowledge, skill, and success of the orthodontist in the treatment of his patients."[10] Well, of course, nothing could be further from the truth, especially in the light of the fact that Angle, and innumerable orthodontists since, made the art base portion of study models parallel to the occlusal plane.

Van Loon, however, whom some with affectionate respect would jokingly nickname, "The Mad Dutchman," would show that such methods clouded the true picture of the stereoscopic significance of the patient's malocclusion. He stated, "It will be clear to the specialists that the main question is not the relation of the upper and lower teeth to each other, but far more the relation of the teeth to the remaining part of the skull and the facial lines." Since this was in the days prior to the advent of roentgenocephalometrics, Van Loon developed a clever, albeit baroque, technique which no doubt was responsible for his pseudonym. He made complete, painstakingly accurate plaster casts of the patient's entire face, similar to the way death masks were made of great individuals. These casts were thin enough to permit plaster study casts of the patient's upper and lower arches to be mounted inside them in direct anatomical relation by means of primitive face bow devices. The cheek sections of the facial casts were laboriously and carefully cut away to permit the oriented casts of the arches in full occlusion to be clearly seen in relation to the rest of the masklike face, nose, and chin. The entire conglomeration was all held together in a primitive (and rather large) articulator-type device called a "cubus craniophor."

One of the most striking features of his setup was the fact that the upper and lower models were entirely removable, and Van Loon trimmed his art bases parallel to the patient's own Frankfort Horizontal plane! This gave the clinician a far better understanding of the stereoscopic aspects of the patient's malocclusion, even when the models were held separately in the hand. It was an ingenious, farsighted, pristine, and comprehensive technique, and, as far as the workaday clinician was concerned, totally impractical. But it represented the genesis of one of the cardinal tenets of all cephalometric endeavors to follow: that of attempting to relate the occlusion to something other than mere teeth.

In the meantime, while Van Loon was fiddling with facial casts and craniophors at Ryks, other great European clinicians of the day were making their own attempts at improving diagnostic techniques. One was the Swiss orthodontist Dr Rudolf Schwarz. In the 1920s he wrote articles

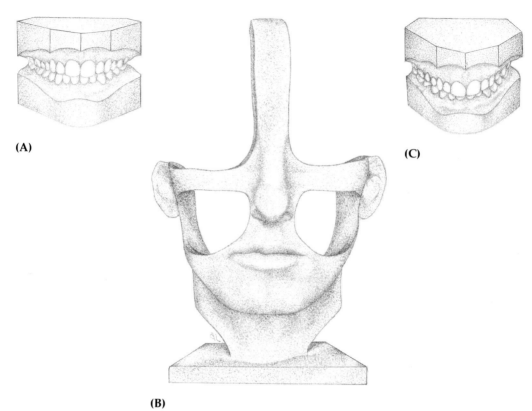

(A)

(C)

(B)

Figure 2–1   Artist's sketch of the manner in which J. A. W. Van Loon of Ryks University, Utrecht, Holland, mounted study models in plaster cast reproductions of the patient's face to better visualize the true nature of the malocclusion in precephalometric x-ray times. Primitive face bow transfer-type devices helped orient the casts to the facial mask. Facial cast and study models were held in place in a device Van Loon called a "craniophor." He trimmed the models so the art base portions would be parallel to Frankfort Horizontal plane. Calipers used to measure the face were called "prosopometers."

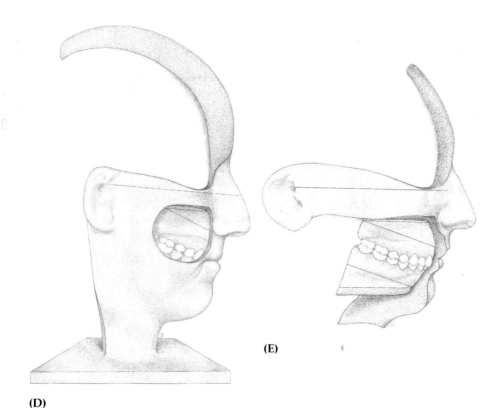

(E)

(D)

describing his method of making lateral profile line drawings of the face and jaws from plaster models that were oriented with special face bows and transferred to a mechanical drawing device called a steriograph.[11-14] He also oriented the art base of his casts parallel to the Frankfort Horizontal plane.

An equally prestigious European was Dr P. Simon of Berlin, whose "gnathostatics" was one of the most widely used methods of analyzing the occlusion of the facial outline prior to the development of the x-ray technique. He wrote a book in 1926 entitled *Fundamental Principles of Systematic Diagnosis of Dental Anomalies*.[15] Sensitive to the anthropological heritage that cephalometrics had spawned from, he developed his system of gnathostatics, which relied upon facial photographs to depict the relationships of the apical bases of the dentures to one another and to other osseous structures in the maxillofacial complex. But since the chief tool of the system was a photograph, accuracy of the surmised position of the bony structures beneath the soft tissues could not be made certain.

Simon also developed one of the earliest and simplest cephalometric analyses. Categorized as a "positional analysis," it was known as the "orbital-canine law." Simon theorized that the orbital plane (a line perpendicular to the Frankfort Horizontal plane passing through orbitale)

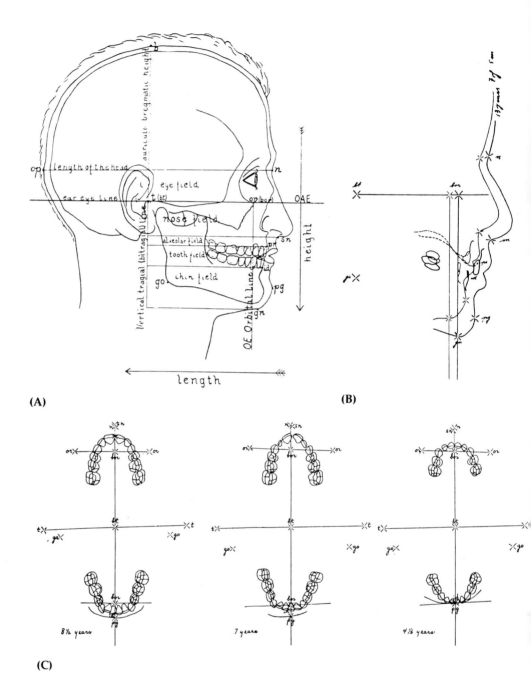

(A)

(B)

(C)

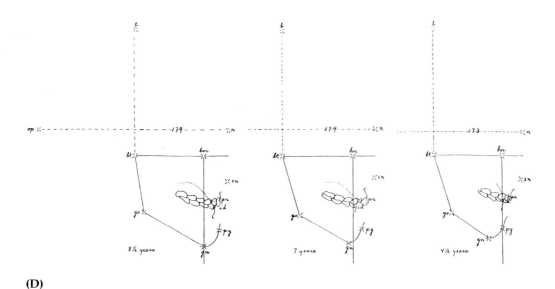

(D)

Figure 2–2 Original drawings of Dr Rudolf Schwarz of Basil, Switzerland, produced in 1923. (**A**) Freehand drawing made using major landmarks as guides transferred to sketch paper from plaster facial casts by a simple stereograph. (**B**) Superimposed facial tracings registered on porion made from two different facial casts of the same individual taken 5 years apart. (**C**) Stereographic reproductions of the teeth and arch form produced from representative dental casts. (**D**) Projections of the median sagittal plane of an individual made at 4 ½, 7, and 8 years of age. The detail available by such methods was obviously scant.

should pass through the tip of the maxillary cuspid. Variance could be measured as the distance from the tip of the cuspid to the perpendicular.[16]. It was an easy and readily understood principle of referencing; but as an analysis of tooth position relative to cranial structures, it would not endure.[17] Nevertheless, the science of cephalometrics was still in its infancy, and further efforts of doing exactly that were still yet to come. The early steps were faltering but undaunted; and they would continue to be made by those ardently striving for a diagnostic standard.

While all this was going on in Europe, along with "the war to end all wars," the United States was making its own contributions to the field. Again, the preradiographic beginnings were founded in craniometry and anthropology. And one of the earliest and most highly respected of the founding fathers of the entire movement was a man who was an expert at both dentistry and physical anthropology, Dr Milo Hellman of New York. He was a full professor of dentistry at Columbia University and a research associate in physical anthropology at the American Museum of Natural History, New York. He began his career prior to World War I, and his contributions to the literature span some 30 years. He had an uncanny knack for keeping things on an academic even keel, especially

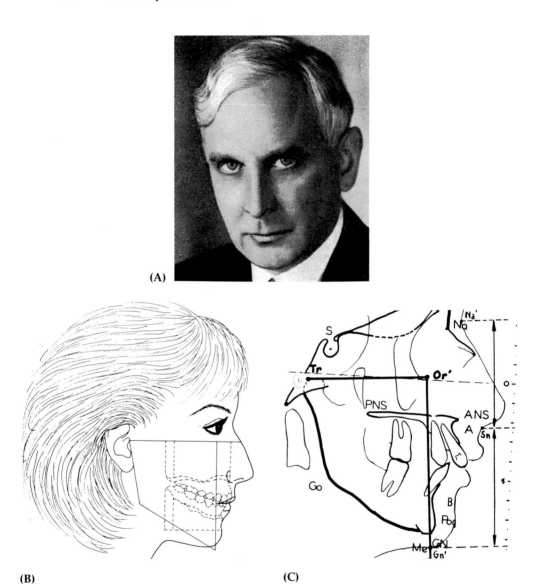

(A)

(B)   **(C)**

Figure 2–3   (A) W. P. Simon, Berlin, Germany. (B) The highly controversial "Orbitale Canine Law" is portrayed here. It stated that a perpendicular to FH through orbitale should pass through the maxillary canines, the corner of the mouth and soft tissue gnathion. (C) Originally Simon's work was cephalometric but later was adapted to roentgenographic cephalometry. In answering criticisms of his analysis system, Simon stated "The orbital law of the canines is not a natural fact, it is a fiction; it is an average won by biometric research, and this was the only way to come to a norm" (1926). In this illustration, since soft tissue gnathion is on the orbitale perpendicular, the mandible is well-situated; however, since the canine is in front of the line, the maxillary teeth are considered protruded.

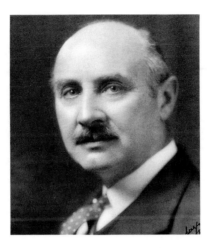

Figure 2—4   Milo Hellman: craniometrician extraordinaire.

through all the wide ranges of infatuations with techniques and theories that orthodontics went through over those years. He was one of the first to stress the study of etiology as well as function in the considerations of malocclusions. In support of such notions he cited studies concerning the role of breast-feeding v bottle-feeding, and the implications of endocrine disorders in the development of malocclusions.[18-20] He also shed light on the role of eruption patterns and their high degrees of variability in the development of malocclusions.[20-21]

Hellman was also one of the first great orthodontists of the time to openly acknowledge and discuss orthodontic failures,[22] and to attack the "myth of 100%." He also repudiated the search for a therapeutic panacea[23] (such as the particular notion of bicuspid extraction).

But the role he is most recognized for from a historical viewpoint is that of craniometrician.[24-30] He was unsurpassed at measuring and analyzing the cranium and associated structures of the maxillofacial complex, with the area of the human face representing his forte. He first gained his craniometric reputation in his studies of dried skulls; he later measured the skulls of living individuals, all without the benefits of the radiographic methods yet to come. Much of what we know about the growth and development of the face and how to reconcile it with artifically induced orthodontic treatment, we owe to the early foundations he laid down so meticulously.

The next great leap forward in the study of cephalometrics was due to the introduction of radiology to the field. The first to be credited with this feat was A. J. Pacini of the Victor X-Ray Corporation. He published a paper in 1922 entitled "Roentgen Ray Anthropometry of the Skull,"[31] in which he described a technique of producing and measuring radiographs of both dried skulls and living patients. He used multiple source/target distances of 15, 20, 30, 40, 50, and 60 in and directed the central ray 1 in above and 1 in to the front of the external auditory meatus. He also pointed out the difficulty of obtaining and deciphering frontal views of either the dried skull or the living human head due to the lack of object definition, because of excessive superimposition of osseous or soft tissue structures. Most clinicians concur with this observation to this day.

To obtain his lateral head plates, Pacini used the awkward procedure of "fixing" the patient's head to the filmholder with wrapped gauze bandages. However, his work was very important in augmenting previous efforts of studying the osteology of the human skull, which merely used anthropometric techniques. He described the following classic landmarks: ANS, gonion, nasion, pogonion, sella turcica, and the external auditory meatus. He also described some of the first measurements ever made on a cephalometric x-ray: the gonial angle, and the degree of maxillary protrusion. His work was so impressive in its day that he was awarded the Leonard Research Prize by the American Roentgen Ray Society.

The door had been opened. From anthropometry to full-fledged roentgenocephalometrics was but a few, albeit somewhat meandering, methodological steps.

Progress was not instant but suffered somewhat from relatively crude equipment and materials. Nevertheless, the frontiers of cephalometrics were steadily pushed back during the 1920s. In 1923 C. O. Simpson of St. Louis presented before a major orthodontic society the first paper describing how to obtain lateral cephalometric x-rays.[32] He used various source/target distances of 6, 10, and 12 ft. The images produced were of poor quality, and anatomical detail was lacking. As an indication of the primitive state of development of the science at that time, Simpson, following the lead of Pacini, held the film cassette against the side of the patient's head by a series of wrapped gauze bandages and employed extra support from the patient's own hand.

Dr M. N. Dewey took profile roentgenograms of the patient's head, aligning the Frankfort Horizontal plane to the horizontal by means of 90-degree-angle leveling techniques while using a source/target distance of 36 in![33] Dewey, in conjunction with Dr S. Riesner, also developed a primitive form of cephalostat or head-clamping device to stabilize the head and film cassette placement.

But in spite of these stepwise advancements to the science there was still a definite lack of order and standardization. The infant discipline of roentgenocephalometrics of the late 1920s had intention but no direction. What was needed was leadership, if you will forgive a play on words, a strong standard-bearer for a strong standard. The science expectantly awaited its needed deliverer to step forward and give radiographic cephalometrics its true definition.

Not only did just such a deliverer soon appear, but two appeared simultaneously, with each individual acting totally independently of the other on two continents. The year was 1931. Dr Herbert Hofrath of Düsseldorf, Germany, published a paper describing a technique to produce lateral cephalometric headplates.[34] On the American side, Dr B. Holly Broadbent of Cleveland, Ohio, published his classic monograph, "A New X-Ray Technique and its Application to Orthodontia."[35] It is this paper which most authorities cite as the point at which true contemporary cephalometric analysis, as we know it today, was born! Broadbent's paper was published in the second issue of the very first volume of the *Angle Orthodontist*, the journal established in memory of E. H. Angle by his co-workers.

The influences of anthropology were still heavily felt by the fledgling discipline of roentgenocephalometrics. The contributions to the field of knowledge of facial bone growth and development made by W. K. Gregory, A. Kieth, G. Campion, and W. M. Krogman dominated the field in the 1920s by virtue of their comparative anatomy and phylogenetic approaches,[36-38] and, coupled with the work of the legendary Milo Hellman, gave the preradiographic cephalometrics of that early era its strong anthropological backbone. Broadbent alludes to such work in his paper: "These men have made us realize the value of their precise methods of measuring biological problems and made us hope we could apply anthropometric techniques to our orthodontic practices." Not only was this a salute to the standards of anthropometrics, but it was also a confession that orthodontic roentgenocephalometrics was taking its first few steps rather timidly. They knew they were working in someone else's shadow!

Broadbent established a standardized source/target distance of 5 ft from the anode to the midsagittal plane of the patient's head, whereas Hofrath used a source/target distance of 2 m. At first, Broadbent used dried skull specimens held in craniostats for radiographic experiments. He cleverly inserted lead implants into various anatomical bony landmarks for direct comparison of the x-ray image measurements with those of the actual skull. Having determined that the x-ray image was a reasonably accurate, albeit slightly magnified, reproduction of the true specimen, it was but a short step to making modifications of the craniostat into a cephalostat for use on living patients.

The device initially developed to stabilize and properly orient the patient's head (or midsagittal plane) 90 degrees to the central beam of the x-ray head was referred to as the Broadbent-Bolton cephalometer. Mrs Chester C. Bolton and her son Charles provided much of the financial support for Broadbent's research work. The Broadbent-Bolton cephalometer oriented the patient's head for the lateral view such that the Frankfort Horizontal plane was parallel to the horizontal borders of the

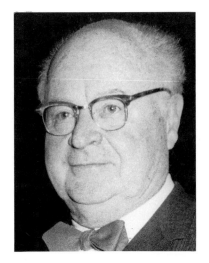

(A)

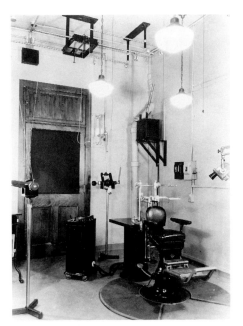

(B)

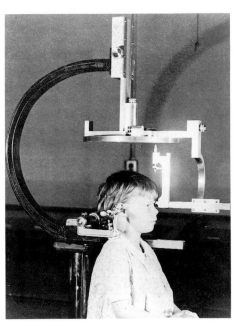

(C)

Figure 2–5   (A) B. Holly Broadbent, Sr. (B) Broadbent-Bolton cephalometric room, Case Western Reserve University Medical School (1928). (C) Broadbent roentgenographic cephalometer c. 1925.

film. This is referred to as having the head or image in "Frankfort relation."

He also developed a method of taking a frontal film by use of a second complete x-ray head, keeping the patient and the cephalostat stationary. Again, this differs from Hofrath's technique, which only took produced films from a lateral view. Hofrath's method stabilized the patient's head with two pairs of wires such that the intersections of the wires lay opposite the respective tragi of the two sides of the head. Broadbent's cephalostat, on the other hand, had ear rods that inserted into the patient's respective external auditory meatuses, which became the source of the famous "machine porion."

Another point of contrast was that Hofrath was primarily concerned with descriptive aspects of clinical significance that could be determined from a lateral cephalogram, whereas Broadbent was primarily concerned with longitudinal growth studies (studies employing sequential radiographs following the same individual over a long time). This differed from the few studies done up to that time, which were primarily cross-sectional in nature; ie, they studied a particular aspect of a cross section of a random or controlled sample of population. The extent of Broadbent's sample in 1931 was about 1700 children. The study had been under way for about 18 months at that time.

In an allusion to its benefactor, the "Bolton study" has compiled cephalometric longitudinal x-ray studies on more than 5500 children (at last count) and has spanned over 20 years! It represents the singular most exhaustive study of growth and development of the human maxillofacial complex ever compiled. Individuals were x-rayed at 3, 6, 9, and 12 months of age. Individuals were then x-rayed semiannually to age 5, then annually thereafter, with some individuals followed to their late teens. Other sample groups were added at various starting ages.

As might easily be surmised, one of Broadbent's chief concerns was the definition of stable reference points, planes, or lines upon which one might superimpose serial tracings of the same individual to analyze growth and development of the maxillofacial complex. There is some misunderstanding about this point; but the very first base reference line Broadbent developed for superimpositional purposes was the S-N (sella-nasion) line. It appears as his frame of reference in his 1931 paper, but he soon abandoned it for the more sophisticated Broadbent-Bolton Registration Point,[39] or R. This geometrically defined landmark is determined by constructing the famous Broadbent-Bolton triangle, which consists of drawing a line from nasion to Bolton Point, and then erecting a perpendicular line from this base line to sella. Bisecting this short perpendicular line gives the Registration Point R (connecting Bolton Point to sella, and nasion to sella creates the triangle). Thus orthodontics made its acquaintance with roentgenocephalometrics as primarily a research tool.

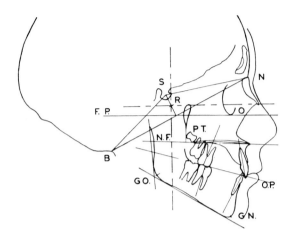

Figure 2−6   Bolton Triangle and Registration Point R. (Reprinted from Brodie AG, Downs WB, Goldstein A, Meyer E: Cephalometric appraisal of orthodontic results. *Angle Orthod* 1938; 8:261−352 with permission.

Yet the coordination of cephalometrics with clinical orthodontics was not only inevitable but imminent, and the first major effort was initiated by Dr Allen G. Brodie of Chicago, Illinois, a city that would become to the development of cephalometrics what St Louis had become to the development of orthodontics. Almost immediately after Broadbent had developed the cephalometric x-ray technique, Brodie pounced on it and started using it to assess clinical results of orthodontics. After a 6 ½-year study, Brodie, in 1938, made the first significant analysis of the clinical effects of orthodontic treatment.[40] He discovered that although orthodontic treatment could change the angulation of the occlusal plane and the axial inclination of teeth, there remained a strong tendency of the teeth to relapse toward the original values.

Growth and development appeared to cause the greatest changes in the occlusion. Any changes that were a direct result of tooth movement seemed to be confined to the alveolar processes only. What lay hidden here in these facts is what forms the very foundations of the FJO philosophy; that is, the tooth-moving fixed appliances are great for moving teeth but do little or nothing to correct the two other major relationships of a malocclusion, bones and muscles. If these are not properly addressed, relapse relegates the fixed appliances to not even being that great at permanent tooth movement. Of course, it must be remembered that in those days when extractions were indicated, it was the bicuspids that were removed, which only compounded the relapse problem. Nobody was taking out second molars yet.

What Brodie's initial findings really meant would take almost a half century to interpret correctly. But in those early days the profession was flush with the ardor of its newfound technique of the cephalogram. Its eyes were looking not for indications of the limitations of its therapeutic approach but rather for other things—things that would indicate they were on the right track all along, things that would help them get the most out of what their limited systems of mechanics could easily deliver, things that would give them an indication of how and when to use those mechanics to obtain a precalculated result, things like cephalometric norms!

Although cephalometrics had fully arrived, the full-scale cephalometric analysis systems that were to be eventually associated with the science had not. It would take almost a generation for them to develop. In their earliest attempts, "smaller" analytical efforts were mounted as soon as clinicians and researchers started deciding just what to do with the cephalogram. In 1940, Dr H. I. Margolis lent additional support to Brodie's concept of recording changes by means of periodic cephalometric x-rays.[41] Thus notions of the "progress ceph" were also born at a very early age. Also in 1940, Dr L. B. Higley stated that the gonial angle or mandibular angle might be analyzed in treatment planning.[42]

In 1941, the famous Dr Charles Tweed began his work, which was eventually to bear fruit in the "Tweed Triangle," with its highly controversial concepts of basing treatment planning around the ideal goal of a 90-degree incisor mandibular plane angle (IMPA).[43–46] At first, Tweed used sagittally sectioned casts to exhibit the anterior interincisal angles, and even as late as 1946 he was measuring the mandibular plane externally on live patients. Yet obviously, the cephalometric x-ray was the key device for such purposes and was quickly applied thereto.

The Tweed Triangle was thought of as a key for unlocking the mysteries of orthodontic cephalometric diagnosis. This was during the time when cephalometrics was still considered as primarily a research tool. In the mid 1940s, the entire focus of the debate over cephalometrics seemed centered around those who supported Tweed's theories[47–49] and those who suspected that too much variability existed[50–51] within a sample of individuals for anything as simple as a single angle or anatomical relationship to be a key to anything. What is important in all this is that it symbolized the genesis of a concept that was to haunt clinical cephalometric diagnosis and treatment planning down to this day, the notion that a given set of norms, numbers, angular or linear relationships, or theoretical cephalometric criteria would serve as a key to indicating just what and what should not be done in treatment planning, and with which appliances or technique. It was as if the orthodontic discipline had become obsessed with the search for a mythical "diagnostic El Dorado," and believed that cephalometrics all but embodied the secret map. If only they could decipher the code!

Hand in hand with this attitude was the desire to seek out the ideal face, an Adonis-like profile that could be used as a standard of excellence against which all other cases might be judged. It was also felt that roentgenocephalometrics would provide the "list of numbers" that would define what was "normal," and could also be used to assist in another obsession of the days, facial typing. Again, this is a reflection of the strong anthropological heritage of the science. The concept of a "standard value" of normality was so strong that it permeates much of the science to this day. In the 1940s, it seemed an adventuresome and noble quest, as it would for three decades to come, and has lured many a clinician and researcher into seeking out its mystical parameters.

But there were others who viewed the problem at that time with a somewhat more perceptive outlook and, if not outwardly, at least inwardly, merely smiled. Theirs was the smile of reason. It too would be ever present, but on a much more muted level, and would act as a moderating influence to the flamboyant escapades of dedicated cephalometricians who would dominate the 1950s and 1960s.

The first to exert such reflective influences on the scene, just as cephalometric analysis was "heating up" in the late 1940s, was a man who also happened to be one of the first to develop an orthopedically oriented analysis system that turned out to be a full generation ahead of its time, Dr Wendell Wylie of San Francisco, California, whose cephalometric analysis first appeared in 1947[52] and concerned itself with appraisal of anteroposterior discrepancies of orthopedic alignment of the bones of the face and jaws. Wylie was part of an ever-growing group who surmised that there was actually no such thing as a "normal" facial pattern and that malocclusions were mostly due to a misalignment of basal components, no one of which of itself was that abnormal in size or shape, but when taken in a random combination was so uncoordinated in light of its surrounding parts that the net result was an imbalance that may be termed the true malocclusion. Wylie was also the first to attempt to subdivide the maxilla and cranial base into sections along Frankfort Horizontal. By analyzing their respective values, he determined not only which linear components were in variance but also how the net comparison with the mandible resulted in the type of malocclusion or "dysplasia" manifested by the case. He was interested in just what the essence of the anteroposterior relationship actually was. This concept was to find a resurgence some 28 years later in the "Wits" appraisal of jaw disharmony, developed by Dr A. Jacobson of Johannesburg, South Africa.

The year 1947 was also when Margolis introduced the "Maxillofacial Triangle" analysis. He felt the disposition of the maxillofacial complex was stable and invariable enough to establish a standardized basic pattern, a pattern that could be outlined by a triangle as a base of reference, each side of which passed (or should pass) through respective anatomical areas or landmarks. He was another "singular-diagnostic-normative-

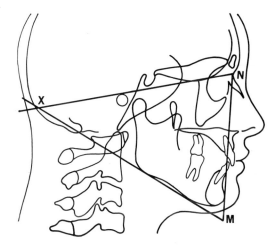

Figure 2—7   Margolis Triangle.

angle" proponent like Tweed, and believed the ideal plane of the lower incisor long axis to the mandible should be 90 degrees plus or minus 3 degrees.

Yet no sooner had Margolis' work been published when the first truly classic full-scale cephalometric analysis system became available in 1948 in the form of the famous "Downs analysis" of William B. Downs of Aurora, Illinois. The components of this analysis system form the bedrock from which many future analysis systems would draw their material. Various components of this system directly appear either modified or completely unchanged in a wide variety of other analyses. Yet the Downs analysis was based on the establishment of an "ideal" norm as the overall standard of desirability. Downs developed his system from the study of only 20 individuals with what were considered "clinically excellent occlusions." He divided his analysis into two sections of five measurements each. Five measurements were used in a description of the relationships of the skeletal pattern, and five for the description of the dentition in its relationship to the skeletal pattern. It was simple, straightforward, easy to comprehend, looked impressive, and took clinical orthodontics by storm!

What Downs had done was to try to alert his colleagues to the dangers of placing too much emphasis on a single value or measurement. He had determined a mean set of values of cephalometric readings to serve as a standard for anatomical relationships that he thought could be judged as excellent. He also contended that a skeletal pattern and occlusion could be judged as "good" or "bad" by the amount of deviation from that mean pattern. In the very last sentence of Downs' classic 1948 paper[52] on his analysis, he cautions,

The ten figures used in the appraisal do describe skeletal and dental relationships, but single readings are not so important: what counts is the manner in which they all fit together and their correlation with type, function, and esthetics.

Now that multiple-value systems had fully arrived, the placing of great diagnostic emphasis on interpretation of mere single values would gradually be abandoned in spite of persistent efforts by Tweed. No longer would clinicians base entire treatment plans on such a paucity of cephalometric criteria. The discipline had come to the realization that the single-value assessment system was not definitive. However, the philosophical approach of the normative ideal had now come to its full influence, and, as a natural consequence, the single-value-analysis approach necessarily become replaced by a multiple-value-analysis approach. The profession seemed less concerned with using cephalometrics as an aid in determining the status of how the patient *was* than it was with determining how the patient *should be*! And in all this, Wylie's simpler approach of merely attempting to evaluate the crux of the problem paled in comparison. Full-blown, multiple-value, normative, idealized cephalometric analysis had bolted out of the starting gate and was gaining speed.

Yet for a while the "smile of reason" seemed to be keeping pace, for there were brilliant observations made at this time as the direct result of the cephalometric technique. The most outstanding example is the work of Dr J. R. Thompson on rest and functional positions of the mandible.[53-57] Thompson showed that the rest position of the mandible was an extremely stable relationship throughout the life of the individual and that it was seldom affected by such things as malocclusions. Therefore, he postulated that a set of trimmed plaster models related in full-contact occlusion may not be truly indicative of the type or severity of malocclusion. One can easily demonstrate this by taking two cephalograms of the same individual, one in rest position and one in habitual occlusion, and superimposing tracings of the two to determine just exactly what happens to the mandible upon full closure. The conceptual seeds of the NRDM-SPDC phenomenon (neuromuscular reflexive displacement of the mandible causing superior posterior displacement of the condyle, possibly past the heel of the intraarticular disc into the bilaminar zone of the temporomandibular joint) were thus sown in the late 1940s, but it would be the early 1980s before they bore fruit. But for the time being, orthodontic considerations rather than orthopedic or myofunctional considerations dominated the minds of most clinicians.

Another important milestone in the development of cephalometrics in 1948 was the work of Dr Richard A. Reidel.[58] The two contributions in which we are most interested are his development of the now famous SNA, SNB, and ANB angular relationships as a form of analysis of the

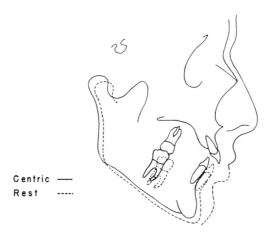

Centric ——
Rest -----

Figure 2—8   J. R. Thompson's comparison of rest and centric positions. This would eventually lead to the notion of the NRDM/SPDC phenomenon 40 years later.

anterior aspects of the maxillary and mandibular apical bases (these relationships would soon become incorporated into the analytical systems of yet another great cephalometrician, C. C. Steiner), and his observation that there was no significant difference between individuals with normal occlusion or Class II—type malocclusions as far as the relative antero-posterior position of the maxilla was concerned. Reidel determined that the component at fault was the relative position of the mandible. This implication that the maxilla was the correct member and the mandible was the incorrect member was completely contrary to the general thera-peutic philosophy of most fixed-appliance-oriented orthodontists of the time who used the lower arches as a basis from which to construct the treatment plan for the case.

   This notion of the correctness of the maxilla was also to reemerge 30 years later in the now classic work of Dr V. Luzi on "the myth of the protruded maxilla."[59] This is another key element in the overall approach of FJO: the concept of developing the mandible forward to meet the correct maxilla and maxillary dentition instead of retracting the maxillary dentition back to meet the incorrect and underdeveloped lower jaw and mandibular dentition. But in those days nobody in the American school of thought believed in the ability to "grow chins." Therefore, the ortho-pedic implications of the findings of men like Wylie and Reidel went either unnoticed or unconsidered by a profession whose attentions were directed to other things. One of its chief concerns, along with making manageable sense out of the new, prolific, and highly confusing science of cephalometrics, was to find a way of determining the best place to put teeth, especially anteriors, once four bicuspids had been extracted (or where to put them even when the bicuspids were not extracted for that matter) in order to obtain the best results with respect to both function and esthetics.

Cephalometrics in the form that Downs had introduced it was thought to hold the answers to this as well as to many other questions. Once the Downs analysis had made its debut, enthusiasm for cephalometric analysis swelled, and many researchers and clinicians were actively engaged in developing all sorts of measurements, analyses, and interpretations. Even university groups were getting into the act. Always having been associated as a research tool that academic institutions used to study growth and development, it was but a short step for the academicians to hop on the bandwagon and apply their efforts to clinically oriented cephalometric analysis. A leading example of this is the analysis system developed at Northwestern University in 1952.[60] It drew heavily from the previously mentioned work of Downs, Reidel, and Thompson and a host of others.[61-66] Like the Downs analysis it is separated into two parts: those measurements concerned with skeletal relationships, and those measurements concerned with dental relationships. Almost all of the analytical systems developed to date since the inception of the Downs follow a similar pattern of both dental and skeletal concerns.

In the years immediately following 1948 a plethora of cephalometric information flooded the scene, actually too much. Almost every conceivable aspect and relationship of the cephalometric x-ray became the subject of the most intense scrutiny (except that most important of structural entities, the temporomandibular joint!). Truly meaningful progress in the field became bogged down in an uncontrolled rush of data and information, much of which was of limited or completely inconsequential clinical value. The mood of the times might best be exemplified by the work of another great, world-class cephalometrician and orthodontist, who stepped forward in a noteworthy attempt to bring some sort of reasonable order to the scene. In 1953, Dr Cecil Steiner presented his famous "Steiner Analysis" in a classic paper entitled "Cephalometrics for You and Me." It was an analysis system of 18 components that represented a composite of many of those who had come before it. Steiner also freely borrowed from Downs, Reidel, Wylie, Margolis, Thompson, and others to produce his composite analysis. It was an analysis that Steiner felt would provide the maximum amount of clinical information with the least amount of recorded measurements, in spite of the fact that it has nearly double the number of measurements of the Downs analysis. It has become one of the most widely used analyses, and almost every clinician is familiar with at least a few of its major components. One aspect of this analysis that made it so popular was the series of precalculated formulas (written in the form of chevrons with linear and angular values written in respective places) for determining just where to place the upper and lower incisors with respect to each other and their common interincisal angle. A series of these formulas, or "acceptable compromises," covered a wide variety of treatment situations providing treatment "goals" for clinicians to strive toward in their completed cases. The system was entirely predicated upon the use of fixed-appliance mechanics.

By the early 1950s, due to the uncontrolled proliferation of the science of cephalometrics in almost every direction, tension over the lack of order and deepening levels of confusion among researchers and practicing clinicians alike reached new heights. In spite of the fact it had been available for over 20 years, there was still an incredible lack of standardization of basic entities such as source/target distance and exposure times. There was also a growing attitude, most likely the result of the individual practitioner's lack of understanding of the methodology, that cephalometrics in some sort of mysterious way held all the answers to the clinician's diagnosis and treatment-planning problems, and that only the most masterful and erudite of individuals could ascend to the level of controlling and interpreting its almost magical powers! The controversy and confusion over the issue had become so great that it prompted one nationally known orthodontic expert to compare the exploits of the members of the orthodontic profession to those of the misadventures of the ancient decendants of Noah at the Tower of Babel![67]

> And lo, confusion grew and multiplied throughout the land. Then arose a cry from the workers: let ivory be brought for the completion of the tower. And it came to pass that the specialists did multiply and did form themselves into lesser groups of specialized specialists until all progress ceased, for there was a strange confounding of language and they understood not one another's speech.
>
> Then were the dentists without unity; then did their common heritage slip from them, and they became scattered like leaves over the face of the earth.

...As a language, cephalometrics was becoming garbled!

By the mid-1950s the orthodontic profession's leadership as a whole realized it had to do something to make order out of its own cephalometric chaos. Thus, in 1956, Dr Philip Adams, then president of the American Association of Orthodontists (AAO), appointed the Special Committee on Roentgenographic Cephalometrics to address these problems. It consisted of A. G. Brodie, L. B. Higley, and W. M. Krogman as key appointees, with J. A. Salzmann as chairman. These outstanding individuals, along with other selected colleagues of equal stature, decided to hold a three-day workshop in 1957 to see what could be done to bring clarity to the subject of cephalometrics. The workshop was held at the Bolton Fund Headquarters at Case Western Reserve University in Cleveland, Ohio. The purpose of the workshop was officially to "define cephalometric points and planes, to standardize technique, to clarify interpretation, and to evaluate clinical application,"[68] a tall order considering the times. The members, in acknowledgment to their benefactor, dedicated the workshop proceedings to "United States Representative

Frances P. Bolton and her son, Mr Charles B. Bolton, who for many years have given aid and attention to the development of roentgenographic cephalometrics, and to B. Holly Broadbent, who pioneered in this field.'' With all due respects paid, the lofty group marched into the Bolton headquarters; orthodontists, physical anthropologists, anatomists, and even a radiologist and an x-ray technician.

Bearing all the figurative pomp and circumstance befitting the dignity of the scene, and flushed with the profound implications of their participation in such an auspicious occasion, the members calmly sat down at the conference table across from each other and, while the orthodontic community anxiously and expectantly looked on, the committee directly proceeded to engage in a veritable three-day academic fistfight over highly controversial and hotly debated cephalometric issues. The original transcript of the meeting numbered some 600 pages (later condensed to 336). All of the participants were in disagreement over one point or another. Many of the various things they disagreed about, such as landmarks, lines, angles, and complete analysis systems, were things the average workaday orthodontist put complete faith in!

Although there was considerable discord, some areas did finally produce a modicum of agreement. It was generally accepted that the desirable source/target distance should be standardized to Broadbent's original 5-ft distance. The radiographs should be taken with the patient's face pointing to the operator's right so that the patient's left side of the face would be closest to the cassette. In such circumstances magnification of objects from the subject averaged 5–7%. It was determined that even with the less sophisticated equipment of that time, up to 50 cephalometric x-rays per year could be taken of the same individual without jeopardizing the patient's safety. The process of tracing films on transparent acetate overlays was explained and accepted as generally accurate enough. A reasonably fair number of landmarks, lines, and angles were defined and suggested as suitable for general all-around cephalometric use, albeit only tentatively so. Obviously the workshop felt a little sheepish over its findings and therefore had not yet developed the courage of its own convictions. Part of this is no doubt due to the vast areas of disagreement that pervaded the meeting. It couldn't make a recommendation as to which of the 44 analyses it had considered was best. As Chairman Salzmann stated in his summary of the events:

> As far as roentgenographic cephalometrics is concerned, after landmarks are decided upon (and they are far from being in a state of final decision at present), there remains the problem of how and what to measure. When these are established (and they are now far from definite establishment), we still have to interpret their significance. As yet, there is no unanimity of opinion as to what they signify. There is still a long road to be traveled in roentgenographic cephalometrics before the technique can be used with a high degree of assurance.

As may be easily surmised, by the end of the workshop tempers were wearing thin. Then somebody suggested that they all go home and cool off a while and try again the next year. So they did.

A second research workshop on roentgenographic cephalometrics was convened in July 1959, again at the Bolton Fund Headquarters. This time even the government got into the act by making its first grant to the AAO for the project through the auspices of the National Institute for Dental Health, United States Public Health Department. Forty-five participants collaborated in this particular exercise, and, again, Dr J. A. Salzmann presided. This workshop, whose output was over 300 pages, was approached with a somewhat different attitude, however, as much experience and wisdom had been gained from the somewhat less than conclusive first session. The committee had come to several realizations, one of which was that in spite of the difficulties arising from the first workshop, man was indeed measurable. It was also realized that measurement is not synonymous with analysis. It is "one thing to measure and quite another thing to classify the things measured." This realization brought about a profound change in the goals that the second conference set for itself. Again, it hoped to discuss and study the relative values of the various major cephalometric analysis systems that existed to date; but the members of the committee were also becoming collectively concerned with the practicability of the entire normative concept. They were also having their attention drawn to just how cephalometrics could be legitimately used in long-term growth studies. The apparent general shift in philosophy may be summed up by stating that they were not as determined to decide what to do, what to measure, or what to think as they were with merely determining what was accurate!

They also drew some incredibly profound conclusions which had far-reaching implications.[69] They all agreed that the individual cephalometric analyses that would best serve the orthodontic discipline would be those which did not require extensive or highly sophisticated training on the part of the average clinician! Such analyses should address the skeletal, dental, and soft tissue profile aspects of a case; and all three should be coordinated not only with each other but also with other more traditional diagnostic aids in order to provide a truly comprehensive diagnosis, for it was unanimously felt by the committee that a cephalometric analysis alone could not stand on its own merits. Another truly aphoristic determination of the workshop was that landmarks are variable. The variability of landmarks changes at different rates during different periods of growth. Some landmarks are less variable than others, depending on the stage of growth of the individual. The determination was also made that cephalometric growth predictions, long a pet project of certain researchers and clinicians, were suspect, and even serial cephalometric records provided at best "only imperfect predictions." A strong objection to this point was raised by Dr Robert Ricketts, an objection not sustained by the committee's chairman. Another finding that had bearing on growth studies was that the workshop felt that no single manner of superimposition to analyze growth or therapeutic changes was completely devoid of merit; yet neither was any one completely accurate. It made its own recommendations as to the most accurate methods of superimposition for analysis of change of respective anatomical entities of the maxillofacial complex.

Yet the most surprising conclusion of the entire conference was something totally unexpected by the orthodontic community. It was agreed that cephalometrics is essentially a "descriptive technique," and it cannot provide information beyond this basic level. However, interpretation of the descriptive information derived from the cephalogram requires that the diagnostician possess an acumen in that field of mathematics concerned with statistics! The concept of comparing the data of the individual to that of standards or norms drawn from samples of what are considered normal or even excellent has *no basis* as a scientifically acceptable procedure from a statistical viewpoint! A patient's own particular deviations from a certain mean or average value is not of itself justifiable cause for treatment. Variability of measurements is a certainty. Therefore, ranges of variability about a mean are more meaningful for analytical interpretation than the mean itself. The diagnostician must know just what it is he wants to find out from the cephalogram. Interpretation should be in the light of the patient's own needs, not in light of a table of numbers! Thus it appears that no diagnostic and treatment-planning El Dorado could be found in Cleveland. Yet others, undaunted by the findings of the two workshops, would faithfully continue the search.

Though the two workshops had a somewhat organizing and clarifying effect with respect to cephalometrics, because of some of the preconceived notions it failed to support it also had a somewhat disconcerting effect on the general populace of clinicians with respect to the overall value of the entire methodology. Yet those who were undaunted by the current developments endeavored to resecure the position of the science, and one of the first, and greatest, was Dr Robert Ricketts of Pacific Palisades, California. Feeling that there was "a need for a restatement of the objectives of so-called cephalometric analysis," he published his own analysis in 1960,[70] and in what would become a characteristic reflection of the level of talents he possessed, he did it in grand style. His data base covered 1000 cases (Downs' original analysis was based on 20!), and his main efforts were in description. Ricketts was quick to point out the descriptive aspects of cephalometrics, which he referred to as "analysis" or "survey," as opposed to the more tenuous areas of inferences that can be made from that description, ie, treatment planning, which he dubbed "synthesis."

The original analysis he devised was composed of five measurements which dealt with a superficial survey of the facial form and position of the denture, and five more measurements concerned with "deeper" structures. The measurements for the superficial survey included (1) the facial angle or Frankfort Horizontal/nasion pogonion angle, (2) the XY axis, an invention of Ricketts composed of the angle formed by the intersection of Downs' S-Gn Y-axis with Huxley's line (Ba-N), (3) the facial contour indicator or the linear measurement of A-point to the N-P facial plane, and (4, 5) the relation of the upper and lower incisors to the A-Po line. These last two measurements have become quite well known to clinicians in the form of the concept of determining "cephalometric crowding" of the anterior teeth, especially lower anteriors. Ricketts himself felt the relation of the lower incisors to the A-Po line was "a key to communication of the problems with the anterior teeth." Though claiming that the original purpose of the analysis was merely descriptive, the rumblings of "synthesis," which would soon become a Ricketts hallmark, were beginning to manifest themselves again. Three years prior to the publication of his analysis (which was the year the first workshop was being held), he had published articles that already indicated he had a profound interest in using cephalometrics as an aid in treatment planning and growth prediction.[71]

The five measurements of deeper structures included (1) the length and angulation of the cranial base, (2) the location of the glenoid fossa, (3) the location of the condylar head, (4) the angulation of the neck of the condyle to the cranial base, and, the old standby, (5) the mandibular plane angle. In all fairness to the genius of Dr Ricketts, this is the first major analysis that has direct measurements of the condyle, condylar neck, and overall glenoid fossa. Finally after 30 years, attention was at least beginning to hover around that heretofore callously neglected, yet most important of structural entities, the temporomandibular joint (TMJ).

In the years to follow, Ricketts would become "the Father of computerized cephalometrics"[72-78] through his association with Rocky Mountain Data Systems, and his analysis would grow to the gigantic computerized analysis, treatment-planning, and growth-forecasting systems with their voluminous computer data printouts of the present day. Many of the measurements and definitions of anatomical landmarks used in this computerized system were invented specifically for this system by Ricketts and his co-workers. Entire booklets of definitions and instructions were provided along with a revolutionary new idea: a computer-drawn individualized set of treatment goals, called a visualized treatment objective (VTO).

The 1960s was the time of the introduction of the marvels of computers to cephalometrics. The movement seemed to stride the orthodontic discipline like a colossus. High-speed, sophisticated, electronic mathematics was being called upon to solve the many questions associated with fixed-appliance-oriented orthodontia, especially the question of whether to extract the long-persecuted, yet innocent bicuspids. Deliverance seemed at hand.

Yet in an ironic quirk of fate, the 1960s was also the age of the full-scale emergence of the maxillofacial orthopedic functional appliances, especially that champion of the functional appliance movement, the Bionator. This somewhat fortuitously precipitated an enormous crack in the ramparts of the presidio of rationale erected by the nonorthopedically oriented analysis systems. But there were also those of a cephalometric persuasion who responded to the implications of the appearance of the functional orthopedic appliance philosophy by designing analysis systems that, though they still included normative standards and treatment goals in them, nevertheless allowed for the possibilities of orthopedic changes that the functional appliances were capable of delivering. Two outstanding examples of cephalometric analysis systems that turn out to be highly compatible with these new potentials in therapy are the analysis methods of Dr Viken Sassouni and Dr James McNamara.

Actually the "archial analysis" of Sassouni was a product of the mid-1950s.[79,80] The beauty of this system, which is predicated on evaluating four major anatomical planes relative to various arcs through certain facial and dental landmarks, is that it does not compare the patient to a set of norms, but to a standard of balance and propriety that comes from the patient's own individuality. Feeling that the final facial form is a combined product of heredity and function (hopefully proper or at least corrected function), Sassouni made a bold statement for the time when he said, "...there is no universal normality; there is no norm which can be applied indiscriminately to everybody." He felt that each individual held within himself his "own ideal type, his optimum." He even went so far as to contend that not only would it be improper to treat malocclusions by referring to absolute norms for a standard, but that it would be "a dangerous mistake." The two separate camps of cephalometric aficionados were beginning to polarize.

Dr James McNamara of Ann Arbor, Michigan, was aware that most of the cephalometric analytical systems developed during the 30-year period after its introduction by Broadbent were systems developed when major changes in craniofacial skeletal relationships were considered not feasible. Yet with the arrival of functional appliance usage and the more advanced and sophisticated techniques of orthognathic surgery, wholesale change in orthopedic maxillofacial relationships became commonplace. He therefore devised yet another "new" cephalometric analysis system that would not only relate the teeth to the teeth, the teeth to the jaws, the jaws to the jaws, and the jaws to the cranial base, but also would be simple enough for every clinician to use and even to be used to explain orthodontic/orthopedic problems to the layman.[81] In a very innocuous way this represented the final step in the aforementioned polarization of the cephalometric discipline into at least two of its major camps.

Dr McNamara is one of the most prolific contributors to dental literature in clinical and, especially, research areas.[82-94] He has evolved his own cephalometric analysis system that reflects his views on possible therapeutics, views which include the potential represented by the ortho-pedically oriented functional appliances. It is not computerized, nor is it concerned with growth predictions, nor predicted treatment objectives; albeit it is normative to what are considered highly acceptable norms. But it does allow for such things as mandibular repositioning via functional appliance treatment.

Thus we have at least two men of enormous expertise who have each developed their own cephalometric analysis system, each of which reflects his own particular therapeutic philosophy. One is more fixed-appliance oriented, the other more liberal in its orthopedic orientation. Both were designed to be normative during a stage of development of the science when the voices of others cried out against the use of any form of norms whatsoever. Needless to say, tolerance of any one of these viewpoints for any one of the others does not exactly approach heroic proportions.

Yet while all the hubbub was going on over what to do with cephalometrics clinically, its original role as a research tool for the longi-tudinal study of growth and development was being forwarded by many great investigators. After the initial studies begun by Broadbent, Brodie, and Thompson, the next truly great researcher to use cephalometrics for longitudinal growth studies was Arne Bjork of the Royal Dental College, Copenhagen, Denmark. Though he may not be the most prolific of dental authors, he is certainly one of the most often cited in the dental literature wherever growth and development of the bones of the face and jaws are concerned.

His most noteworthy research concerns the long-term cephalometric study of the growth of facial and jaw structures longitudinally with the aid of metallic implants.[93-97] Bjork surgically inserted small titanium metal implants into various bony locations of the maxilla and mandible of growing individuals and recorded changes in their relative locations during the growth years via serial cephalometric x-rays and various superimposition techniques. These methods revealed much important information with respect to vertical development of the facial complex and the methods of eruption of the teeth. Bjork's contributions to the field of study of the maxillofacial complex spans nearly three decades.[89-99]

Another contributor to cephalometrics was the great German ortho-dontist Hans Peter Bimler.[100-102] Bimler's analysis represents the culmi-nation of over 35 years of clinical observation and is one of the most elaborate of the orthopedically oriented systems. Like Sassouni and others of the time, Bimler was not a believer in treating to the normative standards, but he believed all patients possessed the potential for their own standard or ideal within their own framework. His cephalometric analysis system, which contains elements totally unique to that particular system, reflects this attitude diagnostically, just as his series of functional appliances reflects his "functional matrix" theories of therapeutics clinically.[103-104]

From the preceding we have seen that the science of roentgeno-cephalometrics has evolved from crude beginnings when patients had their heads stabilized against film cassettes with gauze bandages to an age where computers trace and analyze cephalograms with pinpoint accuracy in milliseconds. This has all taken place over the last half century, but the real "explosion" is yet to come. Where that will take us, no one knows. But the state of the art in our time owes much to those in the past who endeavored to push back the frontiers of the science and to others who still continue to do so.

"...even the most imposing human faces are but made-over fishtraps, concealed behind a smiling mask, but still set with sharp teeth inherited from ferocious pre-mammalian forebears."
William K. Gregory 1929
Our Faces from Fish to Man

BONE GROWTH: THE BEGINNINGS

Since cephalometrics is concerned with the study and interpretation of x-ray images of the human skull and facial complex, and a major portion of that image is a representation of the bones of that area, a basic knowledge of the general mechanisms of skeletal development overall is critical if the clinician wishes to gain better insights into the growth and development of the bones of the maxillofacial complex in specific. This is especially true now that the more orthopedically oriented treatment results are clinically produceable due to the full-scale arrival of modern functional appliances. For the clinician who plans to advance mandibles, rotate down premaxillas in anterior open bite cases, or split midpalatal sutures, a working knowledge of the nature of the bones he is moving becomes essential. It also becomes equally essential that he possess such a working knowledge for the sake of the diagnosis, a diagnosis that is greatly augmented by the analysis of these bones as represented by their image on the lateral cephalogram. It must also be remembered that in most instances these bones will belong to a growing individual. Therefore, a working knowledge of the general growth patterns that these bones follow, and how they interrelate during growth also becomes essential for a proper interpretation of what the clinician sees in the diagnosis and what will be planned into the treatment.

Fortunately, the gaining of such a working knowledge is not difficult, provided one applies the standard approach of breaking the subject down into its component parts and dealing with them individually. Once this is done, an individual may then more easily reassemble the parts to construct a clear overall picture in the mind. This is exactly what we shall endeavor to do here. It is not within the scope of this text to elucidate a detailed study of the nature and growth of the bones of the maxillofacial complex. Scientists and researchers have devoted entire careers to this subject for generations. Yet a brief and practical review of the skeletal development of this area is handy for the clinician who wishes to better understand the diagnostic significance and treatment-planning implications of the x-rays taken of it.

As with any discussion of an involved subject, we must first start with some basic definitions of terminology used. It is generally accepted that the term *skeletal system* implies the bones themselves, the associated cartilage, the internal and external supporting tissues such as endosteum, periosteum, marrow tissues, muscle attachment sites, the sutural sites, perichondrium, and synchondroses. *Growth* of these components generally denotes an overall increase in size of the organ or system concerned as a direct result of tissue proliferation. Growth is an easily measurable process, requiring little subjective interpretation. *Development*, however, is quite another thing. This term is used to denote a particular organism's overall change in size or structure as well as several things the cephalometrician becomes very interested in: the relative positions and stereoscopic relationships that parts of this organism undergo during the life cycle. This is referred to as *topogenesis*. It may be now seen that to analyze development, where individual component parts are not only changing with respect to themselves but also with respect to each other, requires methods of interpretation in light of the knowledge of these individual contributions to the overall picture. This is the very heart and soul of cephalometric analysis, especially in the evaluation of change.

Other than the teeth, there are two basic types of hard tissue formed by the body: cartilage and bone. Cartilage is formed from a loose connective "mother tissue" by the process of chondrogenesis. It may remain as cartilage or, acting as a latticelike precursor, go on to become bone. Bone itself is also formed via transformations of precursor tissue in the counterpart process of osteogenesis. In order for a bone to form either directly or indirectly through a cartilaginous precursor, several other phenomena are manifested. The first is morphogenesis, or the overall development of the outer size and shape of a bone. Genetic factors, as well as hormonal, have an important effect here. An individual may be tall due to inherited height as a genetic trait, or short due to pituitary dwarfism. Nutritional factors such as vitamin D have an effect also.

Hand in hand with this goes the internal development of the compact and spongy portions of the bone. This is more related to function and external stimuli such as mechanical stress. Trabecular patterns in the stress-bearing areas of such bones as the mandible are a well-recognized example of this principle. As a bone grows and undergoes these changes, "transformation" is said to take place. Thus growth and transformation are integral parts of the overall developmental process of bones. Transformation, or changes in the internal trabecular structure, can be an ongoing process for as long as the individual is living and stimulated. However, morphogenesis usually ceases once the individual stops growing, at which point the bone is said to have reached maturation.[105]

It is the manner in which bones grow—more correctly, the type of tissues from which they grow—that determines the classification to which they are assigned. There are three basic types: cartilage bones, membrane bones, and cartilage-membrane bones. All three appear in the maxillofacial complex.

Cartilage Bone Development

Cartilage bones develop from a cartilaginous primordial precursor. Endochondral ossification takes place at primary diaphyseal centers and secondary epiphyseal centers through intramembranous ossification at the periosteal areas. This process is responsible for most of the skeletal development of the entire human specimen, as all of the bones of both the axial and appendicular skeleton (excluding the clavicle) develop from such cartilaginous precursors. One of these cartilaginous precursors is Meckel's cartilage. This famous cartilage primordial has a long and familiar phylogenetic history. Eons ago, it began as a primitive gill substructure. It then evolved to the level of a component of the jaw skeleton of fishes and reptiles, and finally became part of the inner ear in the form of the malleus and part of the sphenomandibular ligament.[106] The bones of the cranial base are an important example of this bone type in the skull. What is unique about them is that they are "sandwiched" between bones of other types above and below.

Membrane Bone Development

Membrane (or integumental) bones develop from a process of intramembranous ossification directly from a fibrous connective tissue source without the benefit of a cartilaginous precursor. Other than the aforementioned bones of the cranial base, all of the bones of the skull and maxillofacial complex (but only a portion of the mandible) are of membranous origins. The process of membrane bone formation is considered the older of the two types of processes phylogenetically. This process is thought to be responsible for the first origins of the dermal plates that formed the exoskeletons of the most primitive vertebrate fishes.[107] The initial shape or form of these types of bones are genetically determined, but they also have a characteristic in which the orthodontist is very interested. In addition to being susceptible to certain naturally occurring internal pressures, such as in the condition of hydrocephaly, they are also very sensitive to external mechanical stimuli. Membrane bones are a plastic type and can be subject to deformations as the result of artificially induced external pressures. The alveolar bone of the mandible and all of the bone of the maxilla are of membrane bone origins, as are the bones of the calvarium.

Interestingly, one of the external stimuli that stimulates membrane bone proliferation is actually an internal stimuli of sorts in the form of the individual developing dental organs of the jaws. As the tooth bed develops, it stimulates the increase of alveolar membrane bone around it.[108] This area of stimulation is observed to be quite localized about each tooth bud. While the tooth is forming and erupting, its surrounding bone is highly formative. Once fully erupted, the bone around the tooth is still pliable to a certain degree to mechanical pressures, but it also tends to become more subject to transformation.

Evidence of the stimulating effect on alveolar bone of embryonic tooth buds is commonly observed in the phenomenon of the retained deciduous second molar as a result of a genetically missing permanent second bicuspid. As the respective adult dental organs of the first permanent bicuspid and first permanent molar induce alveolar bone proliferation, the alveolar crest increases in size, width, and height and generally becomes more robust. However, in the intervening retained deciduous second molar area, there is *no* adult dental organ to induce extra alveolar growth. Hence the permanent molar and bicuspid "rise" to a higher occlusal level than the remaining deciduous tooth, which remains in the characteristic stepped-down position of such instances, giving the appearance that all the other adult teeth are erupting around it. It may also now be seen that the increase in vertical dimension brought about by such functional appliances as the Bionator is a truly orthopedic transaction, as the stimuli provided to the alveolar (membrane bone) processes in a roundabout way induce not only vertical movements of the individual teeth but also the entire alveolar process in which they reside.

Membrane bones are also ideal for forming the calvarium because they will assume any shape dictated by the neural growth of the brain. Nature has considerately placed a built-in safety factor into the skeletal system for the sake of both the patient's brain and maybe even the patient's orthodontist, or at least it seems that way!

Combination Cartilage-Membrane Bone Development

Only two bones derive their phylogenetic lineage from both cartilaginous and membranous sources: the clavicle and the mandible. Modern orthodontists are not too concerned with clavicles, but mandibles are where they pitch their therapeutic tents. As previously discussed, the alveolar process of the mandible is a membrane-type bone, whereas the corpus is of cartilage bone type. Then there is that truly unique and mysterious entity, the mandibular condyle, which assumes an almost paradoxical role in skeletal development.

The behavioral differences between cartilage v bone in specific are also reflected in the overall behavior of cartilage bones v membrane bones in general. First, with respect to growth, cartilage grows both interstitially and peripherally. Bone, on the other hand, grows by a combination of deposition and resorption on both external and internal surfaces. Bone deposition is restricted almost exclusively to accretion on existing surfaces, however. The internal changes in bone growth are often concerned with trabecular transformation, usually a response to external mechanical stress load. Second, the shape of the cartilage portions of the skeleton are more a product of genetic control than is the case with membrane bone. Third, chemical influences, such as hormonal influences (growth hormone stimulates proliferation and thyroid hormone influences resorption) and nutritional considerations affect cartilage, and hence cartilage bones, much more than membrane bones.

Another key difference, and one that at first might seem paradoxical to functional orthodontists, is that cartilage is relatively unresponsive to mechanical stresses and stimuli, especially of a compressive or restrictive type. The ramus portion (and only the ramus) of the mandible is an example of a cartilage-type bone that is so governed. Surprisingly, cartilage bones do seem to show some response of a proliferative nature to tensile stresses, the reaction being an increased activity at endochondral ossification sites.[109]

We need two more definitions: growth site and growth center. A *growth site* is an area usually associated with the external-force-sensitive membrane bone formation and usually takes place at interosseous sutures or along periosteal sections of a bone. *A growth center*, on the other hand, signifies an area of endochondral activity where bone growth of the axial and appendicular skeleton (as well as the cranial base) takes place. These centers, such as the epiphyseal cartilages of the long bones or the synchondroses of the cranial base, have a growth potential of incredible power[110] since they follow mostly the genetic dictates of the individual. They can physically displace bones on either side of the intervening cartilage. This process of bones moving away from each other because of the growth activity of a powerful, genetically governed cartilaginous growth center is exactly what happens in the cranial base, and no orthodontic appliance, nor any other mechanical force known to man, will stop it.[111] Except for hormonal influence (pituitary growth hormone, estrogens, thyroid hormone, etc) and a slight proclivity for increased activation due to tensile forces, the entire endochondral growth center process obeys the orders of the DNA.

With these facts in mind, we now return to consideration of that most unique component of the skeletal system and one in which the functional orthodontist is most interested, the TMJ. The head of the condyle or capitulum is, like all articular surfaces, covered with cartilage. However, the condylar cartilage develops in a way that is different from most endochondral growth centers. Cartilage formation takes place only peripherally in the fibrocartilaginous covering. There are no secondary ossification centers. Another important difference is that the condylar cartilage possesses a growth potential that is not lost once the mandible goes through its process of maturation! Hormonal control is greatly diminished compared with epiphyseal cartilage centers, and the big thing, condylar cartilage, is highly responsive to mechanical stimuli.[112] This response is age-related, which is why younger patients are more likely to have increased growth of the condylar areas and induced growth changes of the related joint structures of the temporal bone due to the tensile stresses and altered mechanical stimuli provided by functional appliances like the Bionator.

Although the phenomenon of bone growth is widely observed, it is not widely understood. The results of bone growth are easily recognizable (to which any mother trying to keep her teenager in properly fitting clothes will readily attest), yet just exactly how a bone changes its three-dimensional topographical shape is an exotic and multivaried process full of seemingly paradoxical events. Bones of themselves, static bones, are important in their own right of course; but the process of bone growth, ie, the ability of a bone to increase and at the same time *change* its size and shape, is absolutely fundamental to the survival of all higher life forms. Banal to the common man, enigmatic to the researcher, they represent on the most philosophical of levels muted biological epigrams of an exquisite and carefully thought out master plan.

One of the apparent paradoxes of bone growth is the process of resorption. Resorption is critical to skeletal enlargement; without it bones could not possibly grow, at least not in the fashion in the species as we know it today. Bones actually grow by a combined process of deposition in one area, usually on one side of a bony cortex, and by resorption in another area, usually the opposite side of that same bony cortex, although not necessarily. The process of anatomical change in an area of bone due to this combination of deposition and resorption is referred to as "drift" and represents the purest form of change in bone structure and relative position due to bone growth in that specific area.

Drift is a primary change. Take the example of a radioactive chip surgically placed on the buccal surface of a bone like the mandible in the area of the apices of the mandibular third molar. As the mandibular bone of that area goes through the primary type of growth or drift in an outward direction, the chip may be seen to rest deeper and deeper in the mandibular bone, appearing as if it were migrating lingually through the distal corpus area of the mandible. Not so. What actually happens is that as the new bone is deposited on the buccal surface of the mandible, the chip becomes buried under progressively deeper layers of bone laid down by the periosteum, just as an object left on the lawn would become buried under progressively deeper and deeper layers of snow. The cortical bone of the mandible in cross section does not get thicker and thicker in that area, but remains at the same relative dimension, because as the external cortical plate of bone (periosteal surface) is being laid down on the buccal portion it is also being resorbed on the inner (endosteal) surface of that same external cortical plate. This would give an observer the radiographic illusion that the radioactive chip was migrating lingually when in fact it has remained stationary with respect to its surrounding cells, which also remain stationary. It merely appears to move lingually through the cortical plate, since the plate and the entire mandibular bone of that area are actually growing buccally.

The lingual cortical plate goes through a similar, albeit opposite, process; ie, the external (periosteal) surface of the lingual cortical plate is resorptive, whereas the internal (endosteal) surface of the lingual cortical plate of that region is depository. Thus we have the primary process of bone growth or drift: deposition on one side, resorption on the other.

Once bone is deposited, more bone can only be deposited on top of it from an external direction (even though it might be the internal plate area of a bone). If one side of a particular area of bone or cortical plate (either internal or external) is depository in nature, its opposite side is resorptive. If a given area of bone or cortical plate (either internal or external) is resorptive in nature, its corresponding opposite side is usually depository. The point is that bone is always laid down from on top of itself; it never grows interstitially. Deposition adds to a surface that already exists, and resorption attacks the opposite side of that surface. Resorption keeps the particular cortical area the same thickness by erosion from "underneath," while deposition merely covers an area with more and more layers from "above." Snow always comes down out of the sky, never up out of the ground.

There are two basic designations of depository bone. Bone which has been laid down by the external covering membrane of the bone itself is called *periosteal bone*. Bone laid down by an internal lining membrane on the inner surface of a cortical plate (the marrow side) is called *endosteal bone*. These soft tissue membranes, or linings, are what actually control the bone growth itself. The hard tissue of bone is merely a remnant of the soft tissue membrane's direction and activity. The hard calcified portion we commonly think of as bone is a form of a biological "leftover."

The external area of a given bone may have depository fields on its *external* surface, as might be expected, but it can, and often does, have resorptive fields on various portions of its *external* surface also. This at first might seem like a contradiction, yet this is what allows the bone to gain its ultimate adult shape. The depository fields lay the bone down and might loosely be thought of as bone "stockpilers"; but by default, and by virtue of what they resorb and do not resorb, the resorptive fields are the "bone shapers." This entire process takes place in a coordinated sequential fashion that results in the phenomenon of remodeling.

Take the example of the change in the size and shape of the mandible from childhood to adulthood. The bone tissue which in the child was initially the distal border of the ramus eventually becomes, due to the consecutive layers of deposition, the bone tissue of the center of the ramus of the adult mandible. The reason is that the distal surface of the mandibular ramus is primarily depository in nature. On the other hand, the mesial surface of the ramus must by necessity become resorptive in nature in spite of the fact that it is an external surface of a bone; otherwise the ramus would become proportionally too wide if its growth were a product of deposition only. Also if the anterior portion of the ramus were not resorbed "out of the way" during the growth of the younger, smaller mandible to the larger, full adult size, no room would appear for additional posterior teeth. It must be remembered that the bone here can only be deposited on what already exists and resorbed from what already exists. It is primary growth or drift. A large and detailed snow sculpture becomes even larger after a heavy snowfall accumulates on it overnight. But a certain portion of that newly deposited snow must be sculpted away (resorbed) to regain the original, albeit larger, detailed shape.

However, bones do not merely "drift" as a product of their changing shape via the process of deposition and resorption. There is another process that also takes place that affects the relative physical location of the entire bone itself and somewhat complicates interpretation of its overall growth. The process is *displacement*, and there are two distinct types. As a bone grows, enlarges, and remodels, it carries its whole overall outline away from other bones in contact with it. This process is referred to as translation or *primary displacement*. As a product of the stereoscopic aspects of bone growth, in the process of primary displacement, which is associated with a bone's own enlargement, as the bone

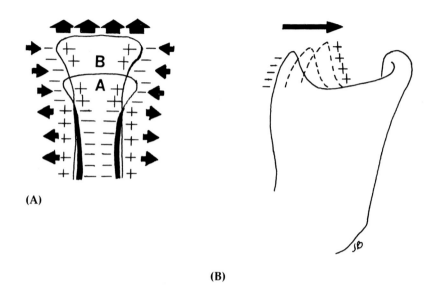

(A)

(B)

Figure 2−9 (A) Since bone growth in the form of "drift" occurs by means of deposition and resorption, external morphological changes occur. In this illustration, the bone at A, which once comprised the end, now becomes part of the shank at stage B. This requires that part of the A area that was once depository (the outer edges) must now become resorptive to obtain the narrower characteristic shaftlike morphology of the shank. (B) Drift of the coronoid process due to resorptive fields on its anterior surface and depository fields on its posterior surface. (Redrawn from Enlow DH: *Handbook of Facial Growth.* Philadelphia, WB Saunders Co, 1975.)

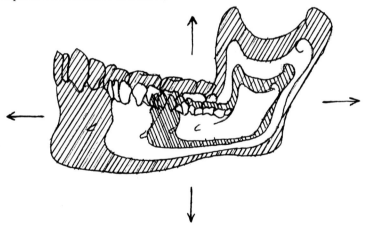

Figure 2−10 "Wrong Way Bone Growth": Bones *do not* grow larger by merely increasing their perimeters by means of universally symmetrical deposition on all surfaces. This would only result in loss of detail and "collision" of intricate surfaces. (Redrawn from Enlow DH: *Handbook of Facial Growth.* Philadelphia, WB Saunders Co, 1975.)

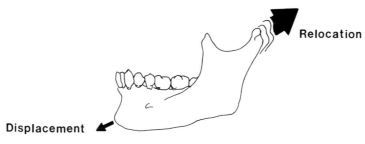

Figure 2–11 Relocation: Since condylar growth (drift) takes place in a superior posterior direction because of the nature of the growth fields present, the entire condyle is morphologically *relocated* (with new bone cell deposition) superiorly and posteriorly. As a result, the pogonial area is correspondingly displaced down and forward.

grows by surface deposition it is displaced to an equivalent degree in the opposite direction from an adjacent bone with which it might articulate. However, the bone does not push itself away from its neighbors because of deposition at its articular surfaces with adjacent bones; instead it is carried by the general overall growth of the entire surrounding matrix. But "pushing" is possible, since it takes place at the epiphyseal growth centers of the long bones. Primary displacement, ie, displacement due to the physical growth of the bone itself, is fundamentally different from the more subtle *secondary displacement* which brings about the physical stereoscopic relocation of an entire bone due to the separate growth and enlargement of the other bones.

Thus it may now be seen after this brief review of bone growth, and the two types of bone displacement due to growth, that the study of both the static (single) or cross-sectional aspects of a cephalometric x-ray, as well as the longitudinal (multiple) aspects of such x-rays, involves more than just a determination of a bone's size, shape, or relative position due to a single factor such as enlargement alone. Hence, consideration of the growth of single components of the maxillofacial complex and their combined overall effect becomes a more manageable matter of interpretation. The net result of these individual contributions make up a "cumulative composite"; that is, a representation of the total result of growth and development. It also helps shed a more definitive diagnostic light over two facets the clinician is very interested in, ie, what constitutes normal *v* abnormal.

A final point to ponder prior to looking at how individual components of the maxillofacial complex develop "normally" is the notion of balance *v* imbalance in growth and development. These terms might be a source of confusion, since during certain stages of the growth of the child into adulthood, some of these imbalances are in fact perfectly normal. The most classic and well-known example of this is the growth of the mandible. In the young child the mandible is often proportionally smaller (usually in a Class II deep bite configuration) in comparison to its fellow components of the maxillofacial complex. However, as the child matures, especially during the adolescent growth spurt, the mandible seems to accelerate its growth rate, thus correcting the state of its temporary imbalance of proportions to a state of more properly balanced proportions once again. Oddly, these multiple and varied growth imbalances throughout the maxillofacial complex may often "cancel each other out," resulting in a net imbalance that varies only slightly from an "ideal" overall picture. Analysis of just which components are of themselves a source of imbalance and what their overall net effect will be with respect to the needs of the individual is an ideal approach to the most comprehensive diagnosis of a given case of malocclusion.

It must also be remembered that a certain modicum of facial component imbalances during growth and development are a perfectly normal state of affairs and are ubiquitous throughout Nature, which accounts for the extremely wide varieties of final facial forms of individuals observable. The diagnostic aspect of orthodontics comes into play once these imbalances have become manifest enough to cause a concern for the esthetic or functional well-being of the patient. The purpose of the diagnostic process is then to attempt to determine which of the individual components are responsible for the overall imbalance in order that the most reasonable method of correcting those imbalances may be devised in the form of a treatment plan. The bony images that appear on a cephalometric x-ray are subject to the scrutiny of just such a process.

Figure 2–12   Area relocation v primary and secondary displacement: (**A**) Although the growth and remodeling in the condylar area causes the morphological relocation of the condyle in a superior, posterior direction, the result is a physical primary displacement of the mandible down and forward. (**B**) This process may also be thought of as the act of the mandible being carried down and forward due to its association with the condylar area growing (relocating) up and back. (C) Secondary displacement between the proximal head of the humerus and the tip of the distal phalanx of the middle finger. The increased linear separation represented by the longer arm (longer line A) over the shorter arm (shorter line B) is *not* due to the primary displacement of the phalanx itself due to its *own* growth, but represents a *total overall* secondary displacement due to the increased growth of all the bones between itself and the proximal end of the humerus. (**D**) Relocation is represented by the forward growth of the frontal bone (resorption on internal surface, deposition on external surface). The maxilla is therefore displaced in a secondary fashion as it is carried down and forward (dashed arrows) by the growth of the frontal bones and anterior portion of the cranial base. But is also displaced in a primary fashion due to deposition at its posterior articular surfaces. This primary displacement (small arrows) is also down and forward. (Redrawn from Enlow DH: *Handbook of Facial Growth.* Philadelphia, WB Saunders Co, 1975.)

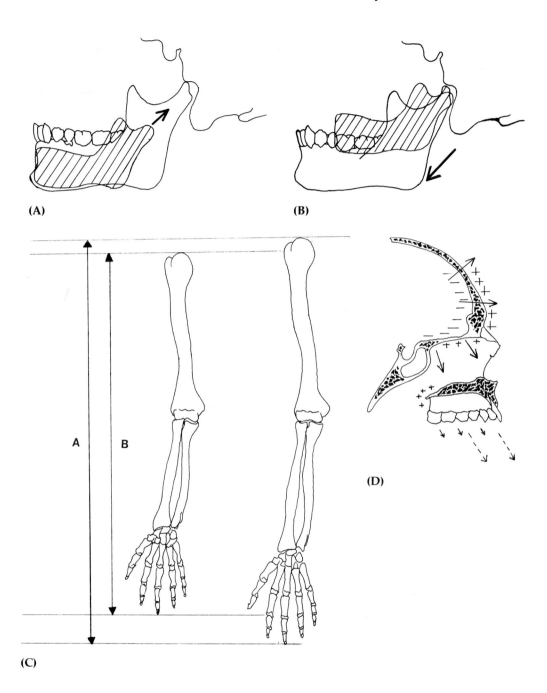

(A)

(B)

(C)

A

B

(D)

However, it must be remembered that some imbalances are, as previously stated, completely normal during certain stages of the growth of the individual. Therefore, a basic knowledge of general growth patterns of these bones is handy in deciphering just what the status of a case actually is at a given point in time. It is easiest to approach this subject by separating the maxillofacial complex into three broad areas of discussion: the cranial base, the maxilla, and the mandible.

BONE GROWTH DIRECTIONS IN THE MAXILLOFACIAL COMPLEX

The Cranial Base

The cranial base is the floor of the brain case upon which the brain sits. It is composed of portions of the occipital, sphenoid, interior portions of the temporal, ethmoid, and orbital plates, and portions of the frontal bones. It actually represents an area—the floor, or base, of the skull. Anatomically, it is divided into the anterior, middle, and posterior terraces or cranial fossae. However, cephalometrically, it has been divided more simply into the anterior and posterior cranial bases. The anterior cranial base is represented by a line from nasion to sella, and the posterior cranial base is represented by a line from sella to basion (or on occasion articulare or Bolton Point). These distances can be expressed linearly, but an angle is also formed by the juncture of the two lines at sella. Thus the angle N-S-Ba is referred to as the angle of the cranial base. It is a concept much easier to describe on a two-dimensional cephalometric x-ray as opposed to an anatomical description of the internal area of the base of the skull on an actual specimen. The cranial base represents the separation between the brain and the facial complex.[113]

The cranial base has always been an area of interest to cephalometricians, but usually only as a source of stable base reference points and lines for the construction of cephalometric analysis systems. Not much attention was given to it as far as what its clinical implications might be.[114] Yet ironically, opinion has come full cycle with respect to the importance of the cranial base in the diagnosis and description of malocclusion. At first, the early researchers attempted to blame the state of a patient's malocclusion on mere arrangements of teeth and improper muscle function. However, as data accumulated, it was discovered that overall facial form, size, shape, and character were also major determinants of the state of occlusion of the teeth, and these turn out to be a direct reflection of the influence of the cranial base.[115-119]

It would be the role of cephalometrics to bear out radiographically what had already been determined empirically. One of the first to do this, in the early 1950s, was Bjork, who pointed out that the size, shape,

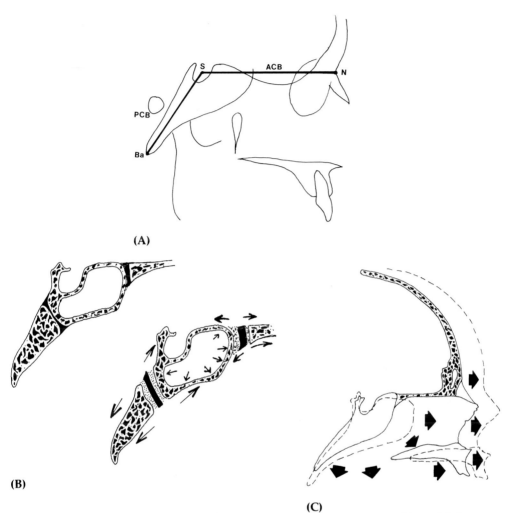

(A)

(B)

(C)

Figure 2–13 (A) N-S-Ba cranial base angle: ACB = anterior cranial base (N-S line), PCB = posterior cranial base (or S-Ba line). (B) Depiction of the growth of the powerful spheno-occipital synchondrosis and the less influential sphenomesethmoidal synchondrosis. (C) Generalized growth directions, primary and secondary displacement of the maxillary complex due to growth of the cranial base.

and degree of flexure of the cranial base had a definite influence on the relative degrees of maxillary and mandibular prognathism.[120,121] There are four basic growth centers of the cranial base, three of which are synchondroses, and as such are remnants of the primary cartilages of the embryonic cranial base (endochrondral ossification centers). The centers are the spheno-occipital synchondrosis, the largest and most powerful; the sphenomesethmoidal synchondrosis; the mesethmoidal-frontal, which is quite restricted; and the frontal bone itself, which is more of a growth site than a center. Now since the calvarium or skull follows a neural growth pattern, which is very rapid during the first 2 to 3 years of life and then falls off at age 7 to 8, reaching about 85–90% full capacity, and since the facial bones follow the slower, steadier pattern of skeletal growth that is independent of the brain (except the adolescent growth spurt), the cranial base might at first consideration be expected to follow a rate of development somewhat representing the average of the two. Not so. This only appears the case when the overall average rate of growth is considered. Individually, the various components of the cranial base follow either the quick-start neural growth pattern or the slower, more steadily paced skeletal rate. The region from nasion to the foramen caecum and the region from sella turcica to basion follow the skeletal rate, whereas the region from the foramen caecum to sella turcica and the distance from the anterior portion of the foramen magnum to the posterior portion follow the neural rate. This stands to reason since the area from foramen caecum to sella turcica is so intimately related to frontal lobe development, and the diameter of the foramen magnum is so closely associated with development of the spinal cord that it could hardly be any other way.

Thus across the entire span of the cranial base from anterior to posterior, bone development is governed by four different growth areas, each of which may be governed by at least two, or maybe even four, different rates of growth! The variance of such a process at once becomes obvious, and a variation of growth rate across a structure that is as curved as the cranial base leads to a phenomenon that has a direct bearing on the status of the occlusion as well as the whole face—flexure!

Flexure of the cranial base, or at least the degree of flexure, has an intimate and orthopedically oriented effect on the jaw-to-jaw relationship anteroposteriorly, and hence the status of the skeletal and dental class of the case. The concept of this flexure is best described by the angle of the cranial base, N-S-Ba (or articulare or Bolton Point as a substitute for basion). S. E. Coben was one of the first to point this out, in the mid-1950s. He noted that a more acute cranial base angle could easily result in a Class III situation if there was not a "canceling out" effect of a correspondingly, naturally shorter mandible. Increased flexure, or a more acute cranial base angle, in this instance would be like the effect of "pulling" the upper part of the maxillofacial complex inwardly while at the same time leaving the normal mandible out in what would be a "high and dry" position, resulting in the Class III arrangement.

Conversely, a relative decrease in flexure, or an excessively obtuse cranial base angle, would be tantamount to bending the upper part of the maxillofacial complex up and away from the base of the neck, leaving the innocent mandible stranded behind in a Class II configuration. Not only could the degree of flexure present or not present bring on such results, but the actual quantitative amounts of absolute linear growth of the individual components could also be influential.[122] An excessively long cranial base could result in a Class II relationship, whereas a relatively short cranial base could result in a Class III relationship, all depending on a normal-sized mandible not canceling out the cranial base imbalance.

Though the lesser synchondroses and growth centers usually solidify early in life, it is now believed that the main spheno-occipital synchondrosis does not close until 13–14 years in females and 16 years in males,[123] as opposed to the 20- to 25-year range as formerly thought.[124] This is well past the time when many children of the adolescent age present with signs and symptoms of malocclusion. It has been shown that the linear distances as well as the cranial base angle were in fact smallest in a range of values for Class III malocclusions and, correspondingly, largest, ie, relatively more obtuse cranial base angles and greater linear lengths, for Class II configurations.[125,126]

In 1968, G. B. Hopkin of the University of Edinburgh corroborated these findings by determining the ranges of values for the linear distances and the cranial base angle associated with the various classes of malocclusion.[127] He preferred the use of articulare as the end point of the cranial base angle. The ranges he determined for the N-S-Ar angles were as follows:

Class III	122.2°, SD±4.7°
Class I	124.2°, SD±5.2°
Class II, Div. 2	125.5°, SD±4.8°
Class II, Div. 1	128.9°, SD±4.5°

There was a standard deviation of plus or minus 4.7 degrees to 5.2 degrees for the various values, which allows for considerable overlap and variation. Yet the general trend is obvious. Flexure of the cranial base has a definite contribution to make to the status of the jaw-to-jaw occlusion. More than just teeth and maxillary-mandibular lengths are involved. In light of such information, it may now be seen why it is more logical to address certain malocclusions with orthopedically oriented techniques that can push out premaxillas or advance whole mandibles where necessary rather than merely tipping teeth in an attempt to mask true bony discrepancies.

With respect to growth, since portions of the cranial base are subject to general skeletal growth rates, the adolescent growth spurt would be expected to have an influence on this area, which it does.[128,129] This is significant because of the effect growth has on two very commonly used landmarks, sella and nasion. During the period of growth, and especially during the adolescent growth spurt, nasion can be expected to move up and away from the center of the maxillofacial complex. Less than uniform consensus of opinion exists, however, as to exactly what happens to sella. Some feel that it rises in conjunction with nasion a sufficient amount to keep the base reference line N-S parallel, albeit relatively higher. Others feel sella (pituitary fossa) rises during earlier growth periods as the sphenoidal sinuses enlarge, but only until about the age of 12 years. Thus it may be seen that the base reference line N-S may not be as stable as the early researchers would have liked it to be. Even if both sella and nasion rise by the same relative amount during the adolescent growth years to keep the N-S reference line parallel, it will still alter analysis of facial height measured to this line by providing slightly excessive estimates of vertical growth, especially with respect to comparisons with horizontal growth.

The Maxilla

Compared to the somewhat complicated development of the cranial base with its combined skeletal and neural growth rates, the growth of the maxilla seems comparatively simple. Yet there are several intriguing paradoxes that envelop this structure with respect to the manner in which it grows. It is of membranous bone origins and is a paired bone. It forms the roof of the mouth, floor of the nose, a portion of the orbit, a portion of the cheek bone or zygomatic process, encloses the antrum or maxillary sinus, and is the base for the entire alveolar process of the upper jaw that contains all 16 of the upper teeth. The maxilla grows in three directions, with its greatest growth increments in height, less so in sagittal depth, and least in transpalatal width.[130-131] It is described as growing mostly down and forward. Yet this may be a confusing over-simplification due to the very nature of its growth. And this very nature of the growth of the maxilla is what lies at the therapeutic heart of what the orthodontic profession has been attempting to address with certain of its techniques for over three quarters of a century, as we shall see shortly.

The concept that bone growth takes place by outer surface deposition and inner surface resorption is over 200 years old. This observation held sway even into the 1920s and 1930s, augmented by the notion that bony proliferation also took place at the sutures. These sutural sites were originally thought to be primary growth centers in the maxilla similar to the epiphyseal cartilaginous growth centers of the long bones.[132] Opinion has since changed on this issue, however, and more current theories still support the concept of bony proliferation at sutural interfaces, but it is felt that the primary suture sites of the maxilla (ie, the ethmoidal, frontal, midpalatal, and zygomatic) are active until about age 7. It is also felt that the developing brain, eye, nasal cartilage, and even tongue are sources, along with other soft tissue growth and development, of separation-type forces that stimulate bony growth along the free margins of the naturally existing sutures. Another theory maintains that this sutural activity diminishes past age 7, after which surface deposition and resorption take over as the main mechanisms of growth.

Another mechanism that all agree is critical to growth of the maxilla is the process of remodeling. Because of its important role in supporting the occular, respiratory, and masticatory systems, the maxilla must maintain the complex, exacting shape in its upper portions while being highly adaptive and forgiving at its "heavy-duty" end, the alveolar process. Remodeling is the phenomenon that controls the processes of either periosteal or endosteal cortical surface deposition that allows the maxilla to adapt to the demands of both the natural dictates of its surrounding soft tissues and the artificial dictates of orthodontic appliances.

The two mechanisms involved in remodeling are deposition and resorption. Both of these processes take place at the surface of a more compact plate of bone or lamella. The external portion of the lamella receives periosteal resorption or deposition, and the internal portion of the lamella, on the inside of the bone, receives endosteal resorption or deposition. Thus the external portion of a particular part of the maxilla may be depository or resorptive. And the internal surface of any of its cortical bony plates may also be depository or resorptive. The sequential resorptive-depository process on a cellular level that reshapes and "moves" the particular surface of bone concerned is referred to as "area relocation"; it is bone movement of a primary type, ie, due to the physical growth of the bone's surface itself. The chief areas of growth of the maxilla are the zygomatic process, palatine process, orbital portion, nasal portion, maxillary alveolar arch, maxillary tuberosity, and premaxillary area. Of these, the last two at first seem the most enigmatic.

The maxilla generally grows down and forward, out from under the cranial base by means of deposition at its posterior and articular margins. As it does so, new bone is deposited at the maxillary tuberosity area, an area of periosteal deposition, which leads to an overall lengthening of the maxilla sagittally. Therefore, even though the growth is by continuous deposition at the posterior and tuberosity areas (ie, growth occurring in a posterior direction), the actual movement or displacement of the maxilla is in an *anterior* direction. It does not push itself away in an anterior direction but is carried in that direction by growth of the surrounding structures of the maxillofacial complex. A portion on the buccal area of the tuberosity is depository also; hence as the maxillary arch gets longer, it also gets slightly wider posteriorly.

In conjunction with the overall downward and forward movement of the maxilla, the palatine processes are depository on the palatal side and resorptive on the nasal side. This allows for general enlargement of the nasal passageways. But the anterior portion of the palate, although

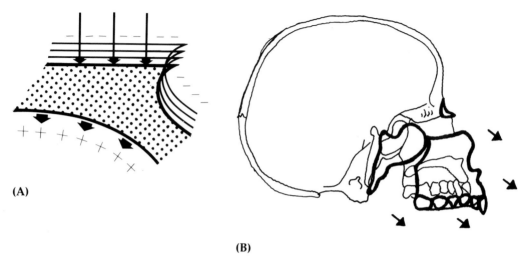

(A)

(B)

Figure 2−14   (A) Growth (drift) in the maxilla is accomplished through growth fields that are resorptive on the superior surface (which represents the floor of the nasal passage) and the anterior surface, and depository on the palatal surface. (B) General growth direction of the maxilla is down and forward with respect to the cranial base. (Redrawn from Enlow DH: *Handbook of Facial Growth*. Philadelphia, WB Saunders Co, 1975.)

depository, is also the underside of the premaxillary area, which has some seemingly contradictory growth patterns of its own.

The premaxilla possesses both a labial cortex and a lingual cortex, each of which has an outer (periosteal) side and an inner (endosteal) side. Now researchers describe the growth of the premaxilla as predominantly downward and slightly inward. Remembering that the predominant direction of growth of the entire maxilla as a whole is down and forward, we might think this to be a contradiction. The anterior external surface of the premaxilla is resorptive, which has also been discovered to be, basically, another seeming paradox! The periosteal portion of the labial cortex is resorptive, the endosteal surface of the labial cortex is depository. Conversely, the endosteal surface of the premaxillary lingual cortex of the nasopalatine area is resorptive, but its external or palatal periosteal surface is depository.

This combination allows two things to happen that effect the general growth of the premaxillary area in a downward and slightly inward direction. First, it allows for area relocation of the entire premaxilla in a downward direction on a primary cellular bone growth level. A point location that started out in the center of the premaxillary medullary area becomes the surface bone of the premaxilla as the external labial lamella or cortex is resorbed down to its level. A point location on the surface of the external lingual lamella or cortex becomes the center of the maxillary bone as deposition buries it under successive layers of new bone. Hence the premaxilla is relocated by its own cellular activity of resorption and deposition on the appropriate sides of its respectie bony lamellae.

Second, since the entire maxilla as a whole is moving down and forward, the facial surface of the maxilla must be resorptive to prevent elongation of the muzzle, which occurs in all other primates. Man's flatter, more erect face is a product of the anterior resorptive fields of the maxilla eroding and remodeling the bone as fast, or faster than, it extrudes out from under the cranial base. Such principles also take place in the mandible as a form of anterior facial control. This is why the degree of facial protrusion of young children may be seen to steadily regress slightly to the flatter, more erect facial outline of the fully grown adult. The failure of this process to take place is what is responsible for the elongated muzzle area of the typically simian profile.[133] It is only a matter of biological coincidence that the slightly more convex facial profile of the young child is reminiscent of the simian profile. Yet considering the principle that "ontogeny recapitulates phylogeny," one wonders if when Shakespeare's doleful Lady MacDuff lovingly addressed her young son in the words, "Now God help thee, poor monkey!" (*Macbeth* 4, ii, 59), she might not have said a real mouthful!

It may now be seen why the forces of mesial and occlusal drift exist with respect to the teeth. Since the alveolar process of the maxilla progressively relocates its position downward and forward, primarily by surface deposition and resorption on a cellular level, and secondarily by the physical displacement of the entire maxilla, the teeth carried in that alveolar process must also follow the same course. But they cannot do so by mere secondary displacement alone, ie, as passengers going along for the ride. A portion of that movement of the entire alveolar process is primary; ie, surface level increases because of depository and resorptive activity on the lamellar surfaces. Therefore, if the individual teeth did not have some compensating factor associated with them to counteract this process, they would gradually become buried in the accumulation of new layers of bone of the primary growth of the alveolar process. Yet Nature has ingeniously provided such compensation by virtue of the forces of mesial and occlusal (incisal) drift, which it incorporates into the mechanism of dental development.

This drift allows the continuance of dental relationships in spite of the shift of the entire alveolar processes of the jaws. Thus teeth have not only an eruptive force to bring them into the oral cavity, but also a drift that helps them maintain their proper relationship with their side-to-side neighbors as well as their opposing antagonists. Mesial drift is not solely for the preservation of tight contacts, more importantly, it maintains the integrity and balanced function of the entire maxillary (and mandibular) alveolar processes as growth carries the bone down and forward.

Additionally, it must be remembered that in the premaxillary area, the labial surface is resorptive and the lingual (palatal) surface is depository, as the premaxilla relocates downward and slightly inward. Because drift takes place on a curve where the forward drift of the two halves of the dentitions on each side of the dental arch would figuratively "collide," certain portions of the anterior maxillary arch gradually shift into more medial positions. The overall effect of this anterior remodeling and surface "condensation" of the labial surface of the premaxilla is to magnify the forces of mesial drift by default from the opposite direction and to impart an uprighting or, more correctly, a slight recession of the permanent anteriors. Attention was first brought to this phenomenon in 1953 by the cephalometric studies of Brodie,[134] who observed that the anterior teeth sometimes exhibited a slight "dropping back" during growth in the premaxillary area.

Now taking into consideration that

1. The general growth and displacement, both primary and secondary, of the maxilla are down and forward due to growth at the posterior and articular surfaces of the maxilla.

2. Mesial and occlusal (incisal) drift exists in the teeth, on top of their eruptive forces, to maintain proper interdental occlusion and contacts in the growing maxilla.

3. The resorptive fields of the anterior areas of the maxilla (and mandible) "erode," remodel, and condense the maxilla (and mandible) as it is "thrust" by growth down and out from under the cranial base, thus intensifying mesial drift as it brings about Brodie's "dropping back" of the anteriors.

4. The thrust of the erupting second molar as it attempts to plow a furrow for the doddering third is powerful.

is it any wonder dental crowding so often appears in the dental arch in the form of shortened anteroposterior arch length?

Crowding is often seen as a result of the posterior segments having drifted *forward* by an excessive amount. And yet, still another consideration of a force of another type sheds light on one of the alternative forms of maxillary arch deformation: the Division 1–type angulation of the anteriors. Here one cannot help but implicate the tongue and its improper function as a contributing etiological agent. For in light of the above considerations, should the balance of forces exerted on the highly bioplastic membrane-type bones of the alveolar processes be tipped in favor of forward forces during the years of growth and development, it may easily be seen how the extra forces of an improperly functioning, forward-thrusting tongue which still operates in the infantile swallowing pattern, sealing itself forward instead of vertically during deglutition, can result in overpowering the resistive forces of the premaxilla.

The tongue, in conjunction with other improper muscle function, is a major contributor to maxillary arch deformations. If the tongue seals vertically, as it should, it helps increase the pressures resulting in the proper development of the vault of the palate. Some practitioners believe that such a process also assists the maxillary arch in attaining its proper complement of width. But with the forces of maxillary growth down and forward to begin with, excessive imbalance of muscle function in that same direction can easily be seen as a primary etiological agent in the resulting Division 1–type narrow or Gothic arch-shaped maxillary dental arch and alveolar process.

It may now be seen how the process of maxillary bone growth covertly lies at the very center of various orthodontic therapeutic philosophies. For one philosophy, it is the focus; for the other, it is a victim.

It has long been common knowledge in the workaday world of clinicians that the fixed-appliance, bicuspid-extraction-oriented American school of thought of orthodontic therapeutics built its case around the mandibular arch. It was erroneously thought that the mandible could not be "artificially grown" or repositioned as a whole. The mandibular position was thought to be immutable; hence it became a treatment-planning standard. All things were made to conform to its pretreatment anatomically stereoscopic demands, even the maxilla. The maxillary teeth were retracted back, and the mandibular teeth were tipped forward in order to resolve severe overjet problems. If this could not be easily accomplished, along with the simultaneous decrowding of arch forms, bicuspids were extracted to facilitate correction of crowding and overjet problems. If a skeletal Class II jaw-to-jaw situation was severe enough, not only were bicuspids extracted and anteriors retracted, but external force in the form of headgear was applied in attempts to provide the extra anchorage to pull everything back. Enough forces were at times applied to attempt to halt the growth of the maxilla, down and forward, from attaining its full potential altogether![135]

In spite of the fact that usually the underdevelopment of the mandible was the chief cause of the skeletal and dental Class II deep bite situations, the correct member, the maxilla, was constricted back to conform to the demands of the incorrect member, the mandible, thus perpetuating and intensifying a naturally occurring orthopedic mistake. This technique fought against everything Nature was trying to do with respect to growth of the maxilla. In addition, second molars were left intact with "everything pulled back upstream" against the natural growth gradients Nature wanted. Relapse descended like a plague. And even when it didn't, what would be the effect of such retruded maxillary arches on the contours of the face, the mandibular arc of closure, and the functional balance of the TMJ? The proponents of the philosophy of FJO look at both growth and therapeutics differently!

The Mandible

Growth of the mandible has long been a subject of interest for researchers and anatomists. Most monographs that appear in the literature cite the classic work first done on the growth of the mandible by the English anatomist John Hunter. By using the vital stain alizarin in the study of swine mandibles, he determined that the mandible grows in a posterior direction, thus elongating itself and displacing itself anteriorly in the opposite direction of its growth. Hunter showed that the ramus grows "backwards" also by means of deposition on its posterior border and resorption on its anterior border. He also discovered that the increase in the height of the horizontal portion of the corpus of the mandible was attributable to alveolar growth and that the mandibular condyle was also a center of active growth.[136] These principles of mandibular growth are as true today as when Hunter first discovered them. That is what is so truly incredible. He published these findings in 1778! The American Revolutionary War was only 2 years old, nobody was President, and the country had no states.

Hunter's findings were corroborated nearly a century later by another Englishman, G. Humphry, who also studied mandibular growth. In a series of ingenious experiments, Humphry inserted small, brass wire rings through the anterior and posterior borders of the rami of young, growing swine mandibles. He found that the rings inserted through the posterior margin of the ramus gradually became more deeply embedded into the body of the ramus during growth, whereas rings inserted through the anterior border of the ramus were observed to "migrate" free, which actually represented abandonment as the anterior surface of the ramus resorbed past them. These studies were reported in 1864.[137]

In 1924, yet another Englishman, J. C. Brash, verified these findings. Brash performed similar growth studies again using the old alizarin vital stain.[138] His work is also considered classic and is nearly always cited in reviews of the literature on studies of mandibular growth.

Contemporary with Brash, and a fellow countryman, S. W. Charles published studies that recognized the mandibular condyle as a critical and major center of growth for the mandible.[139] It was deemed responsible for the predominantly downward and forward growth of the mandible as a whole and felt to be vital to maintaining orthopedic balance during growth of the jaws by governing the rate of growth of the mandible. Modern research has indeed borne this all out. Yet it must be remembered that these findings were all made prior to the introduction of roentgenocephalometrics. The precephalometric history of the study of the growth of the mandible is indeed long and impressive and undoubtedly belongs to the British. However, once the cephalometric x-ray made its debut, the output on the subject shifted to the "three B's," Broadbent, Brodie, and Bjork. Then soon it seemed as if everyone got into the act as cephalometric studies of jawbone growth blossomed.

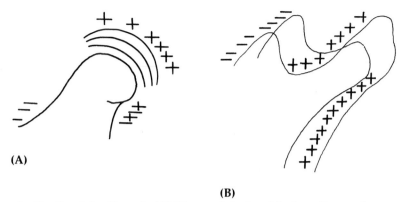

(A)

(B)

Figure 2–15   Condylar Growth. (**A**) The condylar head is depository, whereas the neck area of the condyle must be both resorptive at times and (**B**) depository at times. (Redrawn from Enlow DH: *Handbook of Facial Growth*. Philadelphia, WB Saunders Co, 1975.)

For our discussion it is handy to discuss growth of the mandible in terms of its various areas: the condylar portion, the ramus, the corpus, the alveolar crest, and the chin. In spite of being a single bone, unlike the paired bones of the maxilla, the mandible is seldom thought of by researchers as a single functioning unit, but is more often divided into at least two major components, the corpus (horizontal part) and the ramus (vertical part). It must also be remembered that the mandible is the direct structural counterpart to the maxilla, not vice versa. In other words, in all vertebrate species, the lower jaw functions against the upper jaw, moves to meet it during function, and is braced against it during full occlusion. The mandible moves to adapt to and meet the maxilla, which is a stationary part of the fixed base of the skull; the maxilla never moves down to meet the mandible.

As previously discussed, the condyle has been shown to be one of the chief centers of overall mandibular growth. Its growth is by means of endochondral-type replacement of condylar cartilaginous tissues by bone. Although the condyle grows both superiorly and posteriorly via the mechanism of area relocation (ie, sequential deposition and resorption), the resultant displacement of the entire bone itself is down and forward.[139–141] Because of this process, a particular bone cell that originally resides in the head of the condyle soon becomes part of the condylar neck. Surface resorption and remodeling produce the characteristic shape of the neck. Further growth in the form of newly activated depository processes causes that same cell to next become part of the superior portion of the ramus. Thus an area of bone in which our subject cell exists was at one time wide (the condylar stage), became narrow (the neck stage), then became wider again (the ramal stage), and all the while the entire bone was going through a stereoscopic primary displacement because of the actual growth of the bone itself. The most important thing to remember is the dual nature not only of the condyle as a growth center but also of the entire TMJ complex itself.

To summarize, the condyle and its companion articulating surface of the temporal bone follow genetic dictates of growth, but due to the special nature of the condylar cartilage and the membranous lineage of the temporal bone, the entire joint structure is extremely adaptable to functional demands. However, this attribute of adaptation has its limits. It adapts well to tensile forces; ie, in the growing child the condyle can be stimulated to grow when held down and forward by appliances such as the Bionator, as functional orthodontists have long known. In the adult, during TMJ decompression procedures with mandibular-advancing functional appliances, more subtle adaptive changes take place that result in wholesale condylar repositioning and joint structure coalescence, as many "TMJ specialists" have more recently discovered.

On the other hand, the condyle does not adapt well to compressive forces—but why should it? It is by design a compression movement articulation. Absorbing mechanical stresses and pressures are what it is biomechanically engineered to do. The entire joint responds poorly to condylar displacement off the back edge of its articular disc in a superior posterior direction. In other words, it will grow if "stretched" properly down and forward out of its articular "cradle," but it won't shrink if compressed up and back past the back edge of its cradle. Condylar head and neck growth and adaptation are a one-way street. But then again, everything else of major consequence in the upper and lower jaws grows down and forward out from under the base of the skull. Why should the condylar growth center be different? Its main job is to see to it that it grows superiorly and posteriorly enough, displacing the rest of the mandible inferiorly and anteriorly enough, to keep pace with the growth in that direction of not only the maxilla but also the rest of the maxillofacial complex. This it will do, but during growth years it seems sensitive to functional inhibitions such as restraining improper muscle balance, and/or the interferences of an arc of closure obstructing, distally locking occlusion. Then it might need a little help! On the most basic and fundamental of biological levels, it seems only logical that such therapeutic help should come in the form of attempts to stimulate and increase growth of the lagging bottom rather than attempting to decrease or stifle normal growth on the top.

The ramus itself follows more chondral-type growth patterns; ie, it is more obedient to genetic dictates and less influenced by functional stimuli. Growth fields on the buccal and lingual surfaces of the ramus are complex, but one thing is clear—the ramus grows posteriorly by deposition along its posterior border and by resorption along its anterior border. This results in an area relocation of the ramus distally. This lengthens the lower dental arch, which is a necessary process to permit the eruption of the posterior teeth.[142] Immediately after the extraction of

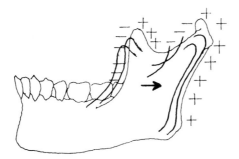

Figure 2—16 Ramal growth: The ramus grows (drifts) posteriorly by deposition on its posterior surface and resorption on its anterior border.

a lower third molar, as the surgeon inspects the socket wall, he is most likely looking at bone cells that were part of the posterior edge of the ramus at an earlier time when the patient was younger.

As the process of distal relocation of the ramus takes place, it serves to lengthen the corpus of the mandible horizontally. Thus posterior growth not only displaces the entire mandible bodily forward in the opposite direction to that growth, but it also lengthens the body or corpus of the mandible posteriorly. Except for the mental protuberance or chin button, the entire anterior surface of the mandible is resorptive. This again seems at first paradoxical; yet, like its counterpart in the anterior maxillary area, this resorptive field serves to control the shape of the anterior portion of the mandible as it moves forward out from the base of the neck due to accumulation of bone at its posterior surfaces. Although the alveolar region of the anterior surface of the mandible is resorptive, the entire inferior border and mental protruberance areas are depository. This deposition in conjunction with the alveolar process growth sites combine to add height to the corpus itself. The growth of the chin button is greater in males because it is a form of secondary sex characteristic.[143]

To compensate for the labial resorptive surface in the mandibular incisor region, the lingual surface of the mandible behind the anterior teeth is depository. The teeth in the mandibular alveolar process have both eruptive forces and mesial and occlusal (incisal) drift forces, as do their maxillary counterparts.[144] These forces, acting in conjunction with the resorptive fields of the anterior alveolar surfaces of the mandible and being on an arc or curve, produce the same condensing effect as in the maxilla, which can lead to an overall flattening of the area with growth. This phenomenon contributes to the principle of relative "dropping back" of the incisors, as described by Brodie. Thus a distant form of condensation is effected in the area which, when combined with the mesial drift effect of the posterior quadrants, can, if imbalanced enough, lead to the commonly observed effect of crowding. This effect is only worsened by

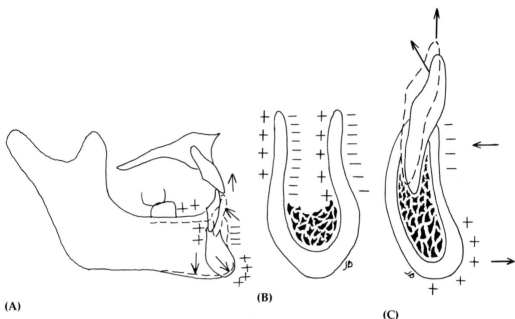

(A)   **(B)**

                                                          (C)

Figure 2−17 (A) Growth direction and displacement of the anterior mandibular area is governed by resorptive fields of the alveolar area and depository fields of the mental protuberance area. (B) Depository and resorptive fields of the symphysis area. (C) Resorptive fields of the alveolar process, depository fields of the mental protuberance area, and general eruptive forces of the incisors. (Redrawn from Enlow DH: *Handbook of Facial Growth*. Philadelphia, WB Saunders Co, 1975.)

the presence of lower second molars. As might also be easily surmised, the failure of either maxillary or mandibular arches to obtain their full size and adequate components of anteroposterior length or transpalatal width due to the constraining effects of imbalanced surrounding muscle function adds to the problems of crowding in the most dramatic fashion.

Another interesting phenomenon of mandibular growth is the effect of growth on mandibular rotation. Rotation of the mandible during growth or treatment refers to the change in the mandibular plane angle as a result of variances in the anterior face height (symbolized by something like menton or pogonion vertically to some reference point or plane in the maxilla or anterior cranial base) and the posterior face height (usually described in terms of gonion vertically to some other reference point or plane that extends to the posterior areas). A change or rotation of the mandibular plane would result from a change in growth rate of either one or both of these areas over a period of growth or treatment. In order for the mandible to grow and at the same time maintain its relative degree of angulation to the base of the skull (as reflected by the mandibular plane), vertical growth in the posterior facial region, governed by the condylar growth rate, must be equal to the vertical growth of the anterior facial region, governed in turn by the combined growth of the maxillary basal and the maxillary and mandibular alveolar areas.

Mandibular rotation, or change of the mandibular plane angle, can take place in one of two ways. First, if the anterior face height in the form of the maxillary base and the maxillary and mandibular alveolar processes were to increase at a faster rate than the *vertical component* of increase in the mandibular condyle, the mandible would in effect be rotated backwards; ie, the mandibular plane would steepen. This is also referred to as clockwise rotation of the mandible (with the profile to the observer's right), or a clockwise grower. (The terms "clockwise grower" and "counterclockwise grower" are popular in America but confusing to Europeans who are used to seeing cephalometric tracings with the profile on the observer's left, as in the Bimler analysis.) The second manner in which a mandible could rotate is when the posterior face height, or vertical component of condylar growth, grows at a faster rate than the anterior face height. This produces a flattening of the mandibular plane angle toward the horizontal and is called forward rotation or counterclockwise growth.

The entire process of mandibular rotation is intimately related to a very important dimensional aspect of the stomatognathic system— vertical. Although many studies addressed the issue of vertical growth changes, the notion that part of the change might be due to an actual rotation of the mandible itself due to differences in anterior and posterior facial height growth rates was a concept considered by relatively few.[145-150] However, there is a reason for this. Mandibular rotations, if not extreme, were somewhat difficult for early cephalometricians to discern. The unequal and imbalanced growth rates in the vertical direction between the anterior and posterior face height areas could be masked behind significant amounts of inferior mandibular border remodeling. Nature has a tendency to want to compensate for irregularities and insufficiencies. This principle is manifest by the example of the attempts made to remodel the inferior border of the mandible in order to recreate former stereoscopic morphology. This process would easily hide a true mandibular rotation behind a blanket of self-correction, making the determination of imbalances in anterior and posterior facial heights more difficult to decipher. For this reason Bjork and others resorted to their famous metallic implants to get a truer picture of what was actually happening to the corpus of the mandible "mandibular-plane-angle-wise" during growth.[151-152]

Several interesting clinical implications have been associated with the relative degree of angulation of the mandibular plane. The more level mandibular planes of the "forward" or horizontal growers are more associated with deep overbites, since there is usually not a lot of height to the maxillary or mandibular alveolar processes and little or no overextrusion of teeth. The arches have a tendency to be wider with less chance of constricted arch form or posterior crossbites, since the diminished vertical causes more flaccidity of the associated facial musculature. Facial profiles also have a tendency to be flatter with less likelihood of severe mandibular retrusion and facial convexity. The more inclined mandibular planes of the "backward" or vertical growers (high-angle cases) have more of a tendency toward skeletal open bites and a more retruded facial profile, especially in the mandibular portion. Such people have a tendency toward longer, thinner faces, more dominant in vertical characteristics as opposed to horizontal characteristics, and often show more of their maxillary anterior teeth upon smiling, since these teeth have a proclivity for overeruption and an increased height to their alveolar processes.

Often the etiological chief offenders, along with less growth of the posterior face height area, are the maxillary molars and their associated alveolar processes. This is why such cases respond so well to techniques of second molar extraction in effort to close down excessive open bites and flatten steep mandibular planes to more desirable levels. Due to the excess vertical, an increased tension is often placed on the associated facial musculature, and it will be seen to manifest itself in the constriction of the maxillary arch form from the more rounded Roman type to the more narrow and pointed Gothic type. Associated with this phenomenon is the bilateral posterior crossbite. Techniques that might increase eruption of posterior teeth in such cases are almost always contraindicated.[153] Thus is seen just one of the many ways rates of growth of various areas of the maxillofacial complex can affect the status of a given occlusion.

For balanced growth to occur, the backward growth of the maxillary posterior articular surfaces and tuberosity area, the amount of corresponding forward primary and secondary displacement of the maxilla, the anterior remodeling (resorption) of the front of the maxilla, the amount of upward and backward growth of the condyle and posterior border of the ramus, the corresponding anterior resorption of the anterior border of the ramus, the resultant corpus lengthening and anterior mandibular displacement (primary), and the anterior remodeling of the front of the mandible and chin-button area must all occur in *relatively equal amounts* to maintain a proper and balanced growth pattern; and all the while the cranial base is also growing and changing, carrying the maxillofacial complex generally forward! Any growth rate disturbance of any of these major components (not to mention a whole raft of minor components) due to constraining (or augmenting) improper muscle function or any of a number of other etiological agents, can produce skeletal malocclusions. It's a wonder so many of us turn out as well as we do!

"Always to excel, and to be distinguished
above others"
Homer
The Iliad

THE FUNCTIONAL MATRIX

Although this has been only a brief overview of bone growth, even in the most cursory discussion of such a subject, it would be remiss not to allude to the singular most exotic and provocative theory of maxillo-facial development conceived to date—the "functional matrix" theory of Melvin Moss. As theories go, its actual supporting experimental scientific evidence makes it one of the most heavily documented hypotheses in all of the dental literature.[154–165] During the 1960s Moss and his associates at Columbia University brought forth a theory concerned with coordinating the then existing theories of sectional growth and development of component parts of the entire cranial complex into an overriding and all-encompassing concept that governs the growth of the unit as a whole. This is how the complete organism develops, as a complete whole; and the functional matrix concepts were proposed as an answer to the question of what could account for such an overall governing mechanism in Nature. It was observed that the head represented an area in which a variety of critical biological functions occurred. Hence it was proposed that each individual function was effected or performed by its appropriate *team* of individual members in the form of a "functional cranial component." These components were composed of two major parts: a functional matrix, which actually did the thing; and its supporting "skeletal unit," which served as the supporting foundation for its respective functional matrix. It was also felt that the latter was always a reflection of and subservient to the demands of the functioning matrix which "led the way" in growth. In other words, in growth and development accepting certain genetic and biofunctional limits, the overall functional matrix develops first in response to more primary demands while the skeletal units correspondingly follow along as a secondary response, not vice versa. The bone follows the tissue; the tissue doesn't follow the bone. All tissues follow the morpho-genetic demands of general life maintenance.

Beginning with the simplest element and working up to the more all-inclusive and more complex, we must start with the definitions of a skeletal unit. This does not necessarily imply a single bone, or even a group of bones, but signifies the entire team of localized bone, carti-lage, tendinous, and generally substantive hard tissues of support of a component. Moss separates these skeletal units into two types: microskeletal and macroskeletal. A microskeletal unit has nothing to do with small size but implies a bone or bones together in a specific unit of

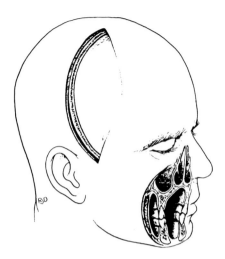

Figure 2−18   The functional matrix theories of Melvin Moss: This illustration appeared in Moss's original paper, "The Primary Role of Functional Matrices in Facial Growth." He uses it to describe the neurocranial and orofacial capsular matrices. The neural capsular matrix is composed of the entire neural mass (including dura mater), and the associated skeletal units are entirely contained within the capsule. Correspondingly, the orofacial capsular matrix consists of the illustrated functioning spaces, and its own respective skeletal units are entirely existent within the capsule. (Reprinted from Moss ML, Salentijn L: The primary role of functional matrices in facial growth. *Am J Orthod* 1969a; 55:566−577 with permission.)

purpose, such as the maxilla or mandible. When a larger area of adjoining bones serves in unison to carry out a larger overall function in the form of a functional cranial component, the "larger" and more complex team is referred to as a macroskeletal unit. The entire cranial base is an example. As examples that clarify these notions further, Moss defines such entities as the microskeletal unit of the coronoid process, angle of the jaw, inferior alveolar neurovascular triad, or the alveolar process. Such microskeletal units may respond jointly in a unified and coordinated manner to a localized demand, or they may respond singly. The gonial angle or shape of the coronoid process might change shape due to the functional and growth demands of their associated musculature without affecting neighboring microskeletal units such as the alveolar process. Yet on a larger scale, the macroskeletal unit, the entire oral skeletal complex, might respond to an overall demand such as natural growth or the dictates of functional-appliance-induced orthodontic/orthopedic treatment. This would be a net summation of the responses of all the associated microskeletal units taken at once.

However, in deference to the concept of a skeletal unit, Moss is quick to point out that the term "functional matrix" should not be thought of as synonymous with soft tissues. Although soft tissues of every conceivable variety can be a part of a given functional matrix, teeth also, by their definitions, may serve as a form of functional matrix. In the specific case of the teeth, their eruption, mesial drift, or orthodontic movement is intimately associated with their own related skeletal units, the alveolar processes. Moss defines two types of functional matrices: the periosteal, which is a smaller neighborhood-type matrix like the temporalis/coronoid process example; and the capsular, the more inclusive, larger neighborhood type, an example of which would be the neurocranial capsular matrix (the entire neural mass of the brain and associated calvarian structures).

A key concept also associated with these theories is that of "functioning spaces." These spaces are critical in such larger capsular matrices as the orofacial capsular matrix. The respective component skeletal units are completely contained within such capsular matrices as the neurocranial and the orofacial. They may be quite independent of one another, since the skeletal units of the neurocranial capsular matrix follow the neural growth patterns dictated by the growth of the brain whereas the skeletal units of the orofacial capsular matrix are subservient to the biomechanical functional and morphogenetic demands of that overall capsular matrix.

To clarify these concepts, Moss cites the example of the case of the skeletal unit of the coronoid process and its associated functional matrix, the temporalis muscle. When the activity of the temporalis muscle is diminished or eliminated altogether experimentally in laboratory animals, its associated coronoid process is equally diminished in size and shape or it may disappear altogether. Conversely, if the temporalis muscle is experimentally stimulated to an excessive level of hyperactivity, the coronoid process may be observed to increase in size and change its shape in response to that hyperactivity. Even imbalances of other muscle activities of associated muscles attached to other "ramal skeletal units" can cause compensatory changes in temporalis muscle function and, therefore, corresponding changes in coronoid process shape. The point is that the responses of all the osseous portions of the skeletal units, by means of resorption and deposition, to demands of their related functional matrices are "direct responses to temporally and morphogenetically prior changes in their specific functional matrices." In other words, with all due salutations to Roux and Wolfe, the bone follows the lead of the muscles, not vice versa. Nature always tries to seek its own level. As the muscles (or any team of soft tissues) grow in response to functional or morphogenetic demands, the bones (or any team of hard tissues) attempt to catch up as their form of response.

Now a functional matrix (like the temporalis) and its associated skeletal unit (like the coronoid process) team up to form what Moss calls a "functional cranial component." Various groups of functional cranial components are organized into the aforementioned larger neighborhoods of cranial capsules. A cranial capsule such as the orofacial is to be thought of as an "envelope" which contains a *coordinated* series of cranial components (functional matrices of muscle and related soft tissues, and skeletal units of bone and related hard tissues). Again, the teeth are an exception because they are a hard tissue functional matrix, their related skeletal units being the alveolar process.

Such capsular matrices as the orofacial, or any other, are also to be thought of as existing in "volumes." A cranial capsule surrounds and protects its cranial components. In the case of the neurocranial capsular matrix, the brain grows and the bones of the skull follow suit in response to its expansion. In the case of the orofacial capsule, which surrounds and protects the oronasopharyngeal functioning spaces, it is the volumetric growth of these spaces that provide the "primary morphogenetic event" that leads the way behind which its localized related skeletal units follow in secondary response. Moss also emphasizes the importance of Nature maintaining the patency of the nasal and pharyngeal airways as well as the oral cavity. These passages are not an accidental leftover after the bone, muscle, and related tissues have had their way as far as growth is concerned. They are believed to be a *primary* response to the biological needs of an individual as a whole, a hypothesis to which other noted experts subscribe.[166,167] Nature assures "from the drawing boards" that these passages remain patent via the stereoscopic musculoskeletal arrangement of the anatomy of the region. It is noted, for instance, that the airway remains patent during the entire range of motion of the head on the spinal column.

This menagerie of facial growth and development hypotheses fits very well into the realm of the functional orthodontist in the specific areas of the growth of the mandible. Considering the above, Moss states that the mandibular condyle is not a primary growth site, but a secondary growth site that responds in a compensatory manner. It has been shown that in both experimental animals and man bilateral removal of the mandibular condyles surgically neither inhibits the overall translation of the rest of the remaining portions (skeletal units) of the mandible, nor does it inhibit in any way the changes in the form of the associated microskeletal units as their related functional matrices change their functional operations. The theory then may be seen to account for why the mandible in such cases still advances, albeit with some compensatory changes, as the rest of the maxillofacial complex grows and develops down and forward out from under the cranial base. It does so because although the mandible in the abovementioned experiments is missing one of the team of its skeletal units, the orofacial capsule still operates in response to the demands of the volumetric expansion of the orofacial functioning spaces and their capsular matrices. This results in the spatial changes in the mandibular position. Under normal circumstances, as the capsular matrix grows, the capsule expands as a whole. All enclosed macroskeletal units (such as a mandible) are progressively and passively translated to different spatial relationships. But as quickly as this happens, the related microskeletal units respond to the changing demands of their associated functional matrices by appropriate alterations of their osseous form; condylar, ramal, alveolar, and all. In the light of the above, the actual growth of the mandible is then described as a summation of translation and changes in form of the associated skeletal units. Growth as a whole is Nature's deliberate coordination of all of these mechanisms. Thus it may now be seen why it is logical according to the functional matrix theories of Moss that changes in function bring about a corresponding change in form. If that change is purposeful and directed as by a functional appliance, the corresponding resultant form thus produced may also be purposeful and directed. This forms the founding premise of the entire FJO movement.

> *"Eppur si muove."*
> *"Yet it does move."*
> Traditional words after being forced to
> recant his theory that the earth moves
> around the sun.
> Galileo Galilei 1564–1642

LANDMARK STABILITY: A SOMETIMES THING

Reflections on growth in the maxillofacial complex soon bring the observer face to face with what may at first seem disconcerting realizations as to the overall value of cephalometrics as it is known in the traditional sense. Since its inception, the science of cephalometrics has been proffered as an ideal medium to enhance diagnosis, treatment planning, normative standards, and, ultimately, growth prediction. Yet surprisingly, each of these acceptably logical divisions of the science has come under fire, with the division of growth prediction receiving such intense criticisms from such a vast number of highly respected authorities that its particular future seems precarious at best! Much of the work of each of the divisions of the science is based on the use of stable points and planes of reference within the facial complex acting as bases against which measurements may be made, compared, and analyzed. Yet this in itself is not an easy task to accomplish, because everything in the head is growing and translating out from some imaginary "center" in all directions at once, even at different rates! It is similar to making astronomical observations of the celestial sphere. The meaning of a particular measurement depends on where the observer stands and is further compounded by the fact that the point upon which the observer stands is also moving. A cephalometric image is a two-dimensional shadow, just as the prolate linear outline of the shadow of an egg is two-dimensional. It is most likely no true indication of the actual three-dimensional topography of the actual subject. It may be seen to resolve itself to a matter of perspective.

Sella.   Just such an issue is brought out in the study of one of the cardinal reference points used in many cephalometric observations, the center of the hypophyseal fossa, sella. We know that the distance between sella and a more anterior part, such as nasion, increases during overall skull growth. We also know that the distance between sella and some posterior point, such as basion, also increases with age. Yet we also know that sella itself moves somewhat relative to overall stereoscopic position during growth in its own right. Describing the movement of sella then becomes a matter of perspective; ie, it depends on where the observer is standing at the time. Dr R. A. Latham,[168] from work done at the University of Liverpool, found that the distance between sella and the sphenooccipital synchondrosis underwent little change after infancy. Others have found similar data.[139,169] Yet since the synchondrosis is known to be an active growth area well into adolescence, Latham interpreted these findings as indicative that growth continues at the sphenoidal surface of the synchondrosis and is accompanied by an upward and backward movement of sella due to remodeling as the size of the pituitary gland itself also grows in volume. Much evidence corroborates the "upward and backward" movement of sella with growth.[121,124,170−172] However, the issue of sella is not without controversy. Excellent studies performed by Dr Birte Melsen[173] at the Royal Dental College in Copenhagen, Denmark, were interpreted to show that sella moves on the average 2 mm *downward* and backward in relation to the tuberculum sella. The planum sphenoidale, the flat area of bone just anterior to the hypophyseal fossa, was considered very stable. Yet it was observed that the distance between sella and the synchondral cartilage did increase through the growth years. Thus, with the observer "standing close," on the planum sphenoidale if you will, sella moves *down* and back. From a greater distance it is interpreted overall to move *up* and back. One thing is sure, it definitely moves backward with growth, and its horizontal stability is a matter of perspective.

Nasion.   Hand in hand with a discussion of the variability of sella should be a discussion of its frequent cephalometric companion, nasion. The famous sella-nasion reference line (S-N) has been a popular base reference line for cephalometric studies since it was first described by Broadbent. Now it must be remembered that sutures represent the boundary between two separate bones. They often are very irregular in course, and the close proximity of the two bones along the sutural lines

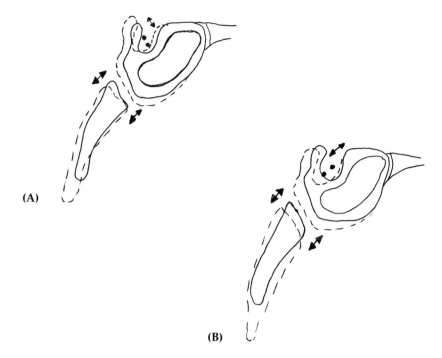

(A)

(B)

Figure 2—19   (A) Sella variability (up and back) due to growth as per the theories of Latham. (B) Sella variability due to growth (down and back) as per the theories of Melsen.

of juncture reminds one of the appearance of a river as seen from an airplane. Nasion is a landmark that is just such a suture; it is defined as the most anterior portion of the juncture of the nasal bones with the frontal bone, ie, the frontonasal suture. A typical bony suture in cross section is composed of first the outer bony edges of each respective bone itself. Next appears a fibrous cellular layer which represents the continuation of a periosteal membrane of each bone. Finally, "sandwiched" in between these is the central layer of tissues which contains both collagenous and vascular elements.[174]

There are two basic categories of sutures, defined by virtue of the way their two bones abut to one another. The first is edge-to-edge type relationship. In this type the edges of the bones may be thought of as reasonably squared off, their respective edges relatively perpendicular to the main bodily edge of the bones. These sutures exhibit growth that is correlated with physical separation of the bony elements. However, growth may take place at one or both sides of the suture, to varying degrees. The second type of suture is the overlapping variety. In this type the edges of the opposing bones are at an oblique edge to the main body. Growth here does *not* necessarily imply bony separation, but it

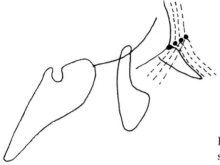

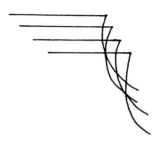

Figure 2—21   Both anterior nasal spine (ANS) and A-point (Downs) travel down and forward along with the general growth of the maxilla. (Redrawn from Enlow DH: *Handbook of Facial Growth*. Philadelphia, WB Saunders Co, 1975.)

Figure 2—20   Nasion travels generally upward and forward during growth.

does imply a physical relocation of the suture itself relative to its respective bones. Extending the previously mentioned analogy, the river changes course, but the land on either side does not move. The frontonasal suture of nasion is of this overlapping variety. As a result, nasion ascends with age. Because of overall growth of the head, nasion moves forward with age. But its upward movement is a combined product of increased anterior face height and actual sutural relocation.[175]

Nasion is closer to the upper margin of the orbit in children than in adults. It is also usually higher than the frontomaxillary suture in adults compared with children. And nasion may also be seen to be some distance above the roof of the nasal cavity in adults, whereas in children it may usually be found at about the same level. Therefore, nasion has an overall movement both forward and upward during growth of the individual due to a combination of primary and secondary factors.

Anterior nasal spine and A-point.   Due to the overall downward and forward growth of the maxilla, such landmarks as ANS and its nearest neighbor, A-point, can be expected to follow a somewhat similar pattern of movement relative to the cranial base during growth. The anterior and posterior nasal spines, which form the limits of the palatal plane, usually descend in unison, thus keeping the palatal plane parallel to former positions throughout growth. Should there be any variance from this pattern, it almost always manifests itself in the form of an accelerated rate of descent of ANS, which would correspondingly increase the steepness of the palatal plane. As the maxilla gains in alveolar height, A-point rises on the anterior surface profile relative to prosthion. It may also have a tendency to "drop in" a little as the adult dentition erupts. Yet at the same time the entire maxilla is being thrust down and out from under the cranial base due to growth at its articular surfaces and at the maxillary tuberosities. The denture, by the way, lags behind somewhat during this process and as a result becomes slightly less prominent relative to the facial profile. This contributes to the slight "dropping back" phenomenon previously described by Brodie. Yet this does not necessarily mean that the anteriors *always* upright themselves more during maturation of the individual. They may become less procumbent, but then again they may become more so or simply retain their original angulation. The net overall movement of A-point is due to the combination of all of these factors.[134]

Mandibular landmarks.   In conjunction with the maxilla, the normal balanced growth of the mandible is down and forward. Most mandibular landmarks follow the same course but with a much greater degree of variation. The occlusal plane and the inferior mandibular border may be seen to develop in a relatively proportional constancy. However there is often a persuasion for both to gradually become more level as posterior face height growth tries to catch up with anterior facial height increases. Less often the former lags behind the latter, and the occlusal plane and mandibular plane may be seen to increase slightly, causing anterior open bite tendencies in what is described as a high-angle case or "vertical grower" (clockwise grower in American orthodontic slang).[176,177] In addition, it must be kept in mind that the mental protuberance, or chin button, also represents an independent growth field and can cause an advancement of pogonion or gnathion without actually being representative of advancement of the entire mandibular denture or body of the mandible itself. This is especially common in males.[143]

In spite of the wide variability of mandibular cephalometric landmarks, they have received the lion's share of attention from orthodontic clinicians over the years, especially with respect to their horizontal discrepancy relative to maxillary landmarks. This preoccupation was due to the belief that mandibular retrusion was essentially unchangeable by therapeutic means. Hence clinicians were concerned with the degree of bony overjet present and how they could correct corresponding dental overjets by retraction of the maxillary anteriors and proclination of the mandibular anteriors to obtain the desperately sought-after anterior coupling and overjet elimination. Needless to say, any amount of mandibular bodily advancement that might come the clinician's way via natural growth was always greatly appreciated. Growth prediction or even ranges of estimates therefore drew paramount attention. Yet in spite of efforts to mask skeletal Class II mandibular retrusions behind such purely orthodontic manipulations, such landmarks as B-point, pogonion, gnathion, or menton showed little change on the horizontal reference plane due to treatments of a fixed-appliance-only nature.

Porion.   It was also observed early in the development of cephalometrics that the key landmark porion, the important "back half" of the Frankfort Horizontal plane, also changed relative to the entire human head due to growth. It moves generally away from the mythological

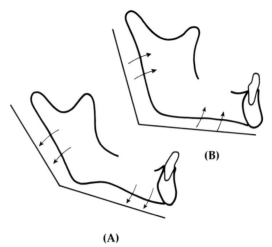

(B)

(A)

Figure 2–22   (**A**) Growth patterns in the mandible that favor a vertical direction, sometimes referred to as a "clockwise grower," result in an elongated mandible and a more open, obtuse gonial angle. This is often the case in Class III and skeletal open bite cases (high-angle cases). (**B**) Growth patterns favoring horizontal development result in more acute or lower-valued gonial angles ("counterclockwise grower"), as is often seen in skeletal Class II deep bite cases. (Redrawn from Enlow DH: *Handbook of Facial Growth*. Philadelphia, WB Saunders Co, 1975.)

center of growth of the human head, and that movement may be straight down, straight back, or anything in between.[134] However, the movement of orbitale with respect to the vertical is felt to be in close enough conjunction with the movement of porion that the Frankfort plane emerges as one of the most reasonably stable reference lines available, although its value has been increasingly appreciated in more recent times only by a process of elimination of others over decades. Regardless of how balanced or imbalanced the growth of the head is, it still has to have a frame of reference as to what constitutes "level," and the Frankfort is it.

Constancy of facial pattern.   From a survey of the above it may now be seen why it was previously stated that such findings might cause some wonder how the early cephalometricians managed to analyze anything. With all parts of the head growing and moving in all directions at once, how could any base reference points, lines, or planes be constructed? Well as it turns out, there *are* reasonably stable points that can be used, provided one understands the perspective from which one is making the respective observations. There is also another factor that gave early researchers in cephalometrics great heart in their attempts to analyze maxillofacial growth—the theory of "facial constancy." One of the theory's first proponents, who developed it only after taking a cue from Broadbent, was Allen Brodie. From a well-documented series of long-term longitudi-

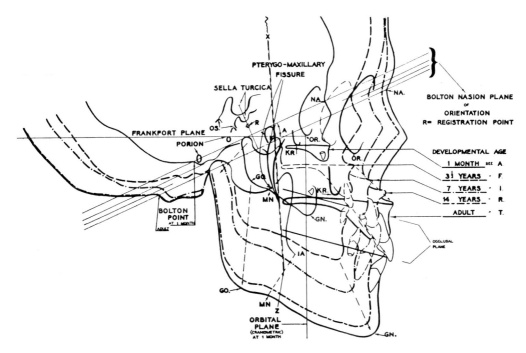

Figure 2–23   Broadbent serial growth study: This famous illustration was intended to depict normal developmental growth of the skull and maxillofacial complex. It is a product of the widely renowned Bolton study. It draws from information gathered from 4000 serial growth studies of children enrolled in the Brush Foundation and Bolton Fund at Case Western Reserve University during the 1930s and 1940s. All the serial tracings were averaged for the ages of 1 month, 3 ½ years, 7 years, 14 years, and adult. The serialized "master" tracings are superimposed such that the Bolton Planes are kept parallel, and each tracing is registered at R point. The concept of attempting to superimpose an entire tracing over another or series of others by registering them on a single registration point for the sake of comparison of growth or treatment changes over the entire maxillofacial complex all at once has become a suspect approach in light of modern knowledge of separate and individual growth directions of maxillofacial components.

nal studies of the same individuals and careful serial superimpositions of cephalometric tracings, Brodie became impressed with two important factors. First he observed that though there are a great variety of different areas of growth in the facial complex, cases exhibiting extreme variations and imbalances in all the areas at once are not seen. In fact he determined that such a circumstance would be impossible because it would place the example totally "outside the human pattern"! The rule instead was for an exhibition of compensation with respect to variations or imbalances. In other words, when a high value for a given measurement existed in one area, a corresponding low value usually existed somewhere else as a form of compensation so that there would exist a sort of anatomical "canceling out" effect as Nature attempted to keep things reasonably balanced. This is why Brodie thought it was "absurd" to attempt to make a complete diagnosis on the basis of a single angle, measurement, or even from small groups of same. The second thing Brodie observed was that facial patterns seemed to remain relatively constant; ie, the original proportions of the case seemed consistent throughout the later years of the subject's growth. This fact is what clinicians had empirically based their treatment plans on for a century. Once a child is well into the adolescent growth years, a skeletal Class II mandibular retrusion, for example, usually remains a skeletal Class II mandibular retrusion. Minor compensatory changes might be observed, but seldom if ever can a miraculous growth spurt of the offending agent be counted upon to spontaneously deliver patients from their plight of malocclusion. FJOs are needed for that.

This only pertains to the older child with the full adult dentition; for as we have previously noted, it is common in the normal pattern of growth and development of the young child for the mandible to lag behind in its development only to attempt to "catch up" with the rest of the face in the late mixed and early adult dentition stage. However, in such cases, the individual usually appears as "borderline" to begin with, as major self-corrections of mandibular retrusions, anterior open bites, bilateral maxillary posterior crossbites, or deep overbites due to spontaneous accelerated growth are rare. Constancy of facial pattern is what allows the tracing of a given cephalometric profile for a given year of the subject's age to fall completely outside, albeit very close to, the tracing for the previous year without crossing over. It is also why serial photographs of a child taken every year of its life allow even a stranger to recognize the resemblance and constancy of facial features from year to year. It is also why to some extent children resemble their parents or siblings.

The above-mentioned factors, in addition to the tendency of most early cephalometricians to gravitate toward base reference lines centered on midline structures of the cranial base (the thing closest to that mythological center of growth for the head), made many feel that diagnosis, treatment planning, normative standards, and even growth prediction were all entirely plausible with the use of cephalometric x-rays. For some, the cephalometric radiograph was thought to be the ultimate medium for such processes. But the hawks of dissension soon spread their wings and descended on the doves of complacent cephalometric pedagogy with a cold and calculated intensity, determined that the sharp talons of scientific reason would dispel methodological illusion where necessary.

As previously alluded to, the concept of making a diagnosis on the status of a single angle, such as Tweed's method of diagnosing off the mandibular incisor angulation with respect to the mandibular plane, met with particularly intense criticisms. Once the degree of variability from individual to individual, and the degree of variability and complexity within the same individual during growth, were fully comprehended, even making a diagnosis from a small group of cephalometric measurements became suspect. It was soon discovered that Angle's old method of classification of malocclusion according to tooth relationships was inadequate and could even be misleading as to the overall skeletal aspects of a case. Class II molar relationships could be found in cephalometrically retrognathic, mesognathic, and even prognathic individuals. Thus, expanded definitions such as "dental Class I—skeletal Class II" started appearing in the jargon of the common practitioners, denoting both dental arrangements and skeletal status of a given case.

Yet though Angle's dental definitions were clear, there were no commonly accepted standards for what would actually qualify an individual as a skeletal Class I, II, or III. The extremes were obvious and well accepted and understood by all. But borderline cases provided some problems. Various individuals defined their notions of skeletal classifications according to parameters of measurements they fancied or were familiar with, and one man's Class I skeletal designation often would turn out to be another man's Class II! This is why somewhat nondescript slang terms such as "a true Class II" appeared for a while, implying a combined dental Class II relationship of the teeth with an accompanying retrusive mandible and retrognathic profile.

Even the most fundamental foundations of the science, the base reference lines, went through a baptism of fire during their cephalometric "coming of age." They are important in that they provide the observer with a symbolic place upon which to stand in order to make the measurements. They are used to orient before-and-after tracings which analyze therapeutic changes. They are used as a "fixed" reference point against which various components of the maxillofacial complex are measured, both linearly and angularly, to determine the status of the case at the time. They also serve as a basis for superimposition of serial tracings in an effort to study long-term growth. Therefore, they should be as stable as possible and allow interpretations made from their use to coincide with what is actually known to be happening in Nature. Due to the fact that everything in the skull moves somewhat in one way or another during growth, their selection and definition over the years have been tantamount to a quest and, as might be guessed, riddled with controversy.

"A PLACE ON WHICH TO STAND"

Frankfort Horizontal-porion. One of the first methods of superimposition of serial tracings of the same individual used by Broadbent to study growth or treatment changes consisted of orienting the overlaid tracings on Frankfort Horizontal with porion (FH-P) as the point of anteroposterior registration. This allowed the parts above and below Frankfort to appear moving away vertically up or down, respectively, from the midline horizontal, and the anterior portions of the face showed movement away from porion. But this was not an accurate representation of what was known to be happening in Nature, for it was known that porion, as well as other portions of the posterior face such as the condyle, gonion, and the body of the ramus, move posteriorly somewhat during growth. The above method also depicted inaccurate changes of the occlusal level such as the maxillary first permanent molars of the later tracing erupting past the level of the deciduous occlusal plane, a process we know does not actually happen in Nature. It also makes the mandibular first permanent molar appear stationary with respect to movement along the vertical plane relative to the mandibular border, something else we know not to be consistent with Nature. It is a well-established fact that the mandibular first permanent molar does move vertically through bone as it erupts. Hence the FH-P base reference line had to be abandoned.

Porion-nasion plane.   Another base line of reference used in those early times was the porion-nasion plane. This technique superimposed serial tracings along this line with the *midpoint* of the line as a registration point. But this method is no more accurate nor truthful than the afore-mentioned FH-P. In the porion-nasion method, sella appears more stationary (in FH-P it appeared to move up), but everything else appears lower because the entire second tracing of the older individual is itself lowered. It also arbitrarily separates the anteroposterior growth in roughly two halves (according to the cosine of the angle of the line with Frankfort), which again may or (most likely) may not coincide with true natural growth. It also forces a slight downward and backward rotation of facial development as it keeps nasion fixed, also not true in Nature. Therefore the whole system is inaccurate.

Porion-nasion on Frankfort parallel.   Another method quite similar to the previously described technique was proposed by Krogman. It consists of orienting the tracings on porion again; but this time nasion of the second tracing is placed on a line drawn through nasion of the first tracing that is parallel to Frankfort. This makes the growth depicted by the second tracing appear more uniform in nature, although with the upward movement of nasion due to growth, the two base reference lines of the separate tracings cannot be superimposed. It also allows sella to appear to move down and back, a suspect finding. One thing all three of the above methods do relate is the overwhelmingly downward and for-ward movement of the maxilla, mandible, and occlusal plane as well as the generally forward movement of the anterior portions of the face, a phenomenon so profound in the growth of the human head that even inaccurate and poorly conceived baseline superimposition techniques can't conceal it!

Nasion-porion on Frankfort.   Yet another method of superimposition developed by T. Wingate Todd is the exact reverse of that developed by Krogman. It consists of using nasion as the registration point and allows the point porion of the second tracing to fall on the *original* Frankfort plane of the first tracing only if the distance between nasion and porion does *not* change in the interval; then both Frankforts are superimposed. However, this method demands a slight rotation of the second tracing if the distance between nasion and porion *has* increased, which it most likely would have done since they both grow out from the center of the head in opposite directions. This rotation incorrectly would be bringing the anterior part of the face down and back. This method assumes the anterior part of the face is stationary while the main body of the face grows down and back away from it. It must be remembered that the highly touted opinions of men like Krogman held sway at the time, which proposed that the face grew "from before backwards," which is not quite the same as the notion of growing posteriorly while being displaced anteriorly. This method is an attempt to reflect these ideas. Close, but no cigar.

Sella-nasion.   As Broadbent pondered the shortcomings of all of the above, he realized a better reference plane had to be devised: one that was accurate, easily reproducible, and reflected changes in the serial tracings that could be interpreted as truthful representations of what was actually happening in Nature. After the "rush" of excitement over the newfound method of cephalometrics had mellowed, Broadbent made the observation that the distance between sella and nasion changed very little during the time span of the first and second radiographs taken in his studies. However, in light of more modern knowledge, we do know that the distance *can* change. Broadbent's observations were probably a result of the short time span between the first and second radiographs (two years), the age of the patient (6—8 years), and the fact that Broadbent selected cases that fit this time and age span. At this age span, the cranial base between sella and nasion is relatively dormant with respect to growth changes.

Still desirous of obtaining base reference lines as close to stable points in the midline of the cranial base as possible, Broadbent hit upon the notion of the S-N line. Representing the anterior portion of the cranial base, S-N would be his new base reference line, outperforming all those previously devised. Under this method the distance between sella and porion shows the greatest increase; and increases are also seen along the inferior border of the mandible, as well as the posterior border of the ramus, all consistent with known facts of facial bone growth. But Broadbent made a serious error of interpretation of changes in the mandible. As the maxillary and mandibular alveolar processes grow and gain in height due to permanent tooth eruption, the inferior border of the mandible and the entire occlusal plane drop with respect to the vertical.

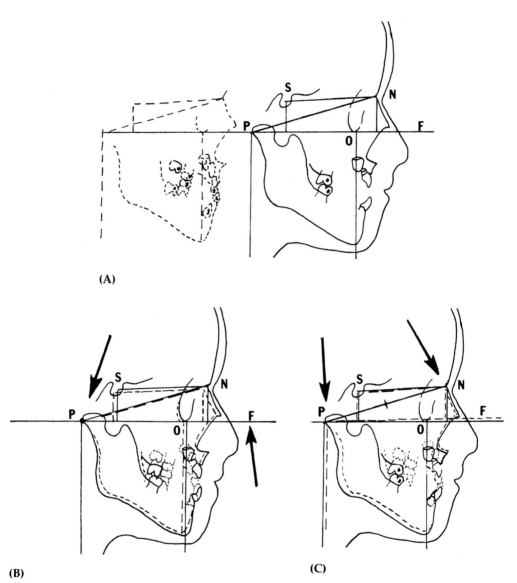

(A)

(B)   **(C)**

Figure 2-24   In this classic series of illustrations by B. Holly Broadbent from over half a century ago, the problems of the various superimposition methods in vogue at the time are made clear. **(A)** Tracings of roentgenograms of the same child taken 2 years apart. It is important to note here the relations of the teeth, maxilla, and mandible to the anteroposterior base lines P-F, P-N, and S-N as well as to the vertical lines P and O. In this series of drawings, Broadbent uses the following symbols: S = sella, P = porion, F = Frankfort Horizontal, N = nasion, O = orbital plane. **(B)** The two tracings in the previous illustrations (A & B) are here superimposed with A on top of B. Both are imposed along the Frankfort Horizontal plane, or in Frankfort relation (arrows) registered at P. **(C)** The two tracings are superimposed on the porion-nasion plane (arrows), registered at their respective midpoints. Note the difference, especially in the ANS, A-point,

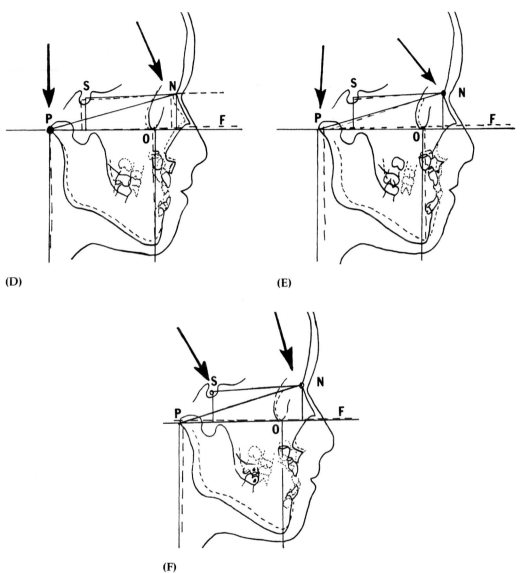

(D)

(E)

(F)

and B-point areas. (D) The two tracings are once again superimposed on the porion-nasion line (arrows), but in this case the tracings are registered on porion (P) and nasion of the second tracing placed such that it falls on a line projected from nasion of the first tracing that is parallel to the Frankfort plane of that first tracing. This was Krogman's method. (E) Yet another method, proposed by Todd, consists of superimpositions along porion-nasion line once again, but this time the tracings are registered at nasion with porion (P) of the second tracing (B) aligned on FH of the first tracing (A). (F) Broadbent's S-N line registered at *both* S and N because there has been no change in the location of the two landmarks of this particular case over the 2-year interim. But he finally abandoned the S-N line in favor of R. (Reprinted from Broadbent BH: A new X-ray technique and its application to orthodontia. *Angle Orthod* 1931; 1:45−66 with permission.)

This causes a slight downward rotation of the entire body of the mandible, a movement Broadbent mistakenly attributed entirely to growth of the inferior border of the mandible alone. Another problem rested with the assumption that both sella and nasion remain fixed. This is not true; yet they are observed in this particular study not to have changed in their linear separation. Forgetting about sella momentarily, if nasion moves forward and upward, the S-N distance must change. If it does not, the only remaining possibility, which then becomes fact by default, is that both sella and nasion move together the same corresponding amount! If this is the case, superimposition along S-N of consecutive serial tracings causes an erroneous and distorted interpretation to be realized with respect to the second tracing, ie, it will be lower all around than it should be. Broadbent finally came to this conclusion and eventually, after about 6 years of use, abandoned the S-N base reference line for yet another.

Broadbent Registration Point R.   Broadbent finally arrived at what he felt was a satisfactory solution to the base reference line problem. Conceding that any anatomical point selected as a reference point for superimposition purposes may itself change or be displaced during growth, and realizing there are no truly fixed areas in the growing individual, Broadbent sought to define a theoretical "space mark" that could be used instead. Since such a mark would only be a matter of definition and a biological nonentity, it could be stationary while everything else around it was growing and moving in all directions at once. The result of his efforts was the Broadbent Registration Point R. It depends on the Bolton plane (BP-N), since this was believed to be one of the most stable available. A line drawn from sella perpendicular to Bolton Plane is bisected at its midpoint. The midpoint of this little perpendicular line is the location of the theoretical space mark R. This allowed the placement of a smaller tracing within the larger, revealing increases of approximately the same size in all directions. Nobody ever planned on bones growing at different rates at different times in this technique! It was pointed out that at the time, the method of growth was believed to take place in a certain hypothetical "even way." This method fit the demands of the originally held hypotheses, but nobody ever questioned the original hypotheses. The theories of growth that prevailed in those times produced a system of registration that agreed with them.

However, it must be realized that this is the opposite of what should have been; ie, the system of registration (if correct) should have generated findings that would have produced the theories of growth. In science we can't force a procedure to fit a preconceived idea. To be scientific we must figuratively let the chips fall where they may and merely record the results accurately, accepting them for whatever they are. The use of Broadbent's R point for superimposition is the cephalometric equivalent to rolling loaded dice. The experiment was "forced" to produce a preconceived result.

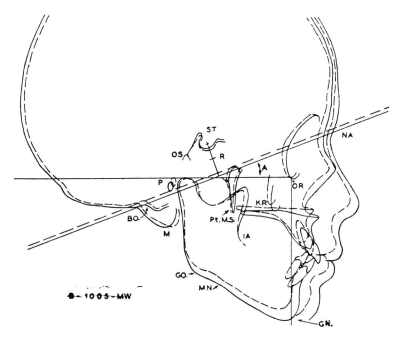

Figure 2–25   Broadbent Registration Point R. (Reprinted from Broadbent BH: The face of the normal child. *Angle Orthod* 1937; 7:183–208 with permission.)

Broadbent also had other problems with this method. The oblique nature of the path of the Bolton Plane through the face made measurements of changes along the occlusal plane awkward. So Broadbent added the old standby, Frankfort Horizontal, to help out in this regard. But then another problem arose. The angle between Bolton Plane and Frankfort Horizontal was seen to change during growth. This left keen observers guessing as to which of the two lines actually *did* change and which remained stable. Quite possibly both could have changed. Thus in spite of the seeming plausibility of registration on point R and the beautiful serial superimposition charts it produces, rivaling the cross-sectional appearance of the consecutive rings of a tree, the system had to finally be abandoned.

Brodie's method, S-N resurgent.   In the late 1940s Brodie pointed out that as the mastoid process enlarges, growing downward, it can obscure Bolton Point and practically obliterate it. This therefore made the use of the R registration point difficult, since it is predicated upon the proper construction of Bolton-nasion line. Consequently, Brodie resurrected the recently interred S-N baseline of Broadbent as his preferred reference line for superimpositional purposes, registering the tracings all on sella. His contention was that after further study it was revealed that the S-N and Bolton Plane maintained a fairly constant angular relation to one another; and S-N was an easy line to construct at any age. Yet Brodie

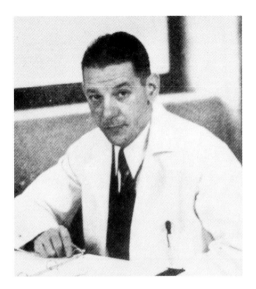

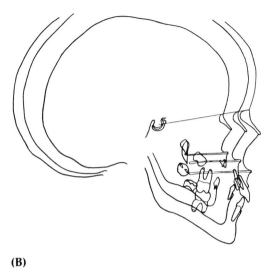

(B)

(A)

Figure 2—26   (A) Allen Brodie. (B) S—N resurgent. (Reprinted from Brodie AG: Behavior of normal and abnormal growth patterns. *Am J Orthod Oral Surg* 1941a; 27:633—647 with permission.)

was one of the first to qualify the use of S-N, or any superimpositional base reference line, with an important caveat that has formed one of the most important and widely accepted principles of bone growth interpretation. He felt that it was erroneous to attempt to superimpose tracings of the entire head or even the maxillofacial complex, in attempts to analyze growth of the entire area all at once. The bones were known to exhibit a wide range of variability with respect to rates and times of growth to which the issues of primary *v* secondary displacement added complications of interpretation.[178] Brodie thought it was much more correct to study contributions of various parts singly as they relate to the whole. He pointed out correctly that in studying the nasal region separately the use of S-N as a base reference line for analyzing growth is acceptable because it acts as a dividing line between the anterior cranial base and the nasal area. However, the line would not serve well in the study of the maxillary alveolar and dental structures because contributions made by the nasal structures (the floor of the nose being the roof of the mouth) would be credited to the alveolar process and/or maxillary teeth. Therefore, the latter should not be measured against the cranial base when anatomical entities that intervene could make their own independent contributions. For such purposes the palatal plane would serve more correctly.

Likewise, with other structures, taking the mandible as an example, relating it to the cranial base or upper facial areas, S-N may serve well. But to study how the mandible has grown with respect to itself, it can only be compared with a former tracing of itself. For analyzing mandibular changes, Brodie suggested superimposition along its lower border, the point being that each independently varying area should be compared separately within its own limited and isolated frame of reference. Bones move too many ways in too many directions during growth to hope that one base reference line could correctly superimpose tracings that would accurately and correctly reveal all the changes at once.

Thus the quest for a single cephalometric base reference line that could serve for universal superimpositional purposes gradually lost champions. Yet others would still try, and in that vein some fairly noteworthy efforts were mounted, but the whole issue would finally resolve itself down to a matter of compromise. In the meantime Brodie had launched the notion of comparing separate parts or areas with each other one at a time. It's a concept that remains with us to this day.[179]

"BRAIN TEASERS"

Other attempts at devising a suitable base reference line were made, and they generally seemed to focus on the midline bony structures that supported the base of the brain, the relatively stable areas along the middle of the cranial base. DeCoster proposed a line for use, the cribriform plane or the plane of the cribriform plate and the jugum sphenoidale, because he, as well as others, had proposed, and research finally showed, this line to be quite stable after the seventh year of life or after the eruption of the first permanent molars.[124, 180-183] However, it was pointed out that a certain portion of the time this area was obscured by overlying osseous structures such that construction of the line was very difficult.[184] This violates the principle of using base reference points or lines that are easy to reproduce.

Another "hawk" that attacked the Broadbent and Brodie methods of superimpositions was A. W. Moore of the University of Washington. He also pointed out that the R registration point and the S-N line were both constructed across areas of growing, hence changing, sutures on either side of the centrally located sphenoid bone. He noted that between the sphenoid bone and point nasion the sphenoethmoidal and the sphenofrontal sutures intervened. Also between the sphenoid and Bolton Point (even when it *was* decipherable) lay the major suture of the sphenooccipital synchondrosis, which remained active throughout the growth years with its penchant for changing the angle between the anterior and posterior cranial bases. He was another believer in the principle of

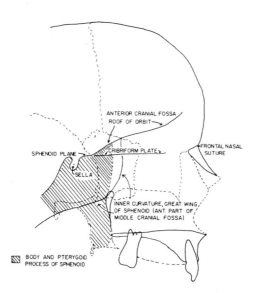

Figure 2–27 A. W. Moore proposed yet another method of registration. He was one of the first to prefer to study facial growth in relationship to one individual bone and its nearest neighbors rather than points on a number of distantly located bones separated by growing areas. His choice for superimpositional purposes was the sphenoid bone, because of its central location and relationship to the surrounding bones of the maxillofacial complex. (Reprinted from Moore, AW: Observations on facial growth and its clinical significance. *Am J Orthod* 1959; 45:399–423 with permission.)

studying a solitary bone and its immediate neighbors relative to either themselves or a localized nearby reference line rather than using distant reference points separated by sutures or independently growing areas.

Like most cephalometricians of the "new wave," he favored use of the sphenoid bone as a localized frame of reference because of its central location and relative degrees of stability. Since the outline of the sella turcica changed somewhat with growth, he felt the space mark sella would serve as an acceptable compromise for a point of registration with further superimposition, as much as anatomically possible, on the profile of the "sphenoid plane and the cerebral surface of the anterior cranial fossa."[185] This incorporates the highly stable midline structures of the DeCoster favorite, the cribriform plate, and the roof of the orbit. This orientation, which he referred to as the "overall" registration, he used to analyze the peripheral bony areas of the anterior portions of the upper face. To this he added two more superimposition techniques, one for the maxilla and one for the mandible, each to be analyzed separately. For the maxilla he proposed registration upon the widely accepted palatal plane and something else quite new, the pterygomaxillary fissure. This new registration point was found to be also quite stable along the horizontal axis. Moore's ideas surfaced in the late 1950s, and this represents one of the first times on the American side of the "Atlantic River" that the pterygomaxillary fissure received major attention for its value as a stable reference point. It had already been in use for over a decade on the European side by Bimler. For study of the mandible, Moore proposed superimposition of the mandibular outlines in the then standard fashion, registering on menton and the line connecting menton to the most posterior inferior position of the mandibular body, gonion.

An interesting viewpoint that resulted in yet another superimpositioning scheme was developed in the late 1950s and early 1960s by S. E. Coben of Jenkintown, Pennsylvania. Coben contended that the superimposition methods developed up to that time tended to "mask" the manner in which horizontal and vertical development of the face unfolds during growth. Therefore, he was determined to develop a method that would reveal the true nature of how growth of the various maxillofacial components would influence these horizontal and vertical developments as well as the facial profile.

Coben preferred to think of the entire head as being composed of two bones: the "craniomaxillary bone" and its counterpart, the mandible. Also, most importantly, he contended that the location of the maxillary arch was not only dependent on the growth of the maxilla itself but also upon the growth of the cranial base to which this complex was attached. He theorized that growth of the cranial base was responsible for carrying the upper arch both upward and forward from the vertebral column, which is what he used as his particular basepoint of reference. Additionally, the growth of the mandible carried the mandibular arch down and forward away from the vertebral column. This represented a somewhat unusual concept of facial growth, quite unlike anything yet proposed up to that time, at least with respect to the idea of the maxilla being described as growing up and forward from some reference point. Thus it may be seen in light of the above theory of growth that maintaining a balanced occlusion, or an entire maxillofacial complex for that matter, becomes a race between the upper and lower two bones of the head, the craniomaxillary and mandibular, and hopefully they will run a synchronized "neck-and-neck" race forward or at least keep close enough to one another on a horizontal plane to permit the teeth to seek out and settle into a reasonably proper dental relationship.

In order to justify his theories of the directions of growth of the two separate components of the "two-bone-head" concept, Coben stated that the growth behavior of the anterior and posterior cranial bases should be thought of separately. This makes for a clearer understanding of the vectors he speculated are responsible for the directional path the maxilla takes in the journey away from the vertebral column during growth. He stated that the anterior cranial base, commonly designated as S-N, is a bit of a misnomer since the sphenoethmoidal suture usually halts its development at the age of approximately 7 years. After that, measurements between sella and the internal plate of the frontal bone show little or no change (0 to 2.0 mm, mean of .5 mm). Changes greater than that are due to external apposition at the outer surfaces of the frontal bone in the nasion area. He made no mention as to any changes in sella. He also agreed with some experts who felt that the pterygopalatine suture is part of the same sphenoethmoidal complex and therefore follows the same bone growth time schedule.

The general consensus of opinion among the experts of the day was that maxillary bone growth results from the maxilla and its passenger teeth being displaced forward by articular sutural growth to make room for the erupting second and third molars. Now we know that alveolar growth has a hand in this too. But Coben disagreed with this theory and in light of the aforementioned material theorized that *two* growth processes are responsible for development of the middle face. First, the maxilla is displaced forward by sutural growth at its posterior articular surfaces to the age of about 7 years. Then the second form of growth takes over which is primarily appositional and resorptive, and it is the normal eruption of teeth that stimulates the development of the alveolar process which makes room, in turn, to allow the eruption of those same teeth.

However, growth at the famous spheno-occipital synchondrosis takes place well on through the pubertal period. It must be remembered that the direction of growth of this synchondrosis is also an important factor to consider. In one case it may be predominantly in the horizontal plane. This would intensify the generalized forward movement of the maxilla and tend to open the N-S-Ar or saddle angle. Conversely, this synchondrosis may exhibit primarily a vertical growth component which would tend to contribute to the vertical development of the face and also have a tendency to slightly close the N-S-Ar angle. (Males generally tend to exhibit more vertical growth tendencies in this area, especially during puberty.) Along with the above, the mandible also expresses both horizontal and vertical growth patterns, and it may now be seen again that to both produce and maintain maxillofacial balance, the "two bones" must be synchronized in their growth vectors.

Accepting all of the above, Coben developed the method of superimposition of serialized tracings that he thought best expressed this divergent two-bone growth concept. It consists of superimposing the tracings on basion while at the same time keeping the S-N lines exactly superimposed, or, if growth changes have taken place at this area, then the two or more S-N lines of subsequent tracings are kept parallel. This then in the superimposition of serial tracings would reflect the divergence of the craniomaxillary and mandibular elements away from the vertebral column. This would show the maxilla to be moving up and away from the somewhat eccentric reference point of basion. However, this approach is not altogether consistent with the overall concepts of growth that select a frame of reference closer to the center of the cranial base. Thus we see how an altered concept of maxillary growth resulted in its own individualized superimpositional methods specifically designed to reflect its premise. Such sometimes happened, for this all took place in the late 1950s and early 1960s when the science of deep bone structure cephalometrics was in its flower. There would be others who would continue to exert their influence on the science.

The late 1950s and early 1960s were the time of the emergence of another individual who commanded enormous respect for his cephalometric prowess, Dr Robert Ricketts. Using computers, Ricketts and co-workers developed a highly sophisticated computerized cephalometric analysis system. Ricketts also separated the cranium from the facial complex, using a cranial base reference line. He avoided the problem of the mastoid process obscuring Bolton Point by using basion instead. Ricketts also used multiple superimpositions for studying various areas. He was a big believer in growth prediction. An interesting point about the Ricketts method is the definition of a new space mark, the CC point, or the "center of the cranium." It is the most recently calculated point that attempts to register tracings on that all-illusive center of craniofacial growth. It is defined as the intersection of the B-N line with a line drawn from gnathion to PT point (the intersection of the foramen rotundum with the posterior wall of the pterygomaxillary fissure). It represents a new form of growth axis. It is also another respectful acknowledgment of the importance of the pterygomaxillary fissure.

But one thing all of the above reflected in common was the efforts to use a *single* line as a reference point to analyze both vertical and horizontal changes in growth or treatment results. It is true that Broadbent originally was sensitive to such "two-way" problems and added Frankfort Horizontal to his system, a near miss that we can only appreciate from hindsight. Upon reflection, if one accepts the concept of the center of growth for the head, all surrounding areas may be assumed to grow out from it in all directions. If one also accepts compromise as a means to an end, these movements of growth may be thought of as divisible into vertical and horizontal components out from a central point. Ricketts alluded to it by virtue of the CC point. Now considering that the chief concern of the cephalometrician is the lateral view, and also considering that growth out from a center is describable in terms of horizontal and vertical, how perfectly reasonable to construct a vertical and horizontal axis or coordinate system similar to the common XY-axis. Such was the view of Bimler. The Frankfort Horizontal plane provided, in his terms, "the best compromise" for a horizontal reference line and for the vertical, a line drawn perpendicular to Frankfort through the crest of the pterygomaxillary fissure. Simple, reproducible, acceptably accurate for clinical purposes, Bimler's orthogonial reference system has served for 40 years as a system for diagnostic purposes, but it has not been used by facial growth researchers.

One of the most recent and truly ingenious cephalometric analysis systems, developed by Dr James McNamara of the University of Michigan, retains only the Frankfort Horizontal and uses several vertical components drawn perpendicular to it for reference purposes instead of the single pterygoid vertical of the Bimler. Thus it may seem that we have come full circle with respect to the never-ending quest for a place upon which the cephalometric observer may stand. The early precephalometric anthropologists and craniometricians started with the Frankfort Horizontal, and now this old standard appears again on the leading edge of cephalometric analysis systems.[186] In the interim, many frames of reference were tried. Some failed, some survived with limited value, and still others required a modicum of compromise and "cephalometric license" for use in diagnostic purposes. In an overall view of the issue, one is reminded again of the words of the Roman poet Virgil, "Non omnia possumus omnes" ("We cannot do all things"). And a single base reference line cannot do all things. Such would require growth to proceed in a univariate fashion, but it does not. Growth proceeds in a multivariate manner and therefore requires multiple frames of appropriate reference if correct and accurate

---

Figure 2–28   (**A**) Coben's concept of the head being two bones, the "craniomaxillary" bone and its counterpart, the mandible, caused an unusual concept of growth to occur. He felt the growth of the *cranial base* carried the maxilla and maxillary arch up and away from the vertebral column, whereas the growth of the mandible carried the mandibular arch down and away from the vertebral column. Thus, balanced growth becomes a "race" between the two. (**B**) Comparing superimpositional methods: "A"—Broadbent's Bolton Triangle registered at R, "B"—Brodie's S-N line registered at S; and "C"—Coben's method of registering at basion while keeping S-N lines parallel! (**C**) Coben's theory of the two-bone head is depicted by means of these illustrations that are superimposed per his method, registering them at basion and either superimposing S-N lines exactly or, if changes have taken place, keeping them parallel. In "A," where S-N lines are able to be exactly superimposed, and in "B," where S-N lines are kept parallel, the mandible obviously grows down and away from the vertebral column (represented by basion). Also in both cases the cranial base may be seen to move either forward ("A") or up and forward ("B") according to Coben's divergence theory. Stimulated alveolar and maxillary growth compensate to move ANS, A-point, and maxillary denture down and forward. (**D**) Ricketts CC registration point: another product of the late 1950s and early 1960s. PT = junction of the pterygopalatine fossa and the foramen rotundum, CF = intersection of FH and pterygoid vertical, CC = the intersection of the basion-nasion plane (Huxley's old line) with the Ricketts facial axis (PT point to gnathion). (Reprinted from Coben SE: Growth concepts. *Angle Orthod* 1961; 31: 195–196 with permission.)

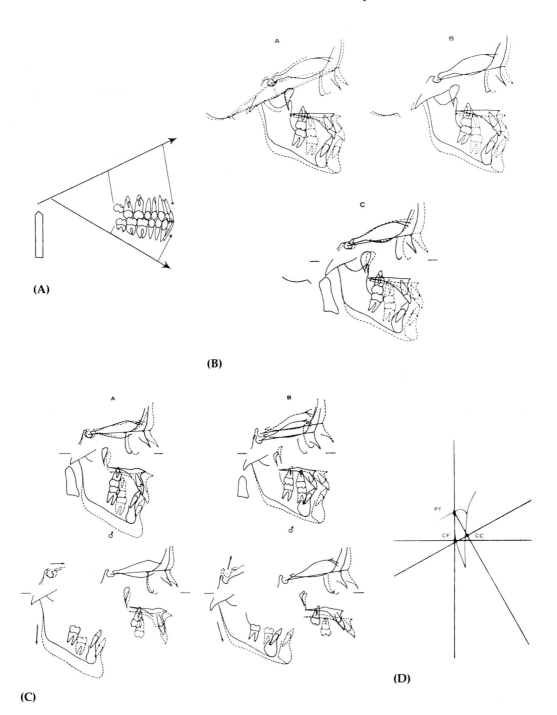

(A)

(B)

(C)

(D)

analysis of bone growth or changes due to treatment are to be performed.

What is also interesting about this process of cephalometric base reference line development is that it took a full generation or better to transpire. This may be due to several factors, the first of which may be jocularly called the "guru complex." As Moore stated, "Too often acceptance of a new philosophy by the profession has been based upon the strength and personality of the person developing it." He also pointed out, as did others,[187] that once new theories gain general acceptance, they are not given up for subsequent new ones easily. In turn, several other factors come to play in this respect. As Sved[179] points out, recent graduates of orthodontic programs find it difficult to reorient their thinking to new ideas or to the folly of old ones, for they might not yet have the experience or confidence to "deviate from accepted procedure." Veterans of the profession may also be guilty of resistance to change in a discipline as dogmatic as orthodontics because of what Sved terms "inertia" and a natural tendency to avoid changes to new procedures, "which always involve additional effort." But the eyes of the hawks never close. Their keen insights inspired by the true scientific spirit ran cephalometric superimposition through an intellectual sieve. But base reference lines were not the only cephalometric pedantries scrutinized. Three other major concepts were also attacked: normative standards, constancy of facial pattern, and that most hapless of cephalometric whipping boys, growth prediction.

A CLARION SOUNDS AT JERICHO

One of the first to suffer swift and sustained criticisms was the concept of normative standards. Early cephalometricians were fond of gathering small samples of handpicked individuals with what were considered "ideal" occlusions and measuring their cephalograms every which way to develop a table of values considered "normal," which loosely translates to "ideal." But this posed problems.[188] Such a table falsely assumes the role of what are held up as treatment goals, since it implies that an individual who varies from such standards is not ideal or, more specifically, is "abnormal." Of course, nothing could be further from the truth.

Brodie himself was quick to attack the normative concept and, as early as 1946, stated that[178]

> My entire plea is for an abandonment of the norm concept. It is time that we ceased to compare each individual we treat with some pattern that has been arrived at either by an inner sense of proportions or by the careful compilation and averaging of large series of measurements of different individuals.

He felt such traditional approaches were a carryover of methods rooted deep in the physical sciences. He was more of a believer in ranges of values within which the normal may fall. This concept of ranges persists and is widely agreed upon to this day. And a full 10 years before the Second Cephalometric Workshop, Brodie was also one of the first to stress the proper use of mathematics in the management of biostatistics. Brodie's contention was that individuals by virtue of their own anatomical makeup held the key to what their own standards should be. What is actually represented by this approach is a simplified way of merely determining what the patient's needs are: What do they need to be balanced and proper relative to their own anatomical frame of reference?

It is important relative to the subject of normative standards to distinguish between description and evaluation. Norms are objective—descriptive of averages of a population. But evaluation of an individual value relative to a mean or average is subjective, and in orthodontics that is the domain of responsibility of the clinician. A mandible may be said to be "long," but when does it become too long? A mandibular arc of closure may be said to be retruded, but when does it become too retruded? (Listen to the joints, they will tell you.)

The enormous number of variations of values possible within a given individual allow for too much overlap for "idealized" norms to be diagnostic or to act as treatment goals. This was held by Brodie and other highly esteemed men of those times. E. H. Hixon pointed out that comparison of a large enough sample of cases revealed that some individuals with malocclusions may possess as many "ideal" values or similar facial patterns as do persons with excellent occlusions.[189] Conversely, an individual may exhibit various values of cephalometric measurements clearly outside the normal range of values for those particular measurements, yet still possess a beautifully balanced and functional occlusion! Hixon further pointed out that the clinician must make use of the norms as descriptive entities that can possibly aid him in his judgmental evaluation. Such judgments are not an integral part of the norms themselves. In fact, Hixon and others, such as the prestigious T. M. Graber, held, at least during the decade of the 1950s when cephalometrics was still coming of age, that plaster models and clinical examination still outstripped the use of cephalometrics as far as value to the clinician in making an accurate and proper diagnosis![190, 191] The net result of such weighty and longstanding derision of the normative concept has come down to us in the form of the singularly most widely acknowledged and accepted dictum in all of cephalometrics: Treat to the patient's needs; don't treat to the numbers!

The theory of the constancy of facial pattern also met with its share of critics, although it is still one of the most widely respected concepts in orthodontics. Evidence of such is obvious every time a clinician constructs a treatment plan. Many clinicians have treated innumerable cases over the years and achieved excellent results without the benefit of any sort of allowance in the treatment plan for additional changes due to growth. Brodie's theory held that regardless of the degree of proportional imbalance of a facial pattern, that pattern will be consistently produced within reason throughout the growth and development of the individual. A Class II, Division 1 malocclusion in a 12-year-old will remain as such throughout the remainder of growth.

There are qualifications to this theory, some of which have already been mentioned. It is common knowledge that in the younger child, the mandible may lag behind the rest of the face in vertical and horizontal development, only to "catch up" during the adolescent growth spurt. At the other end of this example, a normal-appearing Class I skeletal and dental arrangement in the young child has at times been observed to "take off" during adolescence to conclude in a full Class III. With respect to the former, it is often heard, "Mrs. Patient, your daughter is a little on the Class II, deep bite, mandibular retrusive side; but don't worry, she's only 6½. We'll keep an eye on her, and when she's 9, 10, or 11 we'll have a better idea of what's really happening." With respect to the latter, the science of cephalometrics has labored long and hard in futile efforts to attempt, by means of observations of various lateral film measurements, to predict such Class III growth spurts in an effort to obviate such orthopedic surprises. Here, certainly, familial history also carries considerable prognostic weight.

Yet the possibilities of variation occurring somewhere along the line must always be kept in mind. This point was clearly brought out in studies of genetically identical twins and triplets. Work done by Bertram Kraus et al[192] of Seattle in 1959 and by S. L. Horowitz et al[193] in New York a year later brought forth some important findings concerning variability of facial patterns. It was determined that genetics did control the size and shape of individual bones; but, surprisingly, strict duplication of facial pattern was not shown! This means that although the individual bony components of the maxillofacial complex were nearly identical in twins or triplets with respect to size and shape, their arrangement and orientation to one another was influenced by environmental factors. The greatest amount of variation was seen in the lower face areas. Thus, even though the skeletal facial patterns would be expected to be identical, variations occurred as a result of external factors. These external factors are neither predictable nor controllable. Yet the variations measurable cephalometrically were not of major proportions.

Another factor noted was the unpredictability of the direction of growth (flexure) of the cranial base at the all-important spheno-occipital synchondrosis. Active well into the growth years, this governing entity of the cranial base angle may easily contribute to variance of facial pattern by increasing or decreasing the amount of flexure with growth.

Adequate methods of predicting what this area will do have not yet been devised.

Yet the aforementioned factors are not sufficient to totally negate Brodie's facial constancy theory. The variations in twins were not major, and often the angle of the cranial base may be observed to run true over the course of years of growth (though not *always*). Therefore the concept of facial constancy emerges reasonably unscathed, albeit with a few dents due to such qualifications.

The sharpest division in cephalometrics is over the issue of growth predictions. Its critics constitute a long and impressive list, and their position on the issue appears to be universally adamant against the usefulness of the method, at least in the forms in which it appeared up through the 1970s. Due to the weight initially carried by the opinions of Broadbent and Brodie on the constancy of facial pattern, the process of growth prediction received less attention in earlier times. Yet it was something the treating clinicians could not ignore altogether. Knowledge beforehand that a particular facial pattern may grow favorably or unfavorably with respect to a given treatment plan would be of great value to the clinician in helping him decide how to modify that treatment plan in relation to such knowledge. A favorable growth pattern can greatly facilitate treatment, such as a "horizontal grower" being treated for a skeletal or dental Class II malocclusion. Conversely, an unfavorable growth pattern can leave the best-laid treatment plan fraught with difficulties. An example would be a "vertical grower" or "high-angle case" being treated for anterior open bite or Class III problems. However, average changes in growth patterns tend to be minimal, but it must be stressed that this is for the *average* case.

One of the first efforts at helping the clinician handle the enormous problems of estimating growth changes was the development of templates. This technique consists of constructing a tracing of a facial profile with all major cephalometric landmarks drawn on a clear plastic celluloid transparency. There are numbers of serialized tracings constructed for various ages. Some may even be individualized for sex. The values used are the mean values derived from cross-sectional growth and measurement tables. Thus it is possible to construct a template of the mean or average 10-year-old cephalometric profile, or any other age desired. The appropriate template, specific for the age of the patient, is then selected and superimposed on the actual tracing of the cephalogram at the appropriate superimpositional landmarks. This allows the clinician to compare the actual case with the calculated and proposed means for that age group. Things like the patient's interincisal angle, the mandibular plane angle, occlusal plane angle, locations of A-point, B-point, etc, may be compared with the mean location represented by the template. If the clinician wants an approximation of future growth increments (according

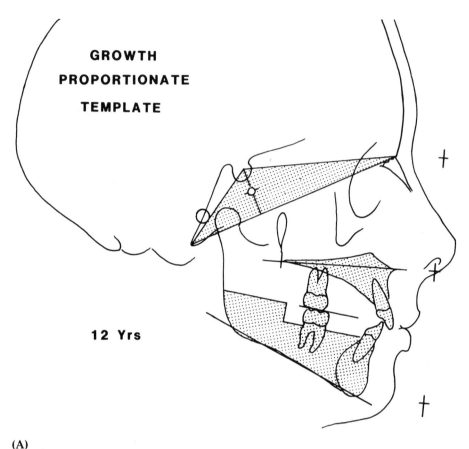

(A)

Figure 2–29 (A) Growth proportionate templates (Jacobson/Kilpatrick) such as this are produced for various age groups on clear plastic cells. They represent average anatomical measurements for that speficic age group. They are placed over the tracing of the patient's cephalogram for analysis. (B) In Example 1 the age-specific template may be placed over the actual tracing to reveal in this case a maxillary protrusion. In Example 2 template superimposition reveals a mandibular retrusion. Both examples register at N and superimpose along the N-Ba line. However, other baseline superimpositions are possible merely by rotating the template over the tracing. (C) Instead of superimposing the entire template all at once on some base reference line, individual portions of the maxillofacial complex may be analyzed separately, such as the maxilla, by superimposing on the ANS-PNS palatal plane and registering on pterygomaxillary fissure. (D) The mandibular changes due to growth or treatment may be analyzed by superimposing on the Go-Gn plane and registering either at "A" gnathion or "B" gonion. (E) Vertical may be analyzed by superimposing on the occlusal plane to check the vertical dimension of the dentition. By using "plus" marks on right-hand margin of template, skeletal vertical may be analyzed, since these represent the distances from N to ANS (upper face height) and ANS to menton (Me) (lower face height). (Courtesy Dr Alex Jacobson.)

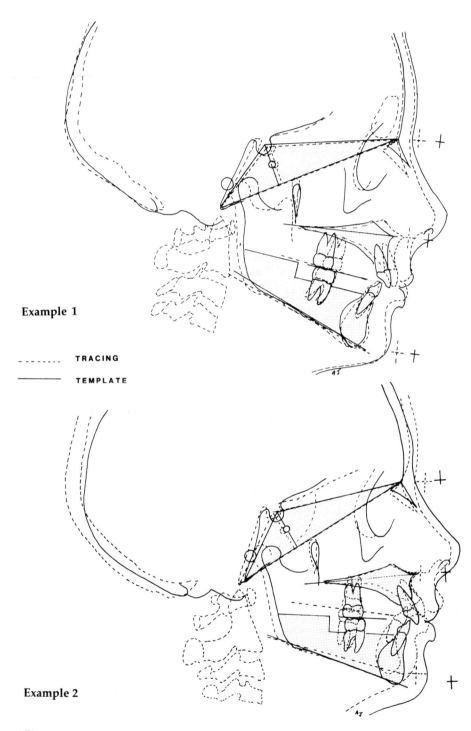

Example 1

TRACING
TEMPLATE

Example 2

(B)

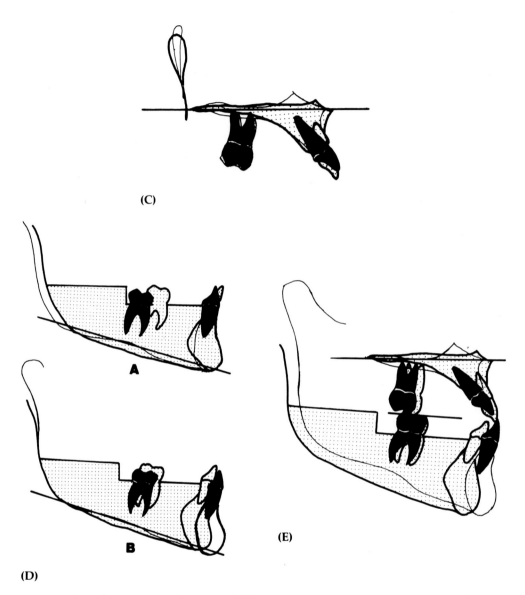

(C)

(D)

(E)

to what the mean values would be expected to do), he may merely superimpose the template for the appropriate year and note the directions and amounts of "projected" growth.

However, of the various types of templates produced by certain investigators, certain limitations are evident. Some are neither sex nor race specific, while others are composed from small selected samples of what were arbitrarily considered "ideal," an obvious mathematical bias. It has been pointed out that still others have been designed in subgroups of predominantly horizontal growers and predominantly vertical growers. These templates pose the problem of correct selection at the onset, for if the clinician guesses wrong as to the type of growth pattern the individual patient actually exhibits and, as a result, selects the inappropriate series of templates (horizontal or vertical), relatively substantial margins of growth prediction error will be generated. Except for age, sex, and predominant growth direction type, these templates cannot be individualized but merely represent the mean of a general sample that may not even be sex specific.

As might be discerned, the enormous amount of data concerned with such a complicated and multivariate process as growth prediction would be all but unmanageable were it not for that marvel of our modern age, the digital computer. Complex mathematical computations may be performed in seconds, and gaining certain types of answers becomes a simple matter of merely translating the pertinent information into the binary language these overgrown counting machines can understand and letting them do their thing. However, like the science of cephalometrics itself, gaining answers is one thing, but interpreting them accurately is quite another.

As previously mentioned, Ricketts was one of the first to undertake the use of computers on a large scale for management of cephalometric data. It might also be remembered that he has long been a keen believer in growth prediction. His use of the computer for growth prediction represents the next step beyond the principles of template use—electronic. The methods initially developed consisted of increasing the patient's existing cephalometric dimensions by an average amount, adjusted for age, sex, and race.[176] This process is not individualized, but merely predicts an average growth increment, according to growth table data, for each facial measurement. The results are close to those obtained by the sex-specific template method (predictionwise, it is like cephalometrically rolling the dice[194]), but still don't alert the clinician to untoward changes in facial pattern development.

By general consensus of many authorities, dating back to the Second Cephalometric Workshop, it is better to have a range of values for prediction of growth or changes of a given cephalometric measurement accompanied by a relative probability rating for those respective ranges. This preference is a result of the fact that all growth table data are derived from cross-sectional studies. Individualized growth prediction probabilities of a high percentage and narrow "confidence limits" can only be obtained from long-term serialized longitudinal studies of that same individual. Predicting growth changes with cross-sectional or average data in turn forces that prediction for the individual toward a mathematical mean, even though individual variation from those means frequently occurs. Hence, mean-value-oriented, cross-sectionally based, computerized growth predictions are generally no more accurate than the assumption of average value changes of facial pattern measurements by methods similar to those obtained with templates.[195-196]

Many researchers have looked into growth prediction, approaching it by one of two possible methods: correlate existing measurements to future values, or correlate past growth rates to future growth rates. So far neither method has revealed relationships that would allow high-percentage-accuracy growth prediction. The amount of leeway on either side of the values generated was simply too wide to give the predictions anything other than a mere statistical significance.[197-204]

Thus, when surveying the general scope of its developmental history, like a scientific Prometheus chained to a rock, cephalometrics has had to suffer the constant attacks of the hawks of criticism, with those critics of growth prediction being the most voracious. Yet, as an important adjunct to diagnosis, it survives. These critical attacks are not a form of punishment for having given the fire of improved diagnosis and treatment planning to clinicians, but they represent a sincere and true form of Herculean deliverance from the shackles of interpretive inaccuracies and theoretical falsehoods.

CHAPTER 3
The Knights of Euclid

CEPHALOMETRIC ANALYSIS

The purpose of the cephalometric x-ray is to establish exact three-dimensional spatial concepts in a communicable, understandable, manageable, two-dimensional language. The lateral view is the one that receives the lion's share of the interest, though the anteroposterior (AP) view is used as a supplement in more advanced analyses, especially those involving computers. But even here, frontal views are not essential. This is no doubt due to the lack of definition of anatomical structures as a result of excessive superimposition of osseous tissues in an AP direction. Thus Pacini's predictions appear to have come true,[31] since the entire scope of cephalometric analysis is in the sagittal plane as revealed by the lateral view and deals with the vertical and horizontal relationships of anatomical landmarks in this plane.

The lateral cephalogram deals with three basic relationships: the amount of flexion of the cranial base; the relationship of the maxilla and the mandible and their respective denture bases to each other; and the relationship of these bases relative to the general profile outline of the face. Conspicuous by its absence to date is the analysis of that anatomical

117

entity which is more important than any of these, the temporomandibular joints (TMJs). These relationships can be measured either linearly or angularly and compared with pre-established clinical norms or ranges of variability for interpretation. The clinician may then select the most appropriate form of treatment for the individual case being analyzed.

A well-founded background in the various treatment techniques will tell the clinician what these techniques can and cannot do. Thus the act of making the "cephalometric analysis treatment-technique capability" comparison helps prevent the practitioner from selecting a treatment modality incapable of satisfying the specific case.

Entire volumes may be dispatched on the numerous methods for obtaining diagnostic information from x-ray analysis. But certain goals exist which the main body of practitioners use to determine what is useful and what is not. Hypothetically one may never have too much information, but, for expediency, most practitioners want the most pertinent and relevant information in the most easily obtainable and manageable form.

FACIAL TYPE

Before entering into the intricate world of detailed cephalometric analysis, let us discuss a method of categorizing patients, which may be useful on a gross anatomic level, that of facial type. Faces are of interest from a treatment standpoint to those of us who must correct malocclusion. Much of what we do in treating the dysfunction and deformity of various malocclusions directly affects the face. The correct technique can help the face, but the wrong technique may detract from it.

Vague terms are used to describe faces, for example, "beautiful." What truly constitutes beauty? Such subjectivity is useless to the measurable-fact-oriented dentist studying malocclusions, and, as far as the orthodontic discipline has been concerned, until recently has been relegated to its traditional resting place, the eye of the beholder. Fortunately, that has changed. Slightly more detailed terms such as long, short, deep, and narrow are also too nondescript to be of much relative value. But here we reach a minor obstacle. To try to start defining faces for orthodontic diagnosis and treatment-planning purposes in a more detailed manner than this approaches mammoth proportions. Yet, a good generalized system of defining facial type is extremely handy, because certain appliances and techniques, or even orthodontic treatment plans in general, are more favorably accepted by one facial type than another and produce better results in one type than another. So sweepingly broad categorizing systems have been evolved with defined descriptions of the more common facial types. But even on a level this broad, the descriptions and definitions, which at first seem simple, clash in overlapping contradiction and confusion. Yet, a simple step-by-step sorting

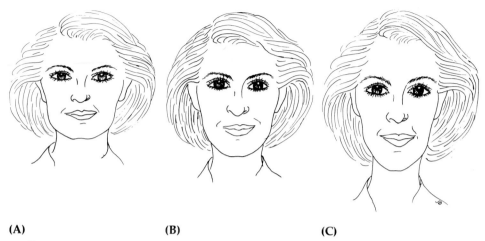

Figure 3–1 **(A)** Euryprosopic (brachycephalic, brachyfacial). **(B)** Mesoprosopic (mesocephalic, mesofacial). **(C)**Leptoprosopic (dolichocephalic, dolichofacial).

out of the material available reveals what is meant by the various definitions and what historical sequence of events (and what turn out to be mistakes) led to the confusion in terminology between anthropologic and orthodontic nomenclature. Knowledge of how these terms and definitions came to be in their present state is essential to practitioners trying to communicate their ideas on orthodontics to their colleagues, *especially* on an international level.

The first category of facial type we shall discuss is the one about which there is generally the least confusion—the "mesofacial" or, more correctly, "mesoprosopic." But already there is a technical problem of an etymological nature. The term "mesofacial" appears to be American in origin and is a bastardized result of the use of the two root words "meso," which is Greek in origin, and "facial," which is Latin in origin: "facia, facies." The term "mesoprosopic" is more accurate because both components of the term are Greek ("prosopic" means "face"). The term is used most often throughout Europe, since Europeans, for about 60 years, have not used terms that combine Latin and Greek roots; such terms are looked down upon among professional circles. Americans are not as concerned over etymological protocol.

The mesoprosopic facial type is also referred to in some major European texts as "mesocephalic," which is also a misnomer. To explain this term, we turn to what Europeans call the "bible" of anthropological anthropometrics, *Lehrbuch der Anthropologie* by Rudolph Martin, a Swiss anthropologist who taught at the beginning of this century, and Karl Saller, a German professor of anthropology at the University in Munich, who published the third edition in 1957. The book gives the skull classification index of Vorschlag von Garson, developed in 1886. Its three main categories of skull or cranium types, considered from an AP aspect viewed from the top, are dolichocran (long and narrow), mesocran (medium), and brachycran (short and wide). But this classification system was for dried skull specimens. To differentiate between dried skull specimens and living skulls, von Garson appended the term "cephalic," to mean a living individual with either a dolichocephalic (long) skull *antero-posteriorly*, a mesocephalic (medium) skull type, or a brachycephalic (short but wide) skull type, *anteroposteriorly*. Hence, the term "meso-cephalic facial type" would literally mean "medium skull facial type," which, if not a contradiction of terms, is certainly confusing. Yet these terms are commonly seen in reference sources![205−208]

Regardless of the terms we use, the mesoprosopic facial type is the average and most common facial pattern. This facial type is associated with equally balanced and proportional maxillomandibular relationships relative to width and height. The dental arches of such facial types are also well-rounded and correctly proportioned relative to arch length *v* arch width, as opposed to the two possible extremes of a long narrow dental arch or a short wide dental arch. The external features of the face are generally harmonious and well-balanced, and the facial outline is symmetrical on the AP plane and within normal esthetic limits on the sagittal plane, especially with respect to the anterior facial profile. As the maxillofacial bones of this facial type grow down and out from under the cranium, their general path is in a straight line at about a 45-degree angle relative to the Frankfort horizontal plane. Growth of the facial complex is evenly divided between horizontal and vertical components.

Class I malocclusions exhibiting simple dental crowding or tooth misalignment are often of this type. Since little orthopedic change is required, the prognosis for a successful conclusion to orthodontic treatment for mesoprosopic facial types is usually quite good. Though the etymological second half of the terms used to distinguish this facial type are different and employed in various usages, the first half is always the same, "meso," and accepted by everyone to mean "middle." However, this is the last point at which all classifying systems of facial type are in confluence. From here on, terms and definitions vary and even contradict one another, so unless each system's particular set of semantic rules is understood, confusion is guaranteed.

VARIANCE IN FACIAL TYPE: THE EXTREMES *V* THE MEANS

With the basic foundations now laid for the sake of our discussions in the commonly accepted ground of all facial typing systems, where "meso" is at least universally accepted by all, we are now prepared to venture forth into the murky waters of conflicting terminologies concerning the two types of extremes on either side of the mesoprosopic facial pattern: the vertically short, sagitally deep, *horizontally dominant* facial type; and the facially long, lean, sagittally shallow, *vertically dominant* facial type. However, just how they are defined, and by whom, and according to what historical precedent is where the facial typing plot thickens.

It must be remembered that the early physical anthropologists of late 19th-century Europe were measuring, categorizing, and defining facial types, as well as every other conceivable anthropometric entity, long before dentists ever took a hard look en masse at orthodontic therapeutics as an organized specialty. It is from these early anthropological foundations that the pioneering orthodontic specialists of Europe drew their material which they used in the formation of their preliminary diagnostic sciences, such as facial typing, malocclusion typing, and cephalometrics. To aid us in our brief sojourn through the evolution of diagnostic terminologies, we will make use of the clarifying influence of two of the diagnostic concepts developed by Dr H. P. Bimler, the *Suborbital Facial Index* and the *Posterior Profile Angle*. Bimler is considered a world authority on cephalometrics, and his knowledge of the methods of the early anthropologists, especially the European physical anthropologists, is weighty to say the least, since his background in these areas is extensive.

Bimler uses his concepts of the Suborbital Facial Index to act as the prime method of defining facial type, which in turn is directly reflective of something the functional orthodontist is extremely interested in, the main directional component of maxillofacial growth. The reason he originated the Suborbital Facial Index was to complement, for *lateral* cephalometric purposes, the already existing Kollmann *frontally* oriented facial indexing system. Kollmann developed his system in 1892, and defined three basic categories of facial osteology. He measured the face frontally in two parameters: height from nasion to gnathion, and width from the most lateral aspect of one zygomatic arch to the other. The middle range of facial types, where the N-Gn height to lateral interzygomatic width was roughly 1 to 1, was defined, as might be guessed, as "mesoprosopic." For the facial type where the interzygomatic *width* was greater than the N-Gn height, Kollmann used the term "euryprosopic," from the Greek root "eury" meaning "broad," which is the dominant parameter in this frontally viewed facial type. Conversely, the facial type where the N-Gn *height* was greater than the interzygomatic width, Kollmann designated "leptoprosopic," from the Greek root "lepto" meaning "lean," a convenience of alliteration for English-speaking practitioners.

Now Bimler wanted a facial typing system that he could apply to a *lateral* projection of the maxillofacial complex, which he was interested in studying cephalometrically for orthodontic diagnostic purposes. So taking his cue from the Kollmann frontally oriented system, Bimler turned the three facial types sideways and, in the early fifties, developed the Sub-

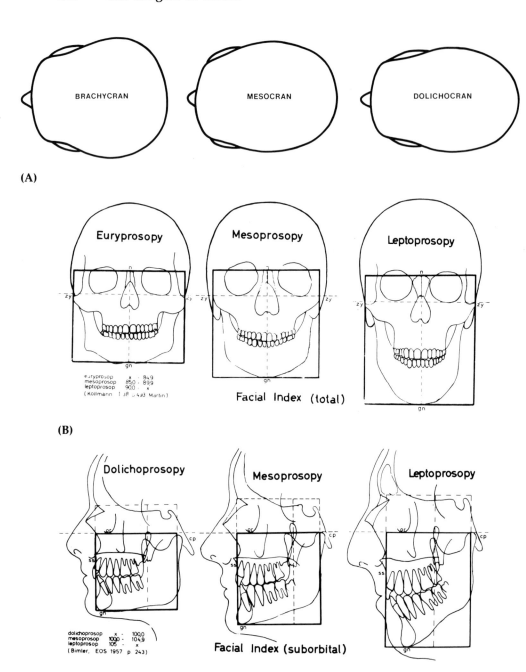

Figure 3-2   (A) Garson index—1886. (B)Kollmann index—1892. (C)Bimler index—1958.

orbital Facial Index. Understandably, Bimler turned the three facial types of Kollmann to the image's right such that the outline of the profile is to the observer's left. This view is completely opposite to almost all American-developed cephalometric analysis systems, which are designed to reflect the profile of the face to the observer's right! However, there is a perfectly logical reason for Bimler's choice. Bimler, who has degrees in medicine and dentistry, also possesses a formidable anthropological background. He was, therefore, quite familiar with the prestigious Martin-Saller text, which depicts most of its graphic material concerning facial or skull profiles oriented to the reader's left. Hence, Bimler oriented his cephalometric profile analysis in the manner in which he was no doubt most accustomed to seeing such profiles.

Bimler retains the term "mesoprosopic" for his laterally oriented Suborbital Facial Index. Bimler accentuates the fact that the Suborbital Facial Index he devised is truly only *facially* oriented and, for the sake of definition, considers the facial bones as those below the inferior border of the orbit, hence the term "suborbital." This also acts as a quite handy reference point for the first of his two parameters, the horizontal component. Bimler uses the ratio of the horizontal to the vertical components of the face to define suborbital facial type. He defines the horizontal component of the face as the distance from the projected perpendicular of A-point along the FH plane to the projected vertical of the center of the mandibular condyle, or capitulare (C-point, Bimler). The Frankfort is the perfect horizontal line because it runs from the inferior border of the orbit, ideal for facial measurement purposes, to the superior border of P. The vertical component runs from the same point where the A-point perpendicular crosses FH perpendicularly down to the horizontal projection of Me to that same vertical line. The Suborbital Facial Index (the actual calculation and scribing of which shall be discussed later) is a simple matter of relating the vertical to the horizontal components. Hence when the two are nearly equal in a well-balanced, *laterally* oriented facial pattern, the term "mesoprosopic" is the most logical choice.

Along with the Suborbital Facial Index, Bimler also developed an angular measurement system to describe in more detail the variations within a given facial type. He did this through what he calls the *Posterior Profile Angle*, which is that angle formed at the junction of a line running tangent to the clivus and the mandibular plane angle. This angle is used not as the primary determinant of facial type but in a supplemental capacity to the Suborbital Facial Index. The Posterior Profile Angle is divided into two subdivisions: the Upper Basic Angle, formed by the line running tangent to the clivus, and the line of the palatal plane (ANS-PNS); and the Lower Basic Angle, or maxillomandibular plane angle, formed by the intersection of the palatal plane and the mandibular plane. The Upper Basic Angle has a variance of about 30 degrees, extending from 50 to 80 degrees. The Lower Basic Angles has a range of variance of

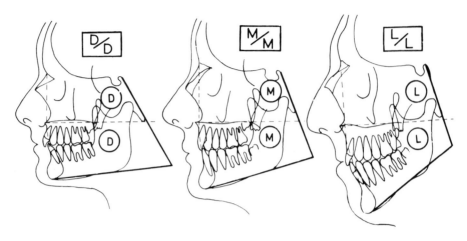

(A)

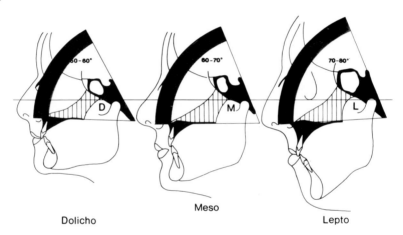

Dolicho   Meso   Lepto

(B)

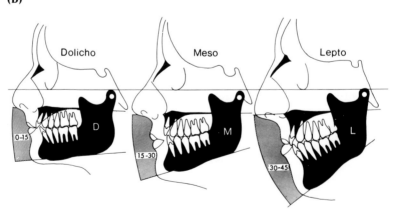

(C)

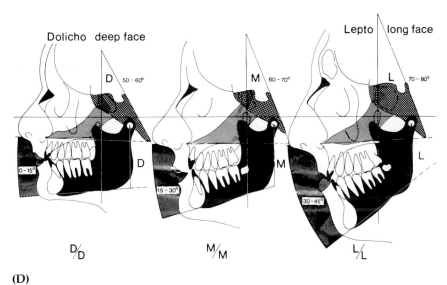

(D)

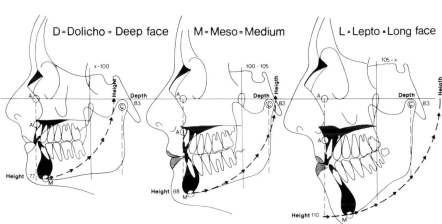

(E)

Figure 3–3   **(A)** Posterior Profile Angle. **(B)** Upper Basic Angle (clivomaxillary angle). **(C)** Lower Basic Angle (maxillomandibular angle). **(D)** Upper and Lower Basic Angles. **(E)** Bimler Suborbital Facial Index: When arc represented by radius A'M (horizontal projection of M on A' perpendicular) passes in front of C, it represents dolicho or deep-face. If it passes between C and the intersection of the clivus with FH, it is meso; and if it passes behind the clivus-FH intersection, it is lepto or long-faced.

nearly 45 degrees, extending from 0 to about 45 degrees. The Upper and Lower Basic Angles are divided into thirds with ranges of 10 degrees for each third on the Upper Basic Angle and 15 degrees for each third on the lower angle. Thus Bimler has divided facial types into upper and lower facial components. He has designated the middle range of the Upper Basic Angle as 60 to 70 degrees and designated the angulations falling in that range as mesoprosopic; he has also designated the middle range of the Lower Basic Angle as 15 to 30 degrees, and angulations falling in that range are also mesoprosopic. He uses the letter *M* to signify meso-prosopic, or medium-faced range, and thus expresses the facial type in terms of the Posterior Profile Angle as the combined relationship of the Upper and Lower Basic Angles, M/M.

Now this all follows a logical sequence of events, because Bimler made his assumptions about his *laterally* oriented *facial* typing index from, in turn, another *frontally* oriented *facial* typing index, the Kollmann. But there were also other Europeans (as well as certain Americans who followed them) who made facial typing assumptions from—and here's the key—*cranial typing* indices! With hindsight, such an assumption appears more tenuous than it would have when such terms were first promulgated. Instead of the Kollmann facial index, some investigators made certain assumptions about human faces relative to the terms and definitions of the old Garson index of 1886 which used dolicho, meso, and brachy for sagittally long (or deep), medium, and sagittally short *craniums*, respectively, when viewed from the superior aspect.

When changing from "cran" to "cephalic" for description of skull shapes in living individuals, some logically assumed that a mesocephalic *head type* went hand in hand with the mesoprosopic frontally oriented *facial type*, which it often does. But this is where the safety of such assumptions of relating head type to face type ends! Taking one ana-tomical aspect, the head, in one plane, the sagittal (from the superior view), with a specific set of terminologies for that aspect alone and attempting to relate it to another anatomical aspect, the face, in a totally different plane of reference, either frontal or lateral, was an unintention-ally deceptive process that has turned out to be a gremlin to haunt cephalometric diagnostics down to the present day.

We now return to the process of defining the extremes of facial type on either side of meso, a problem Bimler faced in dealing with the lateral rotation of the Kollmann euryprosopic facial type, where the width lat-erally, zygoma to zygoma, nearly exceeds the height, nasion to gnathon. When such a face is turned to its lateral profile, the distance representing the *horizontal component* of the Suborbital Facial Index along the FH from A perpendicular to capitulare's projected perpendicular (C-point, Bimler) is *greater* than the vertical component from the intersection of A perpen-dicular and FH to the horizontal projection of Me to that perpendicular line. With the horizontal component greater than the vertical component, the face is deeper sagittally than it is high vertically. Hence, Bimler uses a term that means "long" or "deep" in a *sagittal* direction, "dolicho," similar to what Garson did nearly 80 years earlier in his Cephalic Index where "dolichocran" signified a cranium which had a sagittal or AP length greater than the width laterally (by at least 20%; ie, $W > .80L$). Therefore, dolichoprosopic is in confluence with this system of terminology and is used to denote the *lateral* aspects of a face where the depth *sagittally* is greater than the suborbital height vertically. Dolichoprosopic describes faces now, not craniums (dolicho=deep, still more convenient alliteration!).

However, at this point those who prefer to think of the euryprosopic, wide, short face in cranial terms like "brachycephalic" (actually meaning wide, short cranium on the AP) make a second, far more serious, misconception in continuing to apply that term to a short, wide skull turned sideways, and the etymological lineage of the descriptive term "brachycephalic" begins to seriously break down.

In anatomical descriptions and measurements, we are faced with the problems of trying to depict a three-dimensional object on a two-dimensional flat surface. Therefore, one of the three dimensions by necessity is automatically nullified to an indescribable value. It is similar to a three-coordinate axis situation projected onto two-dimensional graph paper. On the dorsal aspect view of the skull, as in Garson's Cephalic Index, only the coordinates of AP depth sagittally and width laterally can be expressed. The third dimension, skull height, is negated as the "zero factor" (for want of a more descriptive term for our purposes). Upon rotating a skull viewed from the top about its width axis 90 degrees, we are now confronted with a new two-dimensional view from the frontal aspect. The dimension of *width remains* when we find the facial skeleton and skull from a frontal aspect. We may still see how wide it is, but now we may also see how long—more correctly, how high—it is. But we pay the price for this new view because the dimension of AP depth sagittally is lost; it has become the zero factor.

Now, remember that the primary meaning of brachycran is "short" in the AP direction and *only secondarily* implies added width ($W >. 80L$). However, now that we have rotated our sample skull to a frontal view and the AP dimension has become a zero factor, only the secondary meaning of *implied* extra width remains in the newly rotated frontal view. It is on this secondary implied meaning of width that those who associate wide faces with wide craniums pin their meaning, still using the prefix "brachy" to associate description of such a face.

Now if that frontal view of the face is again rotated, this time about its *vertical* axis to a lateral view, the dimension of lateral width now becomes the zero factor, AP sagittal depth once again appears, dominant by default over the diminutive vertical height, and "brachy" is still tacked on for the ride, but this time with a new suffix—"facial." Thus the new term is "brachyfacial" and is supposed to mean, to some, a facial profile where the AP *depth* sagittally dominates the height vertically. And, in the irony of ironies, the root word "brachy" implies such a dominating horizontal depth in the complete opposite context of its original meaning, "short," in the AP sagittal plane! Now, after this double transformation process, consisting of two separate unqualified assumptions, it has now come to mean, to some, "long," in the AP or horizontal sagittal plane and short in the vertical plane! Thus a short, square lateral face deeper than it is high may be seen in literature from two parts of the world as either "dolichoprosopic" (deep-faced sagittally) or "brachyfacial" (short-faced vertically)! Bimler fortifies his definition of the AP sagittally deep dolichoprosopic facial type, where the Suborbital Facial Index of height *v* depth is dominated by the horizontal component, with the additional particular information provided by the Upper and Lower Basic Angles of the Posterior Profile Angle. The angulations of the *Upper* Basic Angle that fall between 50 and 60 degrees are referred to as dolichoprosopic; and correspondingly the angulations of the *Lower* Basic Angle that fall between 0 and 15 degrees are designated dolichoprosopic. In terms of the total Posterior Profile Angle, the combined relationship of two such angles indicating a "closed bite" or low vertical facial situation is written D/D.

A somewhat easier path may be followed in deciphering how Bimler came to name that lateral facial type profile that is vertically higher than it is deep on the sagittal plane. Once again referring to the facially oriented indexing system of the Kollmann, Bimler took the lean, narrow, leptoprosopic, frontally viewed facial type and rotated it 90 degrees about its vertical axis. The facial type of such a proportion so rotated may still be seen to be higher or longer vertically than it is deep on the AP sagittal plane. The *vertical* component is dominant here. Hence, it would be perfectly logical to continue to think of this vertically high facial type as leptoprosopic, which is exactly what Bimler does. "Lepto" means "lean" or "thin." Again, Bimler fortifies the findings of the Suborbital Facial Index which would reveal a dominance of height vertically over AP depth sagittally with the particulars of the Upper and Lower Basic Angles of the Posterior Profile Angle. Upper Basic Angles in the 70–80-degree range and Lower Basic Angles in the 30–45-degree range are designated leptoprosopic, and the relationship of the two angles indicating a high vertically dominant face is written L/L. With these Upper and Lower Basic Angle combinations, *visually observed* clinical phenomena may be basically described from a lateral aspect cephalometrically. For example, the maximum bite-closing effect would be signified by the Posterior Profile Angle formula L/D. Correspondingly, the maximum bite-opening effect would be depicted as D/L.

What is interesting, and even more disconcerting in the final result, is the manner in which the same misconceptions that generated the seemingly conflicting terminologies of the first "brachy-dolicho" incident occur a second time to produce an equally conflicting terminological result for the long, thin, vertically high facial types!

Those who mistakenly form conceptions of the frontally high, somewhat narrow leptoprosopic frontal face of Kollmann in inappropriate cephalic terms instead of facial terms observe the sagittally deep, laterally somewhat narrow skull type when viewed from the top in the Garson Cephalic Index and know it is designated "dolichocran" ($W<. 80L$).

Transferring that term to a description of that skull type in the living, the term becomes "dolichocephalic," still denoting the two cranial dimensions of AP depth sagittally (primary) and transcranial width laterally (secondary). Now rotating *this* descriptive plane of reference for craniums 90 degrees about its *lateral* axis brings the frontal aspect of the facial skeleton again into view. The dimension of diminished lateral width remains, the dimension of facial height comes into effect, but the dimension of dominant sagittal depth is lost and becomes negated as a zero factor.

Now the dolichocephalic head type, which is somewhat narrow in lateral width by implication when viewed from the newly rotated frontal aspect, reveals only this remaining secondary dimension of narrowness laterally as the sagittal component is negated; yet the dolichocephalic designation term remains. Now the high, narrow facial type shows its dominance of height over lateral width when viewed from the frontal aspect and may be easily *assumed* to be associated with a narrow skull type also, though not always. Hence the dolichocephalic skull type with its *cranial*-index-oriented term became associated with the high, laterally narrow, or lean, face when that face is viewed frontally, a face Kollmann would list in his facially oriented index as leptoprosopic. Yet we still have some reasonable degree of semantic compatibility here, because a dolichocephalic-type cranium could conceivably be perched atop a leptoprosopic facial pattern. Viewed frontally, this combination would *accentuate* the narrowness of the face as opposed to its vertical height, due to the secondarily narrow dolichocephalic nature of the skull.

However, once the frontally viewed face of this type associated with a term describing it of cranial origins is rotated 90 degrees about its vertical axis to reveal its lateral aspect, the integrity of the etymological lineage of the cranial-index-oriented term "dolicho" can be seen once again to break down. As the frontal facial view is rotated to the lateral view, the relatively diminished lateral width, which was responsible for bringing the "dolicho" root from the top view to the frontal view, now becomes lost and negated as a zero factor. The dominant sagittal aspect or lateral plane once again becomes expressed; yet the "dolicho" root term tags along for the ride, but this time with a new suffix, "facial." Thus "dolichofacial" evolves to mean a high face viewed laterally, where, by necessity for such vertically dominant facial types, the vertical height, when viewed laterally, exceeds the depth sagittally on the AP plane. Once again, we see how through a series of tenuous assumptions, and as before, a process of double transformation, a Greek root meaning a skull deep sagittally becomes changed to the point where, to some, it signifies a face deep vertically and, by default, shallow or short on the AP sagittal plane! Not only does the term "dolichofacial" signify the complete opposite of its original usage with respect to reference plane coordinates, but it is used when a previously existing term with the same root, "dolichoprosopic," signifies a facial type that is its direct opposite extreme relative to ratios of depth v height of the lateral aspect! Hence the source of many confusions becomes obvious.

"Mesoprosopic," "dolichoprosopic," and "leptoprosopic" appear throughout prestigious orthodontic and anthropologic texts and scientific literature across Europe. "Mesofacial," "brachyfacial," and "dolichofacial" also appear in equally prestigious American orthodontic and cephalometric texts. "Brachyfacial" and "leptoprosopic" signify opposite facial types when viewed laterally. This may be somewhat etymologically readily discerned. However, "dolichoprosopic" and "dolichofacial" also signify opposite facial types when viewed laterally. As might be imagined, the unqualified use of *these terms* can lead to gigantic mis-understandings. When used among practitioners unfamiliar with the nature and history of their usages, not only can confusion be generated, but also one individual may wonder whether the other one knows what he is talking about!

Sorting out the various systems of naming facial types may seem tedious, but it is vital to the all-important clarification of the communi-cation of orthodontic ideas between one colleague and another and in the critical selection of treatment parameters, especially in the selection of standards of arch width, as in the use of the Schwarz facially corrected indices. Language is a tool and can mean whatever those who use it want it to mean. This is especially true when language usage is governed by the dictates of commonly accepted regional conventions. Maybe this whole confusing business of lateral facial typing could be solved by simply describing facial types as either horizontal or vertical growers. But that would be too simple!

The Suborbital Facial Index is determined by placing the point of a compass on the FH plane at a point directly over and perpendicular to A-point (subspinale) and drawing an arc from menton up to the Frankfort plane again. If this arc passes in *front* of the point C (capitulare or dead center of the body of the condyle of the mandible), then the facial depth as viewed horizontally from a lateral view is greater than the height. This makes it dolichoprosopic (deep-faced in Bimler's way). If the arc passes *behind* the clivus, it qualifies as leptoprosopic, or long-faced, be-cause the height is greater than the depth. Anything in between is simply considered mesoprosopic or medium faced. Linearly, these may be expressed simply as height equals the perpendicular from FH to menton, depth equals the distance between anterior vertical through A-point to posterior vertical through C, both points of which are projected to their intersection with the FH plane.

Thus, we can see that we may describe a particular facial type by simply lumping all the characteristics into one of three groups defined by a single term, or we may use three separate designations: the overall Posterior Profile Angle, its two subdivisions the posterior Upper Basic Angle and the posterior Lower Basic Angle, and the Suborbital Facial Index.

The determination of facial type is an important adjunct to the diagnosis and treatment of malocclusions. It is the broadest and least specific of the general categories of classification, and represents the first step in interpreting what type of patient and attending treatment problems the clinician is encountering. Since there are only three basic categories of facial type, Bimler's facial formula notwithstanding, this system of classification is highly generalized. A more specific definition of the anatomical situation the patient exhibits is needed by the diagnostician before he recommends a type of treatment regimen.

The next, more specific, level of classification of malocclusion one will necessarily make is to that of class according to Angle. This step is not as easy as it might appear. Here again the cephalometric x-ray becomes definitive. Clinicians are concerned with more than just teeth in this modern day.

DETERMINATION OF CLASS

The most universally known and accepted classification system of dental malocclusion has been that of Edward Angle. First described in 1899, it has served for nearly a century as the system whereby all malocclusions have been relegated to either Class I, II, or III. Class I was defined as that type of malocclusion where the upper first molar was in its normal relationship with the lower first molar, the mesiobuccal cusp of the upper first molar occluding with the mesiobuccal grove of the lower first molar. Other teeth may exhibit rotations or malalignments in this classification of malocclusion, but the first molars are in normal occlusion, and Angle therefore somewhat presumptively reasoned that the upper and lower jaws were in their normal maxillomandibular relationship with respect to the AP plane, a gigantic mistake!

Angle believed that the maxillary first molar was nearly always in its correct position and that Nature seldom, if ever, erred in the positioning of this particular tooth in the jaws. Since that time, however, cephalometric studies have shown that the maxillary first permanent molar's position in the jaw is not quite as regular as Angle originally thought. The term "Class I," or neutroclusion, also leaves open to question the relationship of the anterior teeth. It does nothing to describe their positioning, which is why their relationship must be tacked on at the end, as in Class I crowded, Class I open bite, etc. The Class I category also assumes the maxillary and mandibular skeletal (structural) components are in proper alignment. This is not always the case. Also in this category would fall the case where the molar relationship is normal, but the entire upper and lower dentures are positioned forward with respect to the rest of the face. This relationship has come to be known as a *bimaxillary protrusion*. Thus the term "Class I" is quite nondescript and sometimes suspect. Is the patient really Class I? What are the bite relationships of the other teeth? What are the relationships of the denture bases to each other and to the skeletal arrangement? Is the maxillary first molar in its true anatomically correct position? These questions may be difficult, if not impossible, to answer from direct observation of the patient or from mere analysis of a set of study models. Cephalometrics answers such questions.

The Class II relationship of malocclusion, or distoclusion, is divided into two divisions by Angle, with a third added later by others. Class II malocclusions exhibit the relationship of the mandibular first molar occluding distally to its normal articulation against the maxillary first molar. The entire lower arch is usually distal to its normal position against the upper arch. The first subcategory is Class II, Division 1, in which all of the above relationships are present, but in addition the maxillary anterior teeth are flared forward, thereby increasing the amount of overjet. The lower incisors may also be flared forward and may or may not be overerupted, increasing the anterior overbite. The upper arch is usually more "Gothic arch" shaped and less like the more desirable "Roman arch" form. Abnormal muscle function is usually a major factor in the etiology of these traits with the musculature contributing to the perpetuation of the deformity through the constant misdirection of improperly coordinated muscle forces, especially those of the tongue and lips. The lower lip usually tenses during swallowing under the protruding Division 1 maxillary anteriors. The tongue usually thrusts forward to some degree during swallowing, or it may flatten out posteriorly over the posterior segments inhibiting their eruption. This, combined with procumbent maxillary incisors and overerupted mandibular incisors, results in deep overbite, loss of vertical, and a deep curve of Spee.

The second subcategory, Class II, Division 2, also exhibits a similar distoclusion of the mandibular denture with respect to the maxilla; but in Division 2 the maxillary centrals are severely retroclined and in deep overbite, while only the upper lateral incisors are flared forward and may or may not be crowded out labially by impinging cuspids. Occasionally, the laterals may also be retroclined, which combined with deep overbite usually leads to some degree of retruded mandibular arc of final closure and, as a result, superior posterior displacement of the condyle (SPDC) in the TMJ upon full contact occlusion, a condition not tolerated well by the joint or associated musculature.

A third category is Class II, Division 3. Here the anteriors are flared forward such that the interincisal angle of the long axes of the maxillary and mandibular anteriors is 120 degrees or less. This would denote the typical bimaxillary protrusion.

But again, the Angle classifications of Class II malocclusion are vague and nondescript about the same questions of denture bases *v* skeletal relationships. Are the dentures at fault with the skeletal bases normal, or are the skeletal bases incorrect, denoting a true structural discrepancy? The same may be said of the Class III or mesioclusion designation. Angle described it as a condition where the mandibular first molar occludes anterior to its normal position against the maxillary first molar. This usually puts the anterior teeth in total anterior crossbite. But is this due to excessive growth of the mandible, an excessively under-developed maxilla, an excessively forward-positioned TMJ (what Bimler describes as a short T-TM), or retarded growth of the maxilla in conjunction with an overgrowth of the mandible? Is it a pseudo-Class III, where only the teeth are malpositioned but the skeletal bases are correct, or is there a true structural deviation?

From the above we can see that there is more to the determination of what Angle classification to assign to a given case than merely eye-balling a set of study models. We must know more than just how the teeth line up with one another cusp to cusp. We also want to know how the bones align with one another. The two bones of greatest interest to us are those in which the teeth reside, the maxilla and the mandible. Their exact positions and relationships to each other and other maxillo-facial osseous structures are critical to our diagnosis and treatment planning, especially if we intend to change their shape or position orthopedically with functional appliances or active plates. Structure and not just occlusion should be before our minds at all times. The terms "structural" and "skeletal" are interchangeable. Thus we want to accurately classify not only occlusal relationships as I, II, or III, but also *skeletal* relationships, for the treatment of these structural relationships is the main forte of FJO appliances. The determination of occlusal relationships is easy enough by simply using Angle's traditional method of direct visual inspection of either the patient or a representative set of study casts. But the determination of the structural or skeletal relationship or class of a given case necessitates the use of cephalometrics. We have to be able to look beneath the dental arches to their foundations. When we do, the cephalometric analysis systems that have been developed over the years help us understand what we see.

THE WITS ANALYSIS

The Wits analysis is a good cephalometric analysis system to begin our discussion with because (1) it is one of the most basic—its sole

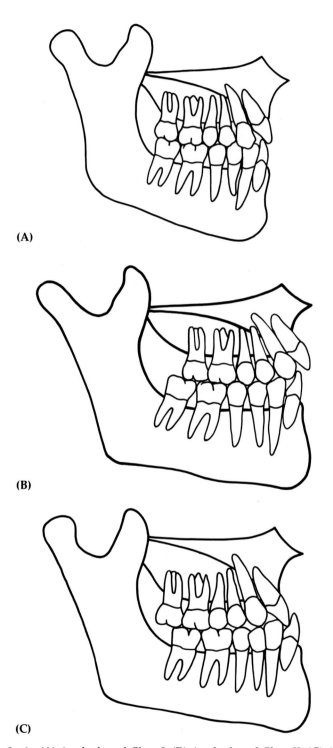

Figure 3-4   (A) Angle dental Class I. (B) Angle dental Class II. (C) Angle dental Class III.

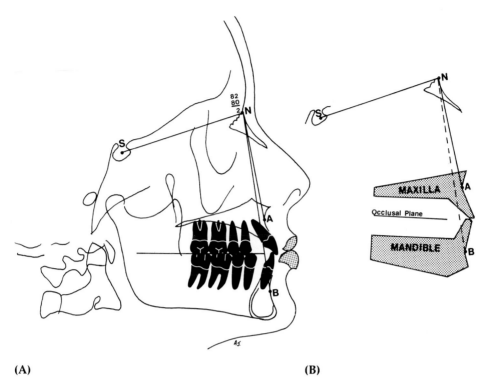

(A)   **(B)**

Figure 3–5 **(A)** Lateral headfilm tracing of patient considered cephalometrically "normal" with ANB angle of 2 degrees. **(B)** Representative drawing to illustrate relationship of maxilla and mandible. ANB angle readings are legitimate for evaluation of apical base relationships only when the occlusal plane or location of sella and nasion are within a certain confined range.
(Courtesy Dr Alex Jacobson.)

purpose is merely for the determination of the structural or skeletal relationship between the upper and lower jaws—and (2) it is a simple, easily used system because it involves only three lines. This ingenious analysis system was developed in the 1970s by Dr Alex Jacobson of the University of Witwatersrand School of Dentistry, Johannesburg, South Africa. It was devised to solve a problem that arose in relating upper and lower jaws to the cranial base, a common procedure of many of the more popular analysis systems. The problems arose when both the upper and lower jaws were juxtaposed to the cranial base or when they were rotated excessively with respect to the cranial base. Such situations result, due to the principles of simple plane geometry, in certain types of cephalometric analysis readings that do not reflect the actual jaw-to-jaw relationship but rather the distorted geometry of the case. This occurs because in many of the analysis systems in use the jaws are related, in unison, to the cranial base rather than to each other.[209–211]

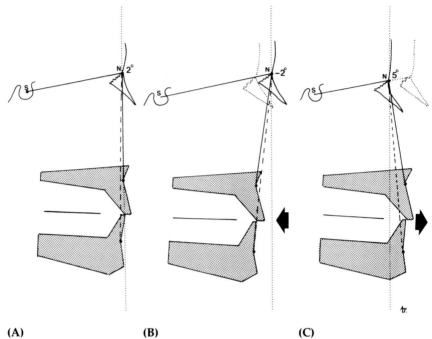

(A)   **(B)**   **(C)**

Figure 3–6   **(A)** Effect of horizontal movement of nasion or jaws themselves on ANB angle. (A) "Average normal" relationship of jaws to cranial base, ANB=2 degrees. **(B)** Effect on ANB angle of forward location of nasion (due to long anterior cranial base SN or retropositioning of both jaws in skull), ANB angle reduced to −2 degrees in this instance, ie, B seems to move closer to A. **(C)** Effect on ANB angle of retropositioning of nasion (due to short anterior cranial base or forward positioning of both jaws relative to cranium). ANB angle in this instance increased to 5 degrees, ie, B "moves" away from A. (Courtesy Dr Alex Jacobson.)

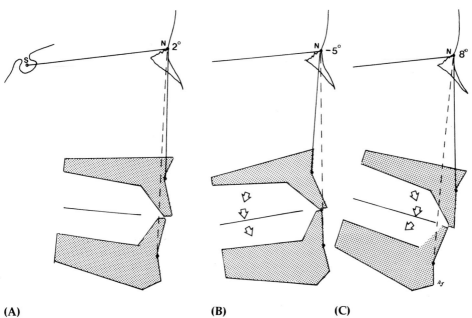

(A)   **(B)**   **(C)**

Figure 3–7   Effects of occlusal plane variance on ANB. **(A)** Average "normal" relationship of jaws, ANB 2 degrees. **(B)** Effect on ANB angle of counterclockwise rotation of both jaws: in this instance ANB angle is reduced to −5 degrees. **(C)** Effect on ANB angle of clockwise rotation of both jaws: increased to 8 degrees in this instance. (Courtesy Dr Alex Jacobson.)

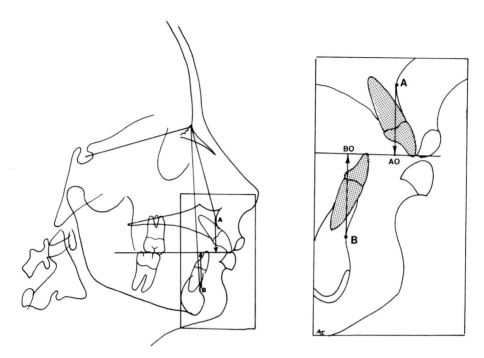

Figure 3–8   The "Wits" appraisal entails dropping perpendiculars from points A and B onto the occlusal plane to intersect at points AO and BO, respectively. The measured distance between points AO and BO represents the Wits appraisal reading. (Courtesy Dr Alex Jacobson.)

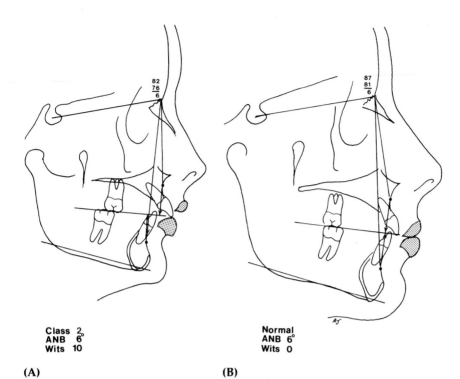

(A)   **(B)**

Figure 3—9   Comparison of Wits *v* Steiner interpretations of two sample cases.
(A) Here a Steiner shows an ANB of 6 degrees but a Wits value of 10, revealing
the case to be more Class II than the Steiner reading would reveal. This results
either from nasion being forward or jaws being retropositioned. **(B)** Here a
Steiner ANB of 6 degrees would indicate Class II, but the Wits reading of 0 shows
the contrary. This is due to a retropositioned nasion or forward-positioned jaws.
(Courtesy Dr Alex Jacobson.)

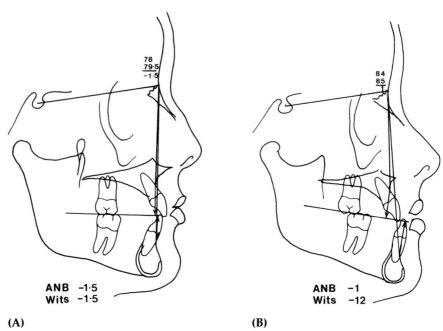

ANB −1·5
Wits −1·5

(A)

ANB   −1
Wits   −12

(B)

Figure 3−10   The extent of the Class III jaw dysplasia is shown in Figure 9. The
Class III tendency in **(A)** is mild, whereas **(B)** represents a major jaw disharmony.
The Wits divulges this clearly, whereas the ANB angle fails to distinguish
between the two. (Courtesy Dr Alex Jacobson.)

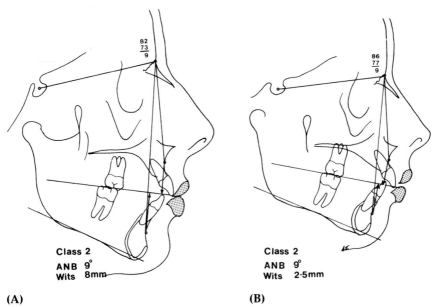

(A) **(B)**

Figure 3−11 **(A) (B)** Application of Wits appraisal to two Class II malocclusions, both having an ANB angle of 9 degrees. The Wits appraisal in **(A)** shows a severe (8 mm) Class II anteroposterior jaw discrepancy. In **(B)** the Class II jaw discrepancy is mild (2.5 mm). Once again the Wits is definitive here. (Courtesy Dr Alex Jacobson.)

The Wits method of appraising jaw relationships concerns itself with the AP positioning of the maxilla and mandible on the sagittal plane. Though it determines cephalometrically the skeletal relationship of the upper and lower jaws to one another, it does not decipher in a malocclusion situation which of the two is at fault; ie, in a Class II it does not indicate whether the maxilla is too long or the mandible is too short. Other systems have to be employed to determine this. But the Wits appraisal is important in that it is quick and easy to use and accurate as to the determination of structural relationships. It may be employed when the limiting parameters of other systems are exceeded, thus negating their efficiency with regard to this aspect. This will be discussed later in the section on the Steiner analysis.

Only A-point (subspinale), B-point (supramentale), and the occlusal plane are needed for the Wits analysis. First, draw the occlusal plane by drawing a straight line through the middle of the intercuspation overlap on the molars forward to a point that bisects the cuspal overlap of the first bicuspids. If the bite is open, bisect the space left between the open incisal edges. A slight angular variation of several degrees in the construction of the occlusal plane is not critical. Next, drop a vertical line from A-point perpendicular to the occlusal plane. This perpendicular is

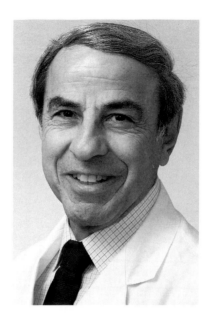

Figure **3–12**   Dr Alex Jacobson.

referred to as AO. Now draw another perpendicular line from B-point up to the occlusal plane. This perpendicular is referred to as BO. The line AO is related to BO such that if AO is more anterior, or to the right of BO toward the front of the patient's face with the profile on the observer's right, the distance in millimeters measured along the occlusal plane between the two perpendiculars is expressed as a positive number. If AO is to the left or behind BO, the distance between the two perpendiculars measured in millimeters along the occlusal plane is expressed as a negative value. The values of this measurement between AO and BO may be expressed and interpreted as in the accompanying table.

Ideal Wits Maxillomandibular Relationships

Class I	Class II	Class III
1 mm±2 mm (male) 0 mm±2 mm (female)	> 2 mm	< −3 mm

The table shows that for both males and females anything more than +2 mm AO-BO distance is considered Class II. If the distance of AO in front of BO expressed as a negative number is beyond −2 mm for females or −3 mm for males, it is considered Class III. The extra millimeter of tolerance for the male Class III designation reflects the fact that males exhibit a slightly more protruding lower jaw than females do and they tolerate more protrusion in this area relative to acceptable facial esthetics.

As stated previously, the Wits analysis is not only an expedient and simple method for determining the structural class of a case as compared with the dental classification, but it also comes into play where the structurally oriented parameters of other analysis systems are beyond certain limits. In cases difficult to diagnose due to unusual physical characteristics, the ability to refer to information derived from various cephalometric systems offers the advantage of comparing individual results to reinforce conclusions drawn about the diagnosis considered. The Wits appraisal offers a quick and handy means of double-checking the structural class of a case when the information derived from other systems seems vague or suspect. Its simplicity makes it easily accessible to all clinicians as one more weapon to place in their arsenal of diagnostic aids.

THE DOWNS ANALYSIS

The Downs analysis system is mentioned here due to its historical importance. Developed in 1948, it serves as the basis in part for some of the more important systems that were to follow it. Both A-point and B-point originated in this system, which is why they are seen written in the literature occasionally as A(Downs) or B(Downs). It also uses the occlusal plane and the mandibular plane, which is tangent to the inferior mandibular border and menton (Me). But perhaps most importantly, it relies on the FH plane as its primary frame of reference. Other important segments are the Y-axis, as a predominant growth direction indicator, and the long axes of the upper and lower anterior incisors. These segments all appear in systems commonly used today. Other lines appearing in this system are N-Po, N-A (nasion to A-point), A-B, A-Po. Of these, the A-B line reappears often, and the N-A appears in the Bimler.

Downs described the facial angle in this system as the internal angle formed from the intersection of FH and the line N-Po. This also reappears in modern systems, as does the mandibular plane angle. The mandibular plane angle is measured as the mandibular plane against FH. In fact, there are few aspects of the Downs that do not eventually show up in one cephalometric analysis system or another. A mere listing of the ten factors analyzed in this system appears as a cephalometric bank from which all subsequently developed systems have freely borrowed. (Normal values are listed as range + mean.)

Facial angle Measured as the inferior internal angle between FH and N-Po; range 82–95 degrees, mean 87.8 degrees. This indicates the severity of protrusion or retrusion of the lower jaw relative to the upper face.

Angle of convexity Supplemental angle formed at the vertex of a triangle, N-A-Po with the line N-Po as its base. If the triangle has its apex in front of the N-Po line, it is positive; if the apex is behind the N-Po line, the vertex angle is negative. The range is −8.5 to +10 degrees with a mean of 0 degree; ie, N, A-point, and Po should appear as a straight line. Specifically it is the angle measured between N-A and the extension of the Po-A line. This angle reveals the degree of protrusion (or lack thereof) of the maxilla relative to the rest of the the face as represented by the line N-Po.

A-B line An angle measured between the A-B line and the facial line N-Po at its intersection at A-point (to the left or behind A-point); range 0 to −9 degrees (indicating B-point to the left or behind A-point), mean −4.6 degrees. With B-point usually being behind A-point, except in Class III cases, the angle is usually negative.

Mandibular plane angle Angle formed between mandibular plane and FH; range 17 to 28 degrees, mean 21.9 degrees.

Y-axis Angle formed internally between the line S-Gn and FH. Used as an indicator of either horizontal, neutral, or vertical growers, its range is 53 to 66 degrees, mean 59.4 degrees. *Note:* The Y-axis is modified in some analysis systems, which may be a point of confusion. Ricketts measures it against Huxley's old line, N-Ba, and calls it the *XY*-axis. In the Jarabak-Bjork system it is still called the *Y*-axis, but is measured as the internal angle between S-Gn and the S-N line.

Cant of the occlusal plane The angle measured between the occlusal plane and FH; range 1.5 degrees to 14 degrees, mean 9.3 degrees.

Interincisal angle The angle formed by intersection of lines through the long axis of upper and lower central incisors, a measure of the procumbency of the anterior teeth; range 130 to 150 degrees, mean 135.4 degrees.

Mandibular incisor angle to mandibular plane This angle measures the relation of the long axis of the mandibular incisor to the mandibular plane, Go-Me. It is indicated as either a plus or a minus number of degrees relative to a perfect 90-degree angle, which is represented by zero; range −8.5 to +7 degrees, mean 1.4 degrees (91.4 degrees). Anything above 90 degrees is plus, less than 90 degrees is minus; 90 degrees is always subtracted from the actual measurement and the remainder expressed as the value for the angle.

Mandibular incisor angle to occlusal plane This angle measures the relationship of the long axis of the mandibular incisor to the occlusal plane. Again, it is read as the remainder of subtracting 90 degrees from the actual measured angle and expressed in either positive or negative numbers. Range is 3.5 to 20.0 degrees, with a mean of 14.5 degrees.

Maxillary incisor inclination (procumbency) The distance linearly between the incisal edge of the maxillary central incisor to the A-Po line; range +5 to −1 mm, mean 2.7 mm.

Even though there were only ten measurements in the Downs analysis, obtaining a manageable mental picture of the entire case is difficult. This would also be true of almost all the multifactored analysis systems to come. Therefore, in an effort to simplify the process of conjuring a

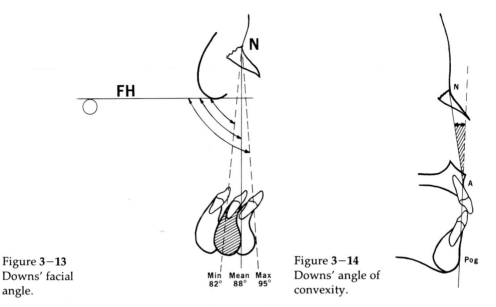

Figure 3–13
Downs' facial
angle.

Min Mean Max
82°   88°   95°

Figure 3–14
Downs' angle of
convexity.

quick "image" of the case, Dr J. M. Vorhies and Dr J. W. Adams, after taking a cue from earlier anthropometric graphs of Hellmann,[212] developed a graph that would give a quick, easy-to-visualize summary of the meaning of the cephalometric values of the case. The graph was constructed along a vertical line with the mean values of each of the ten

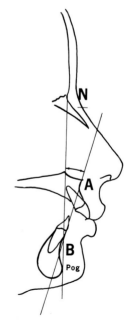

Figure 3–15   A-B plane. This is the angle formed between the A-B plane and the N-Pog line. Range 0 to −9 degrees, mean −4.6 degrees. Angle expressed as negative number of degrees when B-point is behind A-point. It represents the relationship of the anterior limits of the apical bases to each other relative to the facial line, and is also used as a gauge for the degree of difficulty involved in acquiring correct axial inclination of the anteriors by means of orthodontic therapy.

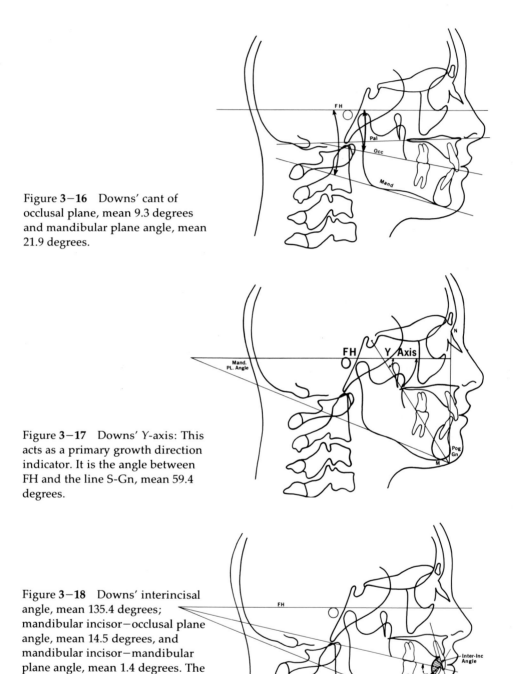

Figure **3–16** Downs' cant of occlusal plane, mean 9.3 degrees and mandibular plane angle, mean 21.9 degrees.

Figure **3–17** Downs' Y-axis: This acts as a primary growth direction indicator. It is the angle between FH and the line S-Gn, mean 59.4 degrees.

Figure **3–18** Downs' interincisal angle, mean 135.4 degrees; mandibular incisor–occlusal plane angle, mean 14.5 degrees, and mandibular incisor–mandibular plane angle, mean 1.4 degrees. The latter two are measured by subtracting 90 degrees from the actual measured angle, which can result in either a positive or negative value.

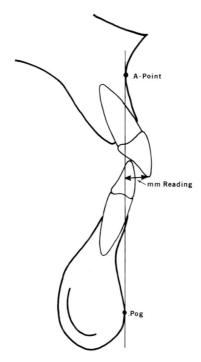

Figure **3–19**   Protrusion of maxillary incisor from A-Pog line, range +5 to −1 mm, mean 2.7 mm.

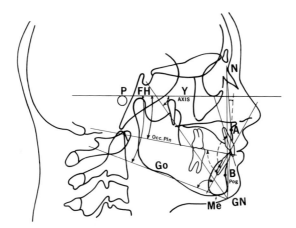

Figure **3–20**   Complete Downs analysis.

retrognathic   prognathic

	Mean	S.D.	
Skeletal Pattern			Facial Plane
Facial Angle	87.8°	3.57	
Angle of Convexity	0	5.09	Convexity
A-B Plane to Facial Plane	− 4.6°	3.67	
Mandibular Plane to F.H. Plane	21.9°	3.24	A-B Plane
Y-Axis	59.4°	3.82	
			Mandibular Plane
Denture Pattern			
Occlusal Plane to F.H. Plane	9.3°	3.83	Y-Axis
$\underline{1}$ to $\overline{1}$	135.4°	5.76	
$\overline{1}$ to Occlusal Plane	+ 14.5°	3.48	Occlusal Plane
$\overline{1}$ to Mandibular Plane	+ 1.4°	3.78	Interincisal
Tip of $\underline{1}$ to A-P Plane	+ 2.7 mm	1.80	$\underline{1}$ to Occlusal Plane

$\overline{1}$ to Mandibular Plane

$\underline{1}$ to A-P Plane (mm)

Figure 3−21   "Wigglegram" (Courtesy C. F. A. Moorrees, Forsyth Dental Center.)

Downs measurements incrementally placed one on top of the other. The top five are the skeletal pattern values; the bottom five are the dental pattern values. Thus everything that falls on either side of the center vertical line represents a value either above or below the norm for that particular measurement.[213] Wylie later modified the vertical graph slightly by adding maximum and minimum values of each measurement to the graph and connecting the extremes to form a polygon.[214] By simple reversal of some of the maximum-minimum values, readings which fall on the left side of the outer limits of the polygon indicate Class II conditions, while readings which fall on the right side of the outer limits of the polygon indicate Class III conditions. Charting the readings of an individual case on such a graph or double polygon produces a wiggle-shaped line that gives such graphs the nickname "wigglegrams."

Another terminological point of interest associated with the Downs analysis is the term "mesognathic." This term was originally used by Downs to indicate what actually should have been more correctly called "orthognathic." Mesognathic actually means a slightly prognathic situation, which is not what Downs wanted to convey. Hence, *mesognathic* may be seen in the original literature. In modern times it has been replaced by *orthognathic*. The two terms signifying the extremes on either side of orthognathic are *retrognathic* and *prognathic*.

One last point must be borne in mind concerning the Downs analysis: its data base. Downs selected ten male and ten female Caucasian subjects with what were considered "ideal" occlusions to serve as a sample for the determination of his norms. The ages of the individuals ranged from 12 to 17 years. Thus with such a small sample that was biased according to the judgments of the investigators, the data base may be criticized as being skewed. Therefore by implication, it holds up what may be an inappropriate ideal which would lead clinicians to force all patients to fit one mold in spite of Downs' admonitions to the contrary.

THE WYLIE ANALYSIS

The Wylie analysis, presented in 1947, is also mentioned because of its historical as well as diagnostic significance. Wylie's work first appeared on the same program as some of the initial work of one of his more famous students, Allen Brodie. What is incredible is that, as Wylie[218] puts it,

> each man chose to present his concept of the fundamental basis of malocclusion and craniofacial disharmony, a sort of synthesis of many different researches. There was no collusion between them and neither one knew the other was presenting a paper. At the same time the two papers said essentially the same thing, and even went so far as to cite from exactly the same passages in the literature.

Both men had discovered quite independently that variation was the rule in the anatomical morphology of the individual.

Wylie's attempts were to develop an analysis system that concerned itself with one dimension, the anteroposterior relationships of the maxilla and mandible of a given malocclusion. He concerned himself primarily in these early cephalometric studies with the Class II, Division 1 maloclusions. He concluded that variations of morphology were quite random. Hence a Class II, Division 1 malocclusion was not a specific pathological condition like pituitary dwarfism or diabetes mellitus, but a chance combination of maxillofacial anatomical arrangements. No specific etiological agent was singled out. Remember this theory appeared when functional influences and muscle imbalances were not of chief concern diagnostically. In his system the mandible is the only component that is not measured as a vertical projection to the FH plane. The remaining measurements are all made relative to perpendiculars projected to the FH plane and, like the mandibular length, are measured linearly. They are perpendiculars drawn from ANS, the maxillary first molar (central buccal grove), the anterior surface of the pterygomaxillary fissure (PTM), sella, and the posterior edge of the condyle.

The historical significance of this system is twofold. First, it shows the wisdom of the early founding fathers of cephalometrics in that, like the Downs, it is another system predicated on using the old FH as its base reference plane. Second, though the Wylie is less popular now and fading into obscurity, its observations of the posterior cranial base length described in horizontal linear measurements again attests to the wisdom of our predecessors. This area of concern has arisen anew a continent away in the exquisite cephalometric system of Bimler.

In the Wylie the mandibular length is measured from pogonion to a line that is both tangent to the posterior edge of the condyle and perpendicular to the mandibular plane. All other measurements are straightforward between the anatomical perpendiculars on the FH plane. This gives the system the ability to compare the mandibular length with the sum total of the depth of the maxilla from ANS to articulare, which makes this system very useful in the evaluation of Class III cases. If the length of the mandible is greater than the depth of the cranial base along the FH plane from ANS to articulare, Class III skeletal patterns are quite likely. The accompanying table gives measurements in millimeters for both males and females.

Measurement	Males	Females
ANS to PTM	52	52
Maxillary 1st molar to PTM	15	16
PTM to sella	18	17
Sella to articulare	18	17
Mandibular length	103	101

Wylie was one of the first to propose the concept that mean values of accumulated measurements should not be equated with normalcy. He states that each of his measurements should not be held up as guides against which the respective individual measurements of the patient should be compared. He even goes so far as to insist that it is not at all necessary that the relative proportions of these measurements be maintained in order for a case to be balanced. These proportions do make a well-balanced facial pattern, but one measurement may markedly vary from the mean without causing a major imbalance if the appropriate compensating area "obligingly" counteracts the abnormal component by varying itself to the appropriate degree.

Wylie was also one of the first to consider a malocclusion, or dysplasia, as nothing more than "...a random combination of craniofacial parts which are in themselves neither abnormally large nor abnormally small, but which when taken together, produce an undesirable combination of parts."

Wylie lists four simple columns of values to determine the extent of dysplasia, in an A-P direction, for a given case. In the first vertical column he lists, respectively, the standard values for glenoid fossa to sella (17 mm), sella to PTM (17 mm), maxillary length (PTM − ANS = 52 mm), PTM to buccal groove maxillary first molar (16 mm), and the mandibular length (101 mm). In a column to the right of these he lists the patient's respective values for these measurements. The next two columns are designated "Orthognathic" and "Prognatic." These terms are confusing to us in more modern times. To Wylie, "orthognathic" equates to skeletal Class II. He merely wished to avoid dental overtones. He preferred to reserve Angle's terminology for dental arch or tooth-to-tooth relationships alone. "Prognathic" implies skeletal Class III tendencies. As these terms are used by Wylie, they are meant to signify also the mere relationship of the mandible to the maxilla without any implication as to which is correct and which is aberrant. They merely describe the maxillomandibular relationship (remember that "orthognathic" in *this* context is different from modern usage). When the difference between the standard value and the patient's value is analyzed, the result for each respective measurement is entered in either the orthognathic column or the prognathic column.

Now, all things being equal, if a particular value is larger than the standard value, it contributes to retrusive or skeletal Class II orthognathic conditions and is placed in the orthognathic column. If a particular value is smaller than the standard value, it implies protrusive skeletal Class III problems and is placed in the prognathic column. There is a major exception to this process—the measurement for the mandible. Here the opposite is true. Values smaller than the standard are interpreted as orthognathic, and those larger than the standard are prognatic. Next add up the two columns. By Wylie's simple formula

(Units of anteroposterior = (Prognathic sum) − (Orthognatic sum)
dysplasia)

The difference is the net score, expressing the degree of anteroposterior dysplasia of the facial pattern from an orthopedic standpoint. Note that except for the A-P location of the molar, not a single measurement is concerned with the dentition. Also note that, like the Wits, the Wylie does not implicate which member—maxilla, mandible, or both—is at fault. It merely expresses the degree of disproportionality on a purely orthopedic basis. Wylie pre-emptively criticized his analysis system by saying it was useless for before-and-after treatment comparisons since only one measurement, PTM to buccal groove maxillary first molar, was believed to be changeable as a result of therapeutics. This was obviously before the age of functional appliances such as the Bionator and their penchant for easy anterior development of retrusive mandibles. If he'd only known!

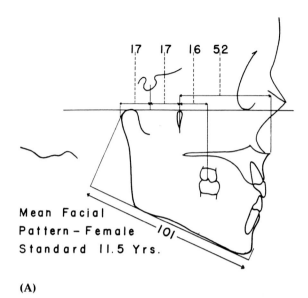

Mean Facial
Pattern – Female
Standard II.5 Yrs.

(A)

Figure 3–22b   Assessment of Anteroposterior Dysplasia
Female

Dimension	Standard	Patient's	Difference Orthognathic	Difference Prognathic
Glenoid fossa to sella	17	9		8
Sella to ptm.	17	22	5	
Maxillary length	52	54	2	
Ptm. −6	16	14		2
Mandibular length	101	98	3	
Totals:			10	10

Units of anteroposterior
dysplasia=prognathic−orthognathic: 0

(B)

Figure 3–22   **(A)** Wylie analysis of anteroposterior dysplasia. **(B)** Wylie dysplasia summation sheet. (Reprinted from Wylie WL: The assessment of anteroposterior dysplasia. *Angle Orthod* 1947; 17: 97–109 with permission.)

THE STEINER ANALYSIS

The Steiner analysis followed right on the heels of the Downs and was developed in the early 1950s as a clinically oriented cephalometric system. Steiner, who came from Beverly Hills, California, first introduced his analysis in a paper read before the Sextas Journadas Ortodoncias, in Buenos Aires, Argentina, in 1952.[215] He intended the system to be used to determine the nature of the malocclusion and to act as a guide or goal toward which treatment modalities could be directed.[216,217] The Steiner analysis compares the existing measured values of the cephalometric aspects of a given case against a predetermined set of norms for those respective measurements. Steiner borrowed heavily fron the Downs system for both his clinical norms and specific dimensions. He borrowed from the systems of other researchers as well, so that the Steiner is actually a composite of systems. It is mentioned here, not because of its particular value, especially in the light of modern FJO techniques, but simply because it is probably the most widely used system to date throughout orthodontics. Whether it will continue in that position with the newer orthopedically oriented systems now available remains to be seen. The sample size of one individual considered subjectively perfect is of course biostatistically laughable.

The Steiner analysis system was one of the first to employ both linear and angular measurements to describe the relationships of the upper and lower anterior incisors. In addition, this analysis exhibits one of the earliest forms of soft tissue profile analysis methods, the "S-line." It was also one of the first to deviate from the use of the old FH plane as a baseline of reference. Steiner felt that the location of points porion and orbitale were sometimes difficult to locate on certain cephalograms, due to asymmetry or superimposition of other osseous structures. He thus substituted the S-N line of Brodie as his frame of reference, a line not altogether as stable as the Frankfort but at least easy to construct. Herein lies one of the problems associated with the Steiner. There are no provisions made for the differences in linear length possible with the S-N line or the variations in its angular inclination relative to other reference lines, such as the Frankfort, during the growth and development of the patient. Another problem associated with the Steiner is the way it is used to determine the Class I, II, or III status of an individual case. This, by Steiner's definition, is a function of the ANB angle, but the ANB angle is also affected by the lower face height. If the mandibular plane is either abnormally steep or shallow, the ANB angle is either exaggerated or diminished, which could affect the interpretation of class, since there is only the single standard of a 2-degree ANB angle for normalcy, and anything greater is considered as exhibiting Class II tendencies and anything less is considered as exhibiting Class III tendencies!

This situation is further complicated because A-point is sometimes difficult to decipher. One simple reason is due to the superimposition of the soft tissue outline of the profile of the cheek. This is still true in spite of modern techniques to increase image quality.[219] This is the reason why alternative A-point definitions have been proposed by various investigators. One alternative is to select a point 2 mm ahead of the apex of the root tip of the maxillary central.[220] But if mechanotherapy is engaged with respect to upper anteriors and the centrals receive any form of root torque whatsoever, this method loses its validity. Since it has been shown that the point of rotation along a root of such a tooth undergoing torquing procedures that changes position the least is about one third of the way down the root from the tip,[221-223] another method has been proposed. It consists of measuring 3 mm forward from a point one third of the way down the root from its tip, a point calculated to be the nearest average center of rotation. The measurement is then made forward along a line parallel to Frankfort. Reasonably unaltered by root torquing, such a revised A-point should be reasonably stable, unless wholesale bodily movement of the entire tooth is affected. Some practitioners believe that this method gives a truer indication of the actual location of A-point.[224] However, Steiner chose his normative values for use with the conventional selection of A-point.

Another problem with the Steiner is that it has no Y-axis determination, as does the Downs. This means there is no reference to the main component of growth—horizontal, neutral, or vertical—of the maxillofacial complex. However, this measurement is easy enough to lift from the Downs and add to the Steiner, as it is often done. Steiner relied on the angulation of the mandibular plane to determine the growth factor, but this somewhat remote and indirect method does not give as clear a picture of the mandibular growth pattern as the Y-axis does.

The Steiner system starts out with the base reference lines S-N from which two lines are drawn at N to A-point and B-point to form the internal angles SNA, SNB, and the angle representing the difference between the two, ANB. Steiner borrowed this part of the system directly from Reidel. The norm for SNA is 82 degrees, for SNB 80 degrees; therefore the ANB angle should ideally be 2 degrees. It is this angle that others have arbitrarily modified to determine skeletal class.

Class I   ANB 0−5°
Class II   ANB⩾5°
Class III ANB<0°

Steiner was not overly concerned with the SNA angle; he believed it was merely an indication of how far forward or backward the face was with respect to the rest of the skull. His two chief concerns in this area were the famous ANB angle, with its maxillomandibular orthopedic discrepancy implications, and its closely associated dental component,

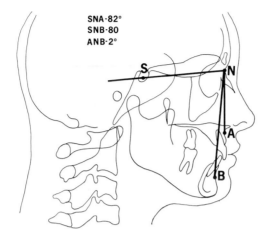

SNA·82°
SNB·80
ANB·2°

Figure 3—23 Steiner SNA, SNB, ANB angles. These famous angles have become very popular in orthodontic diagnosis with norms of SNA = 82 degrees, SNB = 80 degrees, and resultant ANB = 2 degrees. Steiner preferred the use of the S-N line simply because it was easy to find.

the equally famous interincisal angle. In those earlier days of fixed-appliance-dominated orthodontic treatments, the greater the ANB angle, the greater the A-P maxillomandibular discrepancy; as a result, the more difficult it was to treat to satisfactory overjet/overbite relationships. This drawback was masked over by manipulating the interincisal angle via the technique of retracting maxillary anteriors back and torquing mandibular incisors forward by precalculated amounts to obtain anterior coupling while still attempting to remember facial profile considerations. All these dental manipulations of the anteriors were a direct result of combating overjet problems that were reflected by the ANB angle. Orthodontics was used in those days to address what at times were essentially orthopedic imbalances when the problem of a large ANB angle presented itself. Fixed appliances only moved teeth, not bones.

The Steiner system starts to lose its validity when the mandibular inclination strays appreciably from the mandibular plane angle norm of 32 degrees. In extremely high or low values for the mandibular plane angle, the mandible, in effect, rotates more open or more closed, respectively. As it rotates more open with greater vertical dimension to the lower face height, Points A and B rotate in an arc about the axis of the condyle, which puts them in a different relationship to N, falsely appearing from the standpoint of N to be linearly farther apart. This tends to increase the ANB angle, even though A and B do not change with respect to their linear distance apart along the equally rotating occlusal plane. This gives a false impression of a Class II structural relationship when, in fact, one may not actually exist.

Conversely, when the lower face height is short and the mandibular plane angle is nearly flat, the A- and B-points move on an arc upward toward N, and, in so doing, B seems to rotate on a bigger arc and appears to travel underneath A, to give the false impression that A and B are aligned with each other, thus making the ANB angle closer to 0 degree or even negative and indicating mandibular protrusion when there may be none. Thus in this particular parameter, when the mandibular plane angle exhibits a considerable degree of variation, either high or low relative to its 32-degree norm, the information derived from the ANB angle becomes suspect. Solution, call on the Wits.

An abnormal location of N or an abnormal cant to the S-N line can also bias the ANB angle. That too is the time, as previously noted, to call on the Wits analysis. The Wits will give a class determination that is unaffected by the proximity, or lack thereof, of A and B points to N or any abnormalities in the location of N or cant of the S-N line. The perpendiculars AO and BO of the Wits are unbiased by such changes in the relationships of A and B as brought about by wide variations in mandibular plane angle. AO and BO remain linearly at the same distance from each other, regardless of the cant of the mandibular plane or of the occlusal plane onto which they are projected.

Intimately related to the ANB angle was Steiner's method of evaluating soft tissue profiles by means of the S line. He theorized that the profile of the lips in a well-balanced face should touch a line drawn from the soft tissue contour of the chin to the midpoint of the soft tissue inferior border of the midnasal septum. The outline of the inferior border of the nose from the base of the upper lip to the tip of the nose forms an S, hence the name. Steiner does not specify the angle that such a line should make relative to a fixed plane of reference such as FH. Thus, a severely retruded profile could theoretically, according to this criterion, be passable as "balanced" as long as the lips touched this line. If enough anterior retraction were affected in severe Class II, Divison 1 cases, the lips often did touch that line. It was proposed that lips that fell short of this line were an indication of the need for advancing, or most likely torquing, teeth forward to fill out the profile. Lips that were beyond this line indicated a need for dental retraction to help offset the implied protrusion. It may be now be seen how using this approach can quickly lead to an obsession with the pretreatment ANB angle and the interincisal angle.

Yet in all this concern with how much anterior tooth movement a clinician might wish to effect to obtain compensating dental arrangements that would couple anteriors that were grossly separated anteroposteriorly due to severe overjet problems (which may have been entirely orthopedic in nature), not a single thought was given to what all this retraction of maxillary anteriors and "dumping forward" of mandibular incisors was doing to the mandibular arc of closure, especially once it was discovered that bicuspid extraction greatly aided the orthodontic compromising

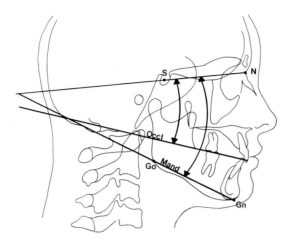

Figure 3—24   Steiner occlusal plane angle (norm = 14.5 degrees) and mandibular plane angle (norm = 32 degrees) are also measured against S-N line, which differs from Downs', who measured these angles against Frankfort Horizontal.

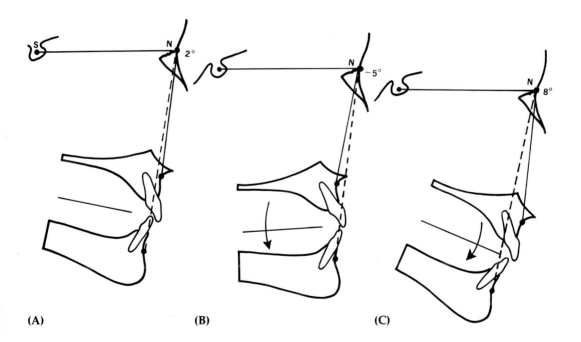

(A)   **(B)**   **(C)**

Figure 3—25   Bias represented by the cant of the Steiner occlusal plane is revealed in these illustrations. The ANB angle can be directly reduced as in **(B)** (from 2 to −5 degrees) by a counterclockwise rotation of the jaws and occlusal plane, or increased as in **(C)** (from 2 to 8 degrees) by a clockwise rotation of the jaws and occlusal plane. However, in all three examples A-point and B-point are relatively in the same position with respect to each other if perpendiculars of each are projected to their respective occlusal planes, as Jacobson points out in his Wits analysis.

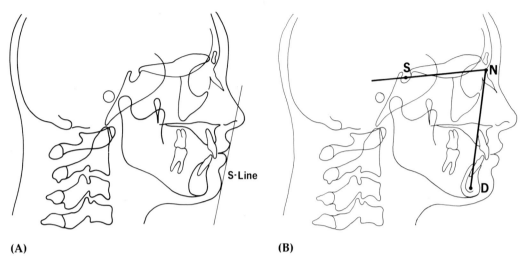

(A)   **(B)**

Figure 3–26   **(A)** Steiner's esthetic line is the S-line. It must be remembered that Steiner was one of the few Americans who drew the tracings with the facial profile to the observer's left. Thus, the outline of the tip of the nose and the upper lip assumed the shape of the letter S. Backwards when the profile is drawn to the observer's right as above, the S still, conveniently, can stand for Steiner. **(B)** Steiner's SND angle (norm 76 degrees) signified the location of the center of the symphysis relative to the cranial base. It received little attention, since the SNB became the traditional favorite.

processes. What was being done anteriorly was not even considered as possibly having an untoward effect posteriorly. The chief concern of the times with respect to severe overjet problems was how to bring the uppers back enough to meet the lowers. Hence the obsession with things like the ANB and interincisal angles and "acceptable compromises." Trapping the mandibular arc of closure behind interfering upper anteriors and thereby forcing condyles to seat superiorly and posteriorly off the heel of the disc upon full closure was an unknown concept. The order of the day was for the clinician to mathematically calculate what combination of upper and lower incisor angulations to select that would give the best orthodontic camouflage to what was quite often an orthopedic problem. In that diagnostic numbers game the famous ANB angle was the key indicator of how severe a compromise would have to be made: the bigger the angle, the more retruded the mandible; therefore, the greater the overjet, the greater the maxillary retraction; the greater the mandibular proclination, the greater the compromise.

A second method Steiner uses to aid in location of the mandible is through the use of the SND angle. "D" is defined as the anatomical dead center of the cross section of the symphysis of the mandible. The norm is 76 degrees. It is obvious that this is nothing more than a modification of

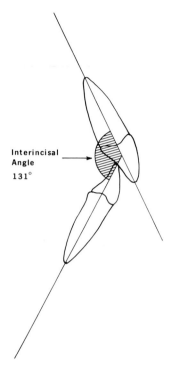

Interincisal
Angle
131°

Figure 3–27 Steiner's famous interincisal angle with a 131-degree norm was 4.4 degrees less (more acute) than the 135.4-degree norm of the Downs.

the old facial angle of Downs. But, again, the SND angle does not take into account changes in the cant of either the S-N line or the occlusal or mandibular planes. No comments were made as to how the SND angle would be affected by changes in vertical, nor were ranges or means determined. Thus, the angle became in effect a cephalometric eunuch.

The other famous and critically important component to this analysis system is the interincisal angle. The interincisal angle is measured internally (on the lingual surface) between the long axes of the maxillary and mandibular central incisors. Though this angle evaluation is often associated with Steiner's analysis, it is borrowed directly from the Downs. However, because of its importance for reasons mentioned above, Steiner greatly expanded its use. Steiner used the value of 131 degrees as the norm. Others have extended this such that in a Class II case, interincisal angles from 120 to 140 degrees are considered Division 1, 140 degrees and beyond are Division 2, and anything less than 120 degrees is considered Division 3 (a Johnny-come-lately among cephalometric terms). These numerical values for the interincisal angle of the long axes of the upper and lower central incisors are easily recognized throughout the field of orthodontics, and Steiner placed such importance on the relationships of these teeth to each other that he used four other measurements to describe their location. In that he excelled.

Because of the therapeutics in use in his day, Steiner obviously wanted to know how the maxillary central incisors were situated relative to the frame of reference he used, the N-A line. The angle of the long axis of this tooth to the N-A line was helpful relative to lip support and to the interincisal angle, but it was not enough. Angulation was not specific as to physical location. For example, a maxillary central could be angulated at Steiner's ideal of 22 degrees to N-A; yet the tooth as a whole could be entirely behind the N-A line, entirely in front of it, or anywhere in between, still at 22 degrees. Therefore, he also incorporated a linear measurement to help physically locate the tooth relative to N-A. The measurement is from the incisal edge linearly to N-A. For the mandibular incisors, he measured the angulation of the long axis of the lower central to the N-B (nasion to B-point) line and measured the incisal edge linearly to N-B.

1. Length 1 to N-A line in millimeters, 4 mm (measured from most anterior portion of crown)
2. Long axis 1 to N-A line, angle 22 degrees
3. Length 1 to N-B line in millimeters, 4 mm
4. Long axis 1 to N-B line, angle 25 degrees

He expressed these four numerical values along with the ANB angle on a chevron:

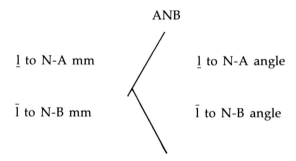

His norms would be represented thus:

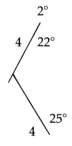

When the most anterior portion of the crown of the maxillary incisor is in front of the N-A line, the value is positive; when the most anterior portion of the maxillary incisor is behind the N-A line, the value is negative. The same holds for the lower incisor relative to the N-B line. If the most anterior portion of the mandibular incisor is in *front* of the N-B line, the value is positive; if it is behind the N-B line, the value is negative.

Steiner has constructed tables of these chevrons listing all the modified, yet acceptable, changes in incisor position and angulation that would go hand in hand with varying ANB angles. Besides the aforementioned norms for an ANB angle of 2 degrees, he has devised nine other chevrons of acceptable relationships for ANB angles from −1 to +8 degrees. But this elaborate system of data for determining incisor position and angulation is predicated upon the mandible remaining stationary throughout treatment, except for the usual changes due to growth and development. However, this is all negated as soon as a functional appliance, such as a Bionator, is inserted in Class II situations, because the ANB angle relationship of the upper and lower jaws is immediately changed.

These data may be used by the clinician at the end of Bionator treatment to check the position of incisors, or at the beginning of treatment to determine the amount of retraction or proclination of anterior teeth that may be needed as indicated by the interincisal angle, but as for planning treatment around existing angulations of teeth relative to a beginning pretreatment ANB angle, the chevron guide system of norms is of little value in an age where wholesale orthopedic changes are possible. If one accepts that the ANB angle can readily be changed, without resorting to extracting bicuspids and retracting premaxillas, the above data may be put to use in their proper perspective only as a mere reference for the positioning of the incisors at the completion of treatment.

Steiner also describes the mandibular plane angle relative to the S-N reference line by the angle Go-Gn (Reidel) to S-N, the norm of which is 32 degrees. He also utilizes the occlusal plane angle measured against S-N, the norm for which is 14 degrees. Steiner borrowed from Wylie his methods of locating the mandible and evaluating indirectly its AP dimension. He projects a line from the most distal point of the head of the condyle perpendicularly to S-N (not Frankfort!). This he calls point E. He also projects a line from the most anterior point on the body of the mandible (pogonion) perpendicularly to the S-N line, the intersection of which he calls point L. He then measures the distance along the S-N line from S to E and from S to L. However, no norms are given. Even if there were such norms, their value would be suspect due to variations in the cant of the S-N line or therapeutically induced changes in the vertical.

The realization of the historical significance of this particular system is important, because being clinically oriented, it has been one of the

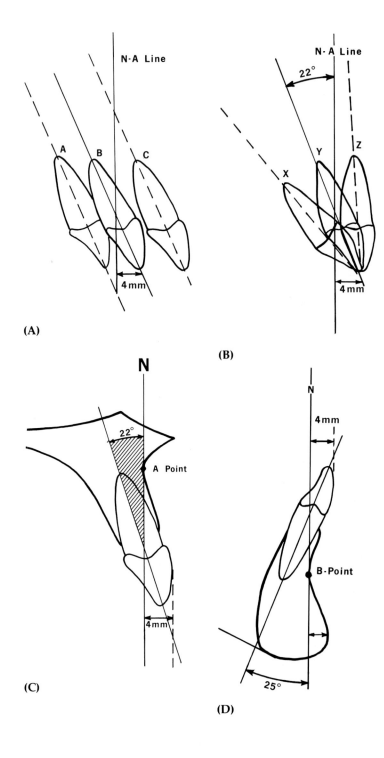

(A)

(B)

(C)

(D)

		Ref Norm		
SNA	(angle)	82°		
SNB	(angle)	80°		
ANB	(angle)	2°		
1 to NA	(mm)	4		
1 to NA	(angle)	22°		
1 to NB	(mm)	4		
1 to NB	(angle)	25°		
Po to NB	(mm)	not established		
1 to 1	(angle)	131°		
Occl to SN	(angle)	14°		
GoGN to SN	(angle)	32°		
Frankfort Horizontal to 1		110		
Y-Axis to FH		59°		

(A)

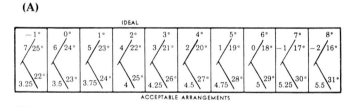

(B)

Figure 3−29   **(A)** Steiner analysis data summation sheet. **(B)** Acceptable arrangements.

Figure 3−28   Both angulation and linear measurements are needed to locate the ideal positions of the maxillary and mandibular incisors. **(A)** Maxillary central may be at norm of 22 degrees to N-A line, but may vary in horizontal location of entire tooth. **(B)** It also may be at ideal of 4 mm of most forward part of facial surface of crown from N-A line, but vary in overall long-axis angulation. **(C)** Therefore, both 22-degree long-axis angulation and 4-mm measurement are needed to locate maxillary central exactly. **(D)** A 4-mm linear measurement and 25-degree long-axis angulation to *N-B* line locates mandibular incisor. These four measurements were varied, since compromises (usually caused by extraction of bicuspids) were necessary when these ideal norms could not be met.

most widely used cephalometric analysis systems in orthodontics. The Steiner is very concerned with the profile, and concentrates on the positioning and relationship of the anterior teeth. But to the practioner in possession of FJO techniques, the Steiner has its drawbacks. It accepts the skeletal relationships as they are, and is interested in what must be done to the individual teeth to improve the situation by purely orthodontic means. Less emphasis is placed on orthopedic information, such as lower face height, relative lengths of the maxilla and mandible, degree of facial convexity, or posterior cranial base measurements. It would remain for men to come later to recognize the importance of these concepts and to devise cephalometric analysis systems designed to express them specifically.

FROM TWEED'S TRIANGLE TO SASSOUNI'S CIRCLES

The best way to properly manage maxillofacial orthopedic appliances is to use the correct appliance for the job at the correct time in the treatment plan. Part of the purpose of the cephalometric x-ray should be to tell the practitioner how and when to apply FJO principles to the case. It should also reveal the status of the case at the beginning and at the end of treatment, serving as a yardstick against which to measure the progress of the finished case and its proximity to certain generally accepted norms or treatment goals. Normative cephalometric standards are merely averages and should not serve as the end goal of treatment, nor should the standards they may represent be the final determination of whether the case is correct. Only the treating clinician is responsible for that decision. Too often, cases are treated to these preestablished norms of cephalometric acceptability simply because the clinicians use them as a mandatory criterion of correctness rather than using their own overall evaluation of the case. The prowess of the practitioner's technical skills in modern-day advanced mechanics allows him to move teeth to just about any position desirable. Thus, it is tempting to use a set of cephalometric norms, rather than the individual operator's clinical judgment, as an end goal. No example more clearly brings this point to the surface than that of the Tweed Triangle.

Conceived by Dr C. H. Tweed of Tuscon, Arizona, in the early 1950s, this cephalometric analysis system was designed to act as a guide to obtaining insight as to what the anatomical relationship of the lower central incisors should be at the completion of treatment and what the chances for a successful outcome for a case would be relative to that final relationship.[44-46] Tweed believed that many malocclusions were the result of discrepancies in tooth size and jaw size that resulted in the teeth being forced mesially in the arches in the posterior sections or having

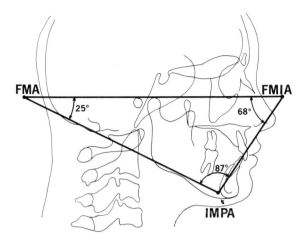

Figure 3–30   The Tweed Triangle.

excessive labial crown torque in the incisor area anteriorly, as if the entire upper and lower dentures were tipped forward over their bases of basal bone. He believed that these teeth had to be properly repositioned over their correct locations on the "basal arches" in order to obtain orthodontic harmony and stability. He felt the key to this stability was the relationship of the anterior teeth, especially the lower central incisors, to this aforementioned basal bone.

Other dental relationships were important too, but less so. The critical factor to Tweed was the axial inclination of the lower incisors. He believed that a certain limited range of incisor angulations relative to the mandibular plane angle would ensure orthodontic balance and stability. But treating teeth to a position beyond this limited range (ie, leaving excessive axial procumbency to the incisors) would result in loss of arch integrity and instability once treatment was complete or retention terminated. If it were not possible to position all of the teeth in the arch orthodontically without exceeding the prescribed limits of axial inclination, dental units would have to be removed to allow the orthodontic retroclination or retraction of the excessively proclined anteriors to the more upright acceptable inclinations required by the theoretical dictates of the system. This gave the practitioner a guide as to whether he should anticipate requiring extractions in a given case, depending on the inclination of the mandibular incisors prior to treatment. But the system was never intented to be a total facial analysis; it was merely an aid to determine the relationships of certain teeth relative to the inclination of the mandibular plane. Yet some practitioners not only used it as a total system, but even made the numbers it represented their exclusive treatment goals.

The analysis is constructed around the Tweed Triangle. This now famous geometric figure consists of a scalene triangle formed by the FH plane, the mandibular plane, and a line extending to each through the center of the long axis of the mandibular incisor. The three internal angles are called the Frankfort mandibular plane angle (FMA), the incisor mandibular plane angle (IMPA), and the incisor Frankfort plane angle (FMIA). The guide to the entire system is the FMA. This single angle determines the relative position of the mandibular incisors and, for some, the ultimate ideal treatment goal and prognosis for success. The accompanying table is a breakdown of the parameters of that angle and the corresponding mandibular incisor axial inclinations recommended.

Frankfort Mandibular Plane Angle

FMA (deg)	IMPA (deg)	Prognosis
16	95	Good
22	90	Good
28	85	Good
29−35	80−85	Fair
>35		Poor

Note: For 28° < FMA < 35°, Tweed recommends that extractions in most cases to allow the arch to be "cinched up" enough to permit uprighting of mandibular incisors with resultant reduction of anterior incisor axial procumbency. For FMA > 35°, Tweed says extractions are contraindicated in most cases.

Though a range of values is represented by this system, Tweed stated that the norms for the FMA and IMPA were 25 and 90 degrees, respectively. Extending the line through the long axis of the lower incisor up to the Frankfort plane forms the FMIA angle. Tweed stressed that this angle be maintained at 65 to 70 degrees. If the FMA were 25 degrees and the IMPA 90 degrees, the FMIA would automatically be 65 degrees (180 degrees−115 degrees = 65 degrees).

Even though the system was not intended for total facial analysis, and even though there is some variance built in, over the years some practitioners regarded the Tweed Triangle as a total system—to some it became an end unto itself. Human nature being what it is, this simple-appearing system soon led some clinicians to use the 90-degrees-lower IMPA as an ultimate treatment goal. All patients were measured by the same yardstick. The results of such treatment were often an excessive bodily translation of the maxillary anterior teeth in a posterior direction, with a fair amount of lingual crown torque imparted also. Lower incisor depression was of reasonable occurrence, as was a reduction of overall arch size. The technique usually consisted of uprighting the posterior teeth first, then tipping them distally to obtain what Tweed referred to as a "toehold" to provide adequate anchorage for the rest of the tooth movements to be performed anteriorly. Mandibular incisors and cuspids were retracted toward anchored molars to close extraction spaces and assist in the achievement of prescribed axial inclinations.

Tweed advocated the use of the mandibular arch as an anchorage for the retraction of the maxillary anterior teeth. The technique involved the extensive use of mechanics on an extremely advanced level. After the posteriors were first tipped distally, a process involving intricate archwire bends and Class III mechanics for anchorage, anterior incisors were retracted bodily with elastics in more conventional Class II mechanics. Other sophisticated and elaborate techniques were also employed in the search for the desired incisor angulation. But in all this noble and concentrated effort to obtain the precise degree of axial inclination of teeth, a perfectly candid assessment of the total needs of the patient at times revealed that the orthopedic considerations of some cases were left wanting. Again, the mandibular arc of closure and its effect on the TMJs were not considered.

What is important to realize in this example is that one must remember to use cephalometric analysis as a tool to help make the most informed and correct clinical judgment of diagnosis, treatment planning, and eventual outcome. But one cannot necessarily "treat to the numbers," since the numbers or norms used in the various systems merely represent populations, not individuals.

The example of the Tweed Triangle illustrates how, on occasion, the total picture of the role of orthodontic care might sometimes become muddled behind the determination of some to let statistical averages become their final treatment end. Each patient is unique, and deserves to have the entire spectrum of his or her needs considered before orthodontic care is initiated. It is obvious that a single angular relationship was never intended to be responsible for the outcome of an entire case. Yet, there has always been the desire in the minds of some individuals to seek an all-encompassing solution to problems that repeatedly plague them in their efforts to reach comforting safety in the harbor of understanding. The science of cephalometrics is no different.

"Order is Heaven's first law."
Alexander Pope 1688—1744
English poet

CHAPTER 4
The Apostles of Charm

It appears that various researchers have been sensitive to the geometric and arithmetic implications of the cephalogram and have searched for a hidden mathematical formula or ratio that would unlock the mystery of anatomical harmony of design behind the maxillofacial complex. The Tweed Triangle is not the only geometric figure that has been superimposed on the lateral head x-ray in an effort to analyze its osseous anatomy. There was also the Margolis Triangle, Koski's Circles, and the Bjork Polygon, a five-sided figure which has the line N-Gn (nasion-gnathion) as its longest base. (The Bjork analysis involves much more than just polygon; many other measurements are included in this fine system.)

An exotic and provocative sidelight to the search for quantifiable mathematical data relative to cephalometric relationships has recently emerged in the work of Dr R. M. Ricketts. Ricketts has taken a geometric principle of a famous mathematical ratio long known to classical antiquity and applied it in an interesting and novel way to frontal facial anatomy and to internal dental and osteological relationships that exist in norma lateralis. This ancient ratio has long been utilized in the arts and architecture throughout the centuries to effect harmony and beauty and

168

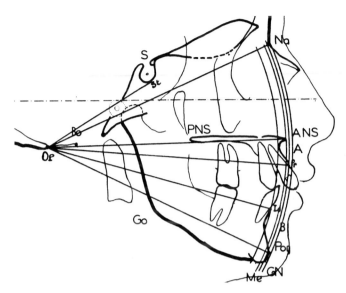

Figure 4–1   Koski analysis: Koski, originally from Helsinki, Finland, developed his analysis in 1953 based on work done in Boston. It utilizes arcs of circles that have opisthion as the center of their radii. Norms consist of a table of linear measurements that are represented as percentages of the Op-ANS linear value = 100 and angular measurements that are represented as percentages of the Na-Op-Pog angle = 100. As a forerunner to the Sassouni, the resemblance is obvious.

to ensure geometric proportion and balance. Ricketts theorized that, in this light, an *anatomical* proportional balance could be obtained between form and function in the maxillofacial complex by the use of what has now become known as the *golden section*.

The term "golden section" is relatively recent in origin. Scholastic writers of the Middle Ages referred to it as the divine proportion, but the problem dates back to the sixth century BC when it was first confronted and solved by the Pythagoreans at Samos. The problem consists of determining an unusual and mysterious numerical ratio brought about by the sectioning of a line segment such that the line is divided into two sections, a larger one and a smaller one, where the ratio of the length of the entire line is as equally proportional to the larger section as the larger section is to the smaller section. It may be diagrammed thus

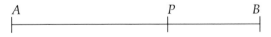

where *AB:AP = AP:PB*. (The symbol : means "proportional to.") The relationship of the larger section to the whole, or the ratio *AP:AB*, is expressed by the fraction 0.618+. Interestingly, the reciprocal of this relationship, or the ratio of the whole section to the larger section (*AB:AP*) and also the ratio of the larger section to the smaller section (*AP:PB*)

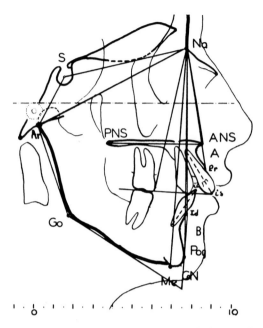

Figure 4–2   Bjork analysis: Developed over a period of years from 1947 to 1953 by Arne Bjork of Sweden; the main geometric figure of this extensive analysis is a polygon running from Na-S-Ar-Go-Gn. The analysis contains over 90 measurements.

works out to the number 1.618. What is astounding about this ratio is the way it may be continued in either direction to infinity.

A simpler way of demonstrating this is

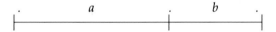

Let *a* represent the major segment and *b* the minor segment of the line divided into golden sections. Then

$$(a + b):a = a:b = b:(a - b)$$

Thus not only are *a* and *b* golden with respect to each other, but *b* and $(a - b)$ are also golden. This process may be continued to form a logarithmic spiral ad infinitum. Such segments are referred to as "incommensurable lines."

The discovery of this ratio had a profound effect. Euclid uses the solution to construct the regular pentagon and decagon. It even influenced Plato and Aristotle. Even though the ratio represents an irrational number, something the Pythagoreans despised and suppressed because it would not fit into their orderly view of the universe or their love of whole numbers, one cannot help but feel it is one of the elemental

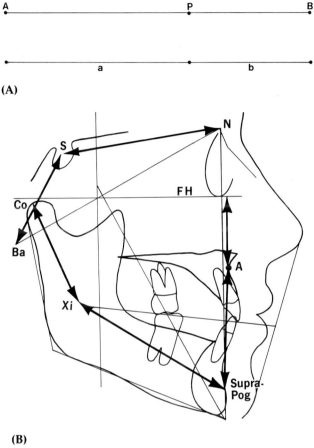

(A)

(B)

Figure 4–3   **(A)** The divine proportion or golden section with the magical ratio of .618 ad infinitum. **(B)** Ricketts' golden sections discovered in the maxillofacial complex.

drafting tools of nature. Ricketts might not be far from wrong in selecting it for cephalometric study and comparison.

Another astounding fact relative to the divine proportion is its close association with the Fibonacci sequence. Ricketts also discusses the relationship of this number series to the golden section in a text he co-authored on cephalometrics,[225] and it is mentioned with good reason. In this numerical sequence, a sample of which is 1, 2, 3, 5, 8, 13, 21, 34, 55, 89, . . ., each number is equal to the sum of the two numbers immediately preceding it. As the numbers become progressively larger, the quotient obtained by dividing one number by the next consecutive one in the series approaches as its limit the value $(\sqrt{5} - 1)/2$, which just happens to work out to be 0.618 $((\sqrt{5} + 1)/2 = 1.618)$!

This fact along with the geometric constructions of Euclid based on his solution to the problem of the golden section (Book VI, Proposition 30) are what make the system suitable to some of the design schemes found in Nature.[226] When a flower possesses either five or ten petals, it is said to express the divine proportion. The simple hydra and the common starfish are examples of this principle. Even something as banal as the common oak twig can be shown to express this concept. Given a long enough stem, the buds are arranged on the twig in a spiral fashion along the length of the branch at regular intervals represented by a ratio 2:5. Other bud arrangements on stems include 1:2, 1:3, 3:8, and 5:13. What is common to all these ratios is that each of the numbers listed with respect to these plants is from the Fibonacci sequence.

Is it any wonder that the good Dr Ricketts might find various anatomical relationships in the face and skull that are related to the golden section or that express the divine proportion? He lists several interesting comparisons of the ratio to a frontal view of the human face. Studying a series of photographs of female professional models, individuals the general opinion of society would accept as beautiful, Ricketts notes that the distance from the top of the center of the forehead to the center of the pupil of the eye is golden to the distance from the center of the pupil to the tip of the chin. Or, on the horizontal level, the width of the pupils of the eyes is golden to the width of the mouth. Dentally, Ricketts states that the width of the lower centrals is golden to the width of the upper centrals, which in turn is golden to the width of the upper centrals and laterals combined. In the lower arch also he states that the cross-arch width of the lower cuspids is golden to the cross-arch width of the lower first molars.

Ricketts admits that more study relative to this mathematical relationship is needed concerning its implications to the lateral cephalogram, but he lists three preliminary findings. First, the corpus of the mandible, Po to Xi-point (a point located at the geometric center of the ramus), is golden to the condyle axis length (condylion to Xi-point). Second, the distance from the FH plane perpendicularly to A-point is proportional to A-point to PM (suprapogonion, the point at the anterior border of the symphysis between B-point and Po where the curvature of the mandibular cortex of bone changes from convex to concave). Third, the anterior cranial base length (S-N) is golden to the posterior cranial base length (S-Ba).

If in fact these anatomical measurements are of divine proportion it has not yet been proven beyond a doubt. But as of this writing, the theory remains unchallenged. In all fairness one must be impressed with the recurrence of this proportional phenomenon in the maxillofacial complex. However, one must also consider the vast number of various measurements that can to be made in an area as anatomically complicated as the human skull. If one were to search long enough, ratios of this type are bound to occur. Given the enormous number available to choose from, one may readily select the most favorable ones that would appear to be compatible with what is approximately a 6 to 10 ratio. The amount of tolerance acceptable in the anatomy of this area allows for a certain amount of poetic license to exert itself in the arbitrary assignment of the golden section principle to certain measurements that approach the 1.618 ratio. Yet, one cannot deny that their existence may be quite likely. It is a ratio that naturally lends itself to harmony and beauty and is therefore appealing wherever observed. As a theory, it exudes a seductive charm that makes one desire that it be a possible key to the design of the maxillofacial complex, a building block devised by a Supreme Intelligence that is used as one of the guides to the proportion and elegance of the form of man. It may well be, but until further proof is compiled, wishing won't make it so.

In all this history of cephalometric analysis systems, we see that a format of comparing existing structures with a preestablished set of norms became common. Also, various baselines were established. Yet researchers accepted that there was some variance to these baselines from individual to individual throughout growth and development. Cases analyzed by different systems could produce different results, depending on which plane of reference was the basis of the system used. The problem seemed to be not what information to record or measure, but what to compare this information with. It was easy to observe and determine what was abnormal. The question remained: What *was* normal for the *individual* patient being treated?

THE SASSOUNI ANALYSIS

One of the first to seriously address the issue of what is normal was Dr Viken Sassouni. He believed that no one cephalometric baseline or angle remained consistent enough to serve as a basis of comparison for all individuals. Proceeding on this premise, he sought to devise an analysis system that was not predicated upon linear baselines between changeable landmarks or upon the comparison of lengths and angles with a set of mathematical averages. Instead he wanted a system based on relationships of anatomical structures to each other within the framework of the individual patient; ie, he wanted to let the patient's own anatomy serve as the clue to what is normal or abnormal to himself. Thus, he developed a system that utilizes a series of circles, or actually portions of circles in the form of arcs, that have a common center formed by the intersection of a composite of anatomical planes to form what has become known as the *Sassouni Archial Analysis*.[227] This system makes allowances for the fact that various landmarks used by other systems, such as sella or nasion, may be superiorly, inferiorly, anteriorly, or posteriorly displaced, thereby affecting the outcome of the particular system in a possibly misleading manner. The Sassouni has its own method of

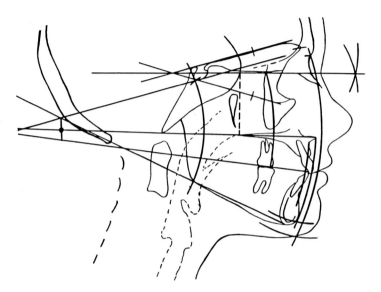

Figure 4−4   Original format of the Sassouni analysis. (Courtesy R. Beistle.)

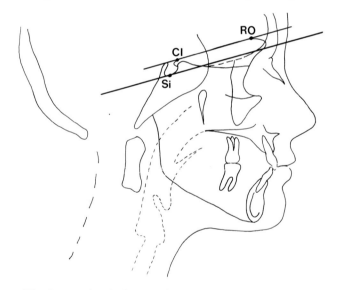

Figure 4−5   The Supraorbital Plane and Parallel Plane.

facial typing built into it. It is a simple system, essentially composed of five lines (planes) and four arcs drawn on easily identifiable landmarks of the lateral cephalogram.[228-238]

Of the five planes used in the system, two are a little less common to cephalometric study. The first is the supraorbital plane, which runs from the most superior point on the roof of the orbit to a point tangent to the most superior portion of the anterior clinoid process (forward lip of the sella turcica). This line merely acts as a reference for parallelism for the second plane that we are really interested in and will use in the analysis. It runs parallel to the supraorbital plane through the lowest point of the inferior surface of the sella turcica, a point denoted as *Si*. Since it has no other particular cephalometric landmark that it connects with, it remains nameless other than being referred to somewhat awkwardly as the "plane parallel to the supraorbital plane." In more recent times it has been dubbed the "Parallel Plane." Thus the supraorbital plane's sole purpose for existence is to act as a directional guide, through the principle of parallelism, to the real plane of interest that only has one fixed anatomical reference landmark.

The other three planes are common to almost every analysis: the maxillary or palatal plane (ANS-PNS), the traditional occlusal plane, and the mandibular plane. As previously stated, there is some variance as to what actually defines the mandibular plane in various cephalometric systems. Some define it as the line Go-Me. The Sassouni is one of the first that defines it slightly differently as extending from menton to the lowest point of the ramus just posterior to the Antegonial Notch! (Another form is defined as extending from menton to the uppermost part of the Antegonial Notch. This is the one used by Bimler.)

Another very important component to this system is the location of yet another spacemark, the locus O. This locus is defined as the area of most common intersection of all four of the major planes, the plane parallel to the supraorbital, the palatal, the occlusal, and the mandibular. In an ideally balanced individual, these four planes should intersect at the common point locus O. In actuality they seldom, if ever, do. As a result there are several different ways of determining this critically important point. When only three of the planes converge at the same point, the remaining plane that fails to meet the other three is considered as being deviant from the general facial pattern. If only two of the four planes intersect at a convergent point, the juncture of the plane parallel to the supraorbital plane and the mandibular plane is considered as point O. If none of the planes intersect at a common point, but do intersect in a generalized area, they will form a geometric isthmus. As the planes converge posteriorly, they reach a common area of intersection, then start diverging from one another again. To locate point O, draw a vertical line through the narrowest point of the isthmus of these converging, then diverging, planes and place O at the midpoint of the vertical line.

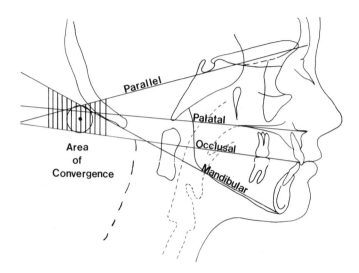

Figure 4-6

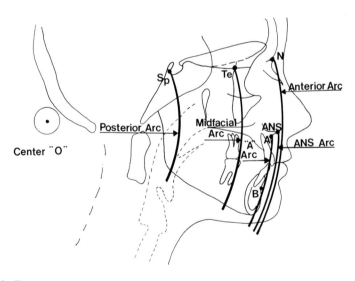

Figure 4-7

Two anatomical points are peculiar to this system and used by it exclusively: (1) temporale (Te), the intersection of the cribriform plate with the anterior wall of the infratemporal fossa, and (2) sella posterior (Sp), the most posterior point on the distal outline of the sella turcica. These points along with A-point and nasion serve as guides for drawing the four major arcs characteristic of the system. The arcs are constructed as follows:

Anterior Arc.   With the point of the compass set on point O, draw an arc from nasion through all four planes. In a well-balanced facial profile, this arc should pass through ANS, the tip of the maxillary incisor, and pogonion. If both ANS and pogonion are anterior or posterior to the Anterior Arc simultaneously, it is customary to draw a second Anterior Arc starting at ANS and passing as far as the level of pogonion. It is called simply the ANS Arc.

Basal Arc   The Basal Arc is used to evaluate the apical bases or "basal arches" of the maxilla and mandible. From center O, construct an arc extending from A-point to the level of B-point.

Midfacial Arc   The Midfacial Arc is used to identify the status of the maxillary dentition (which then in turn denotes the status of the mandibular dentition by default). Again from center O, construct an arc from Te to the occlusal plane. In normal dentitions the mesial surface of the maxillary first permanent molar should be tangent to the Midfacial Arc.

Posterior Arc   The Posterior Arc is used to evaluate the relative position of the mandible. From center O construct an arc from Sp down to the mandibular plane. It should normally pass through gonion.

To these major arcs are added the anterior and posterior vertical dimension arcs. They are very small sections of arcs from which the linear distance to the maxillary (palatal) plane (ANS-PNS) is measured. The palatal plane is considered as the boundary line bisecting the face into upper and lower face height measurements in this system. These vertical dimension arcs are easily scribed as follows:

Anterior vertical dimensions   The anterior vertical dimensions are determined by measuring the distance from the intersection of two small sections of arc with the large Anterior Arc. Place the point of a compass on the tip of the ANS, and inscribe an arc at the point where the plane parallel to the supraorbital plane (sometimes referred to as the cranial baseline) intersects with the Anterior Arc. Sassouni later substituted the nearly identical point supraorbital or SOr. Rotate the compass at that exact distance to the area of the symphysis of the mandible and inscribe a second small arc across that area of the Anterior Arc. Measure along the Anterior Arc 10 mm, open the compass by the corresponding amount, and inscribe a third small arc across the major Anterior Arc. This gives the range for lower face height as compared with upper face height. At 4 years of age the upper and lower face heights so designated by this method would be equal in the normal individual. Between 4 and 12 years of age, the lower face height (ANS-Me) will usually appear about halfway between the two lower arcs. At adulthood the normal patient's menton is at or near the lower of the two small arcs.

Posterior vertical dimensions In addition to a measurement for anterior face height, the original Sassouni Analysis has a posterior face height measurement. This dimension is determined by first placing the point of the compass on the tip of the PNS and opening it to inscribe a small arc at the intersection of the Posterior Arc with the plane parallel to the supraorbital plane (cranial baseline). Transfer this distance by rotating the compass to inscribe a small arc at the point on the Posterior Arc closest to gonion. Opening the compass 10 mm, inscribe a second small arc across the Posterior Arc. Generally, the upper and lower posterior face heights should be equal.

Another oddity of this particular system is that it has a means of determining maxilla size built into it. To determine the size and relative cephalometric location of the maxilla, first drop a perpendicular line from Cr (Cribriform Point, the point where the greater wing of the sphenoid intersects the planum sphenoidale) down through the Frankfort plane to the palatal plane. This denotes where PNS *should be*. If PNS falls on this line, the length, or size, of the maxilla may be denoted by the position of ANS. If ANS is on the Anterior Arc, the maxilla, or palate, is of normal size. If ANS falls short of the arc, the maxilla is short anteriorly. But if ANS is anterior to the arc, the maxilla is long anteriorly. However, these dimensions cannot be taken at face value, but must be corrected. This is relatively simple to do. When ANS falls short of the Anterior Arc, the linear distance from ANS to the arc is transferred to the posterior area and added to it. The palate size is then reevaluated from the new more posterior position of this perpendicular and hence the ideal hypothetical location of PNS which this line implies. Comparison may then be made with the actual location of PNS on the cephalogram. When ANS is anterior to the arc, the reverse procedure is followed. This is more revealing since it allows the clinician to determine both size and position of the maxilla relative to the cranial base. For example, if ANS is short of the Anterior Arc but PNS is posterior to the noncorrected Cr perpendicular, the maxilla is of normal size but merely bodily displaced posteriorly. If ANS is short of the Anterior Arc but PNS falls on the noncorrected Cr perpendicular, the maxilla may be assumed to be short anteriorly. However, if PNS is anterior to the perpendicular and ANS is on the Anterior Arc, the palate is short posteriorly, a condition of relatively little clinical significance.

The final plane used by Sassouni in his system is the optic plane formed by bisecting the angle formed by the intersection of the supraorbital plane and the infraorbital plane (a line from the lower border of the outline of sella turcica to a point tangent to the inferior border of the

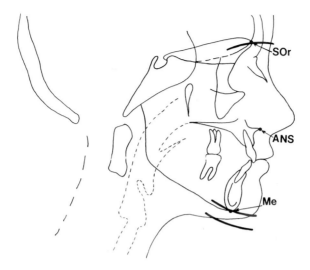

Figure 4–8   To construct the inferior arcs for evaluating individualized vertical dimension, the tip of the compass is placed on ANS and extended to SOr. This distance is transferred to the mandibular symphysis area where a small arc is scribed. The compass is then opened 10 mm, and a second small arc is scribed. The area between these two small inferior arcs represents the range of normality for vertical position of menton for this individual.

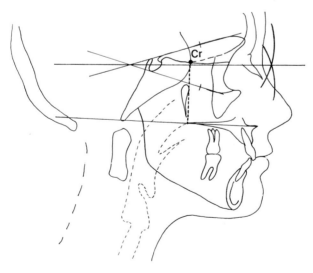

Figure 4–9   Cribriform perpendicular: A perpendicular dashed line is dropped from cribriform point (CR) to the palatal plane where it should denote the location of PNS.

orbit where the floor of the orbit forms its lowest depression, ie, where water would puddle if poured into the eye socket). Generally confluent with the path of the optic nerve, the optic plane is used as a reference for parallelism for the maxillary (palatal) plane, both of which are ideally parallel to the "old standby," the Frankfort horizontal.

INTERPRETATION

Several factors become immediately obvious upon initial inspection of a cephalogram traced with the original Sassouni Archial Analysis system. If the planes all converge rather quickly toward point O posteriorly, creating a large angle between the plane parallel to the supraorbital plane and the mandibular plane, the greater is the tendency toward a skeletal open bite. This would also indicate the vertically dominant leptoprosopic (Bimler) facial type, or what is commonly called in America a "clockwise grower" or "high-angle" case. The vertical component of growth in these types is usually relatively greater than the horizontal component. But if the planes are of more parallel tendency such that they converge very slowly posteriorly forcing point O "a yard off the page," the greater is the tendency to a skeletal deep bite. This indicates the horizontally dominant dolichoprosopic (Bimler) facial type, or what Americans call a brachycephalic facial type or "counterclockwise grower." In this facial type the horizontal component of growth of the jaws is relatively greater than the vertical component. If point O (or center O, as it is also called) is driven low posteriorly by the convergence of the planes, the greater is the tendency to Class II skeletal jaw relationships. But if the planes converge such that point O is high posteriorly, there is more of an indication of Class III relationships. Thus it is seen that the location of point O is one of the single most critical determinants of this particular system.

One consideration that must be made relative to evaluating the Anterior Arc is that there is a certain variation among a sample of individuals with respect to the location of nasion. It varies in position either forward or backward. If the other three anatomical landmarks, ANS, tip of the maxillary incisor, and pogonion all fall on the same arc and only nasion varies from it, either to the front or back, the arc is reevaluated from ANS instead of N. In these circumstances the case is

---

Figure 4–10   **(A)** Construction of infraorbital plane. **(B)** Construction of optic plane: It bisects the angle formed by the supraorbital plane and the infraorbital plane. **(C)** The seven primary planes of original Sassouni format.

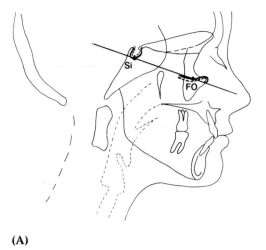

(A)

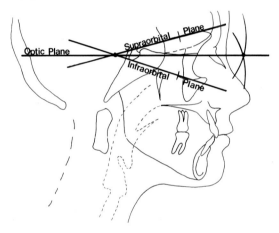

(B)

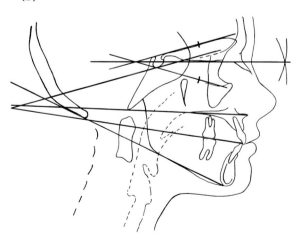

(C)

sometimes referred to as either prearchial or retroarchial, depending on the location of nasion relative to the newly oriented Anterior Arc.

The location of pogonion on or near the Anterior Arc also provides important diagnostic information. Sassouni originally defined an 8-mm leeway space, 4-mm anterior, and 4-mm posterior to the Anterior Arc in which pogonion may lie and still qualify the case to be Class I skeletally. But if pogonion falls more than 4 mm posterior to the Anterior Arc, the case is considered skeletal Class II. If it should fall more than 4 mm beyond or anterior to the Anterior Arc, the case is considered skeletal Class III. Within this 8-mm leeway space, the case is said to merely have Class II or Class III tendencies relative to the location of pogonion being either ahead of or behind the arc.

The position of the maxillary central incisor is also important relative to its location on the Anterior Arc. If it is behind or posterior to the arc, the case is considered as needing labial crown torque, as in Class II, Division 2 situations. On the other hand, if the tip of the maxillary incisor is ahead of or anterior to the arc, it indicates maxillary dental protrusion. The same may be said for the lower incisor with the slight amount of correction allowed to keep it in contact with the lingual surface of the upper incisor at proper overbite and overjet.

We have discussed how the alignment of pogonion to the Anterior Arc reveals either mandibular protrusion or retrusion. But the converse is also true relative to the location of ANS. If all the other landmarks—pogonion, tip of maxillary central incisor (although less important when obvious dental protrusion exists in the form of excess labial crown torque), and nasion—all fall on the Anterior Arc but ANS is behind or posterior to it, it indicates maxillary skeletal retrusion. But if ANS falls anterior to the arc, the case is said to exhibit a maxillary skeletal protrusion. However, some experts feel this particular condition is almost never seen by the rank and file of practitioners.[59]

The Basal Arc (sometimes referred to as the A-point Arc or the A Arc) concerns itself with the position of the maxillary and mandibular denture bases. In the normal orthopedically well-balanced case A-point and B-point should fall on the Basal Arc. If B-point falls posterior to the Basal Arc, the case is expressive of a mandibular apical base retrusion. If B-point falls anterior to the Basal Arc, a mandibular apical base protrusion is evidenced, as in a Class III jaw relationship.

In the Midfacial Arc, the mesial surface of the upper first permanent molar should just touch the arc. Anterior or posterior to this arc, the tooth is said to express an anterior or posterior positioning, which would help determine whether one would want to distal drive the molars in an effort to relieve arch crowding or, conversely, to develop the arch anteriorly against stationary molars. (This consideration is also predicated upon the status of the arch width; ie, narrow arches should be developed laterally first before relieving arch crowding further by expanding the arch either posteriorly or anteriorly.)

There are two important corrections to keep in mind when evaluating the position of the upper first permanent molar on the Midfacial Arc. Both are simple concepts and easy to implement. If ANS falls in front of or behind the correctly established Anterior Arc, the linear distance by which it is offset is transferred to the Midfacial Arc, which is in turn moved anteriorly or posteriorly by the same amount. The position of the upper first molar is then evaluated from this new ANS-offset corrected position. Second, it must be remembered that in the mixed dentition stage, when the deciduous second molars are still present, the upper first permanent molars are about 2 mm further back distally than they will eventually be in their final position in the adult dentition. This location distally is due to the extra mesiodistal width expressed by the deciduous second molar and is called the *leeway space of Nance.*

The Posterior Arc is used to assist in the study of the position of gonion. Here a rather interesting anatomical coincidence of Nature may be observed. Roughly speaking, in the average 12-year-old the distance from S to N (anterior cranial base length) should equal the distance from gonion to pogonion (corpus length of the mandible). There is 6-mm variation with respect to this from age 4 to adulthood; ie, at 4 years of age the length of the mandible may be up to 6 mm short of the length of the S-N line, and at adulthood the length may be up to 6 mm longer than S-N. This extra length in the adult shows up posteriorly as gonion moves distally away from the Posterior Arc. This is consistent with what we know to be true about how bone growth actually takes place in the ramus.

It should now be easy to see how Dr Sassouni organizes facial types into his four basic categories, all descriptive of skeletal types: open bite, closed bite, Class II, and Class III skeletal relationships. These four types are predicated primarily on one factor, the relative position of center O.

The deep bite and open bite facial types, are determined by the variance of center O about a horizontal direction. The Class II and Class III types are determined by the variance of center O along a vertical direction. Each type has a set of characteristics that one would expect to be associated with that particular occlusal relationship.

The Open Bite Category (Center O Close to Profile)

Open bite exhibits a large angle between the plane parallel to the supraorbital plane and the mandibular plane. This would be the leptoprosopic facial type (after Bimler). This large angle is the result of the steep inclination of these two planes, which, as a result, intersect quickly behind the posterior facial area. This is what causes the center O to be "pulled" in close to the facial area. Because of the steep mandibular plane, the gonial angle is more open and usually accompanied by a shorter ramus height. With the palatal plane of a more opened inclination

(ANS higher than PNS), the lower portion of the anterior face height (ANS-Me) has greater dimension than the upper face height (N-ANS).

The Closed Bite Category (Center O Far from Profile)

Closed bite exhibits near-parallel planes in the cranial base and mandible that drive their intersection and resultant point O far to the left of the facial profile. This is the dolichoprosopic (Bimler) facial type. The angle between the cranial base and mandibular plane is smaller, and the resultant gonial angle must also be more closed. The anterior face height tends to be more diminished and will usually tolerate the services of bite-opening-type appliances quite well. The lower face height is usually more deficient than the upper face height. This is the reason why these cases respond so well to Bionator or similar functional appliance treatment.

The Class II Category (Center O Low on Posterior Facial Area)

Class II also exhibits a large angle between the cranial base (plane parallel to the supraorbital plane) and the mandibular plane, but in this case the mandibular plane exhibits a more horizontal tendency, with the cranial base line being steeper. This forces the intersection of the two planes and point O downward behind the posterior facial area. The palatal plane usually follows suit, with PNS tipped down inferior to the level of ANS. Common to such cases are the Division 1 maxillary incisor protrusion and mandibular retrusion often associated with Class II mal-occlusion. As might be expected, B-point almost always falls posterior to the Basal Arc.

The Class III Category (Center O High on Posterior Facial Area)

Class III exhibits a more parallel cranial baseline but a much steeper mandibular plane. This forces their intersection and point O upward in the posterior area. The palatal plane also usually follows suit, with PNS higher posteriorly than ANS. Because of the steep mandibular plane, the gonial angle is larger, but, unlike the open bite category, the corpus length of the mandible is *long* instead of short. The ramus is also usually longer and is of more acute angulation with the Frankfort plane, or, conversely, more open with respect to the vertical plane. The maxilla is shorter, and typical Class III mandibular protrusion is evidenced. The mandibular incisors are usually lingually inclined due to pressure from the orbicularis oris. The occlusal plane is also often quite steep. B-point may be seen to fall beyond the Basal (A-point) Arc.

There is no special "magic" to this organization system or its accompanying characteristics. It is merely the logical application of "common sense." What is expected by reason of observation usually proves out with the application of the measuring methods. The human head after all is a sphere. Arcs just naturally lend themselves better to round objects than do straight lines.

Sassouni also analyzes such things as orbital, zygomatic, maxillary, gonial, upper molar widths, and the parallelism of their respective connecting lines across the face of the anteroposterior (AP) view of the x-ray of the head. He also discussed the use of "wigglegrams," as did Vorhies and Adams in earlier times. (A wigglegram is a vertical list of values with their mean values in direct vertical alignment and ranges of normal variance posted to the right and left of these values. The actual clinical values of SNA, SNB intermaxillary angles, etc, are plotted on this column and connected by a zigzagging line, hence the name. This line is then evaluated relative to the listed norms.)

What is important about the Sassouni Archial Analysis system is that it clearly shows a movement in diagnostic thought away from a concern for numerical values (not a single numerical value need be used) and toward an overall evaluation of maxillofacial relationships. This is far more valuable to the individual with the abilities to effect full scale orthopedic change by the use of FJO techniques. The Sassouni is an excellent system for evaluation purposes, but it does offer some difficulties due to the level of complexity associated with it, and it has by now become obvious that the determination of an accurate location of center O is critical to the system. Sometimes in more difficult cases this can be of some concern to the diagnostician. It may also be mechanically difficult to obtain correct arc tracings when point O is far off the edge of the film, as in severe deep bite cases. But it is the somewhat arbitrary location of center O that occasionally makes one feel insecure about the accuracy of the placement of the major arcs. When center O is easily determined by the confluence of at least three of the major planes to an identical point location, the case is usually already in excellent balance orthopedically. It is when the case is very unbalanced orthopedically that the planes fail to meet in a common area, yet this is when the assistance of a system of this type is most required. This may lead some practitioners to doubt the ability of the system to provide the clearest and most well-defined set of treatment goals. Also, there is no proof the human face is actually archial.

But the importance of the Sassouni analysis cannot be overestimated, since it is truly an orthopedically oriented system concerned not only with teeth but also the jaws and the entire face. It allows for the fact that not only the teeth, but their supporting bony structures as well, may be repositioned with the properly applied techniques. This system opens the door for a more complete and total anatomic approach to the treatment of the malocclusion. Doctor Sassouni was a great pioneer in his field, and his contributions to the development of cephalometric diagnosis will no doubt serve as a milestone in the history of the science. Being one of the first to reveal the gradual change in thinking in orthodontics toward orthopedic as well as orthodontic considerations, his system of analysis reveals his concern for the balance of the total face. He was one of the important founders of a philosophy of analyzing the harmony not only of teeth, but their skeletal bases and surrounding facial structures as well. Relative to the establishment of defined orthopedic treatment goals for the clinician to consider in the treatment plan, he represented one of the early clarifying influences.

"SASSOUNI PLUS"

Like most cephalometric analyses, the Sassouni has gone through several modifications since its inception in 1955. Sassouni possessed a degree in dentistry from the University of Paris, France, and degrees in orthodontics and physical anthropology from the University of Pennsylvania. His strong anthropological background links him academically with the great craniometricians that came before him. He brought his analysis to the discipline of cephalometrics in the mid-1950s during a time when other analyses such as the Downs and the Steiner were enjoying great popularity.

After Sassouni's death in 1983 a new champion of the archial analysis, Dr Richard Beistle of Buchanan, Michigan, arose to continue the work of teaching and promoting this great analysis. Beistle recognized the value of the Sassouni Analysis by virtue of its orthopedic implications during a time when orthopedics was coming to the forefront. He had embellished the analysis system, at first somewhat profusely, and subsequently refined it to the form in which he now teaches it. At first Beistle was somewhat of a doubting Thomas and did not have complete faith in the prowess of the original analysis, and as a result supplemented it with a variety of other cephalometric analysis components from other sources until he realized their redundancy with respect to supporting findings already made manifest by original Sassouni precepts and condensed his method into that 11-point marvel of geometric cephalometric simplicity that has now become known as the *Sassouni Plus*. Beistle lists the 11 points of his version of the Sassouni Plus Analysis, in what he calls his cephalometric "bottom line" as follows:

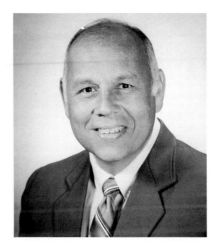

(A)

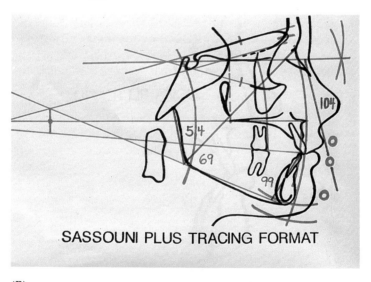

(B)

Figure 4–11   **(A)** Dr Richard Beistle. **(B)** Beistle's format of his Sassouni Plus.

1. Skeletal AP alignment
2. Skeletal vertical dimension
3. Maxillary incisor position
4. Maxillary AP length
5. Maxillary AP position
6. Maxillary first permanent molar position
7. Mandibular AP length
8. Mandibular AP position
9. Mandibular incisor position
10. Growth direction indicator
11. Upper lip angle

The first eight components of the analysis are from the original Sassouni; the last three, which form the "Plus" part of the analysis, were added by Beistle. Two components Beistle formerly used as a part of the analysis are the anterior face height (AFH) ratio and the posterior face height (PFH) ratio. The AFH *ratio* concerns the ratio of the *lower* face height (LFH) to the *total* face height, ie, the linear distance in millimeters from ANS to Me (or lower AFH) divided by the linear distance from N to Me (or the total AFH), ie, ANS-Me/N-Me. The AFH ratio is utilized as a backup or "cross-checking factor" which indicates the skeletal vertical dimension, with "normal" vertical defined as the 54 to 58% range.

Similarly, the PFH *ratio* is calculated by dividing the linear distance from S to Go by the linear distance from N to Me, or S-Go/N-Me. Thus total PFH (or S-Go) is divided by the total AFH (or N-Me): PFH/AFH. The dividend of this ratio may fall into one of the categories listed in the table and may be interpreted as shown.

Sex	PFH/AFH (%)	Grower
E	54–60	Vertical
F	61–64	Vertical
M	61–64	Neutral
E	65	Neutral
F	66–69	Neutral
M	66–69	Horizontal
E	70–80	Horizontal

E = either; M = male; F = female.

Beistle contends that although there is nothing wrong with these components, they are redundant, since AFH may also be analyzed by the location of Me (which we shall discuss shortly), and the growth direction indicator may be analyzed by the split gonial angle (also discussed shortly). As a result, in the effort to keep the analysis as simple as possible, the AFH and PFH ratio comparisons were deleted to keep them from cluttering up the tracing sheet. However, on occasion their use may

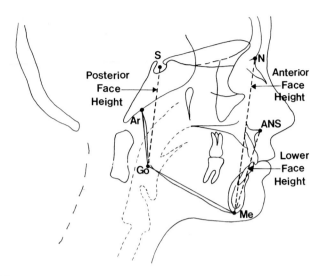

Figure 4–12

be handy to verify findings of the other components. Following is the evaluation of the 11 components of the Sassouni Plus according to Beistle.

Skeletal AP alignment   The Anterior Arc from N is the reference arc that permits the evaluation of ANS, the tip of the maxillary central incisor, and Po. These three landmarks should all fall on the Anterior Arc in an ideal situation. B-point is evaluated relative to its location with respect to the Basal or A-point Arc. Thus, both the maxilla and the mandible are evaluated on the AP plane by combined use of the Anterior Arc and the smaller A-point Arc. Barring for the moment any discussion of the range of acceptability for the maxillary central incisor, there are a series of combinations of locations of these landmarks that Beistle believes are significant.

If ANS and Pog are both posterior to the Anterior Arc by an equal amount, the profile is considered "retroarchial." This situation is considered somewhat normal and may be due to the fact that (1) N could possibly be too far anterior, (2) the entire lower face could be too far posterior, or (3) a slight combination of both.

If ANS and Pog are both anterior to the Anterior Arc by an equal amount, the profile is considered "prearchial." This situation may be due to (1) N being positioned too far posteriorly, (2) the entire lower face being too far anterior, or (3) a combination of both.

If ANS is situated on the Anterior Arc but Pog is abnormally located, two possibilities exist:

1. Pog is located anterior to the Anterior Arc. This would be either merely a chin point protrusion or an entire mandibular protrusion.

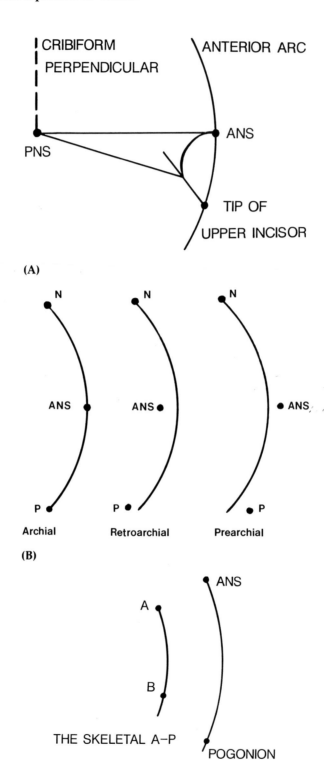

(A)

(B)

(C)

2. Pog is located posterior to the Anterior Arc. This indicates the absence of an adequate chin button or it could signify a full-scale mandibular retrusion.

If Pog is located on the Anterior Arc but ANS is not, two possibilities exist.

1. ANS is anterior to the Anterior Arc, which indicates a maxillary protrusion (rare).
2. ANS is posterior to the Anterior Arc, which indicates a maxillary retrusion (not uncommon).

A-point Arc and evaluation of B-point: B-point ideally should be located on the A-point Arc (Basal Arc).

1. Any combination of *maxillary protrusion* and *mandibular retrusion* of more than 3 mm, which is confirmed by the relationship of B-point to the A-point Arc, is categorized as a skeletal Class II.
2. Any combination of *maxillary retrusion* and *mandibular protrusion* of more than 3 mm, which is confirmed by the relationship of B-point to the A-point Arc, is categorized as a skeletal Class III.

Note: This represents a 6-mm range. Sassouni originally used a 4-mm measurement, which gave a somewhat wider and less specific 8-mm range.

Skeletal vertical dimension   As previously noted, the AFH is demonstrable in the form of the ratio of the ANS-Me LFH linearly to the total AFH N-Me. However, it is also expressible much more easily in the manner in which it appears in the most current edition of the Sassouni Plus—ie, the relative location of Me with respect to the two lower arcs. The two lower arcs are scribed in the usual manner by placing the tip of the compass on ANS and opening it to supraorbital (SOr, the intersection of the most anterior part of the roof of the orbit with the lateral wall of the orbit). Then by rotating the compass, this dimension is transferred to the area of Me, and the first short lower arc is scribed. The compass is then opened 10 mm linearly, and the second lower arc is scribed. These

Figure 4–13   Skeletal anterior alignment. **(A)** A properly positioned maxilla and maxillary central incisor would have ANS and the tip of the upper central incisor on Anterior Arc and PNS on cribriform perpendicular. **(B)** The location of ANS and Pog (P) posterior to Anterior Arc, is designated as a retroarchial profile; if they are in front of the Anterior Arc, they are designated as being in a prearchial profile configuration. **(C)** In addition, B-point should fall on the A-point (Basal) arc.

two lower arcs serve to demarcate the "range of normality" for the vertical position of Me *for this particular individual.*

Vertically, the upper face height (UFH or SOr-ANS) should equal the LFH (or ANS-Me) *at age 4.* But from here on the LFH starts gaining on the UFH as both the maxilla and the mandible grow down and forward out from under the cranium. The LFH should surpass the UFH, by 6 mm at age 12 and by 10 mm at adulthood. The general rate of increase in LFH from age 4 is about 3 to 4 mm per year. This would place Me on the more superior of the two lower arcs at age 4, and even though growth takes place at both UFH and LFH areas simultaneously, if growth is proportionally balanced, Me will ideally fall on the more inferior of the two lower arcs at age 18 to adulthood. The reason is that the two lower arcs are scribed 10 mm apart and are proportionally a product of the distance from ANS to SOr transferred to the symphysis area. Thus, the proportion of LFH to UFH increases by the addition of an age-dependent factor. The accompanying table lists the ideal relationship of LFH to UFH.

Age	Facial Dimensions (mm)
4	LFH = UFH + 0.0
6	LFH = UFH + 1.5
8	LFH = UFH + 3.0
10	LFH = UFH + 4.5
12	LFH = UFH + 6.0
14	LFH = UFH + 7.5
16	LFH = UFH + 9.0
Adult	LFH = UFH + 10

Therefore, if the location of Me is aberrant *for the age of the patient,* either closer to the superior or inferior lower arcs, it may be interpreted only as insufficient or excessive vertical *tendencies,* respectively, as long as it falls within the two arcs. These tendencies are expressed simply as open bite or closed bite, because Me still falls within the two-inferior-arc 10-mm range of normality proportional to age. However, if Me falls completely outside the two lower arcs, it is no longer within the normal range.

Maxillary incisor position   In the maxillary incisor position an "extra" arc, the ANS Arc, might have to be drawn if needed. In a balanced profile, ANS should fall on the Anterior Arc. When it does, the tip of the anterior incisor should also fall on the Anterior Arc (from N), but it has a range of 0 to +3 mm ahead of the Anterior Arc for normal upper incisor angulation. In more modern times, the tooth-positioning trend for the sake of both lip support and mandibular arc of closure purposes is to favor a slight protrusion in the maxillary incisor region. Nevertheless, 0 to +3 mm ahead of the Anterior Arc is the range of normality, but *only* when the ANS is *on* the Anterior Arc. If it is not, a separate ANS Arc is

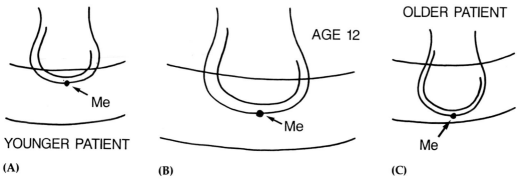

Figure 4–14   In evaluation of vertical, menton should be (A) nearer the upper of the two inferior arcs in the younger patient, (B) midpoint in the adolescent, and (C) nearer the lower of the two inferior arcs in the adult.

drawn, from which the analysis of the maxillary central incisal tip is made, following the same range 0 to +3 mm ahead of the *ANS Arc*.

Maxillary AP length   The evaluation of both the length and the position of the maxilla involve the use of the Anterior Arc and the cribriform perpendicular. The cribriform perpendicular is composed of a vertical line dropped perpendicular to the optic plane from Cribriform Point (Cr, the intersection of the planum sphenoidale with the greater wing of the sphenoid). This perpendicular line is drawn to the level of the palatal plane (ANS-PNS). Three combinations of location of ANS and PNS exist, which determine the interpretation of the *length* of the maxilla.

1. If PNS is on the Cr perpendicular and ANS is on the Anterior Arc, the maxilla is of normal length.
2. If PNS is on the Cr perpendicular and ANS falls behind the Anterior Arc, the maxilla is short anteriorly. If ANS is anterior to the Anterior Arc, the maxilla is long anteriorly. But this rarely, if ever, happens.
3. If PNS is anterior to the Cr perpendicular and ANS is on the Anterior Arc, the maxilla is short posteriorly.

Note: If ANS is posterior to the Anterior Arc, the distance from ANS to the Anterior Arc *is transferred* posteriorly to the Cr perpendicular, and the length evaluation is made with respect to the *newly adjusted* Cr perpendicular point in all cases.

Maxillary AP position   Regardless of the size of the maxilla itself, concern also exists as to its overall relative location with respect to common base reference structures such as the anterior cranial base. In the Sassouni Plus Analysis, maxillary overall position is again analyzed by virtue of the location of ANS and PNS with respect to the Anterior Arc and the Cr perpendicular. Once relative size or length of the maxilla is assessed, its location is also evaluated relative to the same boundaries.

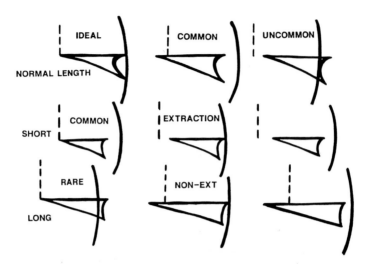

Figure 4—15   Evaluations of maxillary AP length.

If ANS and PNS are both in back of the Anterior Arc and Cr perpendicular by the same amount, the entire maxilla is retruded. If the reverse is the case, ANS and PNS are both ahead of their respective reference lines by the same amount; the entire maxilla is protruded, a condition considered by most practicing cephalometricians as quite rare.

Maxillary first permanent molar position   The upper first permanent molar is evaluated such that its mesial surface should be tangent to the Midfacial Arc. The Midfacial Arc extends from Te down to the level of the occlusal plane. There is a *correction factor* associated with this component, however, and it is a result of the *relative* position of the maxilla. The purpose of the evaluation of the upper first molar is to see how it sits in the maxilla. But the entire maxilla may be positioned abnormally one way or the other relative to the cranial base (usually posteriorly, if not normal). Therefore, a correction factor must come into play to allow proper evaluation of the molar relative to its position in the maxilla alone. This occurs only when ANS is not on the Anterior Arc, and it takes the form of transferring the distance from ANS to the Anterior Arc back to the Midfacial Arc.

If ANS is posterior to the Anterior Arc, the distance from ANS to the Anterior Arc is transferred posteriorly to the Midfacial Arc, and the molar is evaluated relative to this newly corrected position of the arc.

If ANS is anterior to the Anterior Arc, the reverse procedure is followed.

In the mixed dentition where the maxillary deciduous second molars are present, the first permanent molars reflect the distal displacement caused by the wider E's by usually being up to 2 mm posterior to the adjusted Midfacial Arc, which is normal for this dental age group; it is a reflection of the leeway space of Nance.

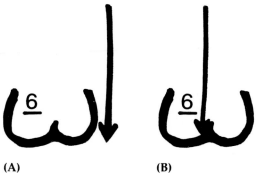

(A)   **(B)**

Figure **4−16**   Evaluation of maxillary first molar position. **(A)** Ideal position of maxillary first molar is mesial surface tangent to *adjusted* Midfacial Arc. **(B)** When mesial surface is anterior to Midfacial Arc, posterior quadrant distalization techniques of one sort or another are usually indicated.

At this point we note what observations Beistle makes relative to the palatal plane. He states that it is normally parallel to the optic plane (as is FH). The palatal plane should pass horizontally through the opening between the tip of the basisphenoid and the odontoid process. In open bite and Class II cases, the prolonged palatal plane will be tipped down in back and thus pass through the odontoid process. In deep bite cases, the palatal plane usually remains quite horizontal. In Class III cases, the palatal plane is quite often tipped up in back and therefore passes through the basisphenoid.

Mandibular AP length   Like the maxilla, the length or size of the mandible as well as its relative AP position with respect to the maxilla and cranial base are evaluated by its own pair of reference arcs, the Anterior Arc and the Posterior Arc. The Posterior Arc is scribed from Sp down to the level of anatomical Go. The Posterior Arc from Sp should pass directly through Go at age 12. This permits AP evaluation of Go. If Go is located on the Posterior Arc and Pog is on the Anterior Arc at age 12, it means that the length of the corpus of the mandible (from Go to Pog) is *equal* to the anterior cranial base Sp-N (the sources of the Anterior and Posterior Arcs). This is a normal situation—*for age 12*. Prior to age 12 the corpus is smaller than the Sp-N anterior cranial base, and after age 12 it becomes progressively larger than the Sp-N anterior cranial base as the mandible accelerates in growth down and forward out from under the facial complex. Shortness of the corpus anteriorly is more influential on malocclusion and the profile than the same degree of shortness posteriorly. At age 4 Go should be 6 mm ahead of the Posterior Arc. At age 16 Go should fall 4 mm behind the Posterior Arc in males. In the adult, Pog should fall 6 mm behind the Posterior Arc in males, but only 4 mm behind in females. This method is concerned with mandibular size or length of the mandible relative to the individual.

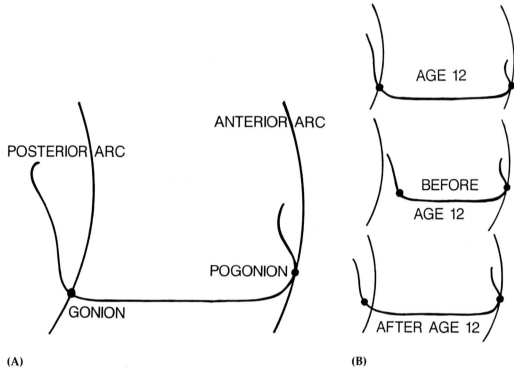

Figure **4–17** **(A)** Ideal mandibular AP *length* at age 12 places pogonion on Anterior Arc and gonion on Posterior Arc. **(B)** *Length* of the mandible may be evaluated by analyzing location of gonion relative to age (provided, of course, Pog is on Anterior Arc).

Mandibular AP position The relative position of the mandible with respect to the AP plane must be evaluated as a function of the age of the patient. For our discussion here we will assume the patient to be 12 years of age, the time when a properly positioned mandible of proper size would have Go on the Posterior Arc and Pog on the Anterior Arc. When Pog and Go are displaced in the same direction, either anterior or posterior to the arcs by an equal amount, the mandible is displaced as a whole by the equal amount. If displaced by unequal amounts, a displaced mandible exists, but also one that is abnormal in size by the difference of the two displacement values. If Go and Pog are displaced in opposite directions, an abnormally large mandible (farther apart) or an abnormally small mandible (closer together) is indicated. The analysis of Pog to the Anterior Arc and B-point to the Basal (A-point) Arc also helps determine the AP position and size of the mandible when the location of Pog and Go vary by unequal amounts. Also, since the Posterior Arc is intimately related to the location of the TMJ according to Beistle, when Go is posterior to the Posterior Arc *relative to age*, it is usually interpreted as a

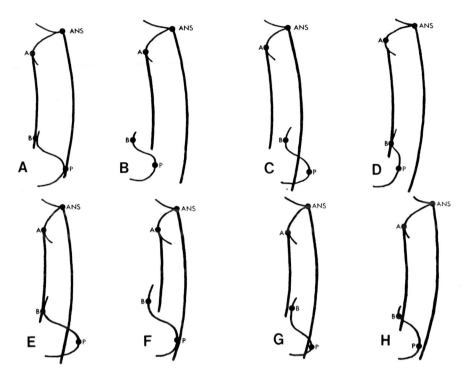

Figure 4–18 Various combinations of location of B-point and Pog (P) in evaluating mandibular AP *position*. (This assumes gonion is correctly located relative to Posterior Arc, considering age of patient.)

posteriorly displaced mandible. TMJ symptoms and transcranial radiography can easily corroborate this.

Mandibular incisor position The mandibular incisor position is the first of the three remaining components of the "Plus" part of the analysis. It is composed of the angle formed by the intersection of the line through the long axis of the mandibular central incisor with the mandibular plane. The angle, read on the lingual surface of the intersection, has as its norm 95 degrees with a range of ± 5 degrees. Thus with a 10-degree total range, the tolerance for proper positioning, which actually is predicated upon the position of the upper incisor and the position of B-point relative to it, is quite broad. This is a reflection of the more modern demands of upper incisor positioning (with its penchant for protecting the mandibular arc of closure), since the Sassouni Plus range of lower-incisor positioning is more protrusive than the more traditional norms of 90 degrees plus or minus 5 degrees. However, once the position of the upper incisors and B-point are balanced, either naturally or by means of therapeutics, the location of the lower incisor is then a dictate of their relationship.

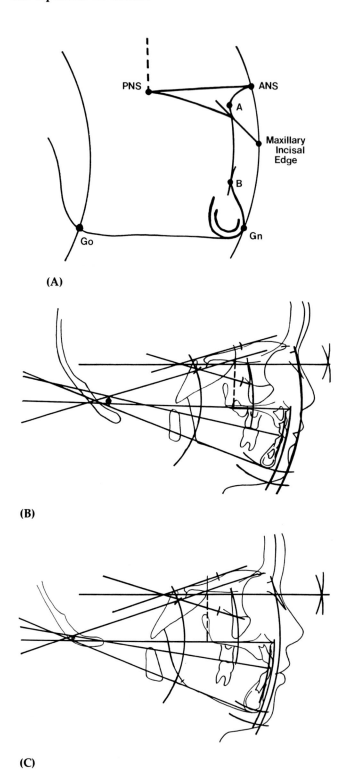

(A)

(B)

(C)

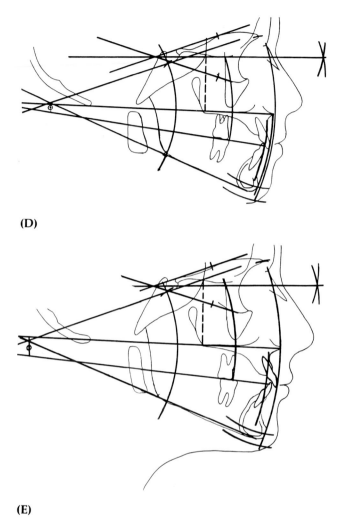

(D)

(E)

Figure **4–19** **(A)** Ideal locations of landmarks ANS, tip of maxillary central incisor and pogonion on Anterior Arc, A- and B-points on A-point (Basal Arc), PNS on cribriform perpendicular, and gonion on Posterior Arc *at age 12.* Appearance of Sassouni analysis of average patient **(B)** at age 4, **(C)** at age 8, **(D)** at age 12, and **(E)** having reached adulthood.

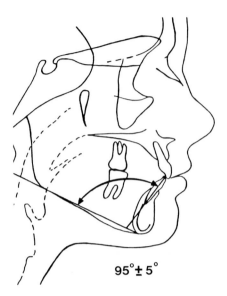

95°±5°

Figure **4−20**   Lower incisor−mandibular plane angle: norm = 95 degrees, range 90−100 degrees.

Growth direction indicator   The growth direction indicator is the component that obviates the use of the PFH/AFH ratio as a growth direction indicator. Beistle determines the main direction of growth by calling the world's attention to a very valuable, yet little-known and little-used, cephalometric calculation originally devised by Bjork. Beistle splits the gonial angle and uses the upper and lower portions of it to evaluate growth direction. It is important to note here that instead of anatomical Go he uses *cephalometric gonion*, which is a space mark constructed at the intersection of the ramal line (articulare to the most posterior point on the posterior surface of the ramus) with the mandibular plane.

To construct the mandibular plane, draw a line from Me to a point tangent to the most posterior part of the inferior border of the mandible. Now as these two planes intersect, *cephalometric Go* is formed. Next, a line from N is drawn to cephalometric Go, thus dividing the gonial angle into upper and lower components. Beistle contends that in order to estimate the main component of growth direction more accurately, the diagnostician must look beyond merely accepting the gonial angle as a single factor in determining mandibular morphology. The manner in which the ascending ramus and the corpus (or mandibular body) are coupled and related to each other to form the gonial angle determines how the mandible will grow. Thus, Beistle splits the gonial angle into upper and lower portions in order to determine the angular relationship governing how the ramus and corpus are put together.

The line from N to cephalometric Go not only divides the gonial angle into two parts, but it is also an indirect indicator of facial depth.

The *upper* portion of the split gonial angle represents the *slant of the ramus*. The *lower* portion of the angle represents the *slant of the body of the mandibular corpus*. The table summarizes these facts.

Angle	Range of Normal (deg)
Total gonial	120–132
Upper gonial	52–55
Lower gonial	70–75

If the upper gonial angle is large, growth will be forward. If the upper gonial angle is small, growth will be downward and backward. If the lower gonial angle is large, growth will be downward. If the lower gonial angle is small, growth will be forward.

Special note   Due to his great insight into the significance of the split gonial angle, Beistle refers to it not only as a growth direction indicator but also as a treatment response indicator! One of the criticisms of functional appliance performance made by those not totally familiar with appliance usage is that the effects of the appliance on the mandible are unpredictable. Not so! The split gonial angle as described by Beistle holds the answer. It serves as a tip-off to the main component of growth that will be manifested during functional-appliance-type treatment of mandibular relationships. This is clearly brought out by the citing of two hypothetical examples.

First, take the instance of a mandible that needs advancement out of its skeletal Class II retrusive position. Let us also assume for the sake of this example that this mandible exhibits a large gonial angle of, say, 140 degrees. If the upper gonial angle is large, 66 degrees (which would be large even relative to the overall 140-degree angle), and the lower gonial angle is small, 74 degrees (which is normal only if the overall gonial angle is normal, but is small relative to the 140-degree angle), the combination adds up to both angles, indicating a strong horizontal component of growth. Thus, mandibular advancement would proceed "like a shot," but the response of posterior quadrants to attempts at increasing the vertical would seem to struggle. This indicates the appropriate alteration of the construction bite for the Bionator to possibly only end-to-end instead of slightly past, and also indicates a greater inter-incisal thickness of the construction bite to provide extra help in the effort to increase vertical, a process somewhat naturally resisted by this type of growth pattern.

Yet, if reversed, the same 140-degree oversized gonial angle could have a small relative upper gonial angle, say 54 degrees, and a large lower gonial angle, say 86 degrees, and this combination adds up to a strong downward and backward grower. This in turn would indicate a somewhat thinner construction bite for a Bionator, since increasing the vertical will come more easily in a dominantly vertical grower. However,

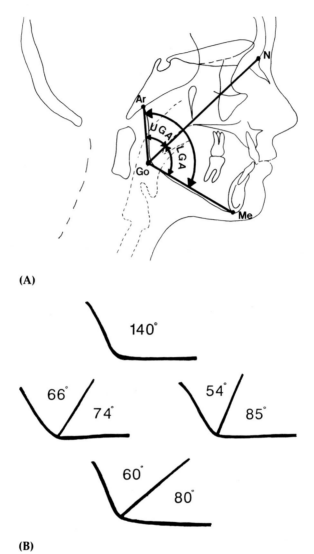

(A)

(B)

Figure 4–21   Does a large gonial angle mean open bite or Class III? Split gonial angle as growth direction indicator: **(A)** Gonial angle Ar-Go-Me is split into upper and lower gonial angles by the line N-Go. **(B)** In this example a large gonial angle (140 degrees) may be representative of several modified growth types. As Beistle points out, a large gonial angle can be indicative of several things, depending on the split. When UGA is large, growth will be forward; when UGA is small, growth is more down *and back*. The opposite holds for the lower gonial angle; ie, if LGA is large, growth will be downward, and if LGA is small, growth will be forward; eg, 66/74 = forward, 54/84 = downward, 60/80 = proportional split.

a more concentrated effort may be needed to advance the mandible horizontally, since this would be against the main vertical growth component. A mitigating circumstance might also take place when the 140-degree angle, which is generally associated with vertically dominant growth, has an equal, albeit large, ratio of upper to lower gonial angles of, say, 60 degrees and 80 degrees. Each is larger than the optimum limits of the ranges of normality, although by the same amount. The large overall gonial angle of 140 degrees is still suggestive of a vertical grower, but not nearly so much as the aforementioned state of a small upper and large lower gonial angle, which would be the most intense combination. When one of the two angles is normal and the other is abnormal, that singular abnormal angle is suggestive of somewhat lesser tendencies to its respective growth direction.

In a second example, a relatively small gonial angle, indicative of a predominance of horizontal growth, may have mitigating components such as a small upper angle and a large lower angle, which are indicative of vertical dominance in spite of the overall horizontal suggestions of the total angle. Construction bites could therefore also be appropriately modified to compensate for the lack of the desired component or counteract the excess of an undesired component. With respect to our second example of a small gonial angle, if it is intensified by a small lower angle and a large upper angle, we have the most intense form of horizontal grower, which would effect rapid mandibular advancement, but in which vertical development would dawdle. Beistle places much more diagnostic weight on the significance of the proportions of the upper and lower gonial angles to their ranges of relative normality than to the "watered down" significance of the less specific overall gonial angle.

Upper lip angle   The upper lip angle (ULA) is constructed by drawing a line tangent to the anteriormost tip of the upper lip, through the point where the upper lip ends and the soft tissue midnasal septum begins (soft tissue subnasale), and extending it upward to intersect the optic plane (or Beistle's "visual horizontal," a quasi-physiological horizontal closely paralleling osteologic Frankfort). The angle is measured inferiorly and posteriorly at the intersection of the upper lip line and the optic plane. It is used as an indicator of the proper esthetic protrusion of the upper lip. See the table.

Angle (deg)	Lip Type
90 or less	Retruded
91–99	Flat
100–115	Normal
116 or more	Protruded

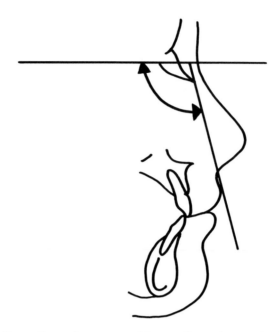

Figure 4—22   Upper lip angle: measured internally against optic plane.

Another important point of difference between Beistle's method and the original Sassouni is that Beistle prefers to use the functional, rather than the traditional, occlusal plane, because he contends that it better indicates overeruption of anteriors, especially the lower incisors. Beistle also uses the angle of the long axis of the upper central to the palatal plane (110—113 degrees=norm) as an indicator of flexure in the premaxilla or angulation (torque) of the upper incisors.

In its current form the Sassouni Plus represents the evolutionary end product of what was one of the first truly great orthopedically oriented cephalometric analysis systems. Created by an individual of true genius, and refined, augmented, and promulgated by yet another clinician of inspired talents, the archial analysis in the Sassouni Plus configuration stands as strong and firm today as it did over 30 years ago, when it was first produced. One of the chief reasons that its precepts are in such confluence with clinical application is that it has not become outdated like so many other "orthodontically oriented" analyses, in an age when clinicians' therapeutic prowess has been so greatly expanded along orthopedic lines. The two most noteworthy examples are the response of the Sassouni to such modern concepts as moving the maxilla orthopedically as a treatment modality and the big thing—TMJ.

In the 1980s the concept of the protruded maxilla took it pretty hard on the chin. Always thought of in older circles as justification for maxillary retraction, headgear, and Class II elastics, the myth of the protruded

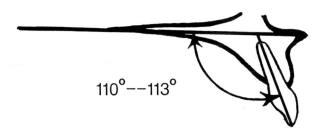

$110° - -113°$

Figure 4-23   Maxillary incisor—palatal plane angle.

maxilla was pretty well debunked, first by Luzi and then by a host of others.[59] It was discovered that 90% of the time the maxilla is either neutral or even retruded! Thus the backward-pulling-type headgears were dumped en masse by the new deciples of the FJO philosophy in favor of forward-pulling headgear (FPHG) in instances when the maxilla was determined cephalometrically (and clinically by the appearance of the upper lip in profile) to be retruded.

Beistle points out that when the location of ANS is behind the Anterior Arc, indicating a maxillary retrusion according to the Sassouni, the system's analytical precepts still stand up by virtue of the treatment options made available by the diagnostic integrity of the analysis. For example, Beistle states that the angulation of the long axis of the maxillary central incisor to the palatal plane should be 110 to 113 degrees as an indicator of the amount of "flexure" between the premaxilla and the palatal plane. Thus, if the angle is more acute and the ANS is only a

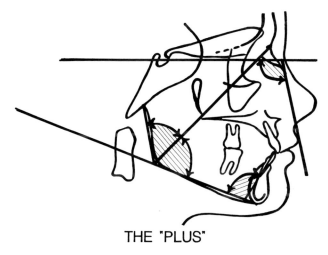

THE "PLUS"

Figure 4-24   The "Plus" added by Beistle to the original Sassouni analysis consists of three additional measurements: (1) ULA or upper lip angle, (2) split gonial angle, and (3) lower incisor—mandibular plane angle.

millimeter or so short of the Anterior Arc, the case might easily be developed forward with conventional Sagittal II techniques. Such information, provided by analysis of the area according to Sassouni's methods, would be helpful in the treatment selection for addressing anterior crossbites or Class III or pseudo-Class III situations. An acute upper incisor palatal plane angle with ANS on or very near the Anterior Arc and a mild toothy anterior crossbite is an obvious indication for Sagittal II techniques to correct. However, if the angulation of the maxillary incisor is already at or near its outer limits of 113 degrees, or the distance from ANS to the Anterior Arc is more appreciable, the clinician may be better off opting for a brief stint with FPHG first.

Again, Sassouni cephalometrics holds the key. For example, in the case of a maxillary first molar that is correctly positioned in a retruded maxilla (ANS behind the Anterior Arc) and an existing Class III skeletal and molar relationship, FPHG is an obvious treatment option. Both the molar and the maxilla need advancement to aid in correction of the case from Class III to Class I. The *corrected* Midfacial Arc would verify that the molar is in its *relatively* correct location in the maxillary bone, and the AP evaluation of the maxilla via the Anterior Arc—ANS relationship and the Cr perpendicular—PNS relationship, if equally displaced posteriorly, would reveal a retruded maxilla. Hence the opting for the FPHG becomes a viable treatment option. Yet in other instances ANS might be short of the Anterior Arc, but PNS might be right on or near enough to the Cr perpendicular to indicate a maxilla short anteriorly (premaxillary insufficiency) while the upper and lower first molars occlude in dental Class I. The FPHG would advance the maxilla, but also the entire maxillary arch, thus creating an unwanted dental Class III. Hence, concerted development of the premaxilla with Sagittal II techniques would be indicated for correction of anterior crossbite, esthetic lip support, or general Class III problems. The tip-off here is again the relative location of the upper first molar to the *corrected* Midfacial Arc.

An even more complicated situation is easily unraveled in a Class III skeletal maxillary retrusion compounded by crowding of the upper arch due to forward migration of the upper posterior quadrants. Here the upper first molar would be ahead of the *corrected* Midfacial Arc. The maxilla could be shown to be retruded by ANS—Anterior Arc/PNS—Cr perpendicular evaluation, but due to the mesial migration of the upper molars in a posteriorly displaced maxilla, they would appear correct in a dental Class I relationship with the lowers. But it is an illusion, and again Sassouni cephalometrics proves it. The upper first molars would need to be *distalized* to their correct position on the corrected Midfacial Arc, which would also relieve crowding and aid in obtaining proper arch form as a result. This would be done by conventional Sagittal I techniques in conjunction with extraction of second molars. Then FPHG may be subsequently enlisted to bring the upper arch and maxilla out of its

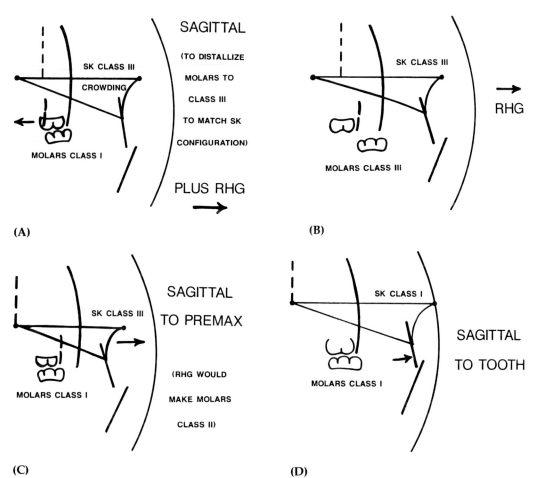

Figure 4–25   Sagittal appliance *v* reverse headgear: **(A)** Indications for *orthodontic* Sagittal II techniques to teeth only, second molars acting as anchorage. **(B)** Full-scale orthopedic forward movement of entire maxilla needed. **(C)** Indications for *orthopedic* Sagittal II techniques to premaxilla and centrals, as premaxilla is short anteriorly, while posterior quadrants are correctly situated. **(D)** Both techniques of first Sagittal I technique (second molars removed) to distalize upper molars to proper position with respect to corrected Midfacial Arc (which reveals them to be the true molar Class III they actually represent), followed by techniques to pull entire maxilla forward with forward-pulling headgear (reverse headgear, RHG) to correct distally displaced maxilla.

retrusive state back to a Class I relationship with the lower arch once again.

Such decisions are a product of the methods of cephalometric analysis in conjunction with clinical examination and model analysis, and the newer orthopedically oriented techniques now made available by FJO principles and philosophies. The technique and the philosophy are corroborated by the diagnostic implications of a cephalometric analysis employed such as the Sassouni; the two go hand in hand and one complements and verifies the other, a pretty good indication things are on the right track.

Another consideration of the Sassouni that shows how well adapted it is (and has always been) to our "orthopedically oriented age," is how it serves as a preliminary indicator of potential TMJ problems. The Sassouni analysis it must be remembered was first developed during the early 1950s at a time when orthodontists had not yet made the association of posteriorly positioned mandibles, posteriorly seated condyles, and posteriorly driven mandibular arcs of final closure with the final manifestations of such, ie, TMJ pain and dysfunction. Now that concern for this relationship is becoming paramount, it is interesting to note that the techniques of the Sassouni archial system corroborate the postulates of the FJO viewpoint on the issue.

Beistle proposes that the location of the Posterior Arc is closely associated with the location of the TMJ.[239] The origin of the Posterior Arc, Sp, and Go show a relationship to TMJ status that Beistle has observed empirically such that he feels the location of Go *relative to age*, to the Posterior Arc is a harbinger of potential TMJ problems. Evaluation of the location of Pog to the Anterior Arc assists in this process also. As previously stated, Go should fall on the Posterior Arc at age 12. Prior to age 12, it is found progressively *in front* of the Posterior arc. Past age 12, Pog is found progressively posterior to the arc. Thus it may be inferred that if Go is already past the Posterior Arc *prior* to age 12 or is considerably past it *at* age 12, a posteriorly displaced mandible may be present, ie, displaced relative to the location of the condyle in the fossa upon full closure (which is when the x-ray is taken). One could conceivably have a normal sized mandible that is grossly displaced posteriorly as in a classic Class II, Division 1, deep bite situation. Another possibility is that one might observe a slightly larger than normal mandible that is in a "housed" Class III situation with its extra length being exhibited "out the back" due to anterior incisal interference trapping the mandibular arc of final closure posteriorly, thereby forcing the condyles to seat posteriorly and merely giving the illusion things are fine anteriorly. This is why, as Beistle points out, a seeming skeletal Class I maxillomandibular relationship can actually "jointwise" be a skeletal Class II TMJ problem in disguise.

Again, Sassouni cephalometrics helps solve the riddle. For example, in the case where the maxilla and mandible are in skeletal Class I relative to A-point and B-point alignment, ie, both on the Basal (A-point) Arc, just because Pog is on the ANS Arc does not obviate TMJ problems of the retrusive mandibular arc of closure type. If ANS is severely retruded enough, even though Pog may lie on the ANS Arc, the condyles may be forced posteriorly enough during occlusion to cause TMJ-type symptoms. Regardless of the source of a mandibular/condylar retrusion, the victimized bilaminar zones do not know the difference in causes; they merely feel the net effects.

In the above example the retruded maxilla (ANS posterior to the Anterior Arc) is to blame. It falsely gives the impression that the mandible is skeletal Class I with respect to it because Pog is on or near the maxilla's own ANS Arc. But the joints suffer because the arc of mandibular closure is experiencing the NRDM-SPDC phenomenon (due to the shorter maxilla with its maxillary dental interfering guiding planes forcing the occluding mandible back). So as far as the joints are concerned, the case is a severely retruded skeletal Class II. It might as well be a Class II, Division 2, deep bite case, for the effects on the joints would be the same. The net result is the same, ie, condyles displaced posteriorly off the heel of the disc upon full closure transmitting all those powerful vectors of shock to the bilaminar zone instead of the shock-absorbing disc.

Alignment of A-point and B-point on the *posteriorly displaced* Basal Arc is no indication everything is fine back in the joint area. Aligning a mandible on the AP plane with a retruded maxilla still results in a retruded mandible, even though they both may appear Class I anteriorly. It is again an illusion, and the joints will say so eventually. In such cases of maxillary retrusion, cephalometrics gives the clinician several treatment options also. First, if the maxilla and mandible are retruded by the same amount, the cause of the Class I illusion, and if the mesial surface of the upper first permanent molar is tangent to the noncorrected Midfacial Arc, the maxilla is probably just short in the premaxillary area. The molars often reflect this by virtue of a dental Class II arrangement of some degree. The maxilla is usually not displaced posteriorly, as indicated by the location of PNS relative to the Cr perpendicular. Therefore, treatment often takes the form of merely developing the premaxillary area forward with conventional Sagittal II techniques followed by advancement of the trapped mandible forward with appliances like the Bionator, much to the relish of both the TM joints and the facial profile.

In a more serious case of maxillary retrusion where the PNS−Cr perpendicular/ANS−Anterior Arc comparison divulges a full scale maxillary retrusion, more powerful orthopedic measures may be needed. The molars may be aligned in dental Class I, further adding to the illusion, but this is due to the severe retrusion of the whole maxilla and maxillary dental arch back past an already retruded mandible (retruded at least as

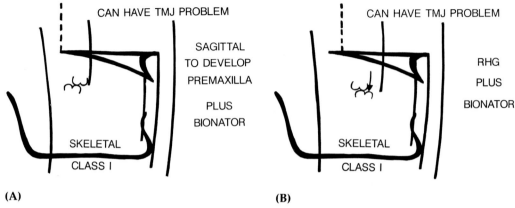

(A)   **(B)**

Figure 4−26   Why skeletal Class I cases can have a TMJ problem due to a retruded mandibular arc of closure. **(A)** Retruded mandible is housed under equally retruded maxilla; therefore, they appear Class I relative to each other, but arc of closure can be retruded enough to force condyle off back edge of disc. Proximity of maxillary first molar to Midfacial Arc indicates need for Sagittal II techniques to premaxilla followed by Bionator to advance mandible to decompress TMJs. **(B)** When maxillary first molar is distal to Midfacial Arc, the above indications call for RHG to move entire maxilla forward to enable mandible to be cleared.

Figure 4−27   Sassouni summaries of various general types of malocclusions. **(A)** In skeletal Class I cases with blocked-out cuspids, the location of the maxillary first molar mesial to the Midfacial Arc is often an indicator to extract second molars and distalize posterior quadrants with conventional Sagittal I techniques to relieve crowding. **(B)** When above situations are accompanied by a retruded mandible (gonion too far distally with respect to Posterior Arc relative to age, B-point distal to Basal Arc, pogonion distal to anterior arc), the above decrowding of the maxilla by Sagittal I techniques to obtain proper arch form (maxillary first molar on Midfacial Arc) is followed by Bionator to advance mandible out of Class II to skeletal Class I. **(C)** In Class II, Division 2 cases, when ANS is on or very near the Anterior Arc, *orthodontic* Sagittal II techniques are needed for the upper anterior teeth to obtain proper relief of Division 2 angulation followed by Bionator to advance mandible and increase vertical. **(D)** *Orthopedic* Sagittal II techniques to both teeth and premaxillary bone are needed when ANS falls 1−2 mm short of Anterior Arc. Second molars are left intact (1) as anchorage for Sagittal II technique, and since (2) upper first molars are correctly positioned next to Midfacial Arc. **(E)** In this example once premaxilla and anterior teeth are correctly positioned by Sagittal II techniques, second molars may be extracted and the remaining crowding can be relieved by distalizing upper posterior quadrants so that upper molars lie tangent to corrected Midfacial Arc.

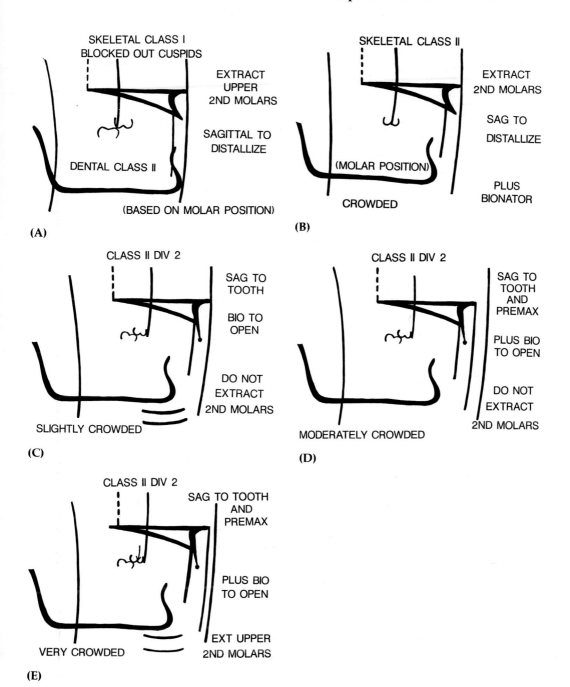

(A)

SKELETAL CLASS I
BLOCKED OUT CUSPIDS

EXTRACT
UPPER
2ND MOLARS

SAGITTAL TO
DISTALLIZE

DENTAL CLASS II

(BASED ON MOLAR POSITION)

(B)

SKELETAL CLASS II

EXTRACT
2ND MOLARS

SAG TO

DISTALLIZE

(MOLAR POSITION)

PLUS
BIONATOR

CROWDED

(C)

CLASS II DIV 2

SAG TO
TOOTH

BIO TO
OPEN

DO NOT
EXTRACT
2ND MOLARS

SLIGHTLY CROWDED

(D)

CLASS II DIV 2

SAG TO
TOOTH
AND
PREMAX

PLUS BIO
TO OPEN

DO NOT
EXTRACT
2ND MOLARS

MODERATELY CROWDED

(E)

CLASS II DIV 2

SAG TO TOOTH
AND
PREMAX

PLUS BIO
TO OPEN

EXT UPPER
2ND MOLARS

VERY CROWDED

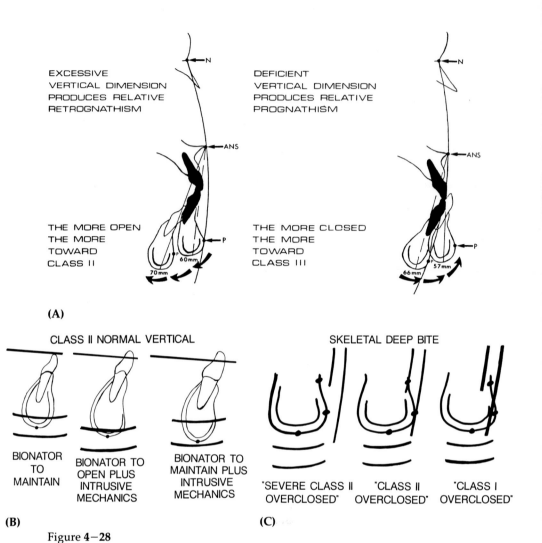

EXCESSIVE
VERTICAL DIMENSION
PRODUCES RELATIVE
RETROGNATHISM

DEFICIENT
VERTICAL DIMENSION
PRODUCES RELATIVE
PROGNATHISM

THE MORE OPEN
THE MORE
TOWARD
CLASS II

THE MORE CLOSED
THE MORE
TOWARD
CLASS III

(A)

CLASS II NORMAL VERTICAL

SKELETAL DEEP BITE

BIONATOR
TO
MAINTAIN

BIONATOR TO
OPEN PLUS
INTRUSIVE
MECHANICS

BIONATOR TO
MAINTAIN PLUS
INTRUSIVE
MECHANICS

"SEVERE CLASS II
OVERCLOSED"

"CLASS II
OVERCLOSED"

"CLASS I
OVERCLOSED"

(B)

(C)

Figure 4—28

far as the condyle/fossa relationship is concerned). The upper molar may also be found to be distal to the noncorrected Midfacial Arc. Here FPHG may be needed initially to (1) align the maxilla properly with respect to the cranial base, (2) to bring ANS out closer to the Anterior Arc, (3) to free up the posteriorly trapped mandible, and, in so doing, (4) to cause the Class II dental and skeletal arrangement to be revealed for what it actually is. Once accomplished, further treatment to advance a mandible that temporarily appears to have been "left behind" delivers the case out of its retrusive condylar state, once again much to the delight of the TMJs and the improvement of the facial profile.

In all the above situations, the location of Go will be more posterior than normal *relative to age* with respect to the Posterior Arc! More specific determinations such as the transcranial radiographic technique are available today for a more definite diagnosis of joint status. But the location of Go with respect to the Posterior Arc, along with analysis of other Sassouni components, may be found to augment the general implications of diagnostic conclusions derived from other clinical means.

Another important consideration comes into play here concerning something intimately related to TMJ problems as well as to mandibular advancement, the vertical. It is here that the unique attributes of the Sassouni arcs again show their value. When the vertical is increased, B-point and Pog will change position, since the mandible rotates back as the vertical dimension of occlusion increases. This would cause them to increase their horizontal distance from a given vertical reference line such as the N vertical, facial plane, etc. This would change the numerical and angular value of their relationships to various points of reference; therefore, the diagnostician would have to reevaluate these changes with respect to the overall status of the case. However, techniques that merely increase the vertical alone have no effect on the relationships of B-point to the Basal Arc or of Pog to the ANS Arc (when used) or the Anterior Arc. If either is "right on," then as the vertical is therapeutically increased these points will usually keep fairly close to their same relative location with respect to their respective arcs as the rotation of the mandible moves down and back on its own arc. Conversely, if they are abnormal with respect to their respective arcs, a change in vertical alone will not usually alter their archial relationship a great deal. This makes for a clearer, more dependable cephalometric "picture" as to what will be involved in treating a given case when orthopedic relocation of the mandible and changes in vertical are needed.

In spite of being developed over 30 years ago, the Sassouni Analysis has a definite contribution to make in modern orthopedically oriented cephalometric diagnosis. It is not a perfect system—no system is. Yet the insights and diagnostic information it is capable of providing make its future in the orthodontic diagnostic world a certainty.

> *"Hats off, gentlemen. A genius!"*
> *19th-century German Romantic composer*
> *Robert Schumann's critique upon first*
> *hearing young Frederic Chopin's set of*
> *variations for piano and orchestra of*
> *Mozart's duet from* Don Giovanni, *"La ci*
> *darem la mano," composed 1827.*

THE MCNAMARA ANALYSIS

The McNamara cephalometric analysis was developed by Dr J. A. McNamara at the Center for Human Growth and Development at the University of Michigan. It is heavily weighted in favor of orthopedic and facial relationships. It is also a composite analysis, since it draws on work of previous investigators. However, important portions of this system were developed by McNamara himself. This fine system relies primarily upon linear measurements rather than angular measurements. The normative ranges have undergone some slight modifications since the original development of the analysis in 1984.[240] One of its main attractions as an orthopedically oriented system is its built-in recognition of the importance of vertical dimension. It also devotes particular attention to the horizontal growth patterns of both the maxilla and the mandible. This is of prime importance to practitioners capable of employing current FJO techniques. It also has methods built into it for determining anterior tooth positioning, yet remains sensitive to the fact that the basal portions of bone in which these teeth reside might change in position as a result of treatment. It is a relatively simple system, easy to use and understand. It relates the teeth not only to each other, but to their respective jaws, which in turn may be related to one another, and the entire tooth-jaw complex may in turn be related to the cranial base.

Its reference norms are also a composite derived from three main samples of excellent research data. The first sample from which data was drawn was the famous Bolton standards of dentofacial growth.[241] The second source of information was a group of "normal" children that composed the longitudinal study of the Burlington Orthodontic Research Centre. The final group consisted of what has become known as the Ann Arbor Group, made up of 111 young adults, all of whom, in the opinion of McNamara and others, possessed good or excellent facial configurations. This selective process aims to produce a standard of normality that will eventually be used as a yardstick of abnormality and even serve as a treatment goal.[242] However, on a purely scientific and statistical level, the sample has a built-in bias, but then sometimes statistical biases are perfectly acceptable. It is a system that will also freely accept additions of other measurements a clinician may wish to incorporate from other analyses. It is concerned with relationships and relative comparisons of ranges of normative values rather than with specific numerical values. For the practitioner looking for an expedient system that is totally compatible with his modern orthodontic treatment capabilities and that will allow him to unleash the full power of his functional appliances and active plates, the McNamara is the ticket.

An ingenious marvel of simplicity, this analysis relies on only three reference lines, seven linear measurements, and one angle, with one small easily performed clinical measurement made directly on the patient. Its main reference baseline is that which has now become the resurrected "darling" of the cephalometric world, the old Frankfort Horizontal. The system does require a very high quality cephalogram. Since the Frankfort plane is predicated on the accurate location of *anatomical* porion, because, as McNamara points out, machine porion may be as much as 1 cm off, and since the two important measurements for the effective lengths of the maxilla and the mandible require the detailed imaging of the TMJ, adequate levels of x-ray penetration of the deep bony structures of the skull are paramount. Hence, the use of a soft tissue shield, either hand-held or cassette-mounted, is mandatory. The soft tissue shield allows the deeper structures of the skull to be properly exposed while protecting the structures of less density such as the nose, lips, and ANS from being "burned out" on the film. Since the amount of radiation absorbed by target objects is strictly additive, it makes no difference whether the shield is held by the patient on either side of the nose relative to the film or attached directly to the exposed side of the film cassette.

The McNamara analysis may be roughly divided into five major categories of cephalometric relationships.

I. Relationship of the maxilla to the cranial base
II. Relationship of the maxilla to the mandible
III. Relationship of the maxillary central incisor to the maxilla
IV. Relationship of the mandibular central incisor to the mandible
V. Relationship of the mandible to the cranial base

In addition, the McNamara also considers the relative lower face height and the relationship of the maxillary central incisor to the upper lip. Of the seven linear measurements, three are major in length: the effective length of the maxilla, the effective length of the mandible, LFH ANS-Me. Of the remaining four, three are measured to one reference line, the N-perpendicular, while the fourth is measured against a line connecting points A and B. The only angle involved is an outline of the soft tissue nasolabial angle and is usually described as either acute or obtuse.

Once class, according to Angle, and facial type are determined by other means, the McNamara may be called upon for determination of what specific areas are guilty of dysplasia. Thus a case may be described not only as, say, an Angle Class II, which is merely a tooth-to-tooth designation, but also as having maxillary skeletal or dental protrusions and mandibular skeletal or dental retrusions with or without LFH discrepancies. The art of classifying malocclusions has come a long way since 1900.

Relationship of the Maxilla to the Cranial Base

The first observation made in the McNamara analysis is that of its only regularly observed angle, the nasolabial angle formed between the soft tissue outline of the inferior border of the midnasal septum and the filtrum of the upper lip in norma lateralis. The measurement of this angle often helps determine the answer to the question, "Is the whole maxilla in the correct location relative to the cranial base?" The general range of this angle is between 90 and 110 degrees, and most of the time the soft tissue outline and the underlying bony structures in this area are responsible for it and will correspondingly coincide. However, when they do not, McNamara feels it is better to use the soft tissue outline as the indicator of whether the maxilla is protruded or not relative to the cranial base. Should the angle be obtuse, above 110 degrees, it is generally indicative of a maxillary prognathism or dentoalveolar protrusion. But if the angle is more acute, falling below 90 degrees, it is often indicative of a wholesale maxillary retrusion. However, maxillary prognathisms turn out to be extremely rare.

The next relationship to be evaluated requires the use of two of the three major reference lines. The first is the base reference line of the system, the FH plane. It runs from the superior aspect of anatomical P to the inferior aspect of the orbit, or a point halfway between the two inferior borders, should both orbits appear on the film. McNamara makes special note of the importance of using anatomical P, not machine P. Because of compression of soft tissues in the external auditory meatuses by the ear rods of the cephalostat, the two may differ by as much as 1 cm.

He also points out a mistake that is often made in locating anatomical P. One must be careful not to confuse the radiographic image of actual anatomical P, which is the outline of the *external* auditory meatus, with that of the *internal* auditory meatus, which is smaller (about half the size) and located posterior and superior to external auditory meatus. As the ear canal travels from the external opening through the side of the temporal bone, it gently curves superiorly and posteriorly as it approaches the tympanic cavity. This is why physicians wishing to examine the eardrum pull the auricle (external ear) upward, backward, and laterally to straighten out the cartilaginous lining of the meatus to make the direct inspection of the tympanic membrane through a speculum possible. It is this curved pathway through the bone that causes the internal auditory meatus to appear superior and posterior to machine and anatomical P. Should it mistakenly be used as the posterior reference point for the Frankfort plane, the entire analysis will be inaccurate, making the patient appear more protrusive in the maxilla and mandible than is actually so. Thus it may be seen that the accurate location of anatomical P is critical to this analysis. Often it is merely a crescent-shaped or semilunar shadow appearing over the top and slightly posterior to machine P. Sometimes machine P obliterates it altogether, in which case, since the two coincide, machine P may be used.

Once the FH plane is established, the next important line to be drawn is the N-perpendicular. A line is drawn from N perpendicular to the Frankfort plane down past the level of Pog. Three important relationships will be analyzed relative to this reference line: the positions of the maxilla, mandible, and maxillary central incisor. Right now, we are concerned with just the relationship of the maxilla to the cranial base.

McNamara relates the maxilla to the cranial base by noting the position of A-point relative to the N-perpendicular. He states that A-point should fall directly on the vertical line in the average 9-year-old, and 1 mm in front of it in the average adult. He assigns a range of ±2 mm in front of or behind the N-perpendicular in which A-point may fall and still be considered reasonably normal. The age of the patient should be a mitigating factor in this range. If A-point falls posterior to the N-perpendicular, the difference, expressed in millimeters, is given as a negative number. If A-point falls anterior to the N-perpendicular, the linear difference in millimeters is expressed as a positive number. This then relates A-Point to N along a standardized vertical line, which is the same as horizontally relating the entire maxilla to the cranial base.

McNamara goes on to point out that Class II patients with maxillary skeletal retrusion often exhibit a steep mandibular plane angle, a more rounded or convex facial profile, a more obtuse or open nasolabial angle, and a characteristic "bump" on the bridge of the nose. This, he believes, is only a result of the maxillomandibular retrusive dysplasia. The nasal osteology remains relatively fixed anteroposteriorly, but as the maxilla and mandible are underdeveloped around it, meaning A-point and Pog are far posterior to the N-perpendicular, the nasal area is left behind relatively "high and dry," causing the characteristic nasal contour. Unless treated, this phenomenon will remain, since both N and A-point move forward at about the same rate during growth and development.

McNamara also points out that there are times when the position of A-point must be corrected before it may be meaningfully analyzed relative to the N-perpendicular. The first is in cases of severe mid- and upper-facial horizontal dysplasia, as in certain Class III types. When this type of facial structure is observed and is obvious clinically, it must be remembered that this will cause N to be retropositioned. This would cause both

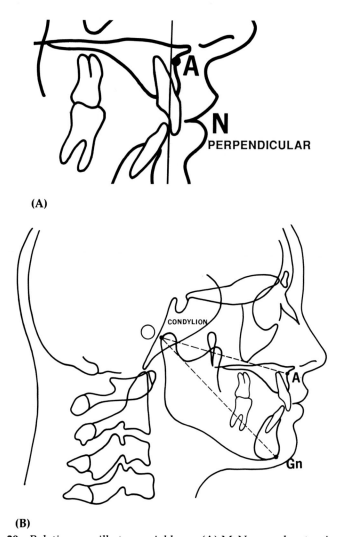

(A)

(B)

Figure **4–29**   Relating maxilla to cranial base: **(A)** McNamara locates A-point or the nasion perpendicular in the 9-year-old and 1 mm in front of it in the adult. Range of normality: ±2 mm in front or behind N-perpendicular. **(B)** McNamara relates the size of the maxilla to the mandible by means of "effective" lengths after Harvold. Here the proportional difference is the key, not the actual lengths per se.

the maxilla, at A-point, and the mandible, at Pog, to appear to be more forward than they actually are. Second, in cases of severe Class II, Division 2 malocclusions, A-point might be forced forward by the severe labial root torque of the maxillary central incisors. This would cause A-point to appear to be located closer to the N-perpendicular than it actually is, giving a false impression that the maxilla is more protruded than it really is. McNamara advises, in such circumstances, correcting the position of A-point by moving it posteriorly by 1 to 2 mm. This is an excellent example of the beauty of this cephalometric analysis system: It is not bound by numerical or pedagogical rigidity; hence in instances such as the two mentioned above, it does not lose its validity. The corrections necessary to compensate for such problems are also extremely easy to effect.

Relationship of the Maxilla to the Mandible

McNamara relates the maxilla and mandible to each other by comparing their effective linear lengths after Harvold.[243, 244] Here the overall relative proportions are what is important, as opposed to comparison with pre-established numerical statistical norms. This represents both scientifically and statistically a sounder analytical approach with respect to these issues. (The recommendations of the Second Cephalometric Workshop finally begin to bear fruit.) So far, the lengths of the maxilla and mandible have been referred to as "effective" lengths, because McNamara defines the effective length as the length measured from *condylion* to A-point for the maxilla, and *condylion* to anatomical Gn for the mandible.

In the average 9-year-old the effective length of the maxilla is established at 85 mm, with a corresponding effective mandibular length of 105–108 mm. In the adult female the proportions are 94 mm for the maxilla and 120–123 for the mandible. In the adult male the proportions are 100 mm for the maxilla and 130–133 for the mandible. But what is astounding about these values is that their relative differences just about stay the same throughout the growth and development of the individual! That is, in the 9-year-old the difference between 85 mm and 105–108 mm is 20–23 mm. This represents the proportional difference between the two measurements for that age group regardless of what the actual measurements are. This allows for size variation from individual to individual. If some 9-year-old's effective maxillary length is 82 mm, the corresponding effective length of the mandible should be 102–105 mm. Or if the maxillary measurement is 88 mm, the mandibular should be expected to be 108–111 mm.

The same holds true for the adult female proportional ratio. The difference between the effective length of the maxilla, 94 mm, and the effective length of the mandible, 120–123 mm, is 26–29 mm. This proportional ratio should be expressed in any well-balanced face. If an adult female has a maxillary measurement of 90 mm, the effective length of the mandible may be expected to be 116–119 mm. If it were a 95-mm maxillary measurement, the mandible should stretch out to 121–124 mm.

In the adult male the difference is 30—33 mm. Thus an adult male's maxillary measurement of 102 mm would predict a mandibular measurement of 132—135 mm, etc. The proportions stay the same; hence relationships, not numbers, are important. These relationships are summarized in the table.

Case	Maxillomandibular Differential (mm)
Mixed dentition	20—23
Adult female (medium-sized person)	26—29
Adult male (large-sized person)	30—33

It is then obvious that should a discrepancy arise between the effective lengths of the maxilla and mandible, the question that presents itself is, "Which of the two is at fault, or are both?" We have already seen how to determine if the maxilla is either retrusive or protrusive by relating A-point to the N-perpendicular. A similar method (discussed later) is utilized for determining the degree of dysplasia in the mandible, if any, involving the relationship of Pog to the N-perpendicular. Thus it may be seen that by determining the cephalometric relationships of the maxilla and mandible to the cranial base, one may determine which of the two, or if both, are incorrect and by a relative number of millimeters when one considers their relative proportional lengths.

Another important factor that has a direct bearing on effective maxillary and mandibular lengths is vertical dimension. This dimension is measured from the ANS to Me and, like the effective lengths of the maxilla and mandible, it increases with age during the periods of growth and development.

McNamara takes special care to point out how critical the LFH is in the significance of the effective mandibular length and the assignment of class according to Angle. The LFH can even mask various problems, resulting in improper interpretation of the cephalogram with resultant incorrect diagnosis. The LFH is nothing more than a way of expressing, to a major extent, the amount of rotation exhibited by the mandible. If a mandible of a given length is in a situation where the bite is very closed with a relatively short ANS-Me LFH, it is, in effect, rotated very far upward on the arc or closure. This would bring the tip of the chin, Pog, out quite far on the horizontal plane. In so doing, it would give the illusion that the chin or whole body of the mandible is longer or more prominent than it actually would be if it were at the increased and more correct vertical dimension of occlusion.

Conversely, if a mandible of the same given length is in a situation where the bite is extremely open with a relatively long ANS-Me LFH, the same sized mandible would be rotated very far downward on the arc of closure. This in turn would bring the tip of the chin, Pog, quite far back

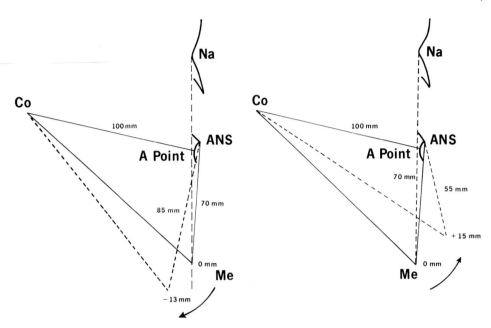

Figure 4−30   Horizontal location of menton can vary with changes in vertical dimension (rotation of the mandible) at almost a 1 to 1 ratio; ie, for every millimeter the vertical is *increased*, menton moves back about 1 mm on the horizontal plane; and for every millimeter the vertical is *decreased*, menton moves forward approximately 1 mm relative to the horizontal plane.

relative to the horizontal plane. This would give the illusion that the chin, or the whole body of the mandible, is shorter or less prominent than it actually would be if it were at a decreased, more correct vertical dimension. This critical vertical dimension is simply measured ANS-Me! (Note: Me is used for these purposes rather than M to avoid confusion with the mandible, which uses this symbol in such designation as the IMPA, as used by Tweed.)

McNamara lists the ideal values for ANS-Me LFH in the well-balanced individual. For the 9-year-old with the effective maxillary length of 85 mm, the ANS-Me should be 60−62 mm. For the adult female with the 93-mm effective maxillary length, ANS-Me should register 66−68 mm. And for the large adult male with the 100-mm maxillary measurement, ANS-Me should be 70−74 mm. Between 9 years old and adulthood the LFH increases steadily from the 60−62-mm range on to the 66−68-mm or 70−74-mm range for adult females or males, respectively.

These three measurements—effective length of maxilla, effective length of mandible, and ANS-Me LFH—are critical to the practitioner intending to employ the services of a functional appliance such as a Bionator in a treatment plan for a given individual. Appliances such as the Bionator affect *both* the horizontal and vertical relationship of the mandible to the maxilla. McNamara was sensitive to these facts, and the methods of his analysis system are constructed in such a way that they reflect this awareness of modern functional appliance potential. The accompanying table summarizes these relationships.

Case	ANS-Me LFH (mm)
Mixed dentition (9-year-old)	60−62
Adult female (medium-sized person)	66−68
Adult male (large-sized person)	70−74

This point is clearly brought out by the example McNamara uses to clarify this phenomenon. In a hypothetical case let us assume A-point and Pog lie directly on the N-perpendicular and that the effective maxillary length is 100 mm. Hence, the normal mandibular measurement should be 130−133 mm. Our ANS-Me LFH is set at the conventional (and proportional) 70 mm to be expected in such a case. Now if the ANS-Me vertical dimension is increased 15 to 85 mm, the autorotation of the mandible about its condylar axis will bring Pog, the chin point, back and downward. It will move posteriorly by about 13 mm on a purely horizontal scale. Conversely, if the ANS-Me vertical dimension is decreased by 15 to 55 mm, Pog will move forward and upward due to this same autorotation of the mandible about its condylar axis. This will deliver the Pog forward by about 15 mm on a purely horizontal level.

Thus it may be seen from analyzing this phenomenon that a change in the vertical dimension, or ANS-Me LFH, has a direct effect on the position of the chin point, or Pog, relative to its position along a horizontal plane. This brings us to what may be termed "McNamara's law of pogonial positioning": For every millimeter of change in the vertical dimension, there is a correspondingly near-equal reciprocal change in the horizontal dimension of Pog. The more the vertical is closed, the more the chin appears forward. The more the vertical is opened, the more the chin seems retruded.

Upon careful reflection it may be seen how this phenomenon could make a skeletal dysplasia appear more innocent than a truly correct analysis, which considers this effect, would reveal. Take the case where an individual has a proportionally correct maxilla, a mandible long enough to place Pog 2 mm short of the N-perpendicular, but an ANS-Me LFH deficient by 8 mm. Initially it appears the mandible has adequate horizontal prominence. Not so. Once the vertical is opened to the correct AFH dimension by a bite-opening appliance such as a Bionator, if the mandible is not purposefully advanced by same, it will reveal the true extent of mandibular insufficiency once correct ANS-Me dimensions are attained. With an 8-mm increase in vertical, the autorotational effect of the mandible down and backward would in effect "pull" Pog a corresponding 8 mm posteriorly relative to the horizontal plane, thus divulging the true degree of severity of mandibular retrusion. Instead of the seeming −2 mm amount of distance from N-perpendicular, which would be perfectly acceptable, Pog is actually −10 mm posterior to the N-perpendicular, a clear skeletal Class II! McNamara emphatically points out that before one should assign a Class I, II, or III skeletal designation to a case, the lower AFH must be considered, so the true relationship of the mandible to the maxilla and cranial base may be realized.

Relationship of the Maxillary Central Incisor to the Maxilla

From the preceding it may be seen that in modern times, when wholesale repositioning of the mandible both horizontally and vertically is possible by the use of functional appliances, a system for analyzing the position of the upper incisors should *not* be predicated upon the pretreatment position of the mandible or even the cranial base.

Nowadays the maxillary central incisor position should actually be determined by the dictates of the TMJ. This concept is concerned not with the limits of protrusion of the maxillary centrals but with the limits of retrusion. An excessive retrusion of maxillary anteriors, or even moderate or no retrusion, coupled with the right amount of protrusion of the mandibular incisors can add up to an untoward combination that effects just enough of a retruded mandibular arc of closure to cause the condyles to slip off the back edge of the intraarticular discs and seat themselves on the anterior edges of the bilaminar zones, thus precipitating the classic TMJ symptomatology. How far anteriorly maxillary anteriors may be acceptably positioned should be governed by esthetics and other factors. But how far lingually they may be safely positioned should be strictly governed by the mandibular arc of closure and its effects on the TMJs.

Now it may be seen why relating the maxillary anteriors to landmarks in the pretreatment mandible, either dental or osseous, is doubly fallacious. McNamara points out correctly that one would be remiss to relate the position of the maxillary centrals to something like the A-Pog line, as does Ricketts, since (1) the mandible may be moved during treatment (forward by functional appliance treatment), and (2) in a majority of cases the mandible is retruded in the pretreatment dental Class II case! Instead the upper centrals should be related to a set of standardized reference points between the dentition and the maxilla as a whole. This is exactly what the McNamara analysis does, and rightly so. The standardized reference point for analysis of the position of the maxillary central incisors is a second vertical line drawn this time from A-point on a perpendicular to FH. This line would, by necessity, also be parallel to the N-perpendicular. Another short line is drawn parallel to the A-perpendicular tangent to the most anterior part of the crown of the maxillary central incisor. The distance measured horizontally from the

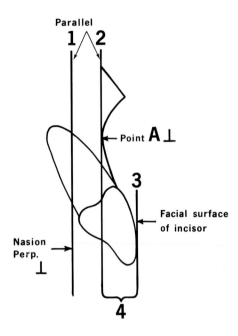

Parallel

1 2

← Point **A** ⊥

3

Facial surface
of incisor →

Nasion
Perp. →

4

Figure 4–31   McNamara norm for linear distance from facial surface of maxillary central to A-point perpendicular, range 4–6 mm. This locates the upper central incisor relative to the maxillary apical base. A-point perpendicular is parallel to N-perpendicular.

facial surface of the central to the A-perpendicular in a well-balanced face should be 4–5 mm. This value is expressed as a positive value. Should the upper centrals be retroclined so severely as to cause the facial surface of the crown to fall posterior to the A-perpendicular, the linear horizontal distance in millimeters between the two is expressed as a negative number.

A second factor concerning the vertical position of the upper central incisor is also considered by the McNamara, but is a little on the arbitrary side, since it must deal with certain anatomical characteristics that are beyond the control of the clinician. According to McNamara, the incisal edge of the upper central should be exposed by 2–3 mm below the edge of the upper lip. But unusually long or short upper lips would bias this factor. Other things such as the level of the occlusal plane and the AFH should also be considered. Another factor to consider is that it is extremely difficult to intrude teeth in some instances, and some practitioners feel that true intrusion is nearly impossible and only root resorption is affected when such is attempted.

Relationship of the Mandibular Central Incisor to the Mandible

McNamara borrows freely from the analysis system of Ricketts for the horizontal determination of the position of the lower incisors.[72, 235] If the mandible is already in a satisfactory position, the facial surface of the crown of the most forward lower central may be compared to a line

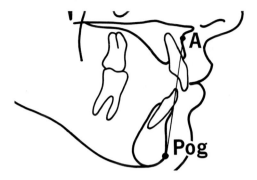

Figure **4—32**   McNamara relates the tip of the lower incisor to the old A-Pog line, range 2—3 mm (2.3—2.7 Ann Arbor, 1—3 Ricketts).

drawn from A-point to Pog (A-Pog line). In a well-balanced face, the facial surface of the mandibular incisor should be 2—3 mm anterior to the A-Pog line. If so, this value is expressed as a positive number. If it falls posterior to the A-Pog line, the value is expressed as a negative number. But this method is valid only if the mandible is to remain in its original pretreatment position. If it is going to be relocated by either growth or functional appliances at some point during treatment, this method of analysis must be modified. There are two ways of doing this.

First, one may use the template method. A tracing of the mandible with its lower incisor is made and repositioned ideally against the maxilla. A new corrected A-Pog line is drawn, and the lower central is evaluated with respect to the "created" A-Pog line in the newer positional relationship. A second, easier, method advocated by McNamara is to estimate the number of millimeters the mandible will be advanced by growth or functional appliance treatment and to move the location of A-point posteriorly along a horizontal plane by the correspondingly same amount. Thus a new A-Pog relationship similar to that which will exist at the end of treatment is effected. A new A-Pog line is drawn and the position of the lower central is evaluated. This method eliminates the tedious process of constructing a mandibular template. Thus whether the mandible is considered stationary or subject to change in position, the horizontal relationship of the lower central incisor may be appropriately analyzed relative to its own frame of reference, the maxilla and the mandible.

The vertical positioning of the mandibular incisors is also a function of the lower AFH as well as the functional occlusal plane. McNamara states that if there is an excessive curve of Spee, a decision must be made as to how to level the occlusal plane. Either the incisors must be intruded (a treatment infrequently seen) or the teeth in the posterior segments must be allowed to extrude. This again is a function of the amount of ANS-Me LFH present. If more vertical would be harmful to the patient, McNamara suggests attempting to intrude the lower incisors. If more

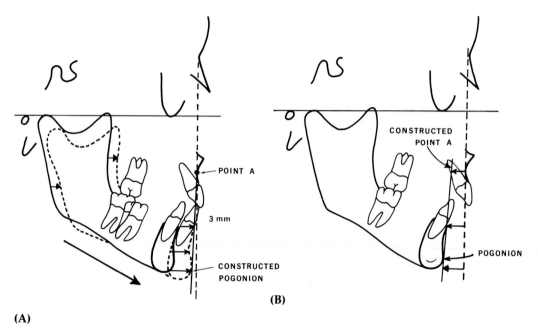

(A)

(B)

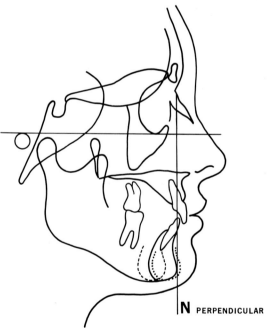

(C)

Figure 4–33   McNamara evaluated lower incisor location, as well as entire mandible, by either **(A)** advancing tracing of mandible artificially to proposed posttreatment ideal location with respect to rest of cephalogram, or **(B)** by construction of artificial A-point (thereby producing new AP line). The artificial A-point is created by moving it posteriorly by about the amount the mandible will need to be advanced by treatment. **(C)** Range of normality for location of pogonion to N-perpendicular is −8 to −6 mm mixed dentition, −4 to 0 mm for adult females, and −2 to 2 mm for adult males.

vertical would be beneficial to the patient because this dimension is initially deficient of the normal amount required due to a deep bite, one would obviously wish to extrude posterior segments with bite-opening appliances such as the Bionator.

Relationship of the Mandible to the Cranial Base

By now it has become clear that one would not want to relate the mandible to a reference point such as the maxilla, which may be long or short and changeable with treatment in this orthopedic appliance age. Instead the mandible should be related to a standardized reference in something far more stable, such as the cranial base. It would also be obvious that one would hope to be able to relate the mandibular position to the dictates of the TMJ. So far we have only been able to do this to a limited extent. Fortunately a cephalometrically proper and balanced mandibular position often goes hand in hand with a proper and balanced TMJ. The status of the joint upon full occlusion of the teeth is a simple product of how retruded or protruded is the all-important mandibular arc of (final) closure. And that is a product of the length and position of the mandible and where the collision maxillary and mandibular teeth force it to go.

At the time the McNamara analysis was devised, the chief concern was merely relating the mandible correctly to the cranial base. Temporomandibular joint demands on the mandibular arc of closure were not given precedence. McNamara analyzes the position of the mandible by relating the chin point of the mandible, Pog, to the standardized N-perpendicular. This reference line is excellent for analyzing the position of the maxilla as a whole and serves equally well as a reference point for the mandible. The linear distance in millimeters is measured horizontally from Pog to the N-perpendicular. The normal range for this value, depending on age and sex of the individual is −8 to +2 mm. If Pog falls posterior to N-perpendicular, the value is expressed as a negative number. If Pog falls anterior to the line, the value is positive. The well-balanced 9-year-old would show a Pog-N-perpendicular distance of −8 to −6 mm. A mid-teen or medium-sized individual may show a value of −4 to 0 mm. And the full-grown, large adult male may have a measurement of −2 to +2 mm. Again, one must consider the ANS-Me anterior LFH when analyzing the value of the position of Pog relative to N-perpendicular. The table summarizes these relationships.

Case	Pogonion to Nasion Perpendicular (mm)
Mixed dentition	−8 to −6
Adult female (medium-sized person)	−4 to 0
Adult male (large-sized person)	−2 to +2

McNamara also analyzes the airway as depicted on the lateral cephalogram. He is an expert on the effects of airway constricture on the growth and development of the maxillofacial complex, and has performed outstanding research in this area on laboratory animals. He looks at two main areas for possible airway problems.

First, he checks the upper pharynx by measuring the distance from a point on the posterior border of the soft palate to the nearest point on the outline of the posterior pharyngeal wall. Should the measurement be 3 mm or less, it is suggestive of a *possible* airway constriction. It must be stressed that this is not definitive of airway impairment, since the cephalogram is only a two-dimensional situation. Only our colleagues in otolaryngology may make such a diagnosis, and only after careful clinical examination. Such may not be accurately determined from a lateral x-ray. Constricture, when it exists, is often due to enlargement of adenoid tissues. These tissues may enlarge steadily until puberty, when they generally regress. But by then the damage to the balanced growth and development of the bones of the maxillofacial complex may have already been done. McNamara has shown experimentally that deliberately obturated airways in rhesus monkeys brought about every type of skeletal malocclusion imaginable. Careful consideration of this problem and consultations with medical colleagues is needed to bring maximum clarity to the situation in an individual clinical case. Caution should also be exerted in the interpretation of this measurement because the patient may have been swallowing when the x-ray was taken. If so, the outline of the soft palate on the film assumes the shape of an inverted V. McNamara warns that this would obviously bias the measurement in this instance to the point where the value expressed may be nullified.

The lower pharynx is analyzed by drawing a line from the point where the posterior border of the tongue crosses the inferior border of the mandible to the closest point on the posterior pharyngeal wall. This measurement should average about 10–12 mm. However, McNamara states that lower values than 10–12 mm are "not remarkable." Should the values be greater than 15 mm, he suggests this represents forward positioning of the tongue due to large tonsils or habit. This would be an important finding in such cases as skeletal Class III's, anterior crossbites, or bimaxillary protrusion.

McNamara is fond of using two other items in his analysis, which he borrows from other analyses: (1) the mandibular plane angle (from mandibular plane to Frankfort plane) and (2) the Y-axis (growth axis). McNamara uses the growth axis of Ricketts,[245] the ideal of which is a 90-degree angle between the base reference line, N to Ba, and a line drawn from the posterior superior aspect of the PTM fissure to anatomical Gn. (This is actually referred to by Ricketts as the XY axis or facial axis. Either method of determining the growth axis angle [from the Downs, the angle between S-Gn and the Frankfort plane or from the Bjork, the angle between S-Gn and S-N] works just as well in this determination because each describes the same concept but uses different base reference lines.)

Expected Changes during Growth and Development

McNamara also lists some of the changes that may be expected during growth and development of the individual. This information is helpful to those studying serial head films and is useful for treatment-planning considerations.

1. The *total* AFH (N-Me) increases at a rate of about 1 mm per year.
2. The effective length of the mandible increases at a rate of about 2−3 mm per year.
3. The effective length of the maxilla increases at a rate of about 1−2 mm per year.
4. The distance from Pog to the N-perpendicular decreases by 0.5−1.0 mm per year.
5. The mandibular plane angle decreases by approximately 1 degree every 3 years.

A handy rule of thumb to remember the rates of growth of various key areas of the maxillofacial complex is the "rule of 1-2-3" of growth of the ANS-Me AFH, maxilla, and mandible. Growth rates vary with age and sex. In females, maxillary and mandibular growth takes place rather steadily until about 13 to 14 years of age, at which time, due to the onset of menses and the appearance of estrogens into the system, growth falls off dramatically. Female hormones such as estrogens have a definite braking effect on the bone growth process. However, in males, growth progresses steadily throughout adolescence into young adulthood with a growth spurt occurring between the ages of 12 and 16. This type of information is obviously important to the orthopedic treatment-planning portions of a case.

McNamara also advocates a particular order for superimposition of tracings to analyze treatment and for growth changes similar to the method of Ricketts. First, he superimposes over the internal structures of the maxilla to study individual changes in tooth position. Second, he superimposes along N-Ba (Huxley's old line) at N to analyze the movement of the maxilla as a whole. Third, he superimposes over the internal structures of the mandible (mandibular canal, lingual border of the symphysis, etc). Fourth, he superimposes along the cranial baseline to check the overall progress of the case. Long gone are the earlier notions that one single reference point or line can serve to superimpose the entire tracing.

Conclusions

The McNamara analysis is a product of our times. It is the result of the fulfillment of a need to expand the horizons of modern orthodontic diagnosis and treatment planning. When men of vision and intellect apply themselves to the task of addressing such needs, inadequacies and obstacles are soon forced to give way to the welcomed consolidation and advancement of understanding. It is one of the hallmarks of our science that its precepts remain dynamic and perpetually open to modifications necessitated by current demands. The McNamara fulfills the requirements of being an analysis system compatible with both fixed and removable orthodontic treatment modalities while being a model of simplicity and expediency. It also delineates between dental and skeletal discrepancies on an individual basis. This is the key to its success and is creditable to the insights and talents of the man who devised it. But others of an equal level of genius have also applied their creativity and perception to the course of events with profound and interesting results. Such a circumstance exists in the lifelong work of another great individual, Dr Hans Peter Bimler of Wiesbaden, Germany.

"Beware when the great God lets loose a
thinker on this planet."
Ralph Waldo Emerson
Essay X, "Circles"

CEPHALOMETRICS SUPREME:
THE BIMLER ANALYSIS

It would be difficult to conceive of any type of diagnostic information relative to maxillofacial orthopedia that would be routinely available on a lateral cephalometric x-ray which could not be gleaned from a case studied under the intensely scrutinizing light of the Bimler cephalometric analysis. It is a system that makes use of angles, linear measurements, arcs, and full scale anatomical relationships, as well as totally new concepts that appear in no other analysis system. Developed just after World War II and carefully cultivated over almost four decades, this analysis is a composite of voluminous amounts of meticulously recorded data that have resulted in the production of some important and well-documented cephalometric relationships.[100–103, 246, 247] Some of these relationships are

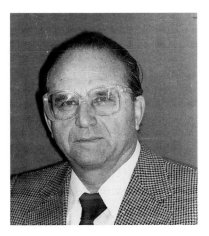

Figure 4—34   Hans Peter Bimler

observed empirically; others are categorized according to detailed mathematical boundaries. Most observations made have been commonly accepted as important and relevant. Some shed a new light on existing situations. Others are common to many other systems. A few have proven over the years to be only vestigial. Yet the main forte of the Bimler is its detailed and comprehensive analysis of skeletal relationships. Though the dental aspects of a malocclusion receive as much attention as with any other system, if not more, it is the determined concentration on individualized as well as conglomerate structural relationships that give the Bimler analysis its brilliance. If controversy and discord were to exist between opposing viewpoints as to the actual status of a given case for diagnostic supremacy, the Bimler appears to control the exclusive rights as to the final definitive statement in lateral cephalometric analytical interpretation. The good Dr Bimler does not merely study a cephalometric radiograph, he attacks it with "furor teutonicus!"

Nomenclature

We have previously alluded to the differences in facial types as described by Bimler's terms (mesoprosopic, dolichoprosopic, leptoprosopic) and the terms used on the American side of the Atlantic (mesocephalic, dolichocephalic, and brachycephalic or brachyfacial). These differing and sometimes seemingly conflicting terms must be kept clearly in mind. Since we are discussing the Bimler analysis in its own context, for this particular portion of the text we shall confine ourselves to the use of its terminology exclusively.

But even before discussing nomenclature, we must be aware of some aspects of the Bimler on an even more basic level, the first of which is the direction of the view of the head when using this system. Bimler has degrees in both medicine and dentistry, and was a physician during World War II before turning his interests to orthodontics. Since he began his studies in this field, when the science of cephalometrics was in its infancy, he was unaware that some of the early researchers first using lateral headplate analysis in America viewed films with the patient's face to the observer's right. However, he views his films with the patient's face to the observer's left. This was common in some of the early anthropological texts of the time.

Bimler has developed all sorts of little terms and symbols used in his analysis system. He also uses many of the conventional terms such as A-point, B-point, N, S, P, M, ANS, PNS, Gn, and PTM (which he symbolizes by T). Terms peculiar to the analysis or not previously mentioned are reviewed here.

Apicale (Ap)   Tip of the root of the maxillary first bicuspid.

Capitulare (C)   The exact dead center of the cross section of the head of the condyle.

Clivus   The sloping portion of the sphenoid and occipital bones that presents itself as an outline on the lateral cephalogram running from sella turcica to the foramen magnum.

Clivion superior (Cls)   A point on the upper third of the clivus which may be either straight in outline or represented by a slight depression in that outline.

Clivion inferior (Cli)   A point on the lower third of the clivus which may be either straight in outline or represented by a slight depression in that outline.

Genion (Ge)   The most inward and everted point on the crest of the curvature of the outline of the interior symphysis of the mandible.

Mandibular plane   Bimler's mandibular plane is defined slightly different from others. He defines it as a line extending from Me to a point tangent to the highest elevation of the outline of the Antegonial Notch.

Mentale   Bimler's term for genion. (Note: Bimler abbreviates it as Me, which should not be confused with the abbreviation for menton, which is often used in American terminology. Context obviously divulges which meaning is intended.)

Notch (No)   The highest point of the outline of the Antegonial Notch on the inferior border of the mandible.

Orthogonal Reference Coordinates

The cornerstone of the entire Bimler analysis is the Orthogonal Reference System of coordinates. This reference coordinate system is composed of two major reference baselines: the vertical line through the

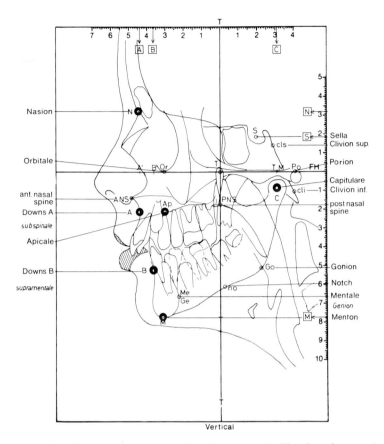

Figure **4–35**   Bimler reference points: Certain anatomical landmarks or points are specific to the Bimler analysis. Ap = apicale; T = superior point of pterygomaxillary fissure; C = center of mandibular condyle; No = superior part of curvature of Antegonial Notch; Cls = clivion superior; Cli = clivion inferior; Ge = genion or mentale, the innermost curvature of the symphysis of the mandible. (Note: Bimler uses Me for mentale, not to be confused with menton, which he symbolizes with M.); A', B' = vertical projections of A-point and B-point on the Frankfort Horizontal; TM = vertical projection of C on the FH. All other landmarks are conventional, except that Bimler uses the German spelling for "Francfort."

pterygomaxillary fissure, and the FH plane. Also included are two accessory vertical lines perpendicular to the Frankfort, one through A-point and one through C-point (capitulare in the Bimler). The vertical line through the pterygomaxillary fissure extends from a point at the center of the upper curvature of the outline of the fissure in both directions, perpendicular to the Frankfort, to the edge of the tracing. The Frankfort likewise extends horizontally across the entire tracing to the edges of the

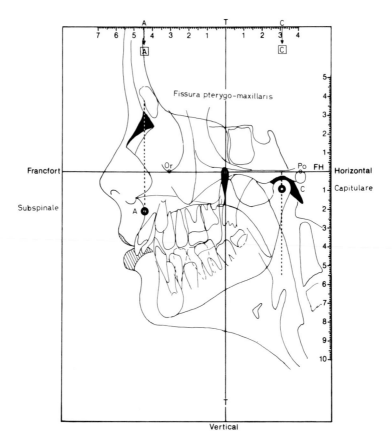

Figure **4–36** The Orthogonial Reference System with FH, PTM, A' and C'
verticals.

tracing paper. The Frankfort plane is labeled FH, and the vertical through
the pterygomaxillary fissure is written as the T vertical line or TV (for
tuber vertical). The accessory vertical line through A-point is written as
the AV and extends from A-point up past N level a short way. The
accessory vertical through C-point is written as CV and extends from FH
down through C to about the level of Go. Both AV and CV are also
perpendicular to the Frankfort plane.

Thus the Orthogonal Reference System contains one major horizontal line (the Frankfort plane), one major vertical line (T), and two
accessory vertical lines (AV and CV). The three vertical lines are all
perpendicular to the FH. The FH and TV are drawn as solid black lines.
The AV and CV are drawn in hatched *green* lines. (The color coding of
lines and its significance will be discussed shortly). The FH-TV coordinate is an ideal reference system for measurement of both angular
and linear measurements as well as superimposition techniques.

Reference Factor Lines

The core of the Bimler analysis revolves around the assessment of a series of ten anatomically oriented reference lines. Bimler calls the inclinations of these baselines "factors" and numbers them 1 through 10. He gives the individual reference lines proper names according to their respective numbers. The factors always connect two anatomical landmarks (except for Factor 6, which extends from one anatomical landmark to an imaginary one, or yet another "space mark"). They are easily constructed on the tracing. Of these ten factors, numbers 9 and 10 have proven over the years to be of no clinical significance. Yet these two vestigial lines are still traditionally included in the analysis. The special Factor 6 that includes the imaginary anatomical landmark "center of mastication" or "Centro-Masticale" (CM) will receive special attention later. But presently here is the list of the ten Bimler Factors and their subsequent designations.

Factor 1. From N to A
Factor 2. From A to B
Factor 3. From menton to a point tangent to the highest curvature of the Antegonial Notch, M-No
Factor 4. ANS-PNS palatal or maxillary plane
Factor 5. A line tangent to the clivus extending from Cli to Cls
Factor 6. From CM to Ge
Factor 7. From N to S
Factor 8. From C to Go
Factor 9. A line tangent to planum sphenoidale (a factor of no clinical significance, no longer used)
Factor 10. A line beginning at N running tangent to the nasal bone (a factor of no clinical significance, no longer used)

Now if we were to draw the Orthogonal Reference System over the tracing, with its four lines FH, TV, AV, and CV, and follow by drawing in the ten Bimler reference factors, we see that the tracing now has 14 lines on it. It may appear a bit complicated, but these lines are all that are needed for the entire system. Short hatch marks are added here and there for various linear or angular measurements, but the basis for the whole analysis is centered around these 14 lines.

Color Codes

As may be seen from the above, the tracing fills up with a considerable number of lines rather quickly in this analysis. Add in the various other incidental little lines and hatch marks, and it becomes difficult to

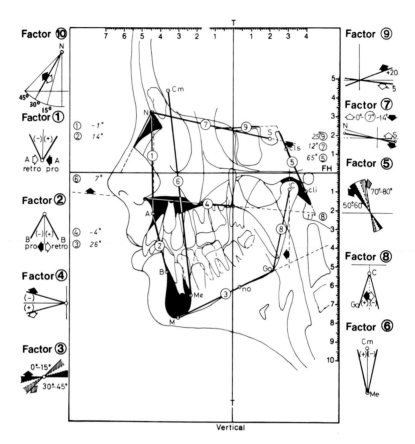

Figure 4–37   Composite drawing of Bimler Factor Analysis system. Note: Of the original 10 factors, the last two, Factor 9, sphenoidal inclination, and Factor 10, nasal inclination, are no longer considered by Bimler as clinically significant.

keep them separated and organized in the mind of the observer. To help delineate these factors, angles, reference lines, etc, more clearly, Bimler devised a color-coding system for organizational purposes. The color-coding system greatly simplifies the interpretation of the tracing. In order to represent a Bimler analysis correctly, its color coding must be strictly adhered to as follows. Initially we shall discuss only major items.

Though at first glance this color-coding system seems only to add to the confusion, after a brief period a certain familiarity is generated about these colors (the same items are always seen in the same color), and the clarity and expediency of organization of interpreting the cephalometric tracing is greatly enhanced.

Special note   The fondness for using a color-coding system for the sake of organizational purposes is not unique to Bimler. Cecil Steiner used it in the early 1950s as a method of keeping his somewhat compli-

Color-Coding System for the Bimler Analysis

Color	Designation
Black	All anatomical outlines plus the FH and TV of the Orthogonal Reference System
Green	The accessory reference lines AV and CV (hatched lines) of the Orthogonal Reference System, the curve of Spee, and the special Factor 6 or "Stress Axis," also the words dolichoprosopic, dolicho, or simply D
Red	All factor lines, except Factor 6 (Stress Axis), all numbers denoting angular measurements and the words mesoprosopic, meso, or simply M
Blue	Numbers denoting linear measurements
Yellow	The point locations of CM, Ge (mentale, Bimler), and Ap as well as the words leptoprosopic, lepto, or simply L

cated analysis system organized. He drew all lines dealing with the teeth in the maxillary arch in red, lines dealing with the mandibular teeth in green, and those dealing with the mandible itself in brown. All others were black!

Color coding also appears in history as an attribute of certain other great nonmedical German men of genius. For instance, the famous 19th-century romantic composer Richard Wagner was also partial to using color coding for a brief period early in his career. Wagner initially had no intentions of becoming a composer but originally fancied himself as a dramatist. Inspired by the works of Shakespeare, he wrote a play, while a student at the University of Leipzig, entitled *Leubald*. It was supposed to be a tragedy, but the audience almost died laughing. It was only then that Wagner decided to try his hand at musical composition. After some initial feeble efforts, he finally composed a Concert Overture. But since his musical training up to that point was less than adequate, he had difficulty managing the orchestration. So to help keep the score organized in his head, he wrote all the sheet music for the string sections of the orchestra in red ink, the brass sections in black, and the woodwinds in green! The work was premiered Christmas Eve, 1830. But as musical humorist Victor Borge wryly quipped, "...the conductor must have been colorblind because it was a flop. In fact, the audience laughed so hard you would have thought they were back at his play." But with all due respect, years later, even without the benefits of color coding, the great composer's heroic four-opera tetralogy, *Der Ring des Niebelungen*, would become a pillar of Western culture and his exquisite *Tristan und Isolde* would change the course of the evolution of classical music on this earth forever.

The Bimler analysis is essentially composed of two basic procedures: analyzing angular measurements and analyzing linear measurements. Whenever possible Bimler trys to avoid comparing the status of these measurements with preestablished norms. (And he never even attended the cephalometric workshops of the Bolton study!) He believes that norms are merely statistical averages of sample groups, which of themselves may be skewed. He questions the value of a mathematical mean relative to a given individual. What he prefers is a range of variability for cephalometric measurements, either angular or linear, and their comparison with the whole individual as to whether these given measurements either lend to harmony or disharmony for the individual patient.

The angular half of the analysis is carried out by means of the ten factors previously listed (only eight of clinical significance). Now the genius behind the use of the Orthogonal Reference System will become clear. All of the factors are lines connecting two points which vary in location. The amount of variation in the position of the two points of any one factor is expressed in the angulation of the line that connects them. But what should this factor line be angulated against? Another factor? If this were done, one could have a situation whereby a certain angle could exist between two factors without the observer being able to determine which of the two, or possibly both, were at variance. What is needed is a fixed reference base to measure factor angulation against, a base which never changes in a given case. What is needed is a standardized base reference system against which factor angulation may be compared that reveals changes or situations of factors which are solely due to their own variation and not to any changes in the base reference system itself. What is needed is a system with hopefully two *base* reference coordinates, one horizontal and one vertical, like the FH and the TV, with maybe a few supplemental lines thrown in for good measure (no pun intended)— hence the Orthogonal Reference lines: FH, TV, AV, and CV. Now factor angulation has meaning!

Not only did Bimler develop this beautiful system for measuring angles, but he even invented a clever little device to expedite the process. Some of the angles measured may be from 1 to 5 degrees and extend over a relatively short linear distance, and this makes for somewhat difficult reading of demarcations very close together on a clear plastic protractor, especially for aging eyes. The gadget Bimler uses to make this process easier is the correlometer. It looks like an ordinary protractor, but it also incorporates the principle of a T-square and millimeter rule. It has a series of concentric semicircles on it used in the determination of Factor 6.

The correlometer has two baselines. Its outermost flat edge is the outer baseline, which is a millimeter rule starting at 0 in the exact center and extending 100 mm in both directions. Above the outer baseline is the inner baseline, which forms the base for the T-square. It is bisected by a small hole directly above the 0-mm point on the *outer* baseline. There is an outer series of protractor numbers and an inner series of protractor numbers. Since the Orthogonal Reference System is itself a

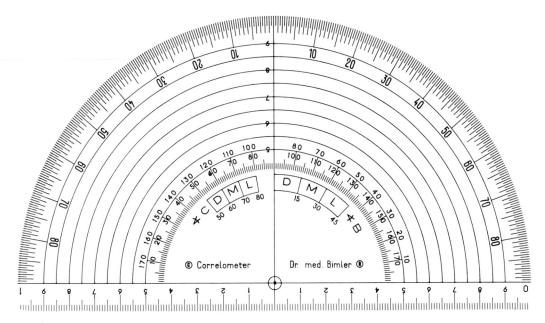

Figure 4-38   Bimler correlometer.

perpendicular set of coordinates, any line that crosses either of these coordinates may be easily measured indirectly by the correlometer and the principle of congruent angles. The principle is quite simple and easy to perform and will be more clearly understood as each factor is subsequently discussed in detail, but the rule for measuring angles indirectly with the correlometer is essentially as follows:

Place the hole of the center of the inner baseline of the T-square of the correlometer directly over the point where the factor line crosses either the FH or TV with the inner baseline directly over and along the factor line. Measure the number of degrees of angulation of either FH or TV from the 90-degree perpendicular vertical line of the T-square on either the inner or outer series of protractor numbers.

Once done, the procedure is extremely easy to repeat, and makes measuring very small angles quite easy. If desired, large angles may be measured directly, but once the observer becomes familiar with measuring angles indirectly with the correlometer and becomes accustomed to its ease of reading, the method is usually utilized for all angles.

Bimler Factor Analysis

We shall now look at the individual factors and their angular assessment, measurement, and interpretation.

Anterior Profile Angle—Factors 1 and 2   The amount of convexity or concavity of the profile of the anterior part of the face is very important with respect to facial esthetics. It is something we would definitely want to know something about, since we know we can change these configurations by orthodontic and orthopedic means. The Anterior Profile Angle, a composite of Factors 1 and 2, is represented by the union of the two factor lines in the composite line NAB and is expressed as the supplementary angle left after subtracting angle NAB (measured distally) from 180 degrees (a straight line). This line represents the extrapolation of the Factor 1 line NA. It may also be obtained by the addition of the individual values of Factors 1 and 2.

Upper Profile Angle—Factor 1   The Upper Profile Angle is expressed as Factor 1. It is composed of the line N to A-point and measured against the vertical line from A-point extrapolated perpendicular to FH up to the level of N. This perpendicular is the AV line and is drawn in green hatch marks; it is one of the aforementioned supplemental reference lines of the Orthogonal Reference System. This angle may be measured either directly, if great enough, or indirectly with the correlometer. Place the inner baseline on the factor line with the center hole of the T-square over the intersection of Factor 1 line with FH. The angle is read on the outer scale between the T-square perpendicular and FH. The Factor 1 line measurement against AV is categorized as follows:

A-point (and therefore AV) in front of N = prognathic = + angle
A-point (and therefore AV) behind N = retrognathic = − angle
A-point in line with N = no angle = orthognathic

The space in the prognathic (+) angle is colored green. The space in the retrognathic (−) angle is colored yellow.

Figure 4–39   **(A)** Bimler Upper Profile Angle. **(B)** Factor 1, or Upper Profile Angle comparison. Prognathic (Factor 1 line posterior to A vertical) is plus.
Orthognathic (Factor 1 line coincides with A vertical). Retrognathic (Factor 1 line anterior to A vertical) is minus.

Aids to Diagnosis and Treatment Planning

I.D.Quick™ superAlginate

Impression accuracy is so very important. It impacts: proper model analysis and treatment planning; the comfort, fit, and function of Appliances; how much time and materials are used up in adjustments; and overall work flow and profitability.

Put the superior qualities of I.D.Quick to work for you:

- Wets out fast — Saves time
- Heavy Body — Excellent soft tissue displacement
- Controlled Flow — Won't slump out of tray to gag patients
- Creamy Smooth Mix — Reveals superb surface detail and is most comfortable for patients—not gritty

- Excellent Strength/High Density — Avoid time lost to re-taking torn impressions
- Pure White Material — No color transfer to models
- Low Dust — Safety

Available **Spearmint** flavored, or select **Unflavored** and use our fine array of Flavoring Concentrates: Makes impression-taking a much nicer procedure for both Patients and Staff!

PACKAGING: Case of 8 1-lb. Containers, $59.10; 12-1 lb. Pail, $66.50; 22-lb. Drum, $111.50

Alginate Flavoring Concentrates

Make impression-taking a much more pleasant procedure for both Staff and Patients! Simply add a few drops to the water before mixing in the Unflavored Alginate powder.

$9.80/bottle

Specials: Buy any 5 bottles, get 1 Free
Buy any 10 bottles, get 3 FREE!

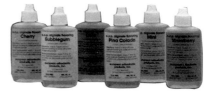

Bubblegum   Strawberry   Pina Colada   Cherry
Raspberry   Grape   Mint

Ortho Impression Trays

Fine perforated aluminum trays with high walls to give impression definition deep into the vestibule, and with non-stick coating for easy cleaning.

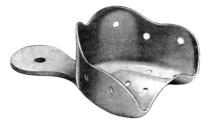

Complete range of 7 sizes each, Upper and Lower. Aluminum may be 'adjusted' to provide ideal shape. These trays work beautifully with I.D.Quick alginate.

$6.85/tray; Full Set of 14 Trays, Reg. $87.50, **Special**: $79.95

FREE BONUS: Free Box of eop Orthodontic Tray & Relief Wax with each Full Set ordered!

Snow White Orthodontic Stone

Beautiful, super strength model material. High surface hardness, low expansion. 11,000 lbs. psi compressive strength.

Ideal for: **Any models shipped** to laboratory—minimized chipping and breakage will reduce technician 'guesswork.' Improved accuracy will slash pre-insertion adjustment time. Better appliance comfort, fit, and function will result in better cooperation!

Permanent Record Models

Display Models

25-lb. Cartons, $18.10 ea.   4 Cartons, $61.40

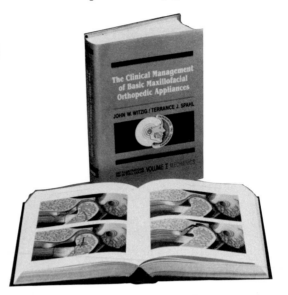

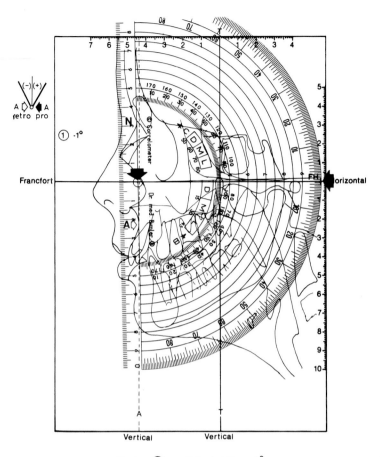

Factor ①   **N A / AV = -1°**

(A)

Prognathic ⊕   Orthognathic ±   Retrognathic ⊖

(B)

Only two circumstances are revealed by the measurement of Factor 1 alone. A high degree of positive value (A-point far ahead of N) obviously indicates a structurally protruded maxilla. (A structurally retruded N would be clearly observable clinically.) A high degree of negative value (A-point far to the rear of N) indicates a structurally retruded maxilla. Where the value of Factor 1 (Upper Profile Angle) lies is in its combined analysis with its cephalometric neighbor, Factor 2 (Lower Profile Angle).

Lower Profile Angle—Factor 2   The Lower Profile Angle is expressed as Factor 2. It is composed of the line from A-point to B-point. This line *must* be extrapolated up to FH so that the angle may be measured between this A-B line (Factor 2) and the AV reference vertical. Also, *without* drawing a line from B-point up to FH, place a small hatch mark on FH directly perpendicular over B-point. This allows for a purely linear difference in millimeters to be expressed on a horizontal basis between A-point and B-point. The point where the AV reference line crosses the FH is called A' and represents the horizontal location of A-point on the FH. Hence the hatch mark representing B-point just described is called B' and represents the horizontal location of B-point relative to the FH. The angle Factor 2 represents is between the extrapolated A-B factor line and the green-hatched AV reference vertical. It may be measured directly or indirectly with the correlometer. Place the inner baseline on the factor line with the hole of the T-square over the juncture of the factor line and FH. Measure the indirect angle between the T-square perpendicular and FH. The Factor 2 line measurement against AV is categorized as follows:

A-point ahead of B-point = + angle
A-point behind B-point = − angle

Figure **4−40**   **(A)** Bimler Lower Profile Angle. **(B)** Factor 2, or Lower Profile Angle comparison. Progenic (Factor 2 anterior to A vertical) is minus. Orthogenic (Factor 2 line coincides with A vertical). Retrogenic (Factor 2 line posterior to A vertical) is plus.

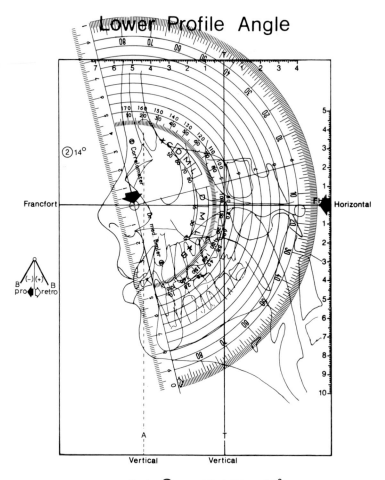

Factor ②   AB / AV = **+14°**

(A)

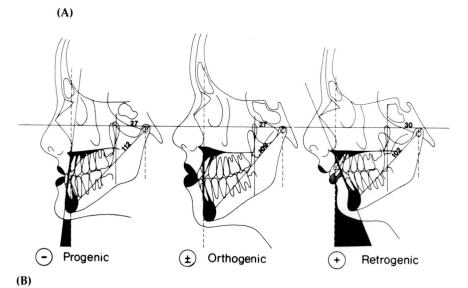

⊖ Progenic   ± Orthogenic   ⊕ Retrogenic

(B)

No color coding is used in Factor 2 angles. Only the maxillary position by itself, described by Factor 1, is color-coded in the Anterior Profile Angle. A high positive value for Factor 2 would indicate B greatly posterior to A and therefore would represent a structurally deficient mandible or skeletal Class II. A high negative value would indicate B greatly anterior to A and would represent mandibular protrusion or a skeletal Class III.

Now we approach an interesting and beautiful mathematical relationship that reveals the interdependency of these factors and the high level of cephalometric insight of the great mind that defined the system. The Anterior Profile Angle may be determined by considering Factors 1 and 2 by simply computing their arithmetic summation. For an example, let us assume Factor 1 = −3 degrees and Factor 2 = +9 degrees. (To save time, Bimler does not use the + sign when values are positive.) The arithmetic summation of −3 degrees and +9 degrees equals +6 degrees. This 6-degree angle represents the same value obtained for the Anterior Profile Angle if the case were measured as the angle posteriorly NAB of the above case subtracted from 180 degrees, the extrapolated NA line! (This is geometrically referred to as a supplemental angle.)

This profile angle may be categorized into four basic groups.

Class I: 0 to 10 degrees—straight facial profile
Class II: 10 to 15 degrees—tendency to convex profile
Class III: 15 degrees and up—fully convex profile
Class IV: 0 degrees and less—concave profile

Thus, we have a determination of the maxillary position (Factor 1), the horizontal maxillary relationship (A'), the mandibular horizontal relationship (B'), the amount of bony overjet (A-B distance linearly on FH), the relationship of the mandible to the maxilla (Factor 2), and the degree of facial profile convexity (the Anterior Profile Angle, Factors 1 + 2). Already we know a lot about the face of our patient.

Posterior Profile Angle—Factors 3, 4, and 5   Nearly every cephalometric analysis system is preoccupied with the anterior profile of the face. Only the Bimler concentrates so much attention on what may be broadly termed the Posterior Profile Angle. This portion of the analysis is concerned with the angulation of certain portions of the osseous anatomy of the deep structures of the maxillofacial complex. We are concerned with this information because a lot of what we do with functional appliances and active plates will be directly affected, either favorably or

---

Figure 4−41   **(A)** Bimler Profile Angle. **(B)** NAB angle: convex profiles have a net positive NAB supplemental angle (180 degrees-NAB), Concave profiles have a net negative NAB supplemental angle.

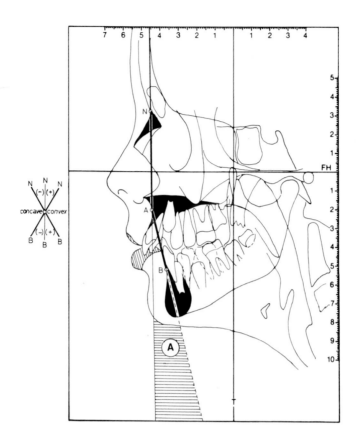

Measured as supplementary angle to 180°

(A)

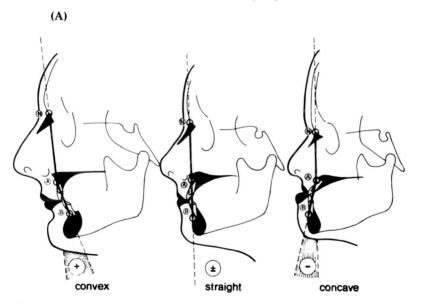

convex   straight   concave

(B)

unfavorably, by what is happening in the posterior part of the face. Sometimes, as we shall see later, certain conditions may be detected that would seriously compromise the best efforts during treatment and could result in a difficult course of therapy if these conditions are undiagnosed or not adequately planned for with properly adjusted techniques.

The Posterior Profile Angle, previously discussed in the section on facial typing, is outlined by a line tangent to the clivus and the mandibular plane. It is divided into an Upper Posterior Angle and a Lower Posterior Angle. We first discuss the three factors individually, before analyzing their interrelationships.

Factor 3—the mandibular plane inclination   In the Bimler analysis the mandibular plane is drawn from menton (M) to the point tangent to the most superior curvature of the Antegonial Notch and is referred to as Factor 3. Its angulation is measured against the FH. The two main facets that affect the angulation of the mandibular plane are the actual anatomy of the inferior border of the mandible itself and the level of the occlusal plane, which acts as the vertical stop on the mandibular arc of closure. Since the vertex of the angle between the mandibular plane and FH would be far off the edge of the tracing paper, even in high-angle cases, the angle must always be measured indirectly against its nearest vertical reference, in this case, TV. The angle is measured indirectly with the correlometer. Place the inner baseline along the factor line with the center hole of the T-square over the intersection of Factor 3 line with TV. The angle is measured in degrees on the outer protractor scale between the perpendicular line of the T-square and the TV. (Note: The perpendicular line of the T-square will always fall to the observer's left of the TV; hence the angulation of Factor 3 is *always* positive, since it would be nearly anatomically impossible for M to be horizontally higher than the Antegonial Notch.) A high Factor 3 value corresponds to what other systems refer to as a high-angle case, ie, a steep mandibular plane often associated with individuals whose vertical component of facial growth is accentuated. A low value indicates a near-horizontal mandibular plane often associated with individuals whose horizontal component of facial growth is accentuated.

Factor 4—Palatal (maxillary) plane inclination   The Bimler Factor 4 serves a dual function. It is of cephalometric diagnostic value in its own right because it represents the inclination of the palatal (maxillary) plane ANS-PNS. But it is also the separating border between the Upper Basic Angle and the Lower Basic Angle, the two components of the Posterior

Figure 4–42   **(A)** Bimler mandibular inclination. **(B)** Factor 3 mandibular inclination (mandibular plane M-No) ranges from 0 to 45 degrees, therefore, is always positive.

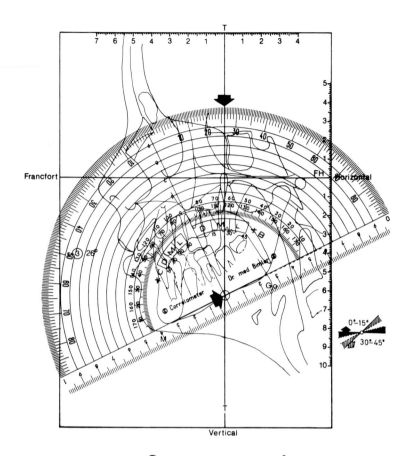

Factor ③   M - Go / FH = + 26°

(A)

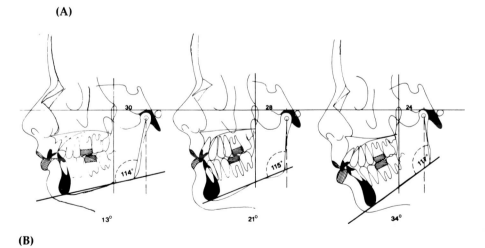

(B)

Profile Angle. Since the angulation of the palatal plane is measured against the FH and is often almost parallel to it, the vertex of the angle ANS-PNS to FH would not only frequently be off the edge of the tracing paper, but probably in the next room! Obviously, such an angle must be measured indirectly, similar to the mandibular plane. To measure the angle indirectly, we again use the correlometer. Place the inner baseline on the factor line with the center hole of the T-square over the intersection of the Factor 4 line with the TV line. Measure the angle in degrees between the perpendicular line of the T-square and the TV on the outer scale of the protractor. The angle is usually very small because palates are seldom, if ever, osteologically deformed so as not to be fairly near horizontal anteroposteriorly. But the value may be either positive or negative according to the following criteria:

ANS higher than PNS—Factor 4 negative
ANS lower than PNS—Factor 4 positive

Now since the Lower Basic Angle is defined as the angle formed between the palatal plane and mandibular plane, it too is an angle with a vertex far off to the observer's right of the tracing and therefore difficult to measure directly. Also since factor line angulations are measured *individually* against their respective reference lines, the comparison of two factors with each other means the correlometer may not be used. The determination of this angle may be easily done mathematically. To compute the Lower Basic Angle, simply subtract the value, positive or negative, of Factor 4 from Factor 3. The following table is an example of two cases, one with a positive Factor 4 and one with a negative Factor 4.

Case 1 (+ Factor 4)	Case 2 (− Factor 4)
Factor 3 = 25 degrees	Factor 3 = 21 degrees
Factor 4 = −(+2 degrees)	Factor 4 = −(−3 degrees)
Lower Basic Angle = 23 degrees	Lower Basic Angle = 24 degrees

Subtracting a positive value *subtracts*. Subtracting a negative value *adds*.

Factors 3 and 4 are measured against the standardized FH, whereas the Lower Basic Angle compares Factors 3 and 4 with each other. Subtracting the value of Factor 4 from the value of Factor 3 gives the true *net*

Figure 4–43   (A) ANS-PNS palatal plane. (B) Bimler Factor 4 or palatal plane is an indicator of increased or decreased vertical development of the middle part of the face. A downward inclination or positive Factor 4 is often seen in Class II, Division 2, or even Class III *closed bite* cases. An upward or negative Factor 4 is often indicative of Class II, Division 1, or Class III *open bite* cases.

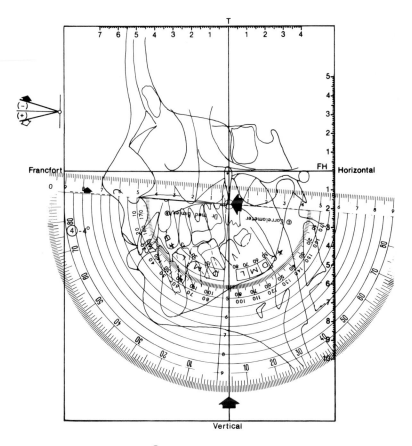

Factor④ ANS-PNS / FH = 4°

(A)

positive   negative

closed bite   open bite

(B)

angulation of the palatal plane–mandibular plane angle as opposed to the angulation of the mandibular plane to a permanently fixed horizontal, Factor 3 alone.

Factor 5—clivus inclination   The anterior cranial base is defined in many cephalometric analysis systems, but Bimler also defines the posterior cranial base by the angulation of a line connecting Cls and Cli or Factor 5. It also represents one of the two lines used to form the Upper Basic Angle, the other line being the palatal plane (ANS-PNS). The angulation of Factor 5 is measured against FH and is *always positive*. But here the diagnostician gets a break, since it is one of the few angles that may be easily measured directly because the vertex of the angle is nearly always within the limits of the tracing and is always a high value. Yet if one insists upon measuring the angle indirectly, it may be done with the correlometer. Place the inner baseline along the factor line with the center hole of the T-square over the intersection of the Factor 5 line with FH. Now here we do something a little different. To measure the angle, read where the FH crosses the *innermost* series of protractor numbers. The range of values extends from approximately 50 to 80 degrees.

This leads us to the final angle measured in this series on the Posterior Profile Angle, that of the Upper Basic Angle. Again, it is another angle that may be measured directly. It is formed by the intersection of Factor 5 line with the palatal plane (ANS-PNS). But, like the Lower Basic Angle, it may be determined mathematically. This time we take the value for Factor 5 and *add* the value for Factor 4 (the opposite of the process for computing the Lower Basic Angle), remembering that adding positives adds and adding negatives subtracts. The following table is an example of two given cases, one with a positive Factor 4 and one with a negative Factor 4.

Case 1 (+ Factor 4)	Case 2 (− Factor 4)
Factor 5 = 57 degrees	Factor 5 = 57 degrees
Factor 4 = +2 degrees	Factor 4 = +(−2 degrees)
Upper Basic Angle = 59 degrees	Upper Basic Angle = 55 degrees

Thus we see that Factors 1 and 2 work together to give us descriptive information about the anterior part of the face and facial profile. Factors 3, 4, and 5 also work together as a sort of little cephalometric family to tell us something about the anatomy and volume of the posterior or deeper portions of the maxillofacial complex.

Figure **4–44**   **(A)** Bimler clivus inclination. **(B)** The Factor 5 or clivus inclination is always positive and merely described by Bimler as flat (50–60 degrees), medium (60–70 degrees), or steep (70–80 degrees). It is also related to the Posterior Profile Angle and Upper Basic Angle representing their upper borders.

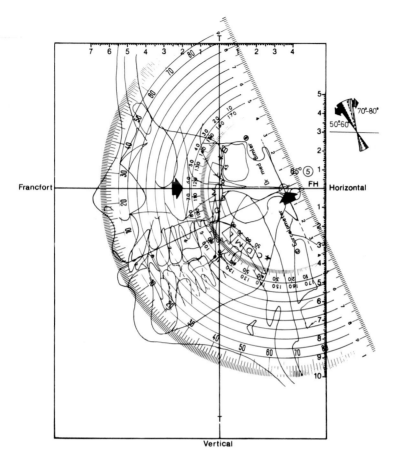

Factor ⑤   **Clivus / FH = 65°**

(A)

flat
50°- 60°

medium
60° - 70°

steep
70°-80°

(B)

Stress Axis—Factor 6   And now we come to one of the most provocative and esoteric concepts of the Bimler system, the Stress Axis or Factor 6. It is a concept totally unique to the Bimler. Even its definition is unusual in that most cephalometric observations involve the comparison of two fixed anatomical landmarks, easily defined by direct visual inspection of the cephalogram. But the Factor 6 involves the use of only one commonly recognized anatomical landmark, and one that is imaginary, that is, not fixed but quite variable in location and which must be determined not by visual inspection but geometrically. This second landmark is found with the correlometer and a somewhat mitigated and forgiving definition of the curve of Spee.

Factor 6 is associated with what Bimler calls the spherical reference system, since the Factor 6, or Stress Axis, represents nothing more than the radius of a circle whose center is the second imaginary coordinate of the line of its path. Bimler noted empirically that the long axes of the posterior teeth, especially in the bicuspid region, seemed to reflect the degree of discrepancy between the arch length required by the anatomical size of the teeth and the arch length of basal bone provided by the jaws in which the teeth are mere passengers. He devised the Stress Axis as a means of more clearly visualizing this discrepancy on a lateral cephalogram. He defines Factor 6 as the radius of a circle whose path approximates as closely as possible the curve of Spee. For the purposes of this particular factor analysis, Bimler defines the curve of Spee as that portion of an arc of a circle which passes through not only the occlusal surfaces of the posterior teeth but also the center of the condylar head, C-point.

The concentric arcs of the correlometer are used in this determination. The arc that best approximates the criteria of this path through the occlusion and, at the same time, capitulare is the one selected. By the way the correlometer is designed, once the appropriate arc is selected, a point is drawn through the center hole at the base of the T-square perpendicular line, which represents the radius center for all the concentric semicircles drawn on the correlometer. This automatically locates the center or origin of the radius for the semicircle of the arc used, and thus we have the second coordinate for the Factor 6 Stress Axis, called *Centro-Masticale* (CM), which is not an actual anatomical location but a hypothetical point of geometric definition.

The other coordinate of the Factor 6 line is Ge (mentale in Bimler) or the inner chin point. Connecting these two points gives us the Factor 6 Stress Axis line. It is always drawn in green, unlike the other factor lines which are drawn in red. There is a second, larger, hole in the correlometer handy for isolating these points more specifically. To make these stand out more, a small circle about 3 mm in diameter is drawn around them and they are colored yellow, as is point C. In well-balanced faces the long axis of the *first* bicuspids coincides with the Factor 6 Stress Axis line.

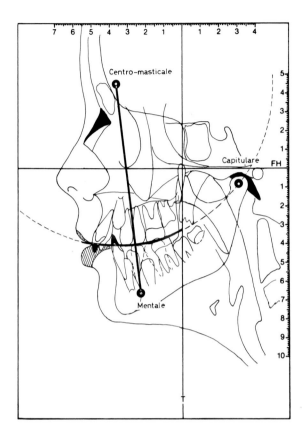

Curve of Spee / Stress axis

Figure 4−45   Bimler's Spherical Reference system employs the use of an imaginary individualized space mark called Centro-Masticale. It represents the center of radius of the circle represented by the curve of Spee and as such is located by the use of the semicircular arcs of the correlometer.

Bimler uses this Factor 6 line to make two assessments: (1) the bicuspid longitudinal axis inclination and (2) the Correlative Classification.

To assist in this assessment, Bimler defines yet another anatomical landmark, the apex of the root of the upper first bicuspid or apicale (Ap). This point is so special in the spherical reference system Factor 6 theater of operations that it too is isolated by the yellow 3-mm dot. [Note: There are only four points so isolated with yellow 3-mm dots: CM, Ge, Ap, and C.]

Bicuspid longitudinal axis inclination   The long axis of the upper and lower roots of the first bicuspids may be in one of three relative positions with respect to the Stress Axis. First, the crown of the bicuspid may be

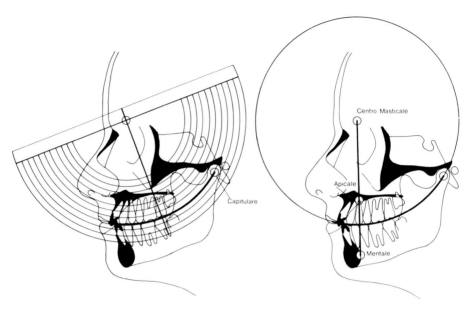

Figure **4–46**   With the correlometer, one establishes the centerpoint of the curve of Spee known as Centro-Masticale by selecting the given semicircular arc that fits the buccal segments of the dentition while passing through C-point (Bimler). The radius from Centro-Masticale to this arc and on to genion (mentale) forms the famous Factor 6 or Stress Axis. It should in balanced cases also pass through apicale, the root tip of the upper first bicuspid.

more forward or mesial than the apex relative to the Stress Axis. This is referred to as proclined and symbolized by the letter P. Second, if the long axis of the tooth is parallel to the Stress Axis, it is orthoclined (symbol O). Third, the crown of the tooth may be more distal than its root apex relative to the Factor 6 line and is termed retroclined (symbol R). The individual teeth, upper and lower, may each have a different axial inclination; hence this facet of the analysis is always represented by two letters, one for the upper and one for the lower first bicuspid, separated by a slash thus: P/P, P/O, O/R, etc.

Figure **4–47**   **(A)** Stress Axis. **(B)** Variations of the Stress Axis or Factor 6 line.

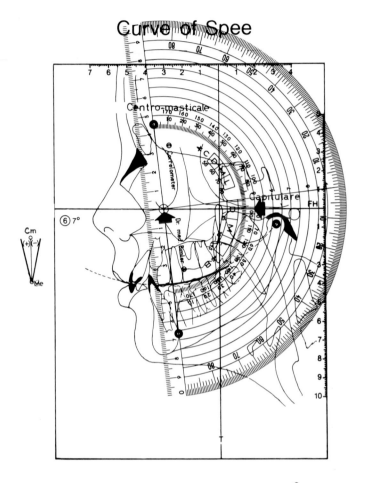

Factor ⑥   Stress axis / TV = **7**°

(A)

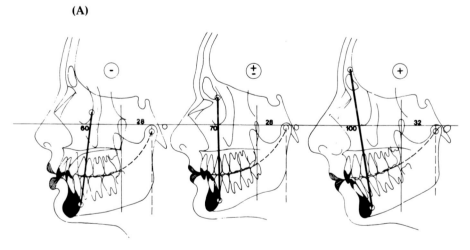

(B)

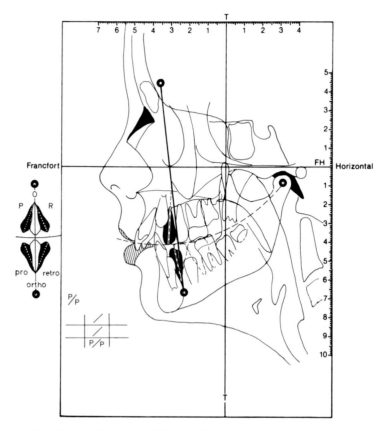

Figure **4–48**   Bimler's Premolar Relationship.

Correlative Classification   This second aspect of the Factor 6 assessment is used to corroborate and supplement the Angle classification. It is determined by observing where the point Ap is relative to the course of the Factor 6 line. Again, there are three possibilities for the location of these two components.

1. Stress Axis line goes through Ap = Pernormal (PER)
2. Factor 6 line passes in front of Ap = Prenormal (PRE)
3. Factor 6 line passes behind Ap = Postnormal (POST)

Figure **4–49**   **(A)** Bimler's Correlative Classification system employs the use of the Factor 6 or Stress Axis and its relationship to apicale. **(B)** The Correlative Classification is given one of three designations: "POST" signifies skeletal Class II status as the Factor 6/Stress Axis line passes posterior to apicale; "PER" indicates a skeletal Class I as the line passes directly through apicale; and "PRE" indicates a skeletal Class III in this system as the Factor 6/Stress Axis line passes anteriorly to apicale.

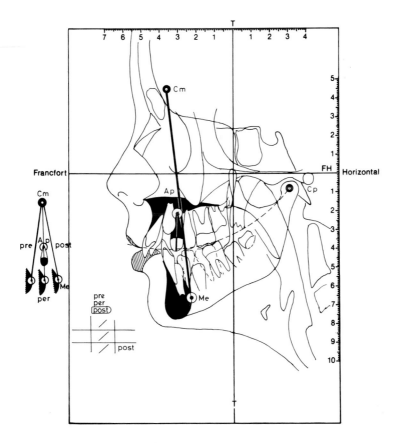

Stress axis / Apical point

(A)

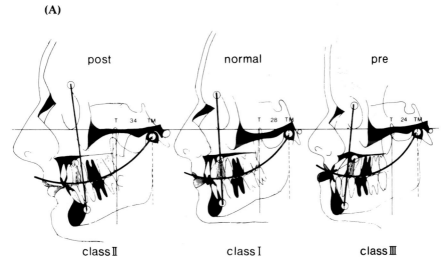

(B)

Often one will see the Correlative Classification followed by its corresponding Angle classification thus: PRE/Angle Class III, POST/Class II, or PER/Class I. Obviously, if the two do not corroborate one another, it is usually the Angle classification that is incorrectly descriptive of the case, since the Correlative Classification is determined cephalometrically, whereas the Angle classification is determined merely by inspection of the relative positions of the upper and lower first permanent molars, which may occasionally both be malpositioned by an equal amount, such that their location becomes deceptive as to the true class of the case (as in a dental Class I, but a skeletal Class II or Postnormal Correlative Classification according to Bimler). Here is a good example of the value of cephalometric analysis, since it clearly points out that if we were to analyze only a set of study models, what we see is not always what we get!

The Anterior Cranial Base—Factor 7   Factor 7 is defined as the line S-N. It is important not so much for the diagnostic value of its angulation, but that it is a reference baseline for many other systems and, more importantly, is the only factor of the ten-factor system that has an important diagnostic contribution to make by virtue of the measurement of its *length*. Its angulation is usually about 7 to 8 degrees with a variance that may extend from 0 to 14 degrees. However, the S-N angulation usually will hover about the 7- or 8-degree mark with an average deviation of ±3 degrees. It may be measured with the correlometer indirectly: inner baseline on the factor line with the center hole of the T-square over the intersection of the Factor 7 line with TV. Measure the angulation in degrees between the perpendicular line of the T-square and TV on the outer series of protractor numbers. The angle is always positive.

But this factor makes its real contribution by assisting in growth predictions and analysis of maxillary positioning. The S-N line, or anterior cranial base, is directly related to the growth of the brain, which sits right on top of it. By age 7 to 8, the brain is approximately 80% full size; hence the S-N line has also developed 80% of its growth by that time, represented by the linear measurement. This S-N length is partially responsible for the status of the maxillary position as defined by Factor 1. Given that, for this example, the maxillary position remains fixed, we have a cephalometrically stationary A-point. Accepting this, it may be clearly seen that since the front component of Factor 7, S-N line, is N, its movement anteriorly or posteriorly can affect the angulation of the Factor 1 line, N-A. The ratio of the length of S-N to the maxillary length (simply determined as the linear distance along FH from A-point to TV) is in an

Figure 4–50   **(A)** Bimler N-S inclination. **(B)** Factor 7, N-S line angulation comparison.

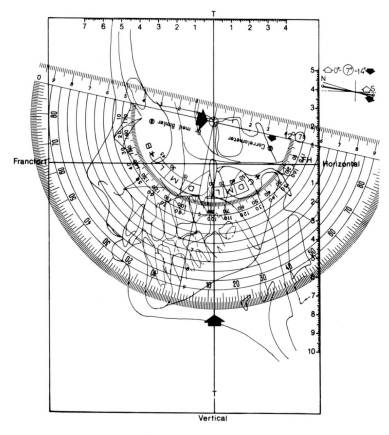

Factor ⑦   N-S / FH =12°

(A)

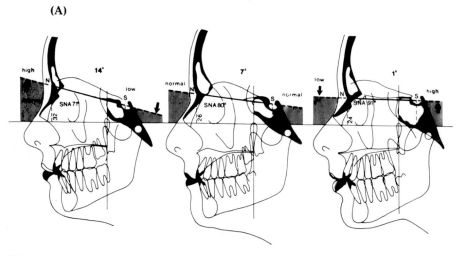

(B)

approximate 7:5 ratio. Thus if S-N were 70-mm, the maxillary length, A-TV, should hypothetically be 50 mm. If S-N were to be short of the 70-mm mark, thus pulling N back posteriorly, this would in effect make Factor 1 a positive angle (green) and make A-point appear more protrusive horizontally than N, a condition defined as prognathic relative to Factor 1. Conversely, if the anterior cranial base length of S-N, Factor 7, were to fall beyond the 70-mm mark, thus pushing N anteriorly, this would in effect make Factor 1 a negative angle (yellow) and make A-point appear more retrusive horizontally than N, a condition defined as retrognathic relative to Factor 1. Now it must be remembered that 70 mm is a numerical value used only for the easily understood arithmetic of this example. *Any* value may be used. The important thing is its proportional relationship (7:5) to the maxillary length, A-TV. Also it must be remembered that the S-N Factor 7 line might be cephalometrically correct while the maxillary horizontal development may be at variance. The consideration of the Anterior Profile Angle and Factor 2 helps clear up this puzzle, as will other facets to be discussed later.

Mandibular Flexion—Factor 8   The last important factor in the Bimler angular part of the analysis is Factor 8 or degree of mandibular flexion. Also referred to as the ramal line, the Factor 8 line is drawn from C to Go. The angle may be positive or negative and is measured indirectly with the correlometer. Place the inner baseline along the factor line with the center hole of the T-square over the intersection of the factor 8 line (which is extrapolated up to the FH) with the nearest vertical reference line (in this case CV) or supplemental green-hatched vertical reference line perpendicular to FH through C-point (capitulare). With the correlometer positioned such that the perpendicular line of the T-square goes out toward the front of the face, measure the angulation in degrees between the perpendicular line of the T-square and FH. If the perpendicular line of the T-square is above the FH, the angle is positive (colored green); if below the FH, the angle is negative (colored yellow). Again, as may be readily surmised, there are three possibilities for the angulation of Factor 8.

1. Hyperflexion = + Factor 8 = Go more anterior than C
2. Orthoflexion = 0 degrees = Go vertically in line with C, usually indicating harmony
3. Hypoflexion = − Factor 8 = Go more posterior than C

Figure 4–51   Bimler evaluation of mandibular flexion: The line Go-C is evaluated with respect to the C vertical. **(B)** The Factor 8 line is also given one of three designations: (1) hyperflexion when the Factor 8 line is anterior to the C vertical; (2) orthoflexion when the line is parallel or coincides with the C vertical; and (3) hypoflexion when it rests behind the C vertical. The Factor 8 line is associated with available freeway space as well as vertical.

Mandibular Flexion

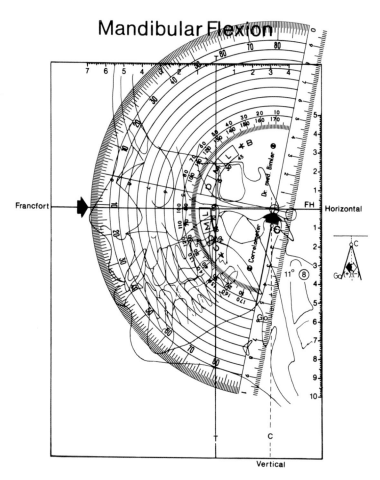

Factor ⑧   C - Go / TV = 11°

(A)

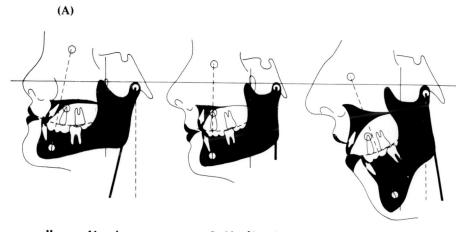

Hyperflexion   **Orthoflexion**   **Hypoflexion**

(B)

What these categories signify is the response of the mandible to the current amount of vertical dimension brought about by the positions of the teeth. It is clear that if the teeth were undererupted, leaving the patient suffering from a gross lack of vertical, the mandible would have to overrotate during its arc of closure in order to bring the teeth into contact. This over- or hyperflexing of the mandible (hyperflexion) would allow Go to rotate in its arc past the CV, thus creating a positive Factor 8 angulation (colored green). Conversely, if the teeth were supererupted, giving the patient an excess of vertical dimension, the mandible would only have to "underrotate" during its arc of closure, since the teeth would hit prematurely due to their excessive height in the alveolar processes. This under- or hypoflexing of the mandible (hypoflexion) would result in Go being unable to travel in its arc of movement past the CV reference line. Remaining posterior to the CV, a negative Factor 8 angulation is created (colored yellow). Thus it may be seen that the degree of flexion of the ramal line of the mandible, Factor 8, is a mere function of the amount of vertical dimension present farther anteriorly in the occlusion of the teeth.

After pondering this phenomenon, we can see that the angulation of Factor 8 is a function not so much of the vertical position of the teeth, but of the amount of freeway space present. A great deal of freeway space would necessitate overclosure to effect occlusal contact, whereas a paucity of freeway space would drive the mandible more open and result in underclosure once occlusal contact has been completed. Clinicians who have the power to easily change the amount of vertical dimension with appliances such as the Bionator are always interested in considerations such as may be gleaned from an analysis of Factor 8.

Factors 9 and 10   As previously stated, Factors 9 and 10 have no clinical significance, but are considered descriptive. Factor 9 is the line tangent to the planum sphenoidale. Factor 10 is the little line from N running tangent to the nasal bone. Some believe in carrying on the tradition of their use, and others believe they only clutter up an already complex tracing with unnecessary lines.

The Bimler Tracing Sheet

The Bimler system is color-coded to help keep the somewhat burgeoning amount of recorded data organized and easily decipherable by the diagnostician. It is also toward that end that Bimler designed his own tracing sheet. This tracing sheet has specific locations for the recording of all the previously discussed factor analysis values, several other supplemental angular values and other important linear measurements (to be discussed next) and facial typing information.

The first thing one will notice on the special tracing sheets used is their relatively small size. They are not much bigger than a common

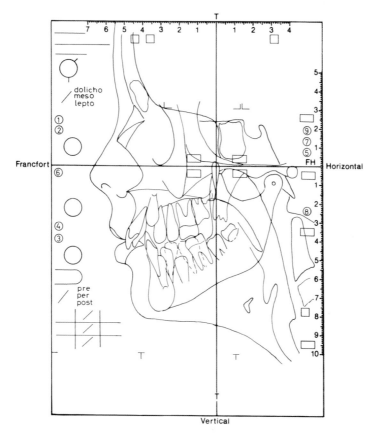

Figure 4–52 Bimler tracing sheet.

5 by 7 inch photograph. The two major components of the Orthogonal Reference System, the FH, and the TV are already printed on the sheet. Where the FH meets the right-hand side of the page, there is a millimeter rule starting at 0 and extending 50 mm up and 100 mm down the right-hand side of the page. Across the top is a similar millimeter grid starting at 0, where the TV intersects the top of the tracing sheet and extends 40 mm to the right and 70 mm to the left across the upper border of the page. These grids are handy for marking things like the vertical level of menton in millimeters. The other markings may appear complicated, but they are really simple. The may be organized into seven types as follows.

   Identification lines   The three lines in the upper left-hand corner of the page are for the patient's name, etc, and the doctor's name. Below these three lines is a large circle with a small slash mark at two o'clock and six o'clock for recording the age of the patient and either an arrowhead at the 2-o'clock mark or a crossbar at the 6-o'clock mark, depending on the gender of the patient.

Facial typing grid Directly below the identification grid is the facial typing grid. The diagonal line is for the Upper and Lower Basic Angle categories M/M, D/L, L/M, etc. Right next to this diagonal are the three words dolicho, meso, and lepto. They symbolize the category for the determination made from the Suborbital Facial Index (height *v* depth). The appropriate word is circled.

Circled factor numbers A series of small circled numbers appears on both left and right-hand margins and represents the corresponding factors. Factors 1, 2, 10, 6, 3, and 4 appear on the left-hand side of the page in descending order and Factors 9, 7, 5, and 8 appear on the right-hand margin. The values for the corresponding angular values of these factors, either positive or negative, are written in red (because they are angles) next to the appropriate factor circled number.

Three large circles On the left-hand margin of the tracing sheet are three larger empty circles for the recording of the Anterior Profile Angle, NAB (upper circle), the Upper Basic Angle (middle circle), and the Lower Basic Angle (bottom circle). Also directly below the bottom circle is an open-ended bullet-shaped demarcation in which is recorded the interincisal angle.

Factor 6 grid Directly below the interincisal angle (bullet) is the Factor 6 grid. Again, a diagonal line is printed for recording upper and lower first bicuspid inclinations relative to the Factor 6 Stress Axis line (proclined—P, orthoclined—O, retroclined—R). Also, directly to the right of this diagonal line are printed the three words PRE, PER, and POST. This is for recording the status of the correlative classification, the appropriate word being circled.

Rectangular boxes Along the FH and along the right-hand margin of the tracing sheet are eight small rectangular boxes for recording linear measurements. (All linear measurements are written in blue.)

Summation grid At the lower left-hand corner of the tracing sheet is a summation grid in which all the information on the entire analysis sheet may be summarized for a condensed overview of the whole case. This will be discussed at the end of this section.

Incidental Angles

Five other angles used by Bimler are incidental to the major angulations of osseous anatomy represented by the factor lines. Four of these angles are concerned with the positions of the teeth, and the fifth is the gonial angle.

Upper Incisal Angle This angle represents the angulation of the long axis of the upper incisor relative to FH. A line is drawn from the tip of the most protruding maxillary central incisor through its apex to the FH. Since the line is *not* a factor line, it is drawn in blue. The angle is

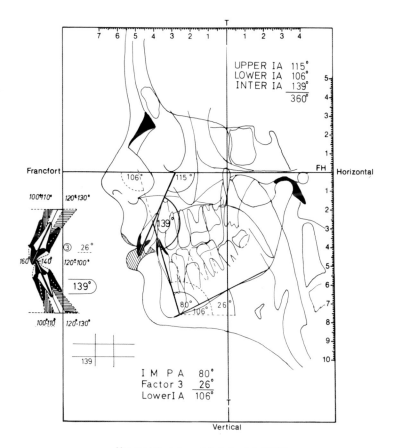

Figure 4–53   Incisor angles used in the Bimler analysis.

measured between the line and the FH on the posterior side and is nearly always obtuse. Be sure to use the outline of the central incisor and not the lateral for this angle since it may actually be more protruded in outline on the x-ray as in a true Class II, Division 2 situation. The angle may be measured with a protractor and written next to the intersection of the line with FH. The value is written in red.

Lower Incisal Angle   The Lower Incisal Angle represents the angulation of the lower central incisor to the FH. A line is drawn from the tip of the crown of the lower central incisor through its apex and on down to the mandibular plane. It is then extended in the opposite direction to its intersection with the upper incisal angle line and from there on extrapolated, without drawing it, to the FH where a half-inch hatch mark is made to represent where the line meets the FH. The angle formed is measured with a protractor as the anterior angle between the line and

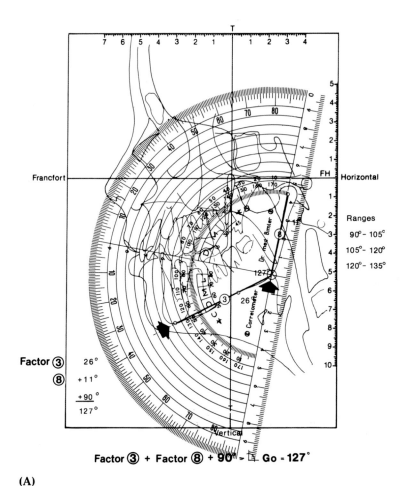

Factor ③ + Factor ⑧ + 90° = ∠ Go = 127°

(A)

Figure 4–54   **(A)** Bimler gonial angle, M-Go-C: This angle may be calculated simply by adding Factor 3 angular value to Factor 8 angular value and adding 90 degrees. **(B)** The gonial angle of Bimler is also given three designations: (1) dolichognathic (90–105 degrees), which is associated with dolichoprosopic facial patterns; (2) mesognathic (105–120 degrees), which is associated with mesoprosopic faces, and (3) leptognathic (120–135 degrees), which is associated with leptoprosopic facial patterns.

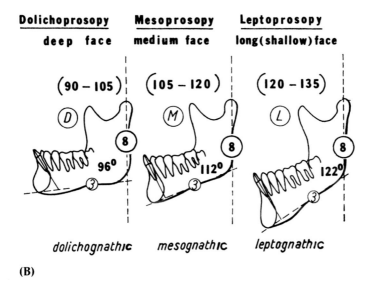

Dolichoprosopy   **Mesoprosopy**   **Leptoprosopy**

deep face   medium face   long (shallow) face

$(90 - 105)$ $(105 - 120)$ $(120 - 135)$

D   M   L

8   8   8

96°   112°   122°

dolichognathic   *mesognathic*   *leptognathic*

(B)

FH. It also is usually obtuse, and the value is written in red just anterior to the intersection of the line with FH.

Interincisal Angle   The Interincisal Angle represents the degree of angulation between the long axes of the upper and lower central incisors and may be measured directly as the angle formed posteriorly between the previous two lines. Its value may also be determined by simple arithmetic. All the exterior angles of a triangle add up to 360 degrees. Since the Upper and Lower Incisal Angles represent these external angles at their intersection with FH (the two lines form a triangle with FH as its base), the value for the interincisal angle would have to equal 360 degrees minus both other angles. Being an angular measurement, it is written in red in the open-ended bullet-shaped bracket on the lower left-hand margin of the tracing sheet. This angle is recognized as being common to many other analyses.

Lower Incisal Angle relative to mandibular plane   The Lower Incisal Angle relative to the mandibular plane is the angle formed by the line through the long axis of the lower incisor at its junction with the mandibular plane. The angle is measured posteriorly. It is the same as the IMPA of the Tweed analysis. The value is written in red within the angle formed.

Gonial Angle   The Gonial Angle is defined as the angle formed internally between the mandibular plane and the Factor 8 or ramal line. The more acute the angle, the more the patient tends toward the dolichoprosopic type. The more obtuse the angle, the more the patient tends toward the leptoprosopic type.

"Life is short and art is long."
Greek Physician Hippocrates
460−357 B.C.

Linear Measurements

So far, the Bimler analysis has been discussed almost exclusively in terms of angular measurements. But Bimler felt that in order to better assess growth and treatment changes, a series of linear measurements should be introduced to the system. There are eight of them, and six are concerned with describing the mandible. The linear measurements are always recorded in blue to keep them separated from angular measurements, which are always recorded in red. Eight small rectangular boxes are reserved for these individual measurements and are printed on the tracing paper along with the Orthogonal Reference coordinates, millimeter grids, etc. Each box is representative of a particular measurement to which it is assigned.

T-TM measurement—temporal position   The vertical coordinate of the Orthogonal Reference System is the line representing the pterygoid vertical and is represented as TV or simply T. As stated previously, a vertical, green, hatched line is also drawn through C-point (capitulare—dead center of the condyle) perpendicular to the FH. Where this green hatched line crosses FH is marked C'. Hence you might think the measurement describing the distance along FH between T and the extrapolated C-point (C') would be referred to as the T-C' distance. Not so. To stress this important measurement's preoccupation with the location of the TMJ, Bimler substitutes the letters TM for C'. Hence the term "T-TM distance." It is one of the most important of the linear measurements made and is recorded in the box above FH and to the right of the TV line. For adolescents this measurement ranges from 28 to 32 mm. But it may easily be seen how this measurement may affect the skeletal class of a given case were it to vary in either direction from this range of normal. An exceptionally long T-TM distance, given an average-size mandible, would bring about a definite Class II situation because it would pull the mandible back under the cranium resultant of the great distance of the TMJ from T. Conversely, the short T-TM distance would tend to drive the normal-sized mandible out from under the cranium to a Class III skeletal situation. This would be due to the close proximity of the TMJ to T. The importance of this measurement is brought to light when one is considering the prognosis of Bionator therapy, especially in the patient approaching the end of the growth period, who happens to have a longer-than-average T-TM measurement. This would make the complete advancement of the mandible slightly more difficult to accomplish before the growth period ends. Concern for this particular form of measurement

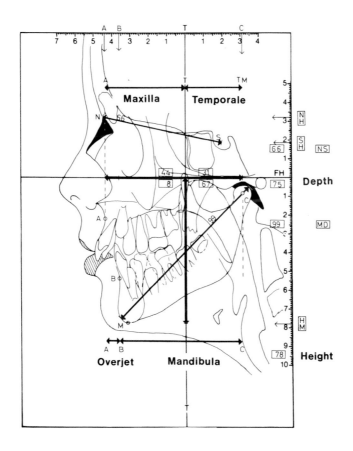

10 Linear Measurements

Figure 4−55   Bimler linear measurements.

is neither new nor unique to the Bimler system. It also appears in a similar form in the Wylie, one of the earliest systems developed.

AT measurement—horizontal length of the maxilla   The first of only two of the eight linear measurements that is not related either directly or indirectly to description of the mandible is the AT measurement or the projected length of the maxilla along the FH. It is not the actual length of the maxilla, but a defined length, which is still quite close, being the length along the FH from the point where the green hatched supplemental vertical line AV crosses the FH, known as A', to the TV of the Orthogonal Reference System. One might think it should be written A'T, but it is merely shortened by Bimler to AT. The rectangular box reserved for it is above the FH and to the left of the TV. The measurement is written there in blue since it is a linear measurement.

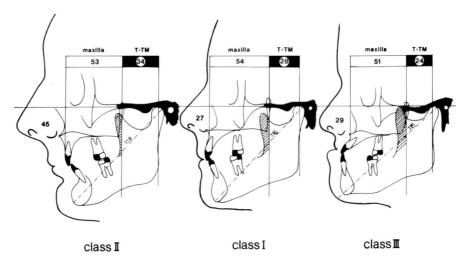

class II   class I   class III

Figure 4−56   Bimler T-TM measurement: Class II cases are often thought of as having large maxillas and small mandibles, and Class IIIs are often thought of as having the opposite combination of small maxillas and large mandibles. Yet the above examples show how important evaluation of the T-TM distance can be. Note that the main difference is *not* the lengths of the maxillas or mandibles. On the contrary, the mandible in the Class II case is only 2 mm longer, obviously not enough to account for the difference. The real difference is in the 10-mm discrepancy between the respective T-TM lengths of the Class II case and the Class III case. The long T-TM distance (34 mm) in the Class II case "pulls" the mandible back far enough posteriorly to make it skeletal Class II despite the extra mandibular length. Conversely, the relatively short T-TM distance (24 mm) of the Class III case forces the mandible out into skeletal Class III configuration even though the maxilla and mandible of themselves are reasonably normal in size.

AB distance—bony overjet   Once the maxillary length AT has been established, the next measurement made is intimately related to it. Rather than record the projected horizontal length of the mandible from an extrapolated perpendicular of B-point on the FH, known as B' and represented only by a short crosshatch at that point, a simple calculation is made by subtracting the length of B'T from the value for AT (AT−B'T). This gives the relative amount of overjet of the maxillary basal bone, represented by A-point, over the mandibular basal bone, represented by B-point relative to the common reference reference line, the FH. It is customary to draw a small zigzag line between the hatch marks A' and B' along the FH. The numerical difference in millimeters is recorded in the rectangular box reserved for it below the FH and to the left of TV just below the box for the AT measurement. In the event B'T is greater than A'T, the difference would obviously be expressed as a negative number. Again, the value is recorded in blue. Rather than perform the calculation, one may simply measure the distance from A' to B' directly, which is usually done. If B' is anterior to A', a negative value must be assumed, by definition, and be applied to the direct measurement. Either way, it gives a quick and easily understood impression of the bony overjet of the basal portions of the maxilla and mandible. Again, rather than write it as the A'B' distance, Bimler simply shortens it to AB.

B-TM distance—horizontal mandibular length   The true mandibular horizontal length is defined as the length along the FH from B' to C', which Bimler prefers to write as B-TM. It is recorded in blue in the rectangular box reserved for this measurement below FH and to the right of TV, just below the box for the T-TM measurement.

Horizontal total length   Once the first four measurements previously mentioned above are made, the horizontal total length of the case along FH may be easily calculated by adding either AT to T-TM or AB to B-TM. This also serves as a system of double-checking the correctness of the originally recorded individual measurements. The horizontal total length is recorded in blue in its rectangular box, which is the second from the top along the right-hand side of the tracing sheet just below the FH.

Diagonal length of the mandible   The diagonal length of the mandible DLM, similar to that seen in the McNamara, is defined as the length of a line from Gn through C-point in the center of the condyle on back to the outermost posterior border of the condyle. It is usually the longest of the eight linear measurements and is extremely useful in clinical situations. It is recorded in blue in its rectangular box along the right-hand side of the tracing sheet, third from the top.

Lower face height   Now that we have measured the mandible horizontally and diagonally, we also include it in a measurement vertically as one of the eight Bimler linear measurements. The lower face height is defined as the perpendicular projection of Gn on the TV, which is then measured to the juncture of TV with the FH. It is recorded in blue in its rectangular box at the bottom of the right-hand side of the tracing sheet. Some also prefer to place a hatch mark at the corresponding point representing the value on the millimeter grid on the right side of the tracing sheet.

N-S linear length (Factor 7)   The last of the eight linear measurements is the linear length of the distance N-S and has already been discussed under Factor 7, which is the only factor that has both an angular value and a linear value. As previously mentioned, the linear value is recorded in blue in the topmost rectangular box on the right-hand side of the tracing sheet.

Alveolar height   Recently an additional accessory linear measurement has been used in the Bimler system that has proven to be of some clinical significance, the alveolar height. The alveolar height is defined as the position of the outline of the mesiobuccal root of the upper first molar, provided it is completely erupted, relative to the palatal plane

(ANS-PNS). If the distance between the two is greater than 3 mm, the bite is considered in the opening range. Between 3 and 0 mm, the effect is considered neutral relative to the vertical, and if the outline of the root extends above the ANS-PNS line, the value is considered negative and of a bite-closing effect. Being a linear measurement, it is written in blue above the Factor 4 angular value on the left-hand margin of the tracing.

Bimler's Ratios: Viggo Andresen Revisited

As previously stated, the chief concern of the Bimler analysis is not to compare the values generated by the cephalogram to a set of mathematical averages or statistical norms, but to help analyze the patient relative to what should be ideal for his or her own morphological circumstances and facial type. This tends to lead one to the use of ranges of values and ratios of proportion rather than single numerical values. Yet even here one must be careful. Sometimes a given assumption relative to a certain set of proportional relationships is presumptively made with respect to one category of facial type which may not necessarily be true in other relative facial types. Such is the case in the well-known "Bimler ratios."

After extensive study of a number of cephalograms of well-balanced and "proportionally normal" individuals, one will soon see that a consistently reappearing set of mathematical proportions is discernible which, though not as exotic or enigmatic as the divine proportions discussed by Ricketts, are nevertheless of limited practical clinical significance. However, this will be so *only* for the mesoprosopic facial type. The length of the Factor 7 line (N-S), the defined maxillary length (AT), the T-TM distance, and the DLM are reported to present in the ratio 7:5:3:11.5.

There is a certain mathematical leeway for the values integrated into this proportion such that, though 70, 50, 30, and 115 mm would represent a perfectly balanced mesoprosopic set of lateral proportions, a reading of 73:51:32:117 would also be considered reasonably proportional for this type of individual. Whereas if the T-TM were on the long side, say in the range 38–42 mm, while the DLM remained at 115, a Class II skeletal (and most likely dental) situation would probably result, even though the mandible would at first appear to be of relatively normal size. It is the degree of *relative* variance of the respective values from the proportional ratio that must be evaluated to determine the degree of clinical significance. In certain cases the accidental appearance of this ratio in the particular mesoprosopic facial category may prove to be of diagnostic value when used in conjunction with all the other accumulated data in the overall assessment of the entire case.

However, the use of this particular proportional set of ratios must always be attended by two important caveats. Number one, it pertains to only the mesoprosopic lateral facial type. Leptoprosopic and dolichoprosopic facial types by their very definition could not fit into this particular set of mathematical proportions. In the leptoprosopic facial type, the Factor 7, AT, and T-TM usually appear as being relatively shorter and the DML is usually much longer. Yet such an individual may still be proportionally balanced relative to his own facial type. The dolichoprosopic facial pattern, on the other hand, may produce values quite close to this ratio, which may lead one to conclude it is merely a mesoprosopic in disguise suffering from a lack of vertical.

The second thing that must be remembered is that this particular 7:5:3:11.5 numerical ratio is *not* a part of the original Bimler analysis. Bimler never developed this ratio as part of his original cephalometric analysis system, nor does he currently use it in any way.[248] He, himself, is uncertain as to its origins even though it is attributed to his system. It most likely crept into the literature on the Bimler from American sources and was inserted by those who brought the system to this country as one of their own clinical observations that became incorporated into the overall analysis. (The same might be said for the alveolar height!?) Though essentially harmless, it merely shows another instance of the prophetic observations of Andresen rising up to echo across the generations and even the continents!

Summation Grid

With the extensive amount of data that accumulates on the tracing sheet of a Bimler analysis, a method of organizing and condensing it would prove most useful. To this end, Bimler developed his summation grid, which appears at the lower left-hand corner of the tracing sheet. Referred to as an "identification grid," Bimler uses it to summarize the cephalometric information derived from the analysis, so that a quick and handy method is available for identifying the problems and characteristics of the case being considered.

The structure of the grid itself is on three tiers with three compartments in each tier such that its overall appearance resembles a "tic-tac-toe" grid. The top horizontal row of three compartments is reserved for data on the *Facial Formula*. The middle three horizontal compartments are for the data concerning the Gnathic Index, and the bottom row contains information referred to as the *Dental Formula*.

Facial Formula   The Facial Formula, or top row of the identification grid, has three compartments. The Anterior Profile Angle is recorded in the upper left-hand compartment and is used to help decipher the skeletal classification of the case according to Ballard as shown in the table.

Angle (deg)	Anterior Profile Angle	Class
0–10	Straight	I
10–15	Transitional	I but tending to II
>15	Convex	II
<0	Concave	III

The middle compartment is reserved for the recording of the Upper and Lower Basic Angles (Posterior Profile Angle) in the conventional fashion: Upper Basic Angle/Lower Basic Angle. The abbreviations used are similar to those on the tracing, such as M/M, D/L, etc. Posterior profiles symbolized by like letters such as M/M, D/D, or L/L are considered as reasonably balanced, whereas posterior profiles symbolized by dissimilar letters are considered unbalanced. The posterior profile with D/L is considered to be the combination producing the maximum bite-opening effect, as in a small upper head and a long lower face height. By contrast, the posterior profile with an L/D designation is considered to be the combination producing the maximum bite-closing effect: a large upper head dominating over a short lower face height.

The final, upper right-hand compartment of the top row of the grid is for recording the Suborbital Facial Index. The words meso, lepto, or dolicho are recorded there as on the tracing sheet. The Suborbital Facial Index is the ratio of the height of the face to its depth. In leptoprosopic individuals the facial height is greater than the depth. In dolichoprosopic individuals (remember to use Bimler's definition of this term now), the facial height is less than the depth.

Thus the Facial Formula is recorded in three items: the Anterior Profile Angle, the basic angular relationship, and the Suborbital Facial Index.

Facial Formula	Anterior Profile Angle	Basic Angular Relationship	Suborbital Facial Index

Gnathic index   The middle horizontal row of the identification grid is referred to as the Gnathic Index. The three compartments of this

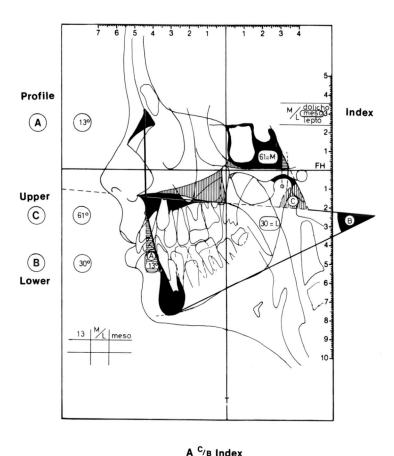

A ^C/B Index

Figure 4–57   Bimler Facial Formula: Profile Angle (anterior)/UBA-LBA/Suborbital Facial Index.

grid are concerned with the skeletal relationships of the jaws to each other and the TMJ. The left-hand compartment is reserved for the recording of the bony overjet of A-point over B-point, the AB distance. An AB distance of 4–8 mm is considered Class I. Anything over 8 mm is Class II, and a negative value represents Class III. Anything between 0 and 4 mm is still considered as Class I, but perhaps should also be thought of as having slight Class III tendencies.

The middle compartment is for recording Factors 4 and 8. Factor 4 is recorded over Factor 8, being separated by a line similar to the Upper and Lower Basic Angles of the Facial Formula. Factor 4 is considered the single most important determinant of vertical dimension of occlusion. A positive Factor 4 contributes to bite-opening, and a negative Factor 4 contributes to bite-closing. The value for Factor 8 indicates Nature's response to the degree of vertical and freeway space present. A positive

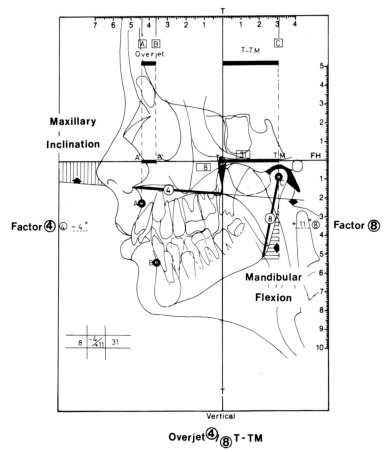

Figure 4−58   Gnathic Index: bony overjet (AB distance)/Factor 4 (ANS-PNS palatal plane angulation)−Factor 8/T-TM distance.

Factor 8 indicates a response to a closed vertical and is referred to as *hyperflexion*, whereas a negative Factor 8 value indicates a response to more open vertical and is referred to as *hypoflexion*. Thus it may be seen that in a severe closed bite situation, the mandible would have to overclose or, since its closing motion is referred to as flexion, it would have to hyperflex in order to bring the teeth into occlusion; hence the term "hyperflexion" for a positive Factor 8. Conversely, if the teeth come into contact quite early in an extreme open bite situation, before the mandible has completed much of a path of closure, it would in effect be "underclosing," or hypoflexing in this case; hence the term "hypoflexion" for a negative Factor 8.

    The right-hand compartment is for recording the temporal position, the T-TM distance. A short T-TM distance (20−24 mm) contributes to a

Class III situation, whereas a long T-TM distance (36−40 mm) contributes to a Class II relationship.

Thus the Gnathic Index, or middle row of the identification grid, is recorded in three items: the bony overjet, the Factor 4/Factor 8 relationship, and the T-TM distance.

Facial Formula	Anterior Profile Angle	Basic Angular Relationship	Suborbital Facial Index
Gnathic Index	Bony overjet	$\dfrac{\text{Factor 4}}{\text{Factor 8}}$	Temporal position (T-TM distance)

Dental Formula   The Dental Formula is depicted by the bottom horizontal row on the identification grid. Here information concerning the dental relationships of the case are recorded. The lower left-hand compartment is reserved for recording the interincisal angle. The middle compartment is reserved for recording the upper bicuspid inclination *v* the lower bicuspid inclination. The letters P, O, and R symbolize proclined, orthoclined, and retroclined, respectively, thus: P/P, O/P, R/R, etc. The final lower right-hand compartment contains two items: the PRE, PER, and POST designation of the Factor 6 Correlative Classification, followed by the Angle classification of I, II, or III, since Angle's classification system is considered primarily of dental relationships and not skeletal relationships. Generally, just the Roman numeral for the Angle classification is written.

Thus the Dental Formula is recorded in four items: the interincisal angle, the upper bicuspid/lower bicuspid inclinations, and the Factor 6 Correlative Classification (Stress Axis) with Angle's classification thrown in.

The entire summation of identification grid may be written as follows:

Facial Formula	Anterior Profile Angle	Basic Angular Relationship	Suborbital Facial Index
Gnathic Index	Bony overjet	$\dfrac{\text{Factor 4}}{\text{Factor 8}}$	Temporal position (T-TM distance)
Dental Formula	Interincisal Angle	$\dfrac{\text{Upper bicuspid inclination}}{\text{Lower bicuspid inclination}}$	$\dfrac{\text{Correlative classification}}{\text{Angle classification}}$

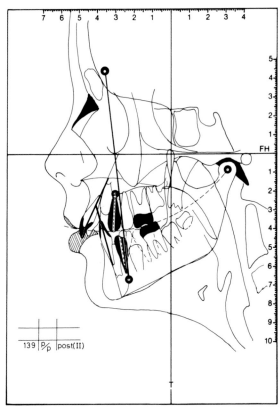

Interincisor angle   **Premolar relationship**
Bimler classification   **Angle classification**

Figure 4–59   Bimler Dental Formula: Bimler Interincisal Angle/upper bicuspid inclination–lower bicuspid inclination/Correlative Classification (Stress Axis status) and Angle's molar classification.

With the information obtained from this grid, it is possible for the experienced individual to envision just about all of the important aspects of a given case without actually seeing the tracing. But this is not its purpose. It merely acts as a quick and condensed summary of the cephalometric aspects of the case and is only an adjunct to the model analysis and clinical examination of the patient.

Incidental coloring   In addition to the above, Bimler is fond of coloring certain portions of the cephalometric tracing to highlight them and add dramatic effect. A summary of color significance follows:

Black: All anatomical outlines
Nasal bone
Maxilla (not roots of teeth)
Mandibular symphysis (not roots of teeth)
Upper and lower incisor crowns
Mesiobuccal half of upper first molar crown
Distobuccal half of lower first molar crown
Outline around condyle
Hyoid bone

Red: All factor lines
Nostril outline
Lips
Cuspid roots (if erupted)
Cuspid crowns (if unerupted)
Angular measurement values
Mesoprosopy letter designation M
(for both Basic Angle and Suborbital Facial Index)

Yellow: Retrognathic Factor 1 angle (negative)
Pterygomaxillary fissure
Positive Factor 8 angle (hyperflexion)
Porion
Leptoprosopy letter designation L
(for both basic angle and Suborbital Facial Index and its
hatched arc)
CM, Ap, Me, C circles (outlined in green)

Green: Prognathic Factor 1 angle (positive)
Factor 6 line
Supplemental AV and CV reference notched lines
CM, Ap, Me, C circles (centers colored in yellow)
Negative Factor 8 angle (hypoflexion)
Dolichoprosopy letter designation D
(for both Basic Angle and Suborbital Facial Index and
its hatched arc)

Blue: Linear measurements
All other lines
Primary teeth (shaded in blue diagonal lines)

"Doch heisse mich das: hat der Wurm ein
Herz?"
"But tell me this: Has the Dragon a
heart?"
Richard Wagner 1813−1883
Siegfried, Act II, scene i

The CCC: Bimler Color-Coded Compact Cephalometric Analytical System

It took Dr Bimler nearly 40 years to gather, correlate, and evaluate the clinical data that he uses in his cephalometric analysis system. Over the years his incisive scientific mind left no stone unturned in his analytical pursuit of diagnostic knowledge obtainable from lateral headplates. He is still exploring and broadening his knowledge in this field today. One of his latest endeavors is the study of the linear distances of N and S from the FH plane and the possible clinical significance of such. He has also evaluated the significance of his own findings on a large scale over the years. Due to his aggressive and dedicated approach to the pursuit of knowledge in the areas of orthodontic diagnosis, his impressive case volume, and the number of years during which he has pursued such knowledge, it is not surprising that his cephalometric analysis system seems to some to approach encyclopedic proportions. Sensitive to this, Bimler analyzed what he thought were the most salient features of the overall system that would be most representative of a given case. Wishing to elucidate such components of a particular malocclusion as facial type, main components of growth, actual linear size discrepancies, skeletal and dental class, and dental angular inclinations of certain key teeth, Bimler recently developed a condensed and simplified method of analyzing a lateral cephalometric headplate, which he has called the Bimler color-coded compact system (CCC).

In seeing numerous orthodontic cases, many of which are often alike, Bimler realized that on occasion some of the busy work and detailing of the more extensive analysis system could become redundant. Such detailing can always be employed where necessary in more marginal cases where a clear diagnostic picture may be at first difficult to grasp with a less detailed system. However, many of the common malocclusions clinicians see on a daily basis follow similar patterns of both etiological development and therapeutic correction. A simple and easy cephalometric analytical system is just the thing needed for such cases. This is the purpose of the CCC. The colors are coded to give the practitioner a visual guide and easily recognizable indication of what major type of case he is dealing with; and the numbers and angles involved in this compact system tell him just how far he will have to go, and in what direction, to correct the case. The Bimler CCC tells the treating clinician just what he wants to know, assuming he has treated cases similar to it hundreds of times. This system also expedites the quick recall of pertinent points of a case in review during the process of treatment and acts as a reminder of the original status of the case in comparison to the actual present in-treatment status of the case as it presently appears before the treating clinician. Bimler uses seven major components to the CCC and four colors, each of which has its own special significance.

I. Orthogonal Reference System
II. Suborbital Facial Index
III. Linear measurements
IV. Gnathic Index
V. Correlative Classification

Orthogonal Reference System   Like the larger, more complete form of the Bimler cephalometric analytical system, the CCC system utilizes the Orthogonal Reference System as its basic frame of reference. As previously stated, it consists of the old FH plane and the major vertical reference line through the center of the pterygomaxillary fissure (TV). It also utilizes the two supplemental verticals through A-point (Downs) up past the level of N and the C-vertical (Bimler) running from C-point up to the FH and down past the level of Go. Since C-point is defined by Bimler as the arbitrary dead center of the condyle, if the outline of both condyles should appear the midpoint of a line connecting the two centers is used as the location for C-point. Due to the simplicity of the system, plain tracing paper may be easily substituted for the more formalized preprinted Bimler tracing sheets of the larger system.

Suborbital Facial Index   As with our discussion of cephalometrics in general, one of the first and most important types of information Bimler wishes to determine relative to a given case is that of facial type. Knowing the facial type that a particular case exhibits aids in the degree of correction one will use in the arch width analysis procedures, such as the Schwarz facially corrected indices. It also aids in determining, along with other factors, something in which the functional orthodontist always has great interest, the main component of growth direction, either horizontal, neutral, or vertical.

Again as previously stated, Bimler developed the Suborbital Facial Index in the mid-1950s as an extension of the Kollmann index, which assessed facial width to facial height from a frontal aspect only. Turning to the lateral aspect, he used the term "dolichoprosopic" to define a facial type where the depth exceeded the suborbital height, which was compatible with the euryprosopic facial type of the frontally oriented Kollmann anthropological index. "Mesoprosopic" indicated generally equal proportions of height to depth sagittally. The term "leptoprosopic" designated faces where the suborbital height vertically was greater than the depth sagittally. This is also compatible with the leptoprosopic facial type of the frontally oriented Kollmann anthropological assessment.

Facial height is the line A'M, or A-point as projected on the FH (Downs) to menton as projected horizontally to the vertical line A. The facial depth is A'C' or A-point as projected onto FH to C-point (Bimler) as projected vertically onto the FH. Now the inscribing compass easily determines facial height. Placing the tip of the compass on A' at its projected location on FH, scribe an arc from menton's horizontally projected position on the A vertical up to the point where the arc would cross the Frankfort plane. If the arc falls in front of C', the case is dolichoprosopic (green) between C' and the intersection of the clivus on FH, the case is mesoprosopic (red). If the arc falls behind the intersection of the clivus on the FH, the case is leptoprosopic (yellow).

Bimler also uses a little color-coded rectangular box in the lower left-hand corner of the tracing paper to simplify this process even further for easy future reference to original facial type. For the balanced, equally proportioned mesoprosopic facial type, Bimler symbolized the case with a small red square. For the sagittally deep-faced dolichoprosopic facial type where facial depth suborbitally is greater than facial height vertically, he uses a horizontal green rectangle, longer horizontally than it is high vertically, to symbolize this facial type. Conversely, for the leptoprosopic facial type where the facial height suborbitally is greater than the facial depth on the sagittal plane or lateral aspect, Bimler uses a vertical yellow rectangle, narrower horizontally than it is high vertically, to symbolize the case. The bony overjet or value in millimeters of the AB difference is usually written within the confines of the Suborbital Facial Index rectangle. (The AB distance appears three times in the CCC.)

Linear measurements   Bimler favors five linear measurements in the CCC.

1. AT length or projected length of the maxilla   The AT length is not an actual anatomical length but is a defined length represented by the linear measurement from the vertical projection of A-point onto the FH plane (A') horizontally to TV. Even though the actual linear line is A'T, it is merely written as AT. The value for this measurement is recorded in its usual place in the small rectangular box in the upper left-hand corner of the four customary boxes reserved for such measurements placed about the intersection of FH and TV.

2. T-TM   T-TM is an important measurement that usually increases during the age of growth and development, carrying the entire TMJ apparatus distally as it increases. In a well-balanced, normally developing

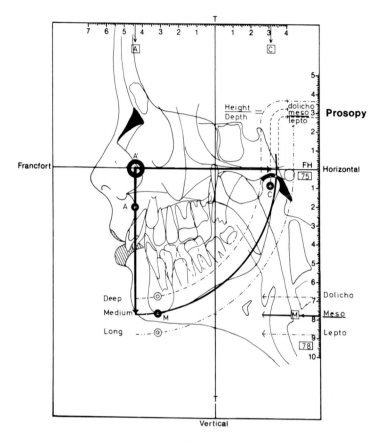

Height A' M / Depth A' C'

Figure 4—60   Suborbital Facial Index of the standard Bimler analysis.

face, as the TMJ increases its distance distally from TV, hopefully the mandible will correspondingly increase in size to compensate lest a skeletal Class II would result. The T-TM is another defined projected measurement along the FH plane from T to C', which is the vertical projection of C-point up to the FH. The normal range for this measurement is 28—32 mm, which usually appears in well-balanced average-sized structural Class I cases. This value is recorded in its traditional place in the rectangular box above FH and to the right of TV. However, in the CCC, Bimler also enlists the added benefit of color-coding to expedite quick and easy recognition of the significance of this measurement. In the CCC, Bimler uses red to signify normal ranges of measurement, those expected in a mesoprosopic facial pattern. He uses green to symbolize a large or excessive degree of measurement as compared with more medium or average values. He uses yellow to signify a deficiency of decreased amount of measurement as compared with more medium values. Therefore, the medium range of values for the T-TM of 28—32 mm would result in the rectangular box in which this value is recorded being outlined heavily in red. A short or low-range value for the T-TM would run from 20—28 mm with the 20—24 mm range of this value almost always resulting in a Class III. Such values would be recorded in the box with a yellow outline. Conversely, a long T-TM from 32—40 mm range with the 36—40 mm or high-end measurements almost always resulting in a skeletal Class II would correspondingly be outlined in green.

3. Bony overjet or AB distance   The bony overjet is the difference along the FH of the vertical projections to the line of A-point and B-point. Since it is defined as the value of A'—B', a range of 0 to +8 is considered in the medium range and therefore color-coded in red. A negative reading where B-point is actually anterior to A-point horizontally, as in skeletal Class III cases, is color-coded in yellow, symbolizing that not only is there very little or diminished overjet but actually none at all (or an underjet), due to the inability of A-point to reside anterior to B-point on the horizontal plane. Conversely, overjets of A over B in excess of +8 are usually confluent with skeletal Class II cases; and this excessive display of overjet is symbolized by coding the value in green. This lends continuity to the color-coding system with respect to the structural characteristics of a given case. A large T-TM (green) would imply a likelihood of some degree of mandibular retrusion even if the mandible may be of normal size relative to its overall length. This T-TM—induced mandibular "retrusion" could easily result in larger than normal overjets which would also be coded green. Conversely, a short T-TM (yellow) combined with even a reasonably normal-sized mandible could easily result in a mandibular prognathism. This would produce negative overjets, anterior crossbites, and negative values for the AB distance, which would also be correspondingly recorded in yellow. These combinations would in turn be expected to corroborate the color-coded rectangles recorded in the lower left-hand corner of the tracing sheet, which denote facial type. The two remaining linear measurements used in the CCC would also fall into suit here.

4. Diagonal length of the mandible

5. AM or suborbital facial height   The AM is nothing more than the horizontal projection of menton onto the millimeter scale to the right of the tracing sheet. Increasing vertical increases its value.

These five linear measurements help the clinician keep tabs on the changes in skeletal size and jaw-to-jaw relationships that take place during treatment and also give him a more firm idea of the course and length of treatment that will be involved in correcting the case.

Gnathic Index   According to Bimler's theories, the Gnathic Index of the larger cephalometric analysis system gives a good indication of the relationship of the upper and lower jaws to one another. Symbolized by the middle horizontal row of numbers of the identification grid of the larger system, Bimler uses almost the entire Gnathic Index, consisting of two linear measurements (the AB difference or bony overjet and the T-TM) and two angular relationships (those of Factors 4); instead of the customary Factor 8, Bimler substitutes Factor 3 in his compact system. The angular relationships of Factors 3 and 4 give an excellent indication of the status of the vertical dimension of the case, and the AB difference and T-TM are already included in the compact system's evolution of linear measurements.

Factors 3 and 4 also easily lend themselves to the use of Bimler's color-coding. As for Factor 4 or palatal plane inclination, it is considered yellow when negative, and green when positive. The line of reasoning for this is clear and predicated on Starck's embryological theories of an "anterior head organizer." During embryological development, the anterior head organizer governs the extent of development of the maxillofacial complex of that area. Interferences in its action in utero are what is believed to be responsible for subtle facial development discrepancies of the microrhinic dysplasia type (discussed later). If insufficient developments were to take place in this area, the results on the palatal plane would be such that the ANS would reside higher on the horizontal plane than the PNS, thus giving the palatal plane a negative value relative to FH. This "deficiency" in normal development of the anterior maxillary area is noted on the CCC by extending a solid yellow factor line along the ANS/PNS palatal plane out to the left-hand edge of the tracing sheet and dashing it in with yellow. Conversely, an abundant expression of the anterior head organizer during embryonic development would result in the ANS residing lower than the PNS relative to the horizontal plane and would cause the Factor 4 to have a positive value relative to FH. This "excessive" development in this anterior maxillary area is noted on the CCC by extending a solid green factor line along the ANS-PNS palatal plane out to the left-hand edge of the tracing paper and dashing it in with green. Neutral or horizontal Factor 4 lines are red.

Now although the Factor 8 has been traditionally viewed as an excellent method of evaluating the extent of vertical dimension present, Bimler abandons it in favor of the mandibular plane angle or Factor 3. This in conjunction with Factor 4 and Factor 7, which he terms as an indicator of "rotation control," is used by Bimler in the CCC to give quick insights to the facial structure. The factor line for the mandibular plane (menton to Antegonial Notch, Bimler's mandibular plane) is colored green for 0 through 14 degrees, red for 15 through 29 degrees, and yellow for 30 through 45 degrees.

The Factor 5 cranial baseline is also color-coded in the CCC. If the clivus inclination is 50 through 59 degrees, it is colored green; 60 through 69 degrees, it is colored red; and 70 through 80 degrees, it is colored yellow.

Though originally designed to be as simple as possible, the Bimler CCC reflects a little of the good Dr Bimler's fondness for some of the more traditional favorite components of the larger system, as they have crept back into the CCC to cause it to appear now in a somewhat more complicated rendition than that which was originally conceived. Carry-overs include Factors 3, 4, and 5 and, as a result, the Upper and Lower Basic Angles these factors naturally generate. They are each coded (written in colored ink or circled on the tracing sheet in colored ink) according to the usual color scheme: green for lesser, flatter, or more dolicho significance; red for meso; and yellow for longer, larger, or more lepto significance. Factor 7 is also carried over and its numerical value, following the lesser-green, meso-red, larger-yellow color designations, is written on the right side of the CCC tracing sheet above the Factor 5 numerical angular value. The Factor 7 line is colored green for 0 through 6 degrees, red for 7 degrees, and yellow for 8 through 14 degrees. The numerical value of the AB distance, the D,M,L/D,M,L designation for Upper and Lower Basic Angle categories, and the Suborbital Facial Index designation of dolicho, meso, or lepto are also written in the upper left-hand corner of the CCC tracing sheet. The angular values for UBA, Factors 4, 3, and LBA, and interincisal angles appear in a vertical fashion in their traditional places along the left-hand side of the tracing sheet, as does the Correlative Classification.

Bimler cephalometric analysis system is founded on two major reference systems: one linear, the Orthogonal Reference System, and one spherical, which employs the determinants for the curve of Spee and the all-important Factor 6 Stress Axis. The Stress Axis is the most sensitive component of the overall Bimler system and is therefore employed in the CCC also. It is interesting to see how intimately related the Stress Axis is to the Gnathic Index. If there is a considerable amount of decreased vertical dimension of occlusion to a given case, mandibular hyperflexion is often associated with it. This has the effect of bringing the Stress Axis line forward past Ap in a PRE designation. In such cases, moving the entire maxillary corpus forward to align Ap properly on the Stress Axis may not be the actual treatment indicated, but common vertical increasing procedures might be required. As McNamara has shown, as the mandible rotates open, the various anatomical landmarks in the mandibular symphysis area, such as pogonion, menton, and mentale, will be brought distally. Thus vertical increasing techniques may be seen to help bring the Stress Axis back more in line with Ap. Similar phenomena have also been previously described that disguise what are actually dental Class II cases into appearing as Class I due to a severe loss of vertical and the seeming forward movement of the mandible due to excessive hyperflexion during occlusion.

Positioning the mandible at its proper ANS-Me LFH of more increased vertical would reveal the true Class II nature of the case as all reference points in the mandible, including the molars, would appear to reside more distally, due to the rotational effect of the arc of opening, as opposed to where they would fall in the pretreatment state during full occlusion. Thus it may be seen that a large positive Factor 8 combined with a parallel or maybe even negative Factor 4, coupled with an advanced Stress Axis in the PRE designation are strong indicators of a reduced vertical and therefore vertical increasing procedures may be indicated in the treatment plan. Also the small AB difference in such cases is only an illusion and the mere result of forward movement of mandibular landmarks due to the hyperflexion or overclosure of the pretreatment mandible to obtain occlusion. Once the vertical is opened to more normal limits, the AB difference would also be seen to increase, thereby revealing the true Class II nature of the case. However, if a Stress Axis in the PRE category is accompanied by a negative Factor 8 and a very positive Factor 4 and adequate vertical appears to be already present, an increase in vertical may be entirely contraindicated, as a true structural Class II situation may in fact exist. In borderline cases, the amount of vertical present, or lack thereof, may confuse the issue and make an accurate diagnosis of the true latent tendencies of the case difficult. A seeming Class I may be actually a Class II in disguise due to a reduced vertical. A pseudo-Class III may also revert back to Class I once adequate vertical is attained. Where the diagnosis becomes even more difficult is in the so-called 1/2 Class II case of nearly normal vertical. Here the Stress Axis along with the Gnathic Index and other factors such as molar drift within the arches may be extremely helpful in determining whether to open verticals and advance mandibles or distal drive posterior maxillary segments to effect correction of Class II to Class I molar relationship.

A POST Corrective Classification in such cases would indicate that the Stress Axis, via mentale, should indeed need to come forward to align the Stress Axis more properly with Ap. However, if a PER situation existed, mentale would be in direct alignment with Ap, and maxillary posterior quadrant distalization techniques may be indicated. The 1/2 Class II molar relationship would be a result of the posterior segments merely tipping or drifting forward a little, leaving the apices of the first bicuspids in their structurally correct Stress Axis alignment position, but merely allowing the clinical crowns to tip forward mesially, effecting the pseudo or 1/2 Class II molar relationship change.

Advancing the mandible, and therefore mentale, and as a result the entire Stress Axis here would be contraindicated because this would pull the Factor 6 line forward past Ap into an introgenic PRE category. For this reason Angle's classification according to molar alignment and Ballard's classification system according to AB difference may at times be suspect. However, the Stress Axis indication may be employed to give a clearer picture of such marginal cases of difficult diagnosis. An easy diagnosis may be made of obvious Class II or Class III cases, but in more marginal cases the Stress Axis determination is the best indicator of latent or hidden tendencies of cases that at first appear to be Class I but may be straining to eventually become Class II or Class III structurally. Such information is of critical importance in an age of functional appliance therapy that is capable of opening verticals and changing mandibular positions and is a great help to the clinician in the overall determination of just which way he may wish to treat a case. Of course, TMJ considerations override everything, even Stress Axis designations!

Bimler defines the Centro-Masticale (CM) as the center of the radius of the curve of Spee. This hypothetical location of a space mark represents the ideal center of the radii of the longitudinal axes of the teeth in the buccal segments and forms the basis of the spherical reference system. Thus a point for comparison results between the long axes of the teeth in the buccal segments and the radius of the curve of Spee (which when placed over mentale also represents the Stress Axis). By evaluating the relationship of the long axes of the buccal teeth to the Stress Axis (the radius of the curve of Spee through mentale), one may evaluate the amount of tooth inclination in either a forward or rearward direction. Bimler believes that the amount of proclination or retroclination of the teeth in this regard is an indication of the body's attempt to compensate for deficiencies in the individual's basal bone arch size or alignment. A short maxillary basal arch would reflect maxillary buccal teeth with their long axes converging to a point posterior to CM. This could mask Class III tendencies when evaluated strictly from a dental standpoint (as does the Angle classification system), since the crowns of the upper posterior teeth might be tilted forward in an effort to compensate for the Class III cuspal alignment, thus making the occlusion appears less Class III to the eye than it really is.

Conversely, in a mandibular basal arch deficiency, the proclination of the long axes of the mandibular buccal teeth would cause the convergence point to be anterior to CM, thus making the occlusion appear less Class II dentally than it really is, due to the forward tilt of the crowns of the lower buccal teeth in their effort to be compatible with the uppers from their basally retruded position. This is a result of the body's effort to compensate for the Class II dental alignment and, hopefully, attain some form of anterior coupling.

But these proclined and retroclined compensations and deviations are not without their price. It is believed that this results in a deviation from the normal functional balance of a proper occlusion as well as an increased susceptibility to attending periodontal problems, because the stresses of occlusion are not absorbed properly down the long axes of

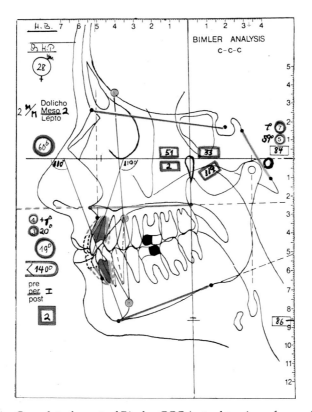

Figure **4–61**   Complete format of Bimler CCC (actual tracing of a case).

such tilted teeth. Again this, along with evaluation of other elements, aids in the determination of exactly which direction treatment will take for a given case. With the vast array of techniques at the disposal of the clinician familiar with both fixed and removable appliance techniques, insights that may be provided by these sophisticated concepts allow the practitioner to generate treatment plans that take advantage of such knowledge to produce the best treatment possible for the case.

The final component of the CCC is the color-coding of the roots of the maxillary and mandibular central incisors. This is the one area where Bimler *deviates* from the red, green, yellow color-coding system, but it is for an important historical reason. The middle range of axial inclinations of the upper and lower incisors *as measured against the FH* in the conventional manner of the larger system is considered to be in the 110-degree to 120-degree range. It is noted in the CCC by coloring red the roots of the teeth in this range of axial angulation. When the angulation is in the range 100 to 110 degrees, the roots of such teeth are colored green, since these angulations are often associated with *dolichoprosopic* facial types or deep bite cases. However, when the axial inclinations are in the range 120 to 130 degrees, relative to FH, the roots of such teeth are colored *blue*! This is due to the fact that blue has been traditionally associated in all Bimler cephalometrics with Class II cases, and since large overjets often involving large axial inclinations are a common trait of structural Class II cases, it is only fitting (and far less confusing for those familiar with traditional Bimler cephalometric analysis) to color code such teeth in the traditional blue. "Blue is for Class II" and its often characteristically proclined, high axially inclined anteriors.

> *"If you can look into the seeds of time,*
> *And say which grain will grow and which*
> *will not..."*
> William Shakespeare
> Macbeth, *Act I, scene iii*

DIAGNOSTIC INTERPRETATION

As may be seen, a fully completed Bimler analysis produces a prodigious amount of information. Though some of its individual concepts may be easily interpreted in a straightforward manner, such as the AB distance, Factor 3 or Factor 4 angulations, and interincisal angle, other relationships require a more distant view covering a broader area of considerations, such as major types of facial disharmonies or future trends of growth. It is on this broadest of scales that Bimler uses his analytical system to describe what have been fairly recently defined as three major types of growth disturbances, or developmental dysplasias, of the maxillofacial complex: microrhinic dysplasia, microtic dysplasia, and leptoid dysplasia. Each dysplasia has its own set of pathognomonic developmental disturbances that are characteristic of them and may appear singly or in various combinations in more complicated cases. Except for the fact that these groups of characteristics are merely growth disturbances and not out-and-out signs or symptoms, these conditions approach the level of syndromes. The theory behind their development, or more correctly *lack* of development, in the individual gives one an insight which enables them to be easily understood and useful in certain diagnostic situations.

Microrhinic dysplasia Microrhinic dysplasia was the first condition to be described and results from an underdevelopment of the anterior

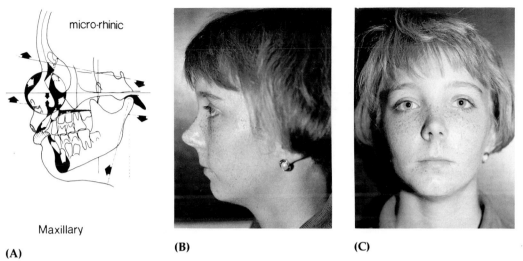

micro-rhinic

Maxillary

(A)   (B)   (C)

Figure 4–62   (A) Microrhinic dysplasia: Bimler defined three basic types of
growth disturbances. In microrhinic dysplasia a small upturned saddle nose with
flared forward nostrils is observed. The *maxilla* is primarily involved, rotating
upward anteriorly so that the Factor 4 ANS-PNS palatal plane is parallel to FH or
at a negative angulation. This is attributed to a disturbance in the embryonic
anterior head organizer during the third week of pregnancy. There is also
commonly an antimongoloid slant to the eyes. Bimler reports observing a
somewhat larger than normal percentage of occurrence of this syndrome in
children of Irish descent. Anterior open bites are commonly observed in this type
of individual. **(B), (C)** Case example.

nasal area embryologically. Some researchers feel that the embryonic
development of the nasal capsule and rhinencephalon is controlled by
what has been theoretically termed an "anterior head organizer." It is felt
that any disturbance of this anterior head organizer during the third
week of embryonic development, such as a temporary hypoxia or virus,
results in the classic malformations of skeletal and facial structures.

Facially, the appearance of an individual with such a condition is
strikingly consistent. Referred to by otolaryngologists as an "adenoid
face," and sometimes by Bimler as the "rotational syndrome," such an
individual exhibits a short, turned-up little nose with the nostrils prominent from a frontal view. The canthus of the eyes may be slanted downward (antimongoloid slant). The upper lip is arched upward incompetent
and provides no unstrained oral lip seal. Adenoids and tonsils are generally enlarged. Skeletally, these individuals exhibit an anterior open bite.
Bimler Factors 4, 7, and 8 are rotated in a clockwise direction. One can
envision this by imagining a normal face instantly suffering an animated
shrinkage in the nasal area. As the nose contracts it displays the nostrils

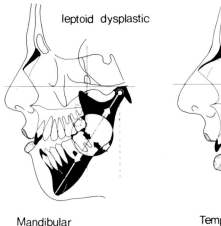
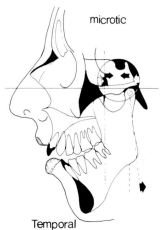

leptoid dysplastic

microtic

Mandibular

Temporal

Figure 4–63   Leptoid dysplasia: This type of growth disturbance primarily involves the *mandible*. It is elongated but weakened in structure through the gonial region. Common in Class III cases, it also appears in certain skeletal open bite cases, which, since the problem is the mandible, are more difficult to treat.

Figure 4–64   Microtic dysplasia: This growth disturbance is believed to result from a disturbance in the embryonic posterior head organizer, which retards development of the temporal region. This results in the chief manifestation, which is an alteration of the normal location of the TMJs.

more, pulls the anterior part of the palate up, and results in a mandibular hyperflexion.

Microtic dysplasia   The same German researchers who theorized the existence of the embryonic anterior head organizer also postulated that a posterior head organizer initiates the embryonic development of the rhombencephalon. Taking a cue from this theory, Bimler surveyed his own records and found a series of patients exhibiting growth disturbances in the otic area. The most glaring developmental disturbances seem to be a short T-TM distance. Also, the clivus appears smaller and more upright. The entire region of the posterior cranial base and adjacent areas of the petrous portion of the temporal bone appear to be slightly under-developed. The short T-TM distance often results in a Class III dental relationship.

Leptoid dysplasia   Bimler defines a third type of growth disturbance that, unlike the previous two, is a result of excessive bone growth rather than a diminished development. He terms it leptoid dysplasia and con-siders it to be of a more generalized nature. The prominent feature of this condition is the increased DLM. The facial height is increased while the facial width and depth are decreased. This would be revealed by the Suborbital Facial Index. The excessive DLM results in a more obtuse gonial angle and either a Class III dental relationship or open bite, depending on the alveolar height.

It must be remembered that these dysplasias may exist individually or in any combination (pandysplastic), and an understanding of their significance helps define the limits of the clinician's ability to deal with them. When cephalometric analysis reveals existing problems that are beyond the scope of certain techniques, more advanced procedures must be called upon. When a practitioner is fully aware of why a given case is beyond a particular technique, he is in the best position to decide what is best for the patient as to more sophisticated treatment modalities or referrals to individuals with, what would be for the patient, more appropriate skills.

CHAPTER 5
The New Breed

THE CONCERN FOR COUNTENANCE

In the diverse and convoluted evolution of cephalometrics as a diagnostic science, great pains were taken to study and evaluate the internal osseous structures made visible by means of the radiographic image. From early on, due to the initial findings of Brodie, the theory that basic bony dimensions were immutable to orthodontic therapeutics became so firmly entrenched that it was almost never questioned. Considering that American orthodontics was totally dominated by fixed appliance mechanics, this is entirely understandable. Once the deep internal osteological anatomy of the maxillofacial complex became exposed to the orthodontic discipline's diagnostic eye, it seemed as if the clinicians had analytically started at the center and gradually worked their way out "analysiswise" in the only two directions possible: toward the facial profile anteriorly and toward the TMJ posteriorly. The former was first to receive attention, while knowledge and even interest in the latter, until only recently, has been sadly lacking!

Concern for the dimension, proportion, and analysis of the face was an area the early anthropometricians and men like Milo Hellman were

294

familiar with to a certain extent. This is partly due to the fact that roentgenocephalometrics had not yet made its appearance on the scene. In the early days, cephalometrics often took the form of osteological measurements on dried skull specimens,[25] although the dimensions of the living face or *soft tissue* profile were also well documented, especially those concerning the subdivisions of the anterior face height AFH.

Early investigators divided and measured the soft tissue AFH of living individuals in a variety of ways. For example: (1) nasion to prosthion and prosthion to menton; (2) nasion to stomion and stomion to menton; (3) nasion to coronal edge of upper incisor, coronal edge of lower incisor to menton; and (4) nasion to subnasale and subnasale to menton.[14, 28, 249-254] However, with the entrance of roentgenocephalometrics, a similar variety of measurements were recorded and analyzed for the osseous component of the AFH.[214, 255-258] Again, great concern was proffered to the vertical aspects of the anterior face and its component subdivisions. It must be remembered, however, that the orthodontic discipline had for all intents and purposes accepted that nothing short of surgery could be done to effect changes in the horizontal aspects of the facial profile except for the relationship of lip position relative to the degree (or lack thereof) of angulation of the anterior incisors.

It is easy to understand the profession's fancy for analyzing AFH, since it is controllable to a certain extent by fixed appliance mechanics. There was a period when concern for vertical reached such heights of intensity that some investigators, such as Dr F. F. Schudy of Austin, Texas, proposed whole new facial typing schemes predicated on the degree of hyper- or hypodivergence of the angle S-N−Go-Gn, which has a direct relationship to the amount of AFH manifest anteriorly.[259] Thus, it may be seen that the concerns and analysis of the facial profile, both bony and integumental, for the most part centered around vertical relationships in "prefunctional appliance" cephalometric times. The horizontal significance of the facial profile relative to such things as the cranial base drew less attention, except for the acknowledgment of the amount of facial convexity and the relative degree of the horizontal position of the mandible.

Studies devoted solely to the facial integumental profile started surfacing in the early 1950s and usually concerned themselves with the relationships of the integumental profile to a variety of the most common cephalometric bony landmarks and their combined significance with respect to "facial beauty."[260] It was concluded that the more convex the facial profile, the more the anterior incisors could be uprighted. The alternative premise was also generally accepted; ie, the more vertically straight the facial profile, the more the anterior incisors could be torqued labially. The latter theory has some merit, but in light of modern knowledge, the former premise can result in devastating sequelae for the TMJs. An example would be an individual whose facial convexity is due to a retrusive mandible in combination with Division 1 angulated maxillary incisors; ie, treating the correct member, the maxilla, to the incorrect member, the mandible, if overdone can result in enough of a retruded mandibular arc of closure to initiate the NRDM-SPDC phenomenon (neuromuscular reflexive displacement of the mandible with superior posterior displacement of the condyle). This could precipitate TMJ-type symptomatology as the condyle transmits the shock of full occlusion to the highly enervated and sensitive bilaminar zone instead of the naturally built-in cartilaginous shock absorber, the intraarticular disc.

The approach to facial esthetics in those days was one of doing everything possible orthodontically to try to get the lips to fall on an arbitrary straight line of one sort or another that only ran from the nose to the chin. The only things amenable to such a concept were the things that could easily be effected through purely orthodontic technique, namely the vertical dimension of occlusion and the degree of procumbency of the anterior incisors, ie, the interincisal angle. Nothing of an orthopedic nature was ever considered. The lines of reference used were never related with respect to their own angulation to the cranial base or the Frankfort Horizontal (FH) plane. The "esthetic" lines, running only from the nose to the chin, could of themselves be biased if the chin were retruded as in skeletal Class II mandibular insufficiencies. Therefore their range of influence was limited.

Of a mere handful of esthetic lines for analysis of facial profile, the most famous are the S-line or Steiner, the Holdaway harmony line, and the esthetic line of Ricketts. Yet these esthetic reference lines all have two major flaws inherent in their basic design. First, they are not oriented with respect to any other frame of reference other than themselves. This means that in a severely retruded facial profile, as in a skeletal Class II mandibular retrusion, if the lips fall in their respective places along the line from nose to chin, the proponents of these esthetic reference lines can claim that the profile is balanced, at least according to their limited and possibly structurally biased frame of reference. This would be the case when the entire face is viewed as a whole and the "fishlike," severely retruded, and weak-appearing chin and high degree of overall facial convexity lends to a less than attractive appearance in spite of the lips conforming to a biased "esthetic" line! Thus orientation (or angulation) of an ideal esthetic profile reference line to vertical frames of reference for themselves as a whole becomes obvious. Formerly, this was not considered important, and the angulation of these esthetic lines with respect to the vertical plane of reference was merely accepted as is, ie, as the position pogonion Pog dictated, regardless of how far retruded it may have been on a given case. This happened because the profession didn't believe mandibles could be advanced in those days.

Second, these esthetic reference lines were simply not long enough. By virtue of merely running from the nose to the chin, they provided

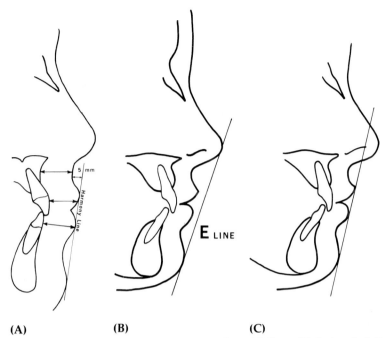

Figure 5-1   **(A)** Holdaway harmony line. **(B)** Ricketts' E-line. **(C)** Steiner's S-line.

only a limited frame of reference for a limited portion of the face, namely the lips alone. However, with such a short reference line the angulation of the entire lower facial profile as a whole, which is a product of the degree of protrusion of the mandible, could not be evaluated as a whole. The lips may fall on the line, but what was the overall angulation of the entire lower face? Thus it may be seen that these earlier esthetic lines merely paid "lip service" to facial esthetics and came up a little short! No profound statements were made, nor were any conclusions drawn, about the general angulation of an ideal anterior profile esthetic reference line to a vertical reference, such as nasion vertical, nor even a horizontal reference such as FH.

But with the coming of the age of orthopedics, mediated by the appearance of functional appliances, practitioners started looking at faces differently, because now they could really start doing something about them on a major structural level. No longer was therapeutic improvement of facial profiles restricted only to positioning the lips relative to a certain limited esthetic line by mere orthodontic angulation of the anteriors. Now whole mandibles could be advanced. Retrusive structural profiles could be filled out and given a fuller, more balanced, stronger appearance in profile.

In the past the notion of studying what were considered "ideal" or attractive faces had crossed the mind of the orthodontic discipline. Charles Burstone, for example, published a report on what was referred to as the "Herron sample," a group of 40 individuals selected as having attractive faces by a panel of three professional artists from the Herron Institute of Art, Indianapolis, Indiana. New emphasis was being placed on facial harmony and beauty from a new and totally unexpected source, as Dr Burstone notes:[261]

> Twentieth century mass media (television, movies, advertising, etc.) have presented to the public, faces that are generally thought of as "good looking" or beautiful. The impact of these media has been so widespread that individuals of varying ethnic and racial groups who ordinarily would be expected to develop their own concepts of facial harmony have come to accept the "Hollywood standard" as the example of a universal ideal of facial excellence. The mean values of the aforementioned Herron sample, either because the artists are part of this culture or because the sample reflects the mean of the population as a whole, simulate the "Hollywood type."

Yet at the time of the Herron study the overall concepts of treating to facial beauty by means of changing retruded mandibular positions was still yet to come, for this study was published in 1958. It also resulted in a facial profile analysis system that was broken down into so many component lines that some 15 angles are used to describe the profile! Although the analysis maintained that the soft tissue profile was intimately related to the hard tissue profile, as did all other studies, it also maintained that tooth position was the only possible therapeutic means of alteration of the profile. The discipline was still stuck in the age of orthodontics. But at least the seeds of the notion of an attractive face being made up of more than just the positioning of lips on a line were starting to take root. Hollywood actually was making a contribution of "redeeming social value" to society!

It was known that the male skeletal profile showed an increase in mandibular prognathism with age,[197, 255, 262] a hint from Nature as to what directions future facial profile analysis would have to take. It was also shown that although Brodie's old theory of uprighting of the incisors and generalized slight flattening of the bony facial profile occur with age, the integumental profile, especially the nose, with age tended to *increase* in convexity.[263] Then the FJO concepts of mandibular advancement came fully onto the scene, and the stage was set for a revolution in the way clinicians would view such things as the facial profile and its relationship to beauty. Yet it would still take a full generation to come to fruition. For as functional-appliance-type treatment techniques made great strides in changing the therapeutic approach the profession would take with respect to addressing malocclusion during the late 1960s, the 1970s, and the early

1980s, the cephalometric appraisal, on the other hand, of such sweeping orthopedic implications and its specific relationship to facial attractiveness and esthetics dawdled. But it was only a matter of time before its tremendous significance would become apparent. That time arrived in the mid-1980s as a movement that represents a whole new wave of facially oriented (as well as orthopedically oriented) treatment approaches for malocclusion made possible by the philosophies and techniques of FJO.

THE BOWBEER ANALYSIS

One of the first and most important to catch and ride the crest of the new wave of FJO-governed facial analysis was the soft-spoken and eclectic Dr Grant Bowbeer of Ann Arbor, Michigan. As an orthodontist, Bowbeer was trained in the "traditional school" of American fixed appliance, four-bicuspid-extraction-oriented orthodontic technique. Aligning anterior teeth by strictly orthodontic means to limited esthetic lines of the Steiner or Holdaway type, cervical and high-pull headgear, and dental class correction with traditional Class II elastics were all a standard part of his daily practice, as well as a status quo for the times.

But a dramatic transformation took place. In the spring of 1983 he attended a seminar, given by the eminent Dr Merle Bean of Des Moines, Iowa, and had his "diagnostic eyes" opened by observing results that he "hadn't seen before." Bean's finished cases exhibited outstanding lateral, vertical, and, especially, horizontal anteroposterior (AP) development, the likes of which Bowbeer never thought possible. And this was all accomplished by Bean without the use of backward-pulling headgear or the removal of bicuspids. When extractions were employed, the second molars were removed. Instead of retracting maxillas and upper anteriors *back* with headgear to meet incorrectly positioned retruded mandibles, those same mandibles were brought *forward* to meet correctly positioned maxillas by means of functional appliance technique (Bionators). Bowbeer was also introduced to what would prove to be a key cephalometric concept, the nasion vertical (NV) as described by McNamara.

In the summer of the same year, Bowbeer went to the office of the American "father" of second-molar-extraction technique, Dr David Liddle, the octogenarian orthodontist from Warren, Ohio, who had been extracting second molars for nearly half a century.[264] Liddle was also treating his patients with a combination of fixed and functional appliances. Again Bowbeer was astounded by what he saw. This visit to Liddle's office only fed the fires of Bowbeer's scientific imagination, which had been kindled earlier by such things as an inspirational address delivered by that firebrand of second-molar-replacement technique, Dr Ira Yerkes,[265] and by the writings of such esteemed authors as D. H.

Enlow, who stated that "it is not the maxilla that protrudes, rather it is the mandible that is actually retrusive."[266] He also came across a series of scientific writings and lecture materials that supported and clarified the basic tenets of the FJO philosophy.[88, 267-270]

Possessing a truly scientific mind that was unfettered from any sort of emotionally based prejudice, Bowbeer decided to return to his practice and start reviewing his own retention patients and those representing nearly completed cases. He was not totally pleased with what he saw. As he candidly states,[271]

> I soon realized I had achieved a good skeletal result in most patients, and some of the faces were outstanding in both non-extraction and four-bicuspid extraction cases. However, many of my cases did not have as good facial esthetics and balance as similar cases treated by Bean, Liddle, and Yerkes. Slowly, it began to dawn on me. It wasn't the removal of bicuspids in itself that led to unfavorable facial changes; it was the direction the teeth had been moved to compensate for skeletal and/or functional problems. How could something so obvious have eluded me for all these years?

He also noted that many cases in which esthetics had been adversely affected as a result of treatment were also found to have TMJ problems "once the right questions were asked." The conversion was complete!

Thus, Bowbeer transcended his traditional orthodontic "upbringing" and concluded that since 80% of maxillas are either neutral or retruded and 90% of mandibles of patients with Class II malocclusions are retruded, techniques that would encourage mandibular growth would represent the treatment of choice much more often than methods that tend to retract the maxilla—the heart and soul of the FJO philosophy! He also concluded that any diagnostic method used in analyzing cases must pay particular attention to the face and the TMJ. But this posed the problem of what to use as an ideal or treatment goal for a beautiful (or handsome) facial contour.

To solve this problem, Bowbeer studied innumerable photographs of professional models, movie stars, beauty contest winners—people the general populace would call attractive in facial appearance. This is nothing new to orthodontic investigations. R. A. Riedel discussed studying photographs of Hollywood stars in 1947.[272] Oddly, Riedel notes that a panel of orthodontists judging the photographs found the facial profiles of the stars to be, in their opinion, somewhat too protrusive! Maybe in those days beauty was in the somewhat prejudiced eye of the beholder.[273]

Bowbeer, however, recognized the full-facial profiles, well-supported lips, and fully advanced mandibles as keys to acceptable or even attractive facial profiles. Therefore, he became determined to develop a method of facial analysis that could be corroborated by supportive cephalometric diagnosis. Like most of the cephalometric hopefuls that came before him, he hoped to keep the analysis as simple as possible, using a minimal number of lines, angles, and measurements. He found too much individual variation to rely on the Steiner ANB angle, the A-PO plane, or the old Tweed Triangle, although he did find a particular fondness for the Frankfort-mandibular plane angle and A-point and B-point. He therefore decided he would invent a new reference line patterned after McNamara. He calls it the BNV (Bowbeer Nasion Vertical) and defines it as a vertical line dropped from the bridge of the nose, the soft tissue equivalent of nasion, perpendicular to FH. The theory he proposed contended that if a correlation could be found between the cephalometric data and the facial data of his patients, then, since numerous studies (such as the Herron) showed that soft tissue facial profiles were a direct reflection of underlying skeletal profiles, certain correlations could be made about the skeletal patterns of the models and movie stars noted for their beauty.

What he discovered after analyzing a large number of cases was that his findings supported the general tenets of the FJO philosophy—ie, rarely was the maxilla protruded; instead it was most often neutral or retruded, and the mandible was retruded in Class II malocclusions. He also determined that by observing the facial profile of an individual, one could "get an idea of the skeletal pattern."

Bowbeer lists five key aspects to facial beauty and TMJ health. They are, in order of importance,

    Key 1 Proper maxillary position
    Key 2 Proper maxillary arch form and arch width
    Key 3 Proper mandibular AP position
    Key 4 Proper vertical dimension
    Key 5 Mandibular symmetry

Keys 1, 3, and 4 are decipherable from a lateral cephalogram. Keys 2 and 5 are intimately concerned with the three-dimensional aspects of the arch forms of the dentures. This is the reason why the entire diagnosis cannot be made from a cephalometric x-ray in norma lateralis alone. Bowbeer contends that the most important key is proper maxillary position, and that if it is not correct with proper arch form (Key 2), no amount of correction of the remaining three keys "can ever achieve proper facial balance."

The use of McNamara's NV for skeletal evaluation in conjunction with Bowbeer's BNV for soft tissue profile evaluation along with a handful of other measurements go into the making up of the Bowbeer Facial Diagnosis system of analysis. It is designed to analyze the facial profile first, then the smile, and finally the teeth last! It is predicated on employment of the above-mentioned Five Keys to be used as both analytical frames of reference and treatment goals. Bowbeer lists both facial and cephalometric criteria for these Five Keys.

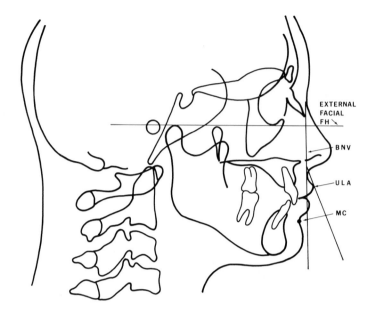

Figure 5–2 Bowbeer analysis, facial criteria: In the portion of the Bowbeer analysis dealing with the face, the external or soft tissue Frankfort Horizontal plane is used. A critical component to the Bowbeer is the BNV, which is a soft tissue nasion vertical. It is parallel to cephalometric or hard tissue nasion vertical. The third line used is the ULA (upper lip angle). The mentalis crease (MC) is an important soft tissue anatomical point that Bowbeer uses to relate the mandible to the BNV.

Key 1:   Proper maxillary AP position
Facial criteria

1. The upper lip should slope forward and curve out slightly from the base of the nose.

2. One third to one half of the upper lip should be anterior to the BNV.

3. The maxillary incisors should also slope forward to provide proper lip support.

Cephalometric criteria

1. A-point should be 0 to 3 mm ahead of skeletal NV. However, there will be some variation here due to the length of the S-N line; therefore, the final criteria of proper positioning of A-point should be based on soft tissue profile criteria!

2. The incisal edges of the maxillary centrals should lie 3 to 5 mm ahead of A-point perpendicular (a line extending from A-point perpendicular to FH).

3. The upper lip will not be well-enough supported (look too thin, flat, or "dished-in") if the incisal edges of the maxillary centrals are less than 3 mm ahead of A-point perpendicular, or if A-point itself is retruded enough. Lack of upper lip support will be manifest if the edges are less than 2 mm ahead of NV.

4. A generally "sunken-in" or flattened facial profile will result if A-point is more than 3 mm behind the NV (McNamara). A "gummy" smile often results when A-point is more than 3 mm behind the NV and the incisal edges of the upper centrals are even behind that.

Key 2: Proper maxillary arch width and arch form
Facial criteria
1. The smile should appear wide, broad, and full.
2. Lips should be fully supported with no flattening or convexity at the canine eminence and no sunken-in look to the corners of the mouth.

Arch form criteria
1. The arch form should follow the generally accepted notions of proper Roman arch shape as opposed to the more pointed or gothic arch outline (a concept best summarized by the concept of the "Leghorn Analyzer").
2. Dental midlines should be centered with respect to each other and the rest of the face.

Key 3: Proper mandibular AP position
Note: This key is predicated on the fact that the maxilla is already correctly positioned.

Facial criteria   The mentalis crease (MC), or the most posterior part of the outline of the curve between the lower lip and the chin in norma lateralis, should lie on or within 2 mm ahead of or behind the BNV. In many beautiful female facial profiles, MC will fall *ahead* of the BNV and have a slight Class III skeletal tendency or a mild bialveolar protrusion. Women just plain look good with a slight protrusion or pout to the lip area, as a careful study of any form of lipstick advertising will show. Many professional female models have a pouty appearance due to a slight protrusion in the anterior dental and alveolar area, especially those selected for cosmetics and lipstick advertising.

Cephalometric criteria
1. Class I alignment anteroposteriorly should divulge the mandibular B-point 3 to 6 mm behind the extension of A-point perpendicular. Many beautiful female faces, as well as handsome male faces, tend to be toward the Class III end of this range.
2. Class II conditions exist skeletally and tend to result in a weak-appearing chin and retruded facial profile when B-point is more than

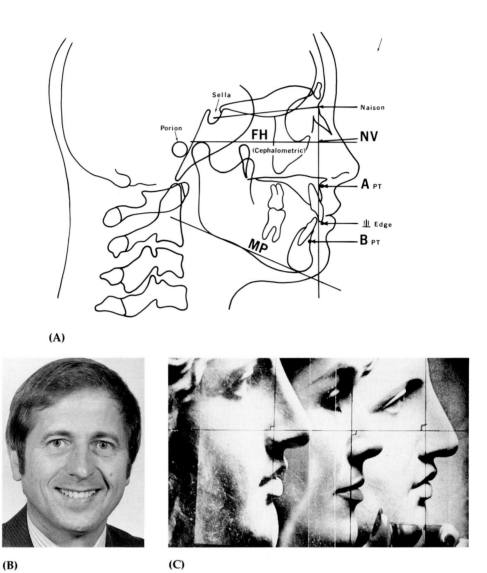

(A)

(B)   **(C)**

Figure 5–3 **(A)** Bowbeer analysis, cephalometric criteria: Bowbeer uses cephalometric nasion vertical, a direct descendant of the McNamara, and relates A-point, B-point, and incisal edge of maxillary central incisors to that line. He also uses the mandibular plane. **(B)** Grant Bowbeer. **(C)** Facial profiles comparing Greek sculpture of ideal profile with modern professional model. **(D)** Michaelangelo's "David." **(E)** Abraham Lincoln.

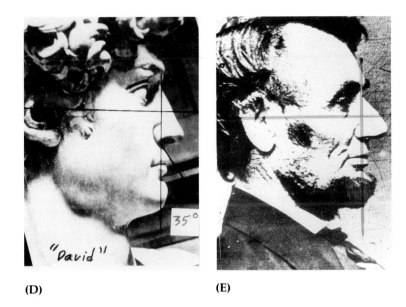

(D)   (E)

6 mm behind A-point perpendicular. Advancing the mandible in such instances usually brings a dramatic improvement in facial profile appearance.

3. Class III conditions exist when B-point is less than 3 mm behind A-point perpendicular, although this condition may often be well-tolerated when B-point is not too far beyond the Class III limiting demarcation.

Key 4: Proper vertical dimension
Facial criteria The lips should be balanced and full and easily sealed at rest with the complete absence of lip strain, or an excessively curled lower lip or accentuated MC.

Cephalometric criteria
1. Mandibular plane angle should fall between 20 and 30 degrees with a mean of 25 degrees. This, however, is also a product of posterior facial height (PFH); therefore the ultimate criteria should be the balance of the soft tissue profile from subnasale to menton as well as considerations of the degree of dental overbite.

2. Lack of sufficient vertical is often exhibited in the form of a "squished" appearance vertically of the lips, excessive curl of the lower lip with its attending accentuation of MC, and possibly a mandibular plane angle of near, or less than, 20 degrees.

3. An excess of vertical dimension is often found in open bite cases and should be a caution against molar distalization techniques that would only serve to increase vertical. Excess vertical often manifests itself in the form of lip strain upon sealing and a "gummy" smile with a mandibular plane angle in excess of 30 degrees.

Key 5: Mandibular symmetry

Facial criteria   The skeletal midline should align frontally. If it does not, the centric relation should be checked to see if either the mandibular deflection is a product of a molar dental interference, such as a slightly constricted maxillary arch that is not of sufficient magnitude to manifest itself as a full maxillary bilateral posterior crossbite, or if the case is one of true mandibular orthopedic asymmetry.[274]

Bowbeer Concepts of Diagnosis and Creation of Attractive Facial Profiles

Finding the maxilla   One of the truly cornerstone concepts that serves as a basis for the Bowbeer analysis is that rarely is the human maxilla protruded; it is either neutral or retruded. The Steiner norm for the proper location of the maxilla is the SNA angle of 82 degrees.

However, more recent studies have pointed out that a marked part of the variation of the SNA angle is to be explained by the variation of the NSAr (nasion-sella-articulare, or Saddle Angle). Since the value of the SNA angle can be affected by the configuration of the cranial base, it should be used with caution. In many cases it will be larger or smaller than the calculated mean value of 82 degrees for a normal face.[275] This supplements the findings of Dr V. Luzi, who is credited with being the first to debunk the myth of the protruded maxilla with his now classic paper: "The CV Value in the Analysis of Sagittal Malocclusion."[59]

From a cephalometric standpont, a clear relationship exists between the SNA and NSAr angles. Their combined value (CV) approaches 204.5 degrees. Thus these two angles, inversely proportional to each other, compensate for one another and therefore maintain the constant combined sum. Bowbeer notes that, in this light, an individual face may look proportionate over a given range of SNA values provided the counterpart NSAr angle can compensate for it. Even though mean SNA values range from 80 to 83 degrees, in many populations of balanced faces these mathematical means are significantly higher.

Therefore, using traditional SNA angular norms of 82 degrees as a yardstick of maxillary position represents a suspect approach. Bowbeer also feels that even McNamara's criteria of maxillary positioning, A-point to NV (mean females = 0.4 mm; mean males = 1.1 mm) can also lead to a misdiagnosis when applied to the individual. After studying many of his best posttreatment profiles, Bowbeer was disconcerted to find there was even more variation (−4 to +3 mm) of the location of A-point to NV than there was variation on the SNA! It is this fact to which he attributed the dissatisfaction many clinicians experience when using these standards in diagnosis and treatment planning. This is the reason why Bowbeer insists that the BNV soft tissue profile approach is the modern-day logical choice for a facial esthetic base reference line.

He contends that 90% of maxillas are either neutral or retruded, no matter how severe the overjet may appear. If a patient has a "flat," vertical upper lip along with vertical or lingually tipped incisors and an attending "gummy" smile, it may be concluded that he or she has a retruded or retrognathic maxilla regardless of what Steiner's SNA or McNamara's A-point to NV may indicate! Bowbeer pays much more homage to the slope of the upper lip and the location of the MC relative to the BNV. He defines the slope of the upper lip as a straight line drawn along the straightest portion of the upper lip from the base of the nose to its vermilion border. This line forms an angle with the BNV, which Bowbeer refers to as the ULA (upper lip angle). It is another critical element in the determination of superior esthetic results.

The ULA Bowbeer has discovered that most fashion models and females with superior facial esthetics have a ULA range of 20 to 30 degrees to the BNV. Attractive females with full lips may have an angle as high as 35 or 40 degrees. If a ULA is less than 15 degrees, the maxilla is usually retrognathic. Although women's lips usually keep their approximate thickness from adolescence through adulthood, men's lips will thin out somewhat during late adolescence and continue to do so into early adulthood. Thus they may possess thin or vertical upper lips even though the maxilla and upper incisors are correctly positioned.

The MC and the BNV In at least 90% of Class II, Division 1 malocclusions the maxilla will be well-positioned but the MC will fall posterior to the BNV. A quick test Bowbeer proposes is to ask the patient to slide mandibles forward so that the incisors are at or near end-to-end in the famous "as if" position, or, more jocularly, in a "poor man's ceph," and then observe the degree of improvement in facial appearance as the lower profile fills out. In most instances it will also be observed that this procedure brings the MC into near-perfect alignment with the BNV. The more severe the mandibular retrusion, the more dramatic this simple procedure appears. However, if the MC is more than 2 mm ahead of the BNV, the patient exhibits Class III tendencies. In such cases it is important to develop the maxilla as much as possible and to avoid extraction of maxillary teeth, for often the Class III facial pattern will become more severe during puberty and on through the teenage years.[276]

Discussion

Articles by many authors, clinicians, and researchers all demonstrate that the maxilla is rarely protruded—in fact, it is often retruded—but the mandible is retruded in Class II, Division 1 malocclusions. Thus, the use of any backward-pulling headgear, Class II elastics, or extraction of bicuspids would be contraindicated in most orthodontic treatment.

Bowbeer found that the standard cephalometric "norms" for determining maxillary skeletal position—the SNA mean of 82 degrees and the A-point to NV mean of 0.4 mm (females) and 1.1 mm (males) are absolutely unreliable for planning treatment for an individual patient.

Unless a cephalometric measurement is clinically accurate 100% of the time, it can never be used as an absolute guideline. Every cephalometric "norm" was based on the "average" of a group of individuals. It wouldn't matter whether the sample size was 20 or 2000, you are still getting an "average" or "norm" for any measurement (ie, SNA) for the group.

But we never treat a group; we treat the individual! Using a group "norm" for a diagnostic decision on an individual patient will frequently lead to a "missed diagnosis" and incorrect treatment. Therefore a group "norm" should only be applied with caution to an individual for a treatment goal!

Determining proper position of the maxilla and mandible Bowbeer finds the position of the upper lip to the BNV the most useful guide in quickly determining the position of the maxilla, and the location of the MC to the BNV is best for determining the position of the mandible.

Maxilla Most movie stars, fashion models, and beauty contest winners with superior facial esthetics usually have at least *one third to one half of their upper lip* in front of the BNV. They will also have a broad, wide smile related to a wide "horseshoe-shaped" maxillary arch form. If the lips are competent (closed at rest), Bowbeer believes the patient doesn't have a protruded maxilla.

Mandible Most movie stars, fashion models, and beauty contest winners with superior facial esthetics usually have their MC lying right on the BNV ±2 mm. This confirms a Class I skeletal pattern. Almost all patients with a skeletal Class II, Division 1 malocclusion will have an MC behind the BNV. The more severe the skeletal Class II pattern, the farther the MC will lie behind the BNV. This will be confirmed by the cephalometric analysis by a difference from A-point to B-point greater than 6 mm (the Class I range is 3 to 6 mm, for a mandibular plane angle of (25 ± 5) degrees).

Cephalometric analysis to achieve beautiful profiles According to Bowbeer, the most significant factor is to assume A-point to NV is "normal" for the individual patient, no matter what its value, as long as the mandibular plane (MP) to FH is within the "norm" of 25 degrees ± 5 degrees. To determine the skeletal pattern, use the following criteria.

Skeletal pattern

1. The A-point—B-point difference determines the skeletal relationship of Classes I, II, and III, but only with respect to themselves.

2. A Class I skeletal pattern will have B-point 3 to 6 mm behind A-point.

3. If B-point is less than 3 mm behind A-point, it reveals a Class III skeletal pattern: the smaller the number, the more severe the Class III (and it will be confirmed by the MC being ahead of the BNV more than 2 mm).

This analysis also works just as well for mandibular plane angles under 20 degrees. The working range is 5 to 30 degrees (MP to FH). If the mandibular plane angle is over 30 degrees, the A-point minus B-point range for Class I malocclusions becomes greater and can be as high as 9 or 10 mm and still be Class I. However, you will almost always see a "longer," lower facial height. Then a Wits analysis may be handy. Usually, the skeletal problem is in the mandible. It is important to never compromise the maxilla in these "longer-face" or "short-chin" patients.

Proper lip support   A-point to maxillary incisal edge difference *should be 5 to 6 mm* (on the A-point plane) for the proper lip support and the best facial esthetics.

Proper lip support will also have an MP to FH of (25 ± 5) degrees and (on the A-point plane) a maxillary incisal edge *5 to 6 mm ahead of A-point* and a B-point only 3 to 4 mm behind A-point (the Class III and of the Class I range). Bowbeer finds the ULA and the smile the two most useful guides in quickly determining the position of the maxilla and the maxillary teeth.

Upper lip angle   There is an important measurable angular relationship between the slope of the upper lip and the BNV that seems to be the key determinant of maxillary facial esthetics. Planning maxillary treatment goals within a certain range of the ULA will lead to superior esthetic results. Most Caucasian female models, movie stars, and beauty contest winners tend to have ULAs as "full" as 40 to 45 degrees. The critical range for the ULA to be displeasing and usually reflecting a deficient maxilla or too vertical maxillary incisors is 10 degrees to the BNV.

If the ULA at the beginning of treatment is less than 10 to 15 degrees and the patient has a "gummy" smile, the maxilla is usually deficient or perhaps in the correct A-point position with the maxillary incisors vertical, but it is *almost never protruded!* In this type of case, retraction of the maxillary incisors associated with the extraction of bicuspids or the use of backward-pulling headgear or Class II elastics will *always* have a detrimental effect on the facial profile because a "normal" or already deficient maxilla is being moved further posteriorly.

Bowbeer lists the following as the most important factors in determining ULA:

Angle of the maxillary incisors   The incisal edges of the maxillary incisors should be at least 5 to 6 mm ahead of A-point on the sagittal plane to give the proper lip support for a ULA of 20 to 30 degrees. If the upper lip is thin, the maxillary anteriors need to be forward even more than 6 mm.

Upper lip thickness   Patients with thin lips will have a lower ULA than average, even though the maxilla and the maxillary incisors may be in the proper position. In general, men have thinner lips than women. There is great ethnic variation in lip thickness. Lip thickness is affected by maturation, vertical dimension, and vertical dimension changes related to treatment.

Maturation   If the lips are thin, there is no way to "plump" them up. Most young children have "thick-appearing" lips that thin out to some degree as they mature in the teenage years. The maturation process never thickens the lips—they either stay the same or get thinner. A female with thin lips at age 11 to 12 will never develop thicker lips. Females tend to keep the same approximate lip thickness throughout the teenage years into adulthood. However, there are enough exceptions that it is better to err on the "full" side. The upper lip tends to be the lip most affected both by maturation and treatment. Men's lips tend to thin out much more than women's in the teenage years, with most Caucasian men having very thin lips and a low ULA as adults.

Vertical dimension   The more overclosed the vertical dimension, the more the lips will appear "squished" because of the lack of "stretch" related to the nose and chin being too close together. This often gives an aged facial appearance due to the "thin" lips and the lack of an adequate vermilion border.

Gummy smile   The gummy smile is one that has more than a 20% gum display when a patient smiles widely. Proper diagnosis of the cause is important, or the treatment will not be effective. Gummy smiles are usually the result of the following factors:

A tipped down premaxilla   This is the most common reason. The easiest way to confirm this problem is to see if the incisor looks too "vertical" or "tipped back" lingually (from the side view). The cephalometric analysis will demonstrate the maxillary central incisor tip to be the same distance from or even behind A-point (related to NV). Proper treatment indicates tipping the anterior teeth and the premaxilla forward and up, not up and back! Keep A-point where it is and rotate the maxillary incisors upward and forward from A-point; the esthetic improvement will be dramatic once the mandible is properly positioned with it.

A short or "lazy" upper lip (very common in females)   Many women, including fashion models, have an open lip posture with the lips at rest. It is important not to misdiagnose this problem as a "protrusion." Lip exercise and/or the use of a functional appliance such as a Bionator can frequently improve lip posture.

Maxillary vertical excess (is fairly rare)   The smile will be very gummy even though the maxillary incisors may have a proper forward slope. There is usually excessive LFH and a steep mandibular plane angle over 30 degrees to FH. When severe, the most effective treatment is orthognathic surgery.

Clinical Application of the Bowbeer Analysis

The impact of the Bowbeer analysis on the orthodontic discipline is multifold. First of all it represents the complete opposite approach to cephalometrics that has been taken since the very beginning. Throughout its entire history, cephalometrics has concerned itself with analyzing the teeth and bones in norma lateralis and determining the significance of their pretreatment relationships and what, if anything, could be done therapeutically to alter those relationships in a desirable fashion. In former times it was felt that the soft tissues could be expected to follow the hard tissue lead and, although considered in the overall scheme of things, they were only secondary to the primary issues at hand, ie, bony and toothy relationships. As previously stated, that form of cephalometric analysis and its resultant treatment planning started from the inside and worked out.

Bowbeer puts the integumental facial profile first, making *it* the standard by which all else is judged and to which all else will be subjugated. The bones and teeth will then be altered to suit the demands of the face, not vice versa. He starts from the outside and works in. This procedure is possible by the wholesale changes in bony jaw-to-jaw, and even jaw-to-skull, relationships as a result of the philosophies and techniques of FJO. It is also predicated upon the principles of the "myth of the protruded maxilla," and here is where one of the real surprises has appeared that represents another major breakthrough in the FJO evolutionary path. It concerns the newly formed attitudes about the location of the maxilla. One of the major FJO concepts that shocked the traditional and conservative fixed-appliance-oriented orthodontic establishment was that of wholesale advancement of skeletally retruded Class II mandibles forward to full Class I by functional appliances such as the Bionator. But at least the shock was mitigated somewhat by the fact that at times the orthodontic establishment would concede that mandibles were retruded on occasion.

However, now an even more revolutionary concept is blossoming forth—the new way of looking at maxillas. The old way of thinking held that often the maxilla was protruded, as in Class II, Division 1 malocclusions, and that the solution was maxillary retraction with elastics and headgear to pull it back and aid in reduction of the gigantic overjets that accompanied such problems. The new way of thinking, the result of extensive cephalometric analysis, holds that 90% of the time maxillas are either neutral or retruded. Treatment of such maxillary retrusion manifests itself in the form of forward-pulling headgear (FPHG) to bring the maxilla into its proper relationship to the anterior cranial base and, more importantly, to its proper esthetic relationship with respect to the soft tissue profile of the face! This is done in complete disregard for the position of the mandible and the mandibular dental arch. For once the maxilla is properly secured with respect to the newfound cephalometric and facial profile standards, the mandible and its mandibular arch may be easily aligned to it, with the "arch aligning appliance" of the new era, the Bionator. Therefore, not only must the conservative establishment accept moving mandibles forward, but they are now also confronted with the concept of moving maxillas forward. This is the direction Nature has always been attempting to develop things in the maxillofacial complex from the start! Only now have we finally started to cooperate.

Bowbeer determined after extensive analysis that the standard cephalometric "norms" for determining maxillary position (SNA mean of 82 degrees, A-point to NV of 0.4 mm for females and 1.1 mm for males) to be "absolutely unreliable for planning treatment for an individual patient."[277] Proper position of the maxilla and proper arch form to the maxillary dental arch may then be seen to be keys to not only facial beauty but also TMJ health. With the maxillary arch properly positioned forward enough relative to the cranial base and facial profile, plenty of space exists in most circumstances to free the mandibular arc of closure from any form of anterior incisal interference and the occurrence of the NRDM-SPDC phenomenon (neuromuscular reflexive displacement of the mandible causing superior posterior displacement of the condyle). Proper position of the mandible is acknowledged by all to be the key to TMJ health and performance. However, in light of the above, it may now be seen that the key to proper mandibular position is *proper maxillary position*! It therefore follows that proper vertical dimension, maxillary arch form, and maxillary position are the three most important keys to the prevention and correction of TMJ problems.

Bowbeer clearly points out that most conventional diagnostic concepts maintain that crowding is due to "teeth that are too large for the size of the jaws they are in." These concepts also state that excessive overjet is due to maxillary protrusion, excessive overbite is due to overerupted incisors, and skeletal growth patterns cannot be modified to any appreciable degree (a concept that goes back nearly a half century, from a cephalometric standpoint, to Brodie). As a result of these suspect diagnostic concepts, treatment of the traditional type took the form of fixed tooth-moving appliances, backward-pulling headgear, Class II elastics, and the extraction of bicuspids to relieve arch-crowding problems. The lower arch was "set up" with mandibular incisors positioned over basal bone to within 1 degree of some standard or another of incisor to mandibular plane angle, and all the teeth in maxilla (and often the maxilla itself) were treated so as to meet the mandibular arch. This was a matter of retracting the correct member back to meet the incorrect member.

The principles of FJO, on the other hand, contend that most crowding is only apparent and is due to a combination of orthopedically constricted dental arches in combination with the compounding thrust of the second molars. Excessive overjet is due to mandibular retrusion, and excessive overbite is due to a lack of vertical dimension, the result of insufficiently erupted posterior quadrants. Skeletal patterns, ie, jaw-to-jaw (and now even jaw-to−anterior cranial base) relationships, are amenable to therapeutic change. As a result, retruded maxillas are developed forward with FPHG. Constricted arches are developed to full potential by a combination of active plate development laterally as well as anteroposteriorly along with second-molar extractions (where indicated), and only then are they finished and perfected orthodontically with fixed appliances. Retruded mandibles are advanced as needed, and decreased vertical dimensions are increased with functional arch-aligning appliances such as the Bionator. The maxilla is secured first; then the mandible is treated to fit it. The TMJs govern the entire operation and are given top priority, with the face coming second and the teeth last! It's a mighty big pill for the conservative orthodontic establishment to swallow, for it's a long way from the chevrons of compromise of Cecil Steiner.

Coda to the Bowbeer—The Sixth Key: Exposing the Illusion!

For St. Paul the Apostle it was the road to Damascus. For Grant Bowbeer it was the road to Toronto. For it was there that his dramatic "conversion" took place, and he began viewing facial profiles and orthodontic methodologies in a new light. The conversion to the FJO viewpoint from the more traditional four-bicuspid-extraction−fixed-appliance-oriented methods eventually manifested themselves in the Bowbeer analysis and the Five Keys. But there was a final component that did not make its initial appearance in unison with the rest but rather took some time to gradually materialize, like a distant object in a slowly lifting fog, the all-important Sixth Key. Its recognition and ultimate definition in the mind of Bowbeer occurred over a four-year period and concerns itself with one of the most fundamental of tenets basic to all orthodontic philosophies, that of mandibular arch form. The Sixth Key to facial beauty, stability, and TMJ health according to Bowbeer lies in the proper uprighting of the lower posterior teeth along with proper mandibular arch form! This must go hand in hand with another important factor, proper vertical!

Bowbeer correctly surmised that there is a major adjustment mechanism inherent in the maxillary and mandibular alveolar processes that automatically compensates (as best it can under the specific circumstances that prevail) for minor discrepancies in the jaw-to-jaw maxillomandibular relationship. To describe this process, he coined the term "alveolar warpage." This alveolar warping is part of the same process responsible for dental eruption and the extrusion of teeth into edentulous areas of opposing arches. It is this adaptive mechanism that functional orthodontists take advantage of in efforts to increase vertical with such appliances as the Bionator. Since such forces are present throughout life, it is for this reason that clinicians, such as John Witzig, emphatically state that these types of functional appliances that take advantage of such eruptive forces will work "as long as the patient is alive."

In light of the above concept of alveolar warping, Bowbeer views Class II skeletal patterns with inadequate vertical dimension as being generally nothing more than a condition where the retruded skeletal Class II mandible forces the upper anteriors forward (due to overclosure, ie, lack of vertical) and subsequently forces the lower anteriors to tip back and crowd up. In Class II, Division 1 problems this results in a more pointed or constricted maxillary arch form with accompanying posterior trans-arch width loss (Leghorn Analyzer fashion). This forces lowered tongue posture (the lower the resting posture, the greater the constriction), an impingement of the airway. It also encourages nearly equivalent mandibular arch constriction. A prime culprit in this condition is "undererupted" posterior teeth. As the maxillary incisors are squeezed forward and flared out, they give an illusion of maxillary protrusion. Mandibular incisors correspondingly must constrict and either flare forward or upright, giving a condition Bowbeer refers to as "apparent crowding," as opposed to actual crowding. He also feels that many Class II, Division 2 cases are actually "Class I overclosed" cases with a trapped mandibular arc of closure (NRDM-SPDC phenomenon). He views the Class III situation as often being nothing more than a hyperpropulsion of the mandible (mandibular arch form) forward due to a constricted maxillary arch. This forms a natural "functional headgear" effect that only serves to displace the maxilla even farther posteriorly. This in turn forces the upper and lower incisors back even farther due to lip pressure.

The significance of all this is that the adaptive mechanism of the

ACCUCEPH™

Cephalometer System

The versatile wall-mounted Accuceph™ Cephalometer system provides valuable diagnostic information by taking precise, high-quality, repeatable cephalograms. Its rigid, durable design ensures stability and accuracy for years of trouble-free use. (See reverse for details.)

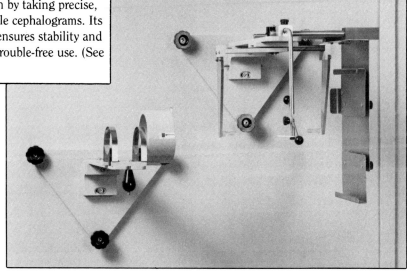

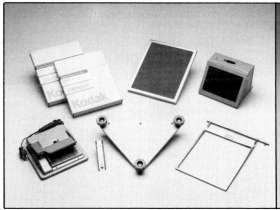

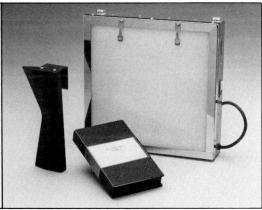

Accessories

The Accuceph Cephalometer System is available with a number of accessories to maximize its versatility and provide the highest quality cephalograms attainable.

A. Accuceph
B. Ortho Film
C. Fluorescent Safelight with GBX Filter
D. 8″ x 10″ Film Hanger
E. Film Processing Thermometer
F. Film Light Imprinter
G. Ortho G Film (for better bone definition)
H. Quick-Release Wall Plate
I. 8″ x 10″ Film Cassette with Rare Earth Intensifying Screens
J. Soft Tissue Shield
K. Tracing Box/Viewer
L. Accuceph Video

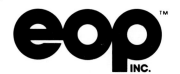

INC.

FEATURES	BENEFITS

Cephalostat:

- Ear post assembly rotates 360° with 45° stops.
- Maintains a constant mid-sagittal reference plane.
- Metal Rings inside plastic ear pieces which appear on the processed film.

- Cassette travel lock allows the cassette to travel with the ear post, keeping the cassette as close to the patient as possible.
- Plastic orbital pointer and nasion rest to establish and maintain proper plane for leveling the patient's head for each lateral shot.
- Cassette adjusts horizontally (8″ x 10″) and vertically (10″ x 8″).

Benefits:

- Accommodates lateral, anterior-posterior, posterior-anterior and oblique views.
- Ensures optimal distance from the focal point of the X-ray beam to the patient.
- Identified external auditory meatus as a reference point for tracings and confirms correct alignment of the cephalostat.
- Ideal magnification and resolution of each cephalogram for viewing and tracing.

- Ensures repeatability of patient positioning throughout progressive treatment.

- Accommodates lateral, A-P, P-A, oblique an cervical area views.

Fixator/Collimator:

- Adjustable cone lock handle.
- Adjusts horizontally (8″ x 10″) and vertically (10″ x 8″).

Benefits:

- Easily adapts to most standard X-ray cones.
- Accommodates lateral, A-P, P-A, oblique an cervical area views.

Accessories:

- Quick-Release Wall Plate.

- 8″ x 10″ Film Cassette with Lanex Rare Earth Intensifying Screens.
- Ortho G Film (pkg. of 100).
- Soft Tissue Shield.

- Film Light Imprinter which places date and patient's name directly onto the cephalogram.
- Fluorescent Safelight with GBX Filter.

Benefits:

- Allows easy removal and storage of one or both parts of the system.
- Reduces standard exposure time approximately 25%.
- Provides better bone definition.
- Enhances tissue definition on cephalograms.
- Provides legitimate legal/medical/insurance documentation.
- Needed for darkroom processing of extra-oral films.

Call to order: Toll FREE Nationwide 1-800-328-8021
MN (612) 572-3757

alveolar processes of the maxilla and mandible react to (and attempt to compensate for) unfavorable maxillofacial anatomical circumstances, which results in an alveolar warpage. This warping of the alveolar process often manifests itself in the form of an illusion of maxillary protrusion and a dental crowding (constricture due to lack of vertical) of the lower arch. Bowbeer, as well as many others, believe that a diminished airway is the chief etiological agent here, and it is responsible for a dominolike effect thus: a diminished airway contributes to forward head posture, which contributes to lowered tongue posture, which contributes to constriction of the maxillary arch, which contributes to retrusion of the mandible, which contributes to constriction of the mandibular arch, which all eventually lead to the big thing, a severe lack of vertical dimension—quite a chain!

Once initiated, a vicious cycle is generated in which the case is worsened by further muscular imbalances and excessive improperly directed occlusal force vectors, which only serve to aggravate the problem, collapsing the arches evermore in on themselves. Into this arena add the mighty thrust of the powerful second molars and their undaunted efforts to make room for the thirds, and it is a wonder patients do not turn out worse than they already are! Thus it may be seen that Bowbeer's Sixth Key fits right dead center into the heart of the FJO philosophy. The unfolding of the flower, ie, arch development, arch form, arch alignment both anteroposteriorly *and* vertically are the basic elements of untangling the stubborn knot of the malocclusion.

From a cephalometric standpoint, Bowbeer discovered that both the facial components and cephalometric components of his relatively simple analysis confirmed the theories of Luzi that maxillas are seldom if ever protruded and that Class II malocclusions are due to retruded mandibles. Both the facial and cephalometric components were found to be not only clinically accurate but also correlated to each other. Since Bowbeer's analysis is not based on norms, it is reliable on each individual patient, being a product of the patient's own anatomical makeup. In comparing his analysis with other major well-known analyses, Bowbeer states,

> When the Bowbeer Facial and Cephalometric Analyses were compared with the Steiner Analysis, the Tweed Analysis, and the McNamara Analysis, it was discovered that there was *absolutely no relationship* between the standard cephalometric numbers and the (patient's) facial profile. The 'norms' of various cephalometric analyses (Steiner's SNA, Tweed's FMIA, and McNamara's A-Point to nasion vertical) have absolutely no relationship to facial esthetics for an individual patient.

It may only be a coincidence, but it seems somehow symbolically appropriate that for the world of orthodontics a great clinician named Dr Larry Andrews developed the Six Keys to proper occlusion and for the world of dental orthopedics another great clinician in the person of Dr Grant Bowbeer developed the Six Keys to facial beauty and TMJ health. As such, Bowbeer's analysis represents a portion of the renewed and intensified concern for the face and the TMJs. But this is only the beginning. More waves are coming.

CEPHALOMETRICS AND THE COMPUTER

A key component in the modern metamorphosis of the status of the science of cephalometrics has been the incorporation of those marvels of our modern age, the digital computers. The computer age has only just begun. Where it will take us in the future is open to even the most extravagant flights of fancy. To comment on their use in cephalometrics at length would require an entire separate text. However, there are some salient features of their history, development, and current usage in cephalometrics that are germane to our discussion here. Due to the nature of the subject and the limited space available in this particular text, we shall direct our discussion not to a detailed discourse of how these sophisticated electronic counting machines are used to augment the academic aspects of cephalometric science but to the overall directions their use has taken over the past decade or so, and to the pioneers who have played an important role in ushering in their use for *clinical* purposes.

No discussion of the use of computers in orthodontic diagnosis in general or cephalometric diagnosis in specific would be possible, no matter how brief, without mentioning the contributions of Dr Robert M. Ricketts, termed by many "the father of computerized cephalometrics." The Ricketts analysis first appeared in 1960.[70] Ricketts produced his analysis for a number of reasons. First, he wanted to provide a method that could be used to adequately describe, classify, and compare the clinical aspects of an individual's given malocclusion. Second, he wanted to clarify the science of cephalometrics somewhat and free it from some of the confusion and misuse that pervaded the discipline. He also wanted to point out that the use of cephalometrics to describe and classify a malocclusion was one thing, ie, "analysis." However, the act of planning a treatment as a result of the inferences of that classification and description was quite another, that of "synthesis." His position was that the clinician could not effectively plan how to treat a case unless it was accurately represented. Therefore, the purpose of his initial analysis was to provide that necessary medium of description. It originally consisted of two parts. The first part, or superficial survey, evaluated the outer gross features. The second part dealt with analysis of deeper structures. Ricketts uses many traditional landmarks for his cephalometric analysis. However, he has also developed some that are unique to his approach, and some which, though they utilize common names, have specific definitions. Those of special interest are discussed below.

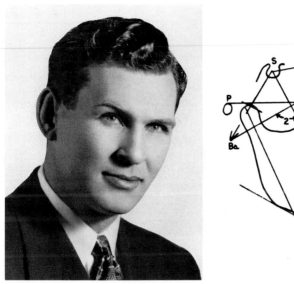

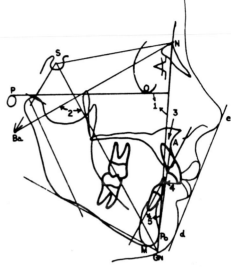

(A)   **(B)**

Figure 5–4   (A) Robert Murray Ricketts. **(B)** Ricketts' original cephalometric analysis: (1) facial angle, (2) *XY* growth axis, (3) facial convexity, (4) linear distance of central incisor to A-Pog line, (5) angulation of lower incisor to A-Pog line, d-e Ricketts' esthetic line (E-line). The original Ricketts analysis consisted of ten criteria. (Figures 5–4 through 5–11 reprinted from Ricketts RM: A foundation for cephalometric communication. *Am J Orthod* 1960; 46: 330–357 with permission.)

Ricketts Analysis (Original)

Superficial analysis—five hard tissue items and the soft tissue profile

Facial angle   The angle formed between the facial plane (N-Pog) and FH. In a 9-year-old it averages 87 degrees and increases 1 degree per 3 years to 90 degrees in the adult. It is used as an indicator of the horizontal position of the mandible.

Facial axis (XY-axis)   The angle formed by the intersection of a line from foramen rotundum (PT) to gnathion (Gn) with the line of the basion-nasion plane. The symbol PT stands for pterygoid point, the intersection of the inferior border of the foramen rotundum with the posterior wall of the PTM fissure. This point (PT) is slightly different from the Bimler point (T). The Ricketts pterygoid vertical (PTV) originates at the PT point, on the *distal surface* of the PTM fissure, and runs perpendicular to FH. On the other hand, the Bimler pterygoid vertical (TV) originates at the *center* of the upper curvature of the PTM fissure and runs perpendicular to FH. The two are quite close, yet distinctly different. The Facial Axis of the Ricketts analysis is measured inferiorly and posteriorly to the intersection of the two lines, PT-Gn and Ba-N, and is used as an indicator of the main component of growth. It should ideally be 90 degrees. This would indicate a balance between horizontal and vertical growth of the facial complex. Less than 90 degrees would indicate mandibular retrusion and vertical growth tendencies. Greater than 90 degrees would indicate a more horizontally dominant growth pattern. It is sometimes referred to as the *XY*-axis and is expressed as such as plus or minus from the ideal of 90 degrees (plus being greater than 90 degrees, minus being less than 90 degrees).

Facial convexity (A-point to facial plane)   Facial convexity is the linear distance between A-point and the facial plane (N-Pog). The clinical norm at 9 years of age was originally recorded at 4.1 ± 2.8 mm. However, this was later modified to ideally be 2.0 mm (at 9 years), and gradually decreases to 0 mm at adulthood. High convexity (plus readings) indicate convex facial profiles and imply a Class II skeletal pattern. Low values are referred to as concavities (negative numbers) and are associated with concave facial profiles and Class III skeletal relationships.

Lower incisor position and angulation   Position of lower incisor relative to A-Pog line. The incisal edge of the lower incisor should fall 1 mm (± 2 mm) beyond the A-Pog line (sometimes seen as AP line). This gives it a rather broad range of acceptability according to Ricketts (−1 to +3 mm).

Inclination of lower incisor to A-Pog line. The inclination of the long axis of the lower incisor should be 22 degrees plus or minus 4 degrees. The A-Pog is also referred to by Ricketts as the "denture plane."

Upper incisor position   Again the denture plane is used here as a base reference line (A-Pog). The distance between the incisal edge of the maxillary central incisor to the A-Pog plane was originally reported to be (5.7 ± 3) mm. This was later refined to a clinical norm of (3.5 ± 2.3) mm.

E-plane   The Ricketts esthetic plane (sometimes seen as E-line) runs from the tip of the nose to soft tissue pogonion. The lower lip ranges from +2 mm to −2 mm from the E-line. Normal for the 9-year-old, however, is the −2-mm reading.

Deep structure analysis—five hard tissue items

Cranial base angle   N-S-Ba angle 129.6 degrees, range 114 to 144 degrees.

Cranial base length   The length of the anterior cranial base S-N was not measured linearly but was expressed as the unusual angle formed by the intersection of lines S-Gn and N-Gn, or the S-Gn-N angle; the mean was 35 degrees with a range of 25 to 42 degrees.

Condyle or fossa position   A line S-Ba was bisected, and this point was called SOR (spheno-occipital reference). Condylion was then measured to that point. Average location of condylion was 1.3 mm upward and 1.9 mm backward from SOR.

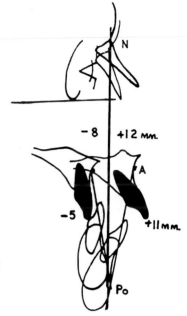

Figure 5−5 Facial convexity and maxillary central incisor position to A-Pog line. This illustration depicts two examples of the facial convexity: one A-point, minus 8 mm behind N-Pog line; the other A-point plus 12 mm in front of it. Incisor position is related to the A-Pog line (unlike A-point, which it must be remembered is related to the *N-Pog* line).

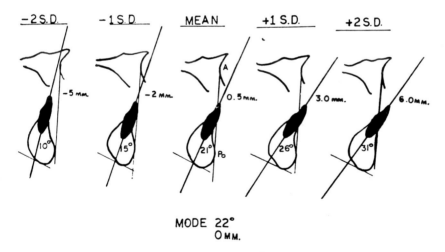

Figure 5−6 Ricketts relates the mandibular incisor both angularly and linearly to the A-Pog line.

Condylar axis (drawn by inspection)   This represents to Ricketts the general growth axis of the condylar neck and hovers around the ideal of 90 degrees to the line S-Ba but is expressed (as is the XY-axis) as plus or minus from the 90-degree ideal.

Mandibular plane angle   The mandibular plane (Go-Gn) as measured to FH should be 26 degrees at 9 years of age and reduces 1 degree every 3 years to adulthood. It has a range of ±4 degrees.

The above represents Ricketts' original analysis with a few of the norms modified to more modern standards. Sometimes the measurement of the location of the maxillary central incisors is incorrectly omitted from reports of the "original" Ricketts analysis. Also, one may occasionally see the inclusion of "Ricketts' rule" of upper first molar positioning reported as one of the original factors of the analysis; but this measurement did not show up until much later. It states that the distance from PTV to the distal surface of the maxillary first molar should equal the patient's age plus 3 mm! The standard deviation is 3 mm, and Ricketts states that at least 21 mm is needed in later years to permit proper eruption of second and third molars. Extracting second molars when indicated obviates concern over this problem.

As stated earlier, the sample Ricketts drew from for this initial study consisted of over 1000 cases. This was one of the first analyses to be developed that included ranges of values for norms and the degree of change expected in that particular norm due to growth over the period from 9 years to adulthood. It is but a short step from such procedures to that elusive goal Ricketts had been seeking ever since the days of the Cephalometric Workshops in Cleveland—growth prediction! However,

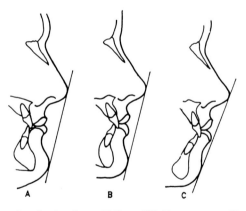

Figure 5–7   Ricketts' esthetic plane, E-line. **(A)** Concave profile. **(B)** Straight face. **(C)** Slight protrusion of lower lip (lower lip to E-line 0 mm at age 11–14, −2 mm at age 15–18, −4 mm in adult).

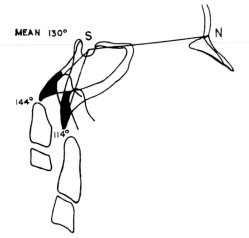

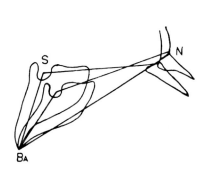

Figure 5—8   Ricketts demonstrated in a survey of 200 cases the variance of the N-S-Ba (Saddle Angle) in the cranial base. Range was 114 to 144 degrees with a mean of 130 degrees. N-S line was superimposed, and tracings were registered at S.

Figure 5—9   Ricketts also demonstrated the extreme variation in S-N angulation in the same example when tracings were subsequently superimposed on N-Ba (Huxley's old line) registered at Ba.

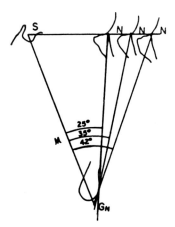

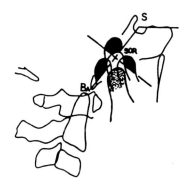

Figure 5—10   Length of S-N line. Ricketts expressed the linear length of the S-N line in the form of an angle S-Gn-N. Range 25 to 42 degrees with a mean of 35 degrees.

Figure 5—11   Condyle/fossa location: SOr.

this would necessitate the management of large amounts of data and require rather sophisticated computations.

In this light is it any wonder Ricketts took advantage of the arrival of the computer to facilitate his methods? He started doing serious work with them in 1965 and his relatively simple cephalometric analysis in conjunction with enormous amounts of data from a wide variety of other sources mushroomed into the gargantuan 50-factor analysis systems of the computerized frontal and lateral cephalometric analysis system now commercially available through Rocky Mountain Data Systems (RMDS). With Ricketts' enormous talents acting as a clinical spearhead, and his research data, along with the data of many other experts, as a foundation from which to launch their efforts, RMDS designed its computerized cephalometric analysis system around the original Ricketts analysis and greatly expanded it in order to facilitate its diagnostic prowess and to enhance the reliability of its growth predictions.

Over a decade, some 150,000 cases were entered into and analyzed by the RMDS computers. The service produces a computer-drawn cephalometric tracing, printouts of the discrepancies present according to the standards represented by the norms assembled and mitigated by the patient's age, sex, and race. It also produces a recommended treatment plan and a visualized treatment objective (VTO), which represents a computer-drawn tracing of the best outcome to be reasonably expected, given the patient's starting condition and *average* growth.

However, it must be remembered that the Ricketts analysis as well as the other efforts undertaken in cephalometrics of that period were devised at a time when fixed appliances and four-bicuspid-extraction technique was still the reigning status quo. Measurements that would be pertinent to such things as a large scale therapeutically changeable position in the location of the mandible were absent, the facial angle notwithstanding. Also missing in those early efforts were the ramifications such orthopedic changes would effect on the facial profile. When arch crowding indicated a need for extractions, the original programs were calculated to consider bicuspid extraction as the solution. Once the concepts of second molar replacement techniques made their assaults on the orthodontic world, modifications were quickly made to original computer programs to include such parameters. Yet the basic premise of the original analysis, and all analyses of the pre-Sassouni era, was that the arch form of the lower arch must be established as ideally as possible in its original pretreatment skeletal position, and the maxillary arch must then be treated to it. (This is the complete opposite of the approach dictated by the FJO philosophy.)

Therefore, as a reflection of this outlook, this was one direction early computerized cephalometrics necessarily would take; for its day it might have been the only direction available to it. It was a movement that began with Downs and Brodie and the early notions of immutability of jaw-to-jaw relationships and went on through the sophistications and intensifications of the Steiner era and culminated in the quintessential form in which it now appears under RMDS. Faces were thought of as merely lips on a line. Treating to improve facial esthetics initially resolved itself merely to a matter of the degree of labial or lingual crown torque imparted to the anterior teeth. The upper lip, lower lip, MC, and soft tissue chin were never related to any form of esthetic reference line that ever extended up past the tip of the nose. Temporomandibular joints were never x-rayed specifically to relate the condyle at rest, and at full occlusion, to the glenoid fossa; and not a single statement was ever made about how the mechanics of the methods used at the time might affect the mandibular arc of closure or where its ending point at full occlusion would force the mandibular condyles to seat.

Treating malocclusions became equated with things like manipulating interincisal angles, exactly determining the relationship of lower incisors to the mandibular plane, bicuspid space closure, directions in which the teeth on either side of the extraction gap should be moved, and what it would take to obtain coupling of the anteriors by means of interarch Class II elastics to reduce huge overjets by pure orthodontic tooth movement. No conclusions were ever drawn as to what effect all this had on that singular entity which allowed the jaws to work in the first place—the TMJs. They were left to shift for themselves. They were far to the back. Concern was concentrated on the front, on the teeth, and getting them to align and couple with each other with only themselves and distorted or limited baselines as a frame of reference. Jaws themselves were never thought of as needing alignment. The cephalometrics of the day was thought to hold the cryptic keys to unlocking the secret numbers that would allow mere fixed appliance orthodontics to successfully use tooth positioning to effect an orthopedic masquerade. But sparked by breakthroughs in removable appliance technique, computerized cephalometrics could also take other directions, and it soon did—not only by RMDS but also by others.

Others on the clinical level also started putting computers to work to deal with the problems of cephalometric diagnosis. Some felt computers could greatly facilitate the physical production of the more complicated analyses, unburdening the clinician or technician from much of the hackwork of producing tracings by hand and making measurements and calculations individually. Computers would not have to make growth predictions or recommend the most likely treatment plans to be used for given malocclusions; they could merely assist with the physical work of doing a given analysis, leaving interpretation and all other "synthesis" to the clinician. One of the first clinicians to employ computers in this way was Dr J. Wellington Truitt of Gainsville, Texas. He and his co-workers developed the first commercially available computerized service capable of performing a complete Bimler analysis, even in color!

The Smith Brothers

Yet there were still those who believed the computer could be put to the work of assisting the doctor on reaching conclusions and obtaining information that would be inaccessible by the human mind alone, or at least not without a great expenditure of time and effort. One of the great pioneers in the field of applying the computer to cephalometric analysis, interpretation, diagnosis, and treatment planning that would be fully compatible with the basic tenets of the FJO philosophy was a professional mathematician and computer expert turned functional orthodontics wizard, the unassuming and rotund Dr D. D. Smith of Painted Post, New York.

Dr Smith brings a truly unique and impressive set of qualifications to the scene of computerized cephalometrics. He earned a bachelor's degree in physics and a master's degree in statistics from Pennsylvania State University in the mid-1960s before entering computer management and statistical forecasting in private industry. Smith's contributions to the literature of mathematics, computers, and statistical analysis includes journal articles as well as coauthorship of a text on the subject of mathematical computerized forecasting techniques (econometric models).[278-281]

After nearly 10 years experience as a mathematician and computer manager, Smith decided to change careers. He earned a DMD degree from Washington University School of Dentistry in St. Louis, Missouri. He quickly became interested in new "functional approaches" to orthodontics and pursued that area of endeavors with a religious fervor. In doing so, Smith realized the overwhelming importance of comprehensive diagnosis as the key to proper treatment planning. He also realized that many of the diagnostic procedures (both two-dimensional and three-dimensional) could be described as nothing more than applied mathematics, and a computer can do anything mathematical. Therefore, he decided to undertake the enormous project of developing computer programs capable of performing much of the tedious mathematical work of accumulating and interpreting two-dimensional cephalometric and three-dimensional model analysis data. He realized that such a system could perform calculations and make predictions with high levels of accuracy totally impossible by the unaided human mind.

For such an ambitious undertaking, Smith's background in physics, computer and statistical management, and his dental education would prove invaluable. But he would need help. And in a stroke of incredible scientific luck, that help was realized in the form of a highly respected individual of national repute in the computer industry, his own brother, Mr Norman Smith of Corning, New York. Norm Smith, a full-time computer programmer, also bears excellent qualifications: He possesses a master's degree in mathematics from North Texas State. Upon graduation he immediately entered the computer field. Though Dr Don provided

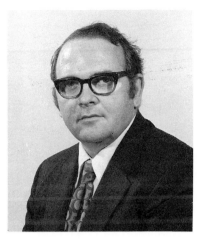
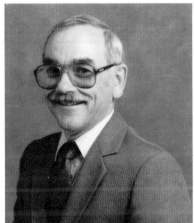

(A)   **(B)**

Figure 5–12   **(A)** D. D. Smith. **(B)** Norman K. Smith.

much of the creative guidance from a clinical standpoint, the Herculean work of converting these ideas into the binary language of computer programs rested with the ingenious efforts of brother Norm. It would require an enormous effort and years of work, but the results of the efforts initiated by these two men and their fellow colleagues are nothing short of astounding.

Together, these two "cephalometric Smith brothers" in conjunction with other orthodontic and computer experts have developed a truly remarkable series of computerized diagnostic programs that represent a turning point in the modernization of the science. These programs, which are now commercially available, have made a wide range of various forms of incisive, comprehensive, accurate diagnostic and treatment-planning information available to the clinician, and have unburdened the orthodontic profession from much of the tedious hackwork of producing cephalometric tracings and analysis. Three-dimensional considerations are also included: Computer program have been developed by the Smiths that are capable of measuring and analyzing information taken directly from representative study models of a given case. In a coup of truly stunning proportions, the Smiths have been able, through a series of intricate and extremely advanced procedures in mathematics and computer technology, to produce extensive computerized output of standard cephalometric analysis components as well as computerized treatment-planning recommendations that are corroborated by the computer's own cephalometric and model analysis findings, and predicated upon fulfilling the basic precepts of the FJO philosophy. With a cephalogram, a pano-

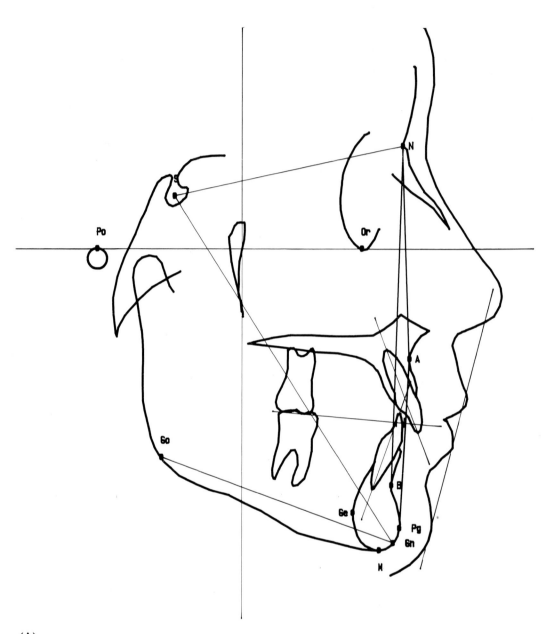

(A)

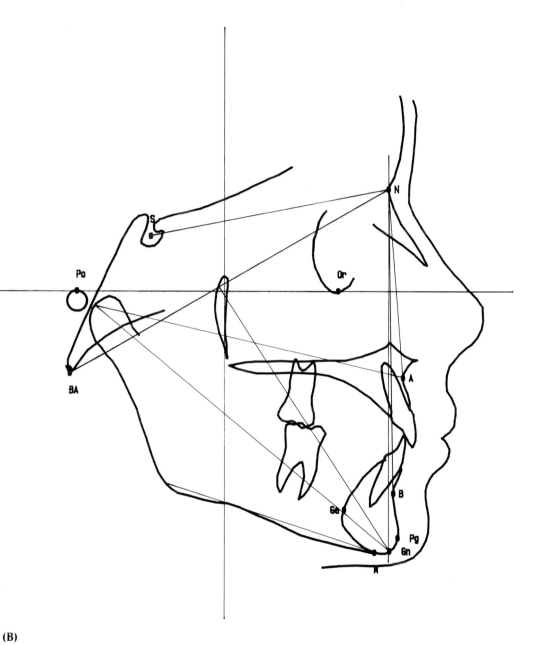

(B)

Figure 5—13   Computerized (modified) versions of traditional cephalometric analysis systems developed by the Smith brothers et al. **(A)** Modified Steiner. **(B)** Functional Orthopedic. **(C)** Modified Bimler. (Courtesy Ortho-Diagnostics Ltd, St Louis, Mo)

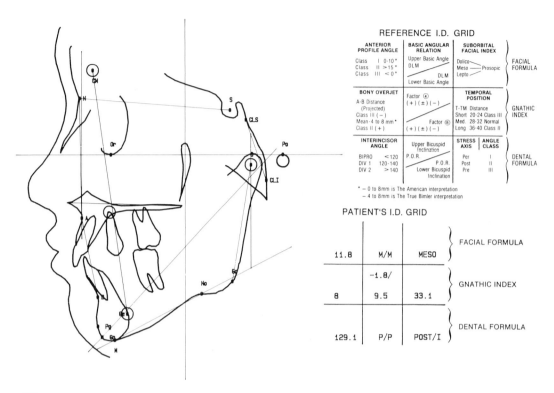

REFERENCE I.D. GRID

ANTERIOR PROFILE ANGLE	BASIC ANGULAR RELATION	SUBORBITAL FACIAL INDEX	
Class I 0-10°	Upper Basic Angle	Dolico	FACIAL
Class II >15°	DLM	Meso ——— Prosopic	FORMULA
Class III <0°		Lepto	
	DLM		
	Lower Basic Angle		
BONY OVERJET	Factor ④	**TEMPORAL POSITION**	
A-B Distance	(+) (±) (−)		
(Projected)		T-TM Distance	GNATHIC
Class III (−)		Short 20-24 Class III	INDEX
Mean-4 to 8 mm*	Factor ⑧	Med. 28-32 Normal	
Class II (+)	(+) (±) (−)	Long 36-40 Class II	
INTERINCISOR ANGLE	Upper Bicuspid Inclination	STRESS AXIS / ANGLE CLASS	
BIPRO <120	P.O.R.	Per I	DENTAL
DIV 1 120-140	P.O.R.	Post II	FORMULA
DIV 2 >140	Lower Bicuspid Inclination	Pre III	

* − 0 to 8mm is The American interpretation
− 4 to 8mm is The True Bimler interpretation

PATIENT'S I.D. GRID

11.8	M/M	MESO	} FACIAL FORMULA
	−1.8/		
8	9.5	33.1	} GNATHIC INDEX
129.1	P/P	POST/I	} DENTAL FORMULA

(C)

ramic x-ray, and a set of accurate study models of a given case, an incredible amount of information is produced by the Smith computer programs. The computerized output covers cephalometric analysis, model analysis, and treatment guides.

Computerized Cephalometric Evaluation (Smith) The first thing the Smiths did was to develop a method of producing computer-drawn cephalometric tracings of the roentgenocephalogram in norma lateralis upon which a variety of analysis systems could be performed. The first three types of analysis systems to be computerized were the modified Steiner, the Functional Orthopedic (which draws heavily on the McNamara analysis), and the modified Bimler. The word "modified" is used because in developing the computer programs for these systems, the Smiths incorporated additional data and calculations from a variety of sources that resulted in more thorough analysis than would have been possible with the individual original systems. This is easy to do from the benefit of hindsight once the shortcomings of a specific analysis have been exposed by critics over the years.

Cephalometric tracings of the radiographic image in norma lateralis are drawn by the computer. After landmark location, the computer quickly (and unerringly) constructs the various reference lines of the particular analysis being performed. It then precisely measures pertinent linear distances and calculates the associated angles involved in the particular analysis. To accompany the cephalometric tracings (produced life-sized by the computer) is the data sheet on which is printed the tabulation of the respective measurements for the analysis being performed. The "norms" characteristic for that given analysis are listed in one column. In addition to the standard measurements, the norms are modified wherever possible by the computer to compensate for age, sex, race, and facial type.

The information and data necessary to produce these mitigating adjustments that help individualize the analysis for a given patient were obtained from the latest available studies of ethnic groups. The enormous data banks for these and other calculations were compiled from a vast array of growth studies and constantly updated electronically by the Smith team whenever new information becomes available.

Adjacent to the column on the data sheet for standard measurements of a given analytical system are listed the respective "actual" values taken (or calculated) directly from the radiograph. This allows for quick and easy comparison. In a third column adjacent to these two are listed any alerts, which are designed to solicit the special interest of the clinician. The appearance of an "alert" is triggered by an "actual" measurement or value that is outside the range of normality for that particular case. This makes the overall cephalometric assessment even easier since it is taken care of automatically by the computer.

To delve into a detailed discussion as to all the various ways the Smith team used computer technology to augment and improve the process of conventional cephalometric analysis would be prohibitive here and could easily fill the pages of an entire separate text. However, one small example of the difference computers (and expert statistical management) can make can be found in how the Smiths dealt with certain aspects of the McNamara analysis. At first, this fine analysis may appear to defy improvement, since it is straightforward, broad-based enough to be both orthodontic and orthopedic, and is based on impeccable research data, or at least so it seems. But there were certain subtle nuances of the analysis that caught the discerning eye of the Smith team. Mathematicians learn to look at things differently. There is a slight problem with the way McNamara arrives at the norms used for effective lengths of the maxilla, mandible, and ANS-Me lower face height (LFH) at a given age. The result of his methods produces a somewhat erratic development of normative standards with respect to age that do not have as reasonable a level of continuity as they might have if the proper principles of advanced and sophisticated statistical management mathematics are employed.

What McNamara did was to use tables like that of the Bolton standards and the Burlington Orthodontic Research Center standards for measurements of the effective mandibular length (Co-Gn), the maxillary length (Co-A-point), the maxillomandibular differential, and the ANS-Me LFH for each sex for the age groups 6, 9, 12, 14, 16, 18, and 20 years, respectively. This makes for a somewhat mathematically "bumpy" plot and a lot of guesswork (one step below what a mathematician would call extrapolation) for patients who fall "between the cracks." Nevertheless, it would still be quite serviceable. But putting computers to work, governed by men who manage statistics for a living, is like adding power steering to an automobile. It smooths things out very nicely.

What the Smith team did was to take these tables and, by advanced mathematical processes dubbed "the bootstrap method," produce a new data base upon which regression analysis procedures were subsequently performed. Two separate formulae were employed at this stage of development. The first predicts the length of the mandible as a function of the length of the maxilla. The second predicts the ANS-Me LFH as a function of the length of the maxilla. This produces a much more refined plot of normative ideal values according to the age of the patient. This allows for a more reasonably probabilistic estimate of what values should be expected as ideal for a given age and sex. This then not only changes the normative values originally used in the McNamara but also makes for a much smoother distribution curve of ideal values for age and sex that have been mathematically "tightened up." Again, this is only possible with the use of computers. Specifically, it is due to a nifty little device built into the computer known as a random number generator. The haunting admonitions of the Second Cephalometric Workshop concerning the proper management of statistics in cephalometrics have come echoing down through the decades to bear witness to their wisdom. A lot of respect must certainly be paid to those who have gone before. How perceptive they must have been.

It is generally known that the average cephalometric x-ray produced by the average practitioner even with proper equipment and exposure technique is of only fair quality at best. To circumvent this problem, Smith et al. employ the use of a highly sophisticated device known as an "enhancer." This device was developed by NASA for photointerpretation of images of distant objects in space. The problem of photographing a distant celestial object such as Venus or Mars was that astronomers had difficulty deciphering the images of such objects, due to the lack of definition of the photographic image. It is easy to imagine what 20 million miles can do to the sharpness of focus of a picture! To solve this problem, NASA developed the electronic computerized image enhancer, which separates a photographic image into 12 separate layers of density ranging from dark to light images. This resulted, to the delight of scientists, in an image of greatly increased clarity, almost approaching a three-dimensional nature. Obviously, such a device is ideal for interpreting the location of the shadowy anatomical landmarks of a cephalogram that are

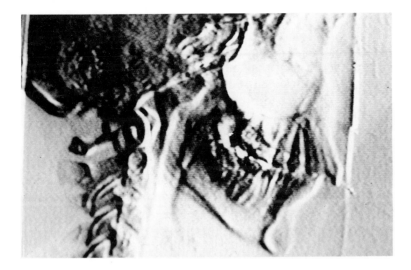

Figure 5–14 Computerized image of standard cephalometric radiograph that has been separated into 12 different layers of density by an enhancer obtained from NASA. (Courtesy Ortho-Diagnostics Ltd, St Louis, Mo)

at times all but totally invisible to the naked eye. Using the enhancer to "read" cephalometric x-rays allows the clinician to locate even the most indiscernible landmarks with a level of accuracy that is unapproachable by the human eye. If they are there, they can be found. This makes for unparalleled accuracy in tracing production. (Remember, Steiner used S-N as a base reference simply because it was easier to find than the much more preferred FH.) Now even the faintest shades of gray may be "electronically picked out" to identify the exact location of a given landmark. Thus, tracing error has been greatly reduced.

In addition, instantaneous cross-checking of landmark location is carried on by the computer programs designed by the Smiths as the information and data are being entered. If any contradictions should appear that may be attributable to human error of entering point location, the computer alerts the operator of a possible mislocation. A light-activated data input system is also employed, which ensures a level of accuracy of data entry into the computer from the radiograph (or study models) never before possible. The days of guessing landmark location and hiding uncertainty behind a thick tracing pencil line are over. Angles can easily be calculated to a tenth of a degree, and lines can be measured to a tenth of a millimeter, all with unerring accuracy in hundredths of a second!

Model analysis (Smith)   As if producing any of the number of cephalometric analysis systems by means of a computer wasn't enough of a boon to the clinician, the Smith-designed programs of three-dimensional model analysis make this component of the work of comprehensive orthodontic diagnosis even easier! Model analysis has always involved the hand measurement of certain prescribed distances across two points, which even on the best of plaster casts may at times be suspect. Once tabulated, the values derived must be interpreted against a table or a formula that gives an idealized single value that only represents the "average" of a sample and, as such, does not exactly represent the most individualized of treatment goals with respect to that specific aspect of the case. However, the computerized model analysis methods developed by the Smiths take the three-dimensional information directly from a set of accurate study models and, by means of the ability of the computer to perform complex calculations drawing on growth information stored in its computer bank, produce much more individualized information and far more specific arch form treatment goals.

With the latest light-activated measurement technology, the arch form and individual tooth measurements are logged into the computer with an accuracy level of one tenth of a millimeter. Obviously, to prevent the "garbage in, garbage out" phenomenon from occurring within the computer, an accurate set of study models possessing sharp detailing of all the teeth is required. The most precise measurement of the size of each tooth is obtained by using the very accurate light-activated measurement system to locate the mesial and distal contact points. This allows the teeth to be measured at the various contact point positions and levels for each individual tooth. If a tooth is missing or only partially erupted, the computer estimates its size relative to the size of the other teeth of that specific case. Once such information, along with the age, sex, and race, are entered into the computer, a remarkable series of calculations are performed that give the clinician an enormous amount of valuable diagnostic and treatment-planning information. The Smiths divide the output data for computerized model analysis into seven categories:

1. Dentition status and teeth widths
2. Computerized Schwarz analysis
3. Computerized arch length analysis
4. Dental midline deviations
5. Overbite, overjet determinations
6. Angle cuspid and molar classification
7. Pont's analysis (Linder-Harth corrected)

Dentition status and teeth widths   As previously stated, the measurements of the teeth are taken directly from the study model and entered into the computer in the stereoscopic arrangement that exists on the model. The mesiodistal widths of each tooth may then be listed. The

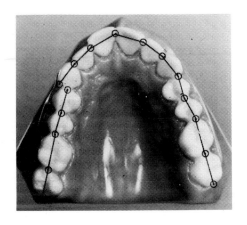
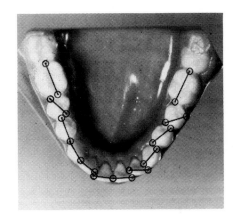

(A)

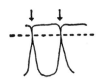
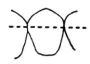
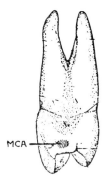

(B)

Figure 5−15 **(A)** Light-activated measurement systems determine the size of each tooth by locating the exact mesial and distal contact points. **(B)** Each tooth has not only its widest mesiodistal measurement recorded but also its position relative to the other teeth in the arch. (MCA = mesial contact area) (Courtesy Ortho-Diagnostics Ltd, St Louis, Mo)

mesiodistal widths of teeth that are only partially erupted or completely unerupted may be estimated by the computer relative to the size of the other teeth.

Computerized Schwarz Analysis The Smiths' programs of model analysis make use of a modified form of the classic Schwarz analysis. In addition to making facially corrected arch width calculations according to traditional Schwarz methodology (where the constant in the famous SI + K formula is varied to 6, 7, or 8 according to facial type), the computer also incorporates dental developmental age, sex, race, and other information to arrive at its final predictions for individualized ideal arch size *after growth*. The computer prints out a table of measurements for actual

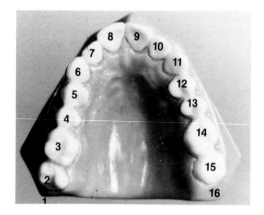
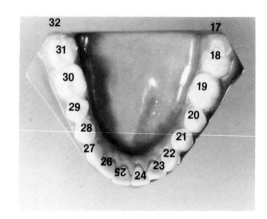

(A)

Model Analysis
Dentition Status and Tooth Widths (mm)

Maxilla

	8.4	9.4	9.2	7.8	7.1	5.1	7.8	8.1	5.2	6.9	7.9	9.6	9.2	8.2	
1	2	3	A	B	C	7	8	9	10	H	I	J	14	15	16

Mandible

32	31	30	T	S	R	26	25	24	23	M	L	K	19	18	17
	10.0	10.7	9.5	7.4	6.8	5.2	5.5	5.2	5.7	5.9	8.1	9.8	10.6	9.9	

Key: Absent   Impacted   Not Erupted   Present

(B)

Figure 5–16   (A) Computerized tooth identification system assigns a number to each tooth. Deciduous teeth are assigned letters of the alphabet, A being the upper right deciduous second molar and T being the lower right second molar. **(B)** The dentition status may then be described with numbers (letters) along with the width (real or approximate) of each tooth. (Courtesy Ortho-Diagnostics Ltd, St Louis, Mo)

pretreatment trans-bicuspid and trans-molar widths for both the maxilla and mandible. The perpendicular linear distance from a line across the distal pits of the maxillary first bicuspids forward to the facial surfaces of the maxillary incisors (LO) is calculated as is the perpendicular linear distance from a line across the mesiobuccal line angles of the mandibular second bicuspids forward to the facial surfaces of the mandibular incisors (LU). The program also calculates the individualized ideals or "should be" values for these dimensions by the methods already described. Three sets of arch width values are calculated. The first is for the "no growth" situation, that is the ideal individualized calculated widths for that individual, assuming no growth will take place past the present condition of the case as represented by the given set of models. The other two calculations are projections of change in these values that might occur in the complete absence of treatment.

The "actual" arch measurements presented in the table of the model analysis report are not simply taken from the stone models "as is." The maxillary bicuspids, for instance, may be considerably displaced from their "correct" position due to migrations, rotations, tilting, or pronounced curve-of-Spee distortions. In order to get more indicative values of *actual arch* measurements, one must take two preliminary steps. First, the actual location of the midline of the underlying apical base is determined and an outline of it is drawn by the computer, even though some of the teeth may not yet be on it. Extremely sophisticated mathematical computations are necessary for this step. (The formulae used to calculate the outline of the apical base would fill four pages of legal-sized stationery!) Second, the teeth are then mathematically moved onto the arch without rotations, diastemata, or curve-of-Spee distortions. Only then can the appropriate measurements be made, thus providing a truer indication of the patient's actual arch sizes.

The "should be" values found in the table in the "no growth" column are based on formulae by Dr Schwarz in which "proper" arch widths are estimated as a function of the sum of the mesiodistal widths of the four maxillary incisors. The classic Schwarz formulae are modified to properly take into account that the ideal is also a function of the patient's head shape. The computer also calculates the handy "discrepancy column" of the table in the "no growth" situation, which provides a clear indication of the basic deficiencies or excesses in arch width at the molars and first bicuspids, as well as arch depth (LO, LU) in the patient as represented at the moment by the study models.

A proper course of treatment will certainly recognize and, insofar as possible, take advantage of the normal growth and development process of the patient. Patients over 18 years of age can be assumed to have completed growth as far as arch width is concerned, and the system operation in these cases will be discussed later. To assist the clinician in evaluating growth in the younger patient, the computerized model analysis next projects the arch measurements to post-growth sizes, taking into account both the chronological and dental development ages of the patient. (For this reason it is important to know the age at which the patient erupted his or her first permanent mandibular incisor.)

Two distinct estimates are made of the post-growth arch measurements: The first, referred to as the "expected" value, represents the average measurements that would be found after growth ceases in a large sample of patients of similar age, with similar starting measurements. This may also be thought of as the set of values that have a 50–50 chance of being reached or exceeded by *growth alone*. Again, the discrepancy

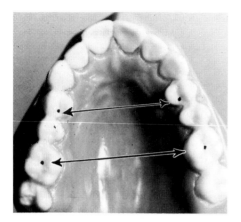
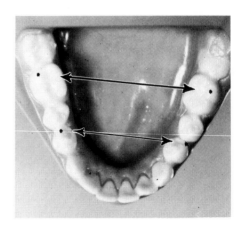

(A)

Schwartz Analysis (Facial type corrected)

	No Growth			After Growth			
				Expected		Optimistic 1 Chance in 10	
	Actual	Should Be	Disc	Proj	Disc	Proj	Disc
Arch width: maxillary bicuspids	36.6	43.2	−6.6	40.1	−3.1	40.4	−2.8
Arch width: maxillary molars	45.3	50.8	−5.5	45.9	−4.8	46.6	−4.2
LO, pre-maxillary size	21.8	20.6	1.3	24.1	3.5	24.5	3.9
Arch width: mandibular bicuspids	36.8	43.2	−6.4	40.2	−3.0	40.6	−2.6
Arch width: mandibular molars	48.1	50.8	−2.7	48.6	−2.2	49.2	−1.5
LU, pre-mandibular size	17.8	17.6	0.2	20.8	3.2	21.1	3.5

All calculations performed assuming teeth are in correct position, ie, no rotations, crowding, missing teeth, or curve of Spee.
The optimistic case projects the growth that will be attained in no more than 1 of 10 similar cases.

(B)

Figure 5−17 **(A)** Values for trans-arch width may be entered for calculation of either Schwarz or Ponts indices for bicuspid and molar arch widths. **(B)** Drawing on the enormous reserve of the computer's data banks, tables of values for present and ideal trans-arch widths may be easily calculated along with projected probabilities of the chances the child will grow out of any shortage of arch width on his or her own. (Courtesy Ortho-Diagnostics Ltd, St Louis, Mo)

column gives an indication of what excess or deficiency can be expected without treatment and hence whether any arch development intervention is indicated. The other post-growth projection, the "optimistic" column, provides the estimated measurements that will be attained in only one of ten similar cases; in other words, this patient has only one chance in ten of reaching or exceeding these values. Clearly then, if this most optimistic result, having only a 10% chance of being realized, is still deficient in arch width, being short of the calculated ideal in either the bicuspid area, molar area, or both, treatment in the form of lateral development most likely will have to be undertaken.

When assessing patients over 18 years of age for whom no more growth is expected, the system will calculate the various arch width discrepancies that may still need correction. In posterior crossbites and Class II malocclusions, lateral arch development may have to be undertaken in order to obtain proper occlusion. Relapse in these situations is more likely unless proper jaw position, good intercuspation, and muscle balance are obtained. Thus, for the nongrowing (adult) patient, the largest pretreatment arch (widthwise) serves as the safest and most conservative standard for individualized arch width values. In these situations the "arch form" column will show whichever is the larger of the maxillary and mandibular actual pretreatment arch sizes, as no more additional lateral growth is to be expected. It should be noted that the maxillary and mandibular numbers listed *are the same* so that the teeth will occlude properly. Therefore, one needs to expand the smaller arch to meet the larger arch. The larger of the two arches in the adult patient 18 years old or older serves as the "Nature-selected" limit of stable arch width, hence the development of the smaller arch to the width of the larger arch. The measurements listed may in fact be greater than those measured by a caliper on the actual model of the largest arch, but it must be remembered that the computer corrects individual tooth position to compensate for tip, drift, curve of Spee, rotations, etc. Therefore, by merely uprighting and placing the individual teeth in their correct nondistorted locations on the arch, the computer may produce trans-bicuspid and trans-molar widths that are different from those on the noncorrected pretreatment model. Thus, some degree of increased arch width is often easily obtained even in the largest of the two adult arches. This width still represents the most stable, most conservative, and "safest" arch width value for that particular adult patient and must be evaluated as such. This process was devised to eliminate overdevelopment problems (relapse) arch-width-wise in the treatment of the adult patient.

Computerized arch length analysis

1. Carey analysis   Section 3 of the Smith-designed model analysis provides an evaluation of the adequacy of arch length anterior to the permanent first molars after taking into account arch growth and the additional space gained by properly aligning and positioning the anteriors, for it must be remembered that rotations in the anterior arch area give up arch length. The form of the computerized output will vary somewhat in the Smiths' version of the Carey analysis, depending on the current developmental status of the patient. If the permanent teeth are already present, then there is no remaining uncertainty about the ultimate sizes of the bicuspids and cuspids: In this case the analysis produced will simply be a standard Carey analysis. An example is given in the table.

Arch Length—Carey Analysis	Upper	Lower
Arch length anterior to molars	66.0	59.3
Tooth mass anterior to molars	73.7	65.9
Space discrepancy	− 7.7	− 6.6

Figure 5−18   With the data on the mesiodistal width of each tooth of a given case stored in the computer, the total existing tooth mass in the arch is easily calculated. However, the calculation of the space available in the existing apical base requires extremely sophisticated mathematics only a computer can perform. Data necessary for such calculations is derived directly from study models. Similar procedures involving computerized prediction of the widths of unerupted teeth, present arch size, and predicted future arch growth are used in the mixed dentition analysis. (Courtesy Ortho-Diagnostics Ltd, St Louis, Mo)

In cases in which permanent cuspids or bicuspids are not yet present, it is necessary to estimate what size they will be. A number of studies have resulted in development of various probability tables and equations which provide predictions of the permanent tooth sizes. Most of these methods use the actual size of some of the other permanent teeth to estimate the cuspid and bicuspid sizes. Usually, as with Moyer, the mandibular or maxillary incisors are used for this purpose. Smith has developed a projection technique which uses an amalgamation of several available data sources and probabilistic projection techniques. Actually, in this case, two projections are made—the *most likely* tooth mass anterior to the molars and, reminiscent of what was done in the Schwarz analysis for arch width and depth, the tooth mass that might be expected in the most *optimistic* case. Note, however, that while "optimistic" in the Schwarz analysis meant that we were looking for arch width development to be as *large* as possible, thus making more space available, "optimistic" in the computerized arch length analysis means we are hoping for tooth sizes to be as *small* as possible so they will naturally fit in the space actually available.

2. Mixed dentition analysis (based on tooth size probabilities and arch growth predicted from development age)   When the patient is still in the mixed dentition stage, the Smiths' computer programs perform a greatly enhanced mixed dentition analysis that incorporates much of the aforementioned data to provide a much more reliable (and probable) estimate of just how the transition from mixed to full adult dentition will turn out. This is possible only through the services of a computer and represents a great leap forward over the old "seat of the pants guess-timate" methods of manual measurement of study models with conventional calipers. The computer produces a mixed dentition analysis data table for both maxillary and mandibular arches. Again, the computer makes several predictions as to the future outcome of the arch in question. First, it predicts what Smith refers to as the "expected arch," ie, the one

Mixed Dentition Analysis

Expected Arch (most likely)	Max	Mand
Arch length anterior to permanent first molars	+76.0	+67.4
Expected mass anterior to molars	+76.6	+67.4
Expected discrepancy (disregarding arch growth)	−0.6	+0.1
Expected arch growth	+5.3	+6.9
Expected discrepancy including arch growth	+4.8	+6.9
Additional space gained (+) or lost (−) from alignment of anteriors	+4.4	−0.2
Additional space gained (+) or lost (−) from labial (+) or lingual (−) torquing of anteriors	+1.0	+1.0
Most Optimistic Arch	Max	Mand
Arch length anterior to permanent first molars	+76.0	+67.4
Expected (10% chance)* mass anterior to molars	+74.0	+64.7
Expected discrepancy (disregarding arch growth)	+2.0	+2.7
Expected (10% chance)** arch growth	+6.1	−7.4
Expected discrepancy including arch growth	+8.0	+10.2
Additional space gained (+) or lost (−) from alignment of anteriors	+4.4	−0.2
Additional space gained (+) or lost (−) from labial (+) or lingual (−) torquing of anteriors	+1.5	+1.5

that mathematical statistics predict as the "odds on" favorite to occur. Second, the computer calculates the size of the arch that would only occur once in ten times, ie, a "most optimistic" category. This represents the best arch form (relative to width) that the clinician can reasonably hope for given the individual patient's own mixed dentition data. Obviously, if even *this* estimate shows a shortage of final arch width compared with the calculated ideal after the most favorable growth that can be expected, treatment in the form of lateral and/or A-P development may be required. An example is given in the tables.

The calculated tooth mass can then be compared with the available space anterior to the molars, taking into account available leeway or "E" space, which may be a shortage (−) or a surplus (+). Growth in arch size as previously discussed will also result in a change in arch length which is computed and represented in the output as "expected arch growth." Other changes in arch length are potentially possible:

1. Space can be gained by closing diastemata among the permanent anteriors.

2. Space can be lost by uncrowding permanent anterior teeth.

3. Space can be gained by proper labial torquing of the anterior permanent teeth, eg, Class II, Division 2.

4. Space will be lost by proper lingual torquing of the upper permanent anterior teeth, eg, condensing flared anteriors.

The arch length changes from these sources are shown in the last two lines of each of the tables in the table of computerized mixed dentition analysis data. Note that the torquing operation may not fully apply to the mandible since there are orthopedic implications which cannot be derived solely from the model analysis. Information about these additional sources of arch length modification is particularly valuable in recognizing the need for *interceptive* orthodontic intervention.

When the existing cuspids and bicuspids are still in transition, ie, some of these permanent teeth have erupted and are measurable, then ultimate tooth size of the as-yet-unerupted permanents can be reliably estimated by the computer from known tooth-size proportional relationships which may be determined from those of which are already present. The overall uncertainty in the total molar-to-molar tooth mass is thus minimized since the unknown tooth sizes are based on the known widths of the patient's own similar teeth. In this case, since the uncertainty is minimized, projections are made only of the most likely outcome.

Dental midline deviations   The dental midline deviation reading can best be made by the dentist at his clinical exam. This measurement made by the Smith computers from the models is a straightforward measurement of the distance between the labial frenum and the dental midline. The mandible and maxilla are measured independently. Skeletal midline deviations can only be measured effectively at the clinical exam.

Transitional Dentition Analysis (based on tooth size projected from permanent teeth)

	Max	Mand
Arch length anterior to permanent first molars	+81.7	+66.1
Expected mass anterior to molars	+74.3	+62.8
Expected discrepancy (disregarding arch growth)	+7.4	+3.3
Expected arch growth	+2.1	+1.5
Expected discrepancy including arch growth	+9.5	+4.8
Additional space gained (+) or lost (−) from alignment of anteriors	+2.6	−3.7
Additional space gained (+) or lost (−) from labial (+) or lingual (−) torquing of anteriors	+0.0	+0.0

Figure 5−19   Transitional dentition analysis: An advantage the computer has in arch form calculations is seen in the transitional dentition analysis. Based on arches that are all but completely grown in their apical bases, and also based on projected tooth sizes of the few remaining unerupted teeth as per the size of the teeth already present, the computer can calculate space gain or loss by rotating, torquing, translating, etc, to obtain an extremely sophisticated arch length analysis that gives the clinician a much more accurate figure representative of space available *v* space needed for arch-decrowding problems.

Pont's Analysis—Linder-Harth Corrected

Arch Width	Actual	Should Be	Discrepancy
Maxillary bicuspids	36.6	41.9	−5.3
Maxillary molars	45.3	54.8	−9.5
Mandibular bicuspids	36.8	41.9	−5.1
Mandibular molars	48.1	54.8	−6.7

Figure 5–20 Computerized Ponts index.

Overbite, overjet determinations Incisal occlusion is calculated by the computer from the cephalometric x-ray. For this reading to be accurate, the x-ray must be taken with teeth together. Negative values are used to indicate open bites or Class III anterior crossbites.

Angle cuspid and molar classification Angle cuspid and molar classification are given based on standard Angle classifications. Whenever an end-to-end molar situation is evident, it is classified as a Class II relationship.

Pont's analysis (Linder-Harth corrected) As with the Schwarz analysis, Pont's analysis is corrected for tooth rotations, crowding, missing teeth, curve of Spee, and growth. The "should be" values are based on Pont's formulae modified by Linder and Harth, since the original values were generally a bit too wide.

Interpretation of arch plots By far, one of the most important developments of the Smith computerized diagnostic system is the ability of the computer to generate plots of the maxillary and mandibular arches. These graphic displays pictorially summarize all of the previously discussed complex calculations and analyses into an easily understood tool for treatment planning. (For the sake of simplicity in discussion, we will restrict our initial explanation to the maxillary arch.)

The actual teeth are indicated schematically by red lines with small circles at each end. Each individual line represents the linear mesiodistal (M-D) width of the respective teeth. The centers of the circles mark the mesial and distal contact points of each tooth. These small circles are used merely to aid in easy visual location of the mesial and distal contact points of each tooth. Although the teeth are drawn to scale, the measurement on the plot will not in all cases be the same as the actual M-D width of the tooth if there is a significant curve of Spee. The computer makes adjustments for the curve of Spee by projecting the actual teeth from the curve to a flat plane, which affects the M-D crown width as displayed.

Actual arch location The computer-determined location of the actual underlying midpoint of the basal arch is indicated by the solid black line. This is tantamount to the average location of the middle of the apical base. Such a tracing requires the most sophisticated mathematical computations. It is this line that requires the four-page mathematical formula for its calculation.

Maxillary ideal arch form   The ideal arch form is determined by the computer from the ideal Schwarz analysis numbers (the "should be" column of Part II of the model analysis). The Smiths, however, found that the LO and LU values as determined by the original Schwarz analysis methods must, in general, be further adjusted to achieve consistency with the required arch form at the bicuspids and the arch length as required by the actual tooth mass anterior to the bicuspids. Therefore, if one were to measure LO and LU on the plots, they *will not* be exactly the same as suggested by the simple formula SI + K/2 of the original Schwarz analysis.

The Smiths make clever use of an innovative way of producing the "ideal" arch form in that the outline of the ideal arch is plotted on a clear plastic transparency so that it may be overlaid on the output sheet on which is plotted the actual pretreatment arch. This can be done by properly aligning the cross marks on the transparency plot, at the upper left and lower right corners, with those of the actual pretreatment plot tracing sheet. The "ideal" arch form is printed in blue.

On the "actual" plot (printed in red), the actual location of A-point is indicated, while the clear plastic overlay of the "ideal" arch indicates where A-point *should be* following treatment (ie, between ±2 mm of the N-perpendicular for the Caucasian). The dentist must keep in mind that the ideal location of A-point is not always attainable with modern mechanics. The Smith-designed computerized diagnostic system assumes that A-point can be moved a maximum of 2 mm anteriorly or 4 mm posteriorly in order to reach or at least approach the desired location. If the clinician feels that further adjustment is possible, he can easily adjust the overlay to compensate for this. It should also be remembered that these limits and assumptions are based on hard-tissue guidelines.

The "ideal arch" also shows the ideal locations of the teeth on the arch. Permanent teeth not currently present are also placed on the arch using computer-calculated proportional estimates of their sizes. Therefore, in summary, the "ideal arch" assumes all permanent teeth present (and that means bicuspids!) with no curve of Spee, no missing teeth, no rotations, no spaces, no crowding, and proper torque on anteriors. The clinician can measure directly from the plots the amount of expansion or distalization needed to obtain an ideal arch form as the arch form plots are printed out in a one-to-one life-size scale!

Treatment-planning output   The material discussed above firmly establishes the great work of Don and Norm Smith as an impressive product of the computer age. Others, of course, will greatly expand the use of computers in the science of cephalometrics. However, the work that firmly establishes the efforts of these two men and their supporters as a product of the computer age and the age of FJO is their totally unique computerized treatment-planning programs. As a result of the overall evaluation of what these programs can be seen to have done so

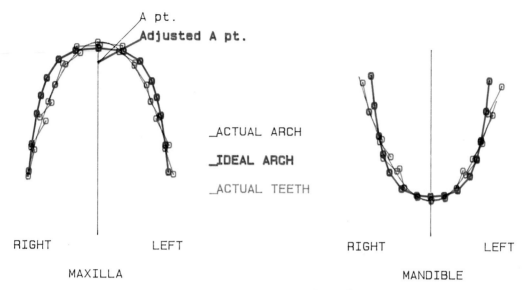

A pt.

Adjusted A pt.

_ACTUAL ARCH

_IDEAL ARCH

_ACTUAL TEETH

RIGHT   LEFT   RIGHT   LEFT

MAXILLA   MANDIBLE

Figure 5–21   Red computerized life-size tracing of actual pretreatment existing arch form. Blue computer-calculated ideal arch form individualized to the specific case. (Courtesy of Ortho-Diagnostics Ltd, St Louis, Mo)

far, the computer is capable of determining with a high level of accuracy some of the most common FJO treatment methods that would be necessary to deliver a given case to its best possible resolution according to modern combined orthodontic/orthopedic standards. The treatment-planning suggestions produced by the Smith programs serve as a guide to the general methods of treatment that the specific information of an individual case dictates, and although they are not intended to map out the exact step-by-step treatment techniques a clinician would most likely employ on the case in question, they certainly come close. The Smiths divide the data of the "treatment plan" into several categories.

Arch preparation and positioning   Under this category the computerized treatment plan makes recommendations. With respect to arch development to the predetermined individually calculated ideal widths, the computer lists the individualized values for the ideal bicuspid and molar trans-arch widths for the given case along with a brief notation to specific arch development appliances of particular value considering the various details of the case. This is done by means of a "comment section" (discussed shortly).

In addition to the size and shape of the individualized ideal arch, the computer is also capable of determining a very important piece of information—the ideal *location* of the maxillary and mandibular arches. It does this by its ability to relate A-point and B-point to each other and even to the cranial base, and, most importantly, to the facial soft tissue profile. In its determination of exactly what location of the arches and their associated apical bases would be ideal for the patient concerned, the computer makes treatment recommendations that (at least as far as the orthopedic ideals are concerned) require the anterior or posterior movements of the respective arches in millimeters relative to FH. Sometimes this may even be out of the range of practical limits of certain treatment techniques, especially with respect to moving the maxillary apical base forward, but at least it will give the clinician an idea of the severity of the imbalances represented by the malocclusion he is facing and of the degree of difficulty he may encounter should he be determined to reach the exact ideal in certain cases.

Advancement of the mandible is easily accomplished with Bionator-type therapy, and maxillary advancement to a certain extent is achievable by FPHG (which moves the dental arch and alveolar process forward more so than the actual apical base or body of the maxilla). Maxillary retraction (rarely needed) requires a bit more sophisticated use of traditional backward-pulling headgear, while retraction of B-point in the form of a true prognathic condition of the mandible in skeletal Class III malocclusions often requires surgery.

Molar position with respect to the respective arches is also directly addressed by the computer. After evaluating (mathematically) a great deal of cephalometric and model analysis data, the computer determines the direction and distance each individual molar will have to be moved (usually distally) to obtain correct position on the arch to within one tenth of a millimeter! Obviously, this process often requires extractions, and when extractions are called for, the computer has been programmed to make its calculations oriented around the second molar "replacement" technique (FJO oriented to the core).

The status of the position and angulation of maxillary and mandibular anterior incisors is also directly addressed (Steiner's old obsession). The dramatic difference here is that instead of calculating teeth positions and interincisal angles that would achieve "acceptable compromises" similar to the older method's attempt to camouflage apical base discrepancies with mere orthodontic tooth tipping, the Smith programs calculate the ideal locations of the incisors from the standpoint of orthopedically correct apical bases, proper lip and facial profile support, and the all-important protection of "the big MAC" (the mandibular arc of closure to final occlusion) from the possibilities of TMJ-damaging, anterior, incisal guiding plane interferences! These treatment-planning programs are quite frankly a master stroke of combined orthodontic/orthopedic computer engineering. Considering the pretreatment position and angulation of the anteriors, the computer makes simplified and extremely practical suggestions as to how far to torque the incisal tips of maxillary and mandibular anteriors in order to obtain the ideal posttreatment location and angulation.

The necessity of space maintenance is also addressed in the event the case is still in the mixed dentition and certain deciduous teeth have been lost prematurely. Overbite and overjet management suggestions are also made, once again with a reference to most favored appliances and techniques specific for the given case.

Temporomandibular joint alerts   As previously alluded to, the computer programs, for both the two-dimensional cephalometric analysis and the three-dimensional model analysis, have been designed to detect certain combinations of physical data that would lead either in the pre- or posttreatment state to the possible occurrence of a TMJ condition due to such things as a retropositioned mandible, anterior incisor interference, excessive distal displacement of maxillary anteriors, excessive anterior displacement of mandibular incisors, or an interfering anterior tooth rotation (ie, the overall NRDM-SPDC phenomenon). When such circumstances are detected, which can result from a wide variety of combinations of anatomical arrangements, the computer takes steps to (1) alert the clinician to these conditions in the pretreatment state, and (2) to "correct" the condition by whatever orthodontic or orthopedic means are necessary.

These measures are not complete and all-encompassing in their "TMJ-detection" abilities, since only a limited number of the most basic (or "drastic" if you will) combinations of anatomical arrangements can be considered in this process. But at least some of the most common varieties have been programmed into the system, even if only on the most basic of levels, and as such will surely detect their "fair share" of potential or actual TMJ problems. Final and complete diagnostic evaluation and interpretation of such problems are still relegated to the far more capable evaluations of the "ultimate computer," the human mind.

Surgical considerations   As previously stated, when pretreatment data indicate that correction of certain landmark locations is in directions or distances outside the commonly accepted limits of modern appliance technique, the computer "kicks out" the posttreatment ideal as unattainable and places it in the "surgical consideration" category. True skeletal Class III prognathisms are the most obvious example.

Comments section   The final part of the Smith-designed programs is a practical addition to an already impressive lineup of accomplishments. The "comments" section refers to given sections of the treatment plan, and it gives more detailed suggestions of appliance type or technique of the most logical choice to attain the specific treatment goal concerned as calculated for that individual by the computer.

Thus it may be seen that the entire series of computer programs as developed by the Smiths and their supporting staff represent both a historic turning point as well as a landmark contribution to the streamlining and modernization of the formidable task of comprehensive orthodontic diagnosis. These computer programs have freed clinicians

Black color -- Actual
Blue color -- Ideal

EXAMPLES OF Ideal vs. Actual arch forms when overlayed

Actual Lateral Relationships	* Arch Relationships Ideal Arch Form & Position of Molars	Interpretation	Possible Treatment
(1)		No Change Necessary	Nothing
(2)		Pre-Maxillary Development (check Ceph for proper torquing of Anteriors)	Sagittal
(3)		Distalization of Posteriors	Sagittal (May Require Extractions of 7's) Crozat straight wire 3-D Wilson Arch
(4)		Distalize Complete Arch (refer to position of "A" point.)	Cervical Headgear Bionator Orthopedic Corrector
(5)		Mesialize Complete Arch (refer to position of "A" point)	Sagittal and Reverse Face Mask or possibly Rapid Patatal Expansion
(6)		Distalize Posteriors and Pre-Maxillary Development	Sagittal and Extractions

* Only location of 1st Molars indicated

(A)

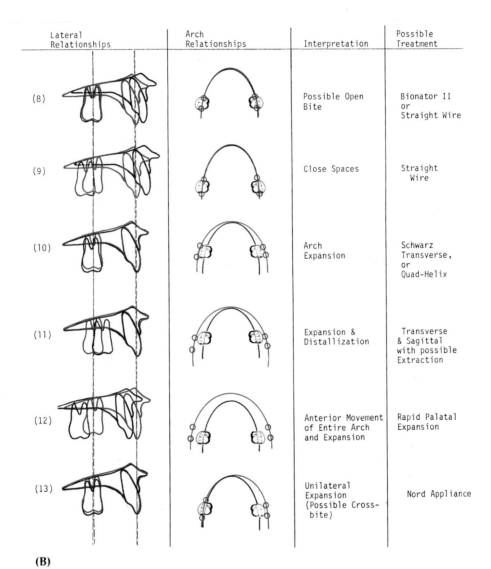

Lateral Relationships	Arch Relationships	Interpretation	Possible Treatment
(8)		Possible Open Bite	Bionator II or Straight Wire
(9)		Close Spaces	Straight Wire
(10)		Arch Expansion	Schwarz Transverse, or Quad-Helix
(11)		Expansion & Distallization	Transverse & Sagittal with possible Extraction
(12)		Anterior Movement of Entire Arch and Expansion	Rapid Palatal Expansion
(13)		Unilateral Expansion (Possible Cross-bite)	Nord Appliance

(B)

Figure 5—22   (A), (B) Example of computer-calculated ideal arch form (blue) overlaid on actual pretreatment arch form (black), both lateral and occlusal aspects. (Courtesy of Ortho-Diagnostics Ltd, St Louis, Mo)

from much of the burdensome hackwork of producing and deciphering cephalometric tracings, and have greatly enhanced their processes of measuring and analyzing representative study models. And they even give guidelines as to the appliances and treatment techniques of choice needed to attain the level of improvements calculated to be appropriate for an individual case.

Just how far computerized diagnostic processes will take us in the future is limited only by our technical prowess and our ingenuity. But one thing is clear. The future will always look back to the 1980s with fond respect for the two men who gave functionally oriented, full-scale, multi-dimensional, orthodontic diagnosis and treatment planning its FJO-oriented, computerized, conceptual birth. It will take the profession a while to fully appreciate the contributions of men like Don and Norman Smith; and no doubt many others will follow in the future. Yet who can fail to owe but a debt of gratitude to these men who took the first pioneering steps in the effort to use seemingly cold and intimidating high technology to give both the clinicians and their patients a better life?

THE BIO-FACIAL MATRIX

As we have seen, the Bowbeer analysis represents the first cephalometric diagnostic system to be developed that it is dominated to a large extent by soft tissue facial profile considerations, although a certain amount of traditional cephalometric components accompany it. Yet the modern wave of concern over therapeutic alteration of the soft tissue profile was taken even a step further by the development of that facial analysis known as the Bio-Facial Matrix, the latest in a series of new ideas to be produced by the energetic and quixotic Dr Jack Lynn of Pittsburgh, Pennsylvania.

Lynn, of "Biofinisher" appliance fame, was very sensitive to the problems of therapeutic alterations, for better or worse, of the soft tissue profile of patients undergoing orthodontic treatment. He realized that until recent times, the great majority of cephalometric analysis systems that had been heretofore developed were primarily concerned with the hard tissue components (bones and teeth) of the maxillofacial complex, and that soft tissue considerations (as well as TMJ considerations) were only accorded secondary status. Like Mark Twain's weather, everybody talked about them, but nobody felt, in pre−functional appliances times, that much could be done about them. However, Lynn points out that for all their precision, theoretical justification, and demanding methods of production, such cephalometric hard tissue treatment goals and standards as those of the Steiner chevrons of anterior incisor angulation, or even such soft tissue criteria as that of the S line or E line, were only viable

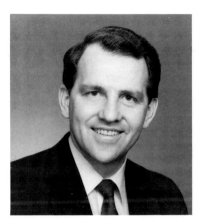

Figure 5−23 Jack Lynn.

if the craniofacial neuromuscular aspects, as well as facial esthetic considerations in the completed case, would be fully adaptable to and tolerable of their final results.

It is common knowledge that for a long time in the discipline of orthodontics a great deal of the treatment effected was concerned only with the problems of mechanically moving teeth to obtain proper arch-to-arch alignment and interdigitation with complete disregard for the posturing of the soft tissues of the face or the hard tissues of the TMJs, as a result of that treatment. Lynn, being aware of such processes, quickly joined in the trend toward making facial considerations a primary goal. His founding premise was that orthodontics should first divest itself of its limited focus on dentition alone (which it already has done to some extent) and, by expanding its pretreatment diagnostic evaluation to include soft tissue or facial analysis (and as a result TMJ considerations), it could produce treatment goals as well as treatment planning that would result in a much more favorable and all-inclusive result. Consideration of the occlusion per se is only a part of the total picture. The "orthopedic age" has changed more than just how we look at teeth.

The genesis of what would eventually become the entirely facially oriented analysis of Jack Lynn began with his concern over the lack of enough facial considerations in standard cephalometric analyses. He was also concerned with the results the tooth-oriented orthodontic therapeutic systems traditionally had delivered. In relation to the area of what orthodontics was producing as a result of its use of traditional cephalometric standards or norms set up as actual treatment goals, Lynn was keenly aware of the work of Park and Burstone.[282] These researchers had analyzed the significance of the use of hard tissue standards for treatment goals and the results such usage had on the soft tissue profile, and found them wanting. They also noted that in spite of their findings, ironically, ortho-dontics had always listed facial harmony as one of its primary goals. They examined the premise that an orthodontic patient treated to a traditional cephalometric standard would in fact exhibit upon completion of treatment an attractive, desirable, and predictable soft tissue profile. The authors noted the following information after studying a limited and select population of "ideally treated" patients, all of whom were treated so that their lower central incisors were positioned 1 mm forward of the A-point/Pogonion (A-Pog) line. This is one of the conservative orthodon-tic establishment's most highly respected norms, as it came from the original work of Ricketts, and represents a mean derived from a sample of 1,000 cases.[70] However, a rather unexpected series of conclusions was drawn.

1. Many of the patients demonstrated what has been referred to as the "orthodontic look" to their facial appearance. This is felt to be a result of treating to cephalometric hard tissue standards instead of the individual demands of a particular patient's soft tissue conditions. Some of the finished cases produced posttreatment profiles that were definitely worse than the pretreatment state. Lips were more retruded and nasolabial angles were more acute in posttreatment conditions. In such instances, further growth of the soft tissue nose through adolescence and into young adulthood would only accentuate and worsen such problems.

2. A large variation in lip protrusion was subsequently observed, along with a variation of other soft tissue measurements as a result of exclusive use of the incisor position as the sole standard for treatment planning.

3. It was concluded that the clinicians would be less likely to make a mistake in treatment planning if *serious* considerations of the needs of the pretreatment facial conditions would be made prior to initiation of treatment.

4. The final conclusion drawn by the investigators was that when hard tissue cephalometric standards are used alone as a source of treatment-planning goals, the clinician is encouraged to ignore critical information that would be available from a soft tissue profile analysis of the radiograph or directly from clinical examination of the patient.

These findings had a profound effect on Lynn and confirmed his assertions that more attention had to be paid to patients' faces. Another important study, by Looi and Mills,[283] also corroborated this notion and reaffirmed Lynn's belief in the importance of combined orthopedic/ortho-dontic approaches to treating malocclusions by the approaches of the FJO philosophy. In this case three groups of patients were studied. All three were classified as having classic Class II, Division 1 malocclusions. Patients in Group A possessed uncrowded dentitions and were treated by func-tional appliances on a nonextraction basis. Patients in Group B had crowded dentitions and were treated with Begg appliance technique on a four-bicuspid-extraction basis. Group C served as a control.

The results showed that upon completion of treatment on the average, Group A (FJO) had the lower incisors 4 mm farther forward than Group B (fixed). A-point was also found to be more retracted in Group B, a major contributor to the "dished in" or "orthodontic look." The generally smaller dental arches, missing the bicuspids at the corners of the mouth, couldn't help but contribute to a collapsed lip line in the canine eminence area. The smile line of the teeth, as to be expected, was greatly reduced and, as a result, narrower-looking in the fixed appliance group. Even though the upper lip tends to be retracted less than the actual amount of anterior incisor retraction, there is still a serious compromise in facial esthetics when such retraction occurs, along with a greatly increased propensity for a posteriorly trapped mandible! This is the result of anterior incisor guiding plane interference upon full occlusion initiating the NRDM/SPDC phenomenon with its resultant "TMJ-type" symptomatology.

Studies like these and others did what they were supposed to do, and the mind of the young man from Pittsburgh bristled with new ideas and new directions that he felt both diagnosis and treatment techniques would eventually have to take. Lynn proposed that not only must the teeth be "straightened," but considerations of the bone and muscle, especially muscle in the form of that soft tissue drape over the bones of the stomatognathic system that is called the face, must be incorporated directly into the diagnostic and treatment-planning process. Not only must they be incorporated, they must be given preferential consideration! Amazing propositions even for the times. Another thoroughly dedicated and enthusiastic convert obviously had been made.

Lynn was also influenced by the theories of Van der Linden, which proposed that the growth of the craniofacial skeleton is naturally adaptive to various types of applied forces, be they natural or artificial.[284] Therefore, the posturing of the muscles—and soft tissue drape of the face over the bones—can have a definite influence on hard tissue formation and development either for the betterment or detraction of the occlusion and even jaw-to-jaw relationships. These notions are further supported by the work of men like McNamara,[285] who showed that deliberate changes in the vertical soft tissue posture resulted in actual reorganization of the affected portions of the facial skeleton and their associated musculature.

The "Functional Matrix" theories of Moss[163] also had a profound effect on Lynn, because they fall in line with this general direction of thinking. In light of such ideas, Lynn developed his basic philosophy of "biologic adaptability." He feels that the body's ability to adapt successfully to the changes the clinician may have in store by way of the treatment plan and its associated mechanics is intimately associated with the proper positioning of the soft tissue drape over the facial bones and the proper balancing of muscles to their physiologic and genetically programmed ideal.

This process can be carried out only by functional appliances, since fixed appliance mechanics are only generally capable of merely moving teeth. They do little if anything to address muscular imbalances. They do little if anything to retrain or reposition musculature. They do little if anything to help the muscles get adapted to a new bone-to-bone or tooth-to-tooth relationship; nor do they assist in the critical retraining of what may be termed the "Class II neuromuscular sling." Functional appliances *can* do these things. They can also dramatically change soft tissue profiles. Fixed appliances can only do that somewhat, but they are still terrific tooth movers. Thus we have the logical marriage of fixed and removable appliance mechanics to make the best effort at addressing a multivariate problem of bone, teeth, and muscle. Now what was needed was a diagnostic analysis system that would be chiefly concerned with the soft tissues, with the face, with the preservation or correction of the soft tissue profile in order that its intimately associated supportive musculature might be corrected and brought to a state of normalcy and physiological balance once again. This would allow the hard tissues, in the form of the teeth and bones, to be placed in *their* proper anatomical balance, with every expectation that they would stay that way. The analysis Lynn devised to provide just such a facially oriented diagnostic system has become known as the Bio-Facial Matrix, and it is predicated upon a revolutionary and totally unique individualized soft tissue frame of reference, the nasal plane!

Lynn realized that an analysis system of a highly facially oriented type would have to employ easily located landmarks and would have to serve as a guide to the relative positioning of the soft tissue profile to a standard derived not from a mathematical mean or table of norms but from the patient's proportional dictates and requirements for his or her specific facial harmony. The analysis system would hopefully be able to analyze each patient's excesses or deficiencies of facial contours and help determine if any existing abnormalities would be amenable to therapeutic correction by orthodontic or orthopedic means. It should hopefully be able to help the clinician decide whether surgical correction (either hard tissue or soft tissue) is necessary. This would be the result of another aspect of the analysis system—its ability to project an individualized ideal profile for each segment of the face based on the patient's structural makeup. It was a tall order indeed, but the revolutionary Bio-Facial Matrix was designed by Lynn to specifically address these issues. And that which allows the Bio-Facial Matrix analysis to stand is the newly devised base reference line of the nasal plane, constructed from a pair of soft tissue landmarks! Lynn selected this soft tissue base reference line for some very important reasons.

"Just Follow Your Nose"

Since the inception of modern roentgenocephalometrics in 1931, obsession with hard tissue relationships have dominated; and up until the 1960s scant attention had been given to the nose either from a hard or soft tissue aspect (except for nasion, of course). The earlier roentgenocephalometric studies that did include nose measurements were usually concerned with the growth and development of skeletal nasal components as opposed to soft tissue profile changes.

J. D. Subtleny did some of the first serious work on making a variety of nose measurements and studying their changes longitudinally.[286] Taking a series of longitudinal cases from the third month to 18th year of life from the files of the Charles Bingham Bolton study conducted over a 20-year period, he followed a sample of 30 subjects. He found that the soft tissue nose increased in length by about the same proportion for both sexes, but the average length for boys was slightly greater at all age levels than for girls. An annual growth rate of 1 to 1.6 mm was found to be fairly constant throughout growth. This was the reversal of what was known to be happening to the face skeletally during growth; ie, convexity of the facial skeletal profile generally decreased through the adolescent growth years.

Thus it may be seen that the corresponding convexity of the soft tissue profile decreased with age (along with the convexity of the hard tissue profile) *if the nose was excluded*. When the facial profile was evaluated *with the nose included*, the convexity of the soft tissue profile was seen to increase markedly with age. This corroborated the findings of earlier studies by other researchers[253] and indicated the growth rate of the nose in a forward direction to be actually greater.

However, the greatest changes were of an increased vertical length as opposed to horizontal growth in both sexes. The tip of the nose (as with so many other anatomical entities of the maxillofacial complex) was observed to steadily grow down and forward with age. Growth spurts were observed between 10 and 16 years of age for boys, and centered around 13 to 14 years of age. Less growth spurt was observed for girls, and it centered around 12 years of age.

After the growth spurt, nose growth seemed to slow a little for both sexes. However, what was important as far as Jack Lynn and the Bio-Facial Matrix was concerned was the finding that the *configuration* of the profile of the nose remained almost the *same* throughout later adolescence, and especially so for individuals exhibiting little or no growth spurt. Other investigators reported similar findings.[287] It is important to remember that the orthodontic discipline had generally felt that the soft tissue drape would always be a direct reflection of the position of the underlying hard tissues.[272] But the later work of Subtleny,[288] along with the findings of men like Burstone,[262] revealed that there is too much variation between the location of hard tissue and the resultant location of the overlying soft tissues, due to variations in soft tissue thickness, to rely too heavily on hard tissue standards for assurance of proper soft tissue positioning.

Further studies during the 1960s confirmed the downward and forward growth of the nose.[289-291] Other findings showed that the nasal bones, as well as the line from the nasal dorsum to the tip of the soft tissue nose in norma lateralis, "swing out from beneath the cranium" during growth. In the late teens the nose tip was found to show a slowing in forward growth as opposed to the nasal bones. This sometimes resulted in a slight elevation (or straightening if previously convex) of the profile of the nasal dorsum.

A superb study providing even more pertinent data on nasal anatomy was conducted by S. J. Chaconas of Los Angeles, California.[292] This work performed by Chaconas earned him the prestigious First Research Essay Award Contest sponsored by the American Association of Orthodontists in 1969. His findings revealed what other researchers had previously noted, but he also discovered that a relationship existed between the lateral profile outline of the nose and the skeletal relationship of the jaws. Class I subjects tended to have "straighter" noses. Class II subjects exhibited a greater tendency toward a pronounced elevation of the bridge of the nose, which McNamara also noted and termed a "Class II bump," which can come from a retruded maxilla or retruded mandible. It has been theorized that this convexity of the nasal dorsum is a result of the facial soft tissue drape being pulled slightly distally by the retruded skeletal conditions, causing a relative tightening of the drape over the nasal bones, thus accentuating them and making the "bump" of the nasal dorsum stand out more. This would also cause the dorsum of the nose to follow the general Class II convexity of Class II facial profiles.

The case for the "nasal dorsum/skeletal class" relationship is further strengthened by the finding that in Class III skeletal relationships, the nasal profile tended toward a concave outline of the dorsum area. The nasal cartilage (not sensitive to pressures) is felt to be responsible for the fact that the nasal bones (membranous in origin) do not resorb or change shape as would be expected in the case of chronic pressure or soft tissue tension exerted over the area as a result of any "pull of the soft tissue drape" that might be a product of the retruded skeletal conditions in the jaws. Chaconas also determined that the convexity of the soft tissue profile increased with age and was directly related to the forward growth of the soft tissue nose. Thus it may again easily be seen why bicuspid extraction, which shrinks maxillary anterior hard tissue support for the lips and often causes retruded lips or the "sunken in" look, can accentuate the convexity of the facial profile and make the nose seem even bigger and longer horizontally than it actually is!

What might be thought of as the coup de grace for building a case for the significance of the nose could be attributed to the findings of more recent studies that showed that 75% of the soft tissue straight profile noses were classified as Angle Class I and an incredible 92% of the convex nasal profiles were found to be Class II! Although the nose becomes larger with growth, it was found that the angle of the nose and its frontal breadth remains quite stable.

In light of the above, it may now be seen why Lynn drew the conclusions that formed the basis for his Bio-Facial Matrix. He concluded that in order to ensure that soft tissue profiles would turn out as desired, hard tissue standards or norms serving as treatment goals could not be fully relied upon. Instead, the soft tissues themselves (and their positioning as represented by the profile view) would have to be used in the analysis of the pretreatment state and evaluation of the success of the posttreatment result. He also concluded that the only thing available on the soft tissue profile to serve as a base of reference for the face was the one thing that would not change to a major extent as a result of orthodontic or orthopedic treatments, the nasal soft tissue profile. He surmised that the dorsum of the nose could be used as a basic frame of reference in the generation of a base reference line for analysis purposes that, unlike more traditional base reference lines of previously developed cephalometric analyses, was completely divorced from any of the internal osseous landmarks of the maxillofacial skeleton. He strongly believes that once the soft tissues are properly treated to a balanced profile, the hard tissues will follow suit by default and also be found to register as acceptable by common hard tissue standards.

In keeping with the theories of Moss, he also feels that properly positioned, correctly functioning muscles and soft tissues will serve to preserve the dental and skeletal arrangements affected by the mechanics of the treatment plan, since he is a firm believer (as are many) that the hard tissues will follow the soft tissues' functioning lead. Stability is a product of both soft tissue and neuromuscular balance, and it cannot necessarily be guaranteed by the achievement of certain hard tissue normative standards alone, especially standards that were devised in the "age of orthodontics" when mere dental arrangement was everything. Combined orthodontic/orthopedic neuromuscular balance and equilibrium in function and rest are the new orders of the day, and Lynn feels that this requires the most exacting attention be justly given to the status of the soft tissue profile.

Construction and Use of the Bio-Facial Matrix

The Bio-Facial Matrix is a gridlike arrangement of lines somewhat reminiscent of the old mesh diagrams introduced to the profession by

Lucien de Coster in the late 1930s. These early, half-century-old rectangular grids, used to analyze cephalometric x-rays, were a modification of methods of using a grid system originally developed by D'Arcy Thompson for the purposes of studying growth. However, the Bio-Facial Matrix of the 1980s is a 16-square grid drawn over the outline of the patient's profile with the one baseline of the square equated with the nasal plane of the dorsum of the nose, the grid's basic base reference line.

What may be one of the most startling procedures concerning the procedure for tracing out a Bio-Facial Matrix is that it is not done on a cephalometric x-ray! Lynn recommends that the diagnostician use a photograph or projected slide (his favorite method) to produce an outline drawing of the patient's profile on white tracing paper. The outline of the eye is also traced on the paper. Since this is all that is required, the production of a tracing for analysis purposes is accomplished with the greatest of ease. Next, the four major anatomical landmarks and the three constructed components Lynn uses are marked on the tracing sheet:

1. Soft tissue nasion (STN)   The STN is the deepest depression of the profile of the nasal soft tissues between the frontal bossing and the bridge of the nose.

2. Pupil of the eye (PE)   For PE to be correctly recorded, the patient should be looking straight ahead with his "visual" FH plane parallel to the floor.

3. Naso labial point (NLP)   The NLP is the deepest depression between the inferior border of the nose and the slope of the upper lip.

4. Nasal tip superior (NTS)   The NTS is the point where the outline of the nasal slope begins its downward turn toward the inferior border. An important additional point is necessary when the outline of the nasal profile is convex. In this instance the second point, nasal tip anterior (NTA), is drawn on the most anterior portion of the nasal profile. Thus two points, NTS and NTA, must be drawn on the convex noses.

5. Nasal plane (NP)   The NP is the base reference line that orients the entire Bio-Facial Matrix grid over the tracing of the facial profile. It is constructed by drawing a line from STN to NTS.

6. Corrected nasal plane (CNP)   When the profile of the patient's nose is sufficiently convex to warrant it, a CNP must be constructed. First, the usual NP is constructed. In so doing it will be drawn from STN to NTS (a convenient reversal of landmark letters for easy remembering). It will also be observed that this line will "slice off" the excess portion of the nasal dorsum responsible for the convexity. A second line is drawn from STN to the second additional point always present on tracings of convex noses, NTA. The angle formed by these two lines (NTA-STN-NTS) is then bisected to form the line we really want, the CNP, or the line associated exclusively with convex nasal profiles.

7. Matrix value (MV)   The MV is a constant derived from the

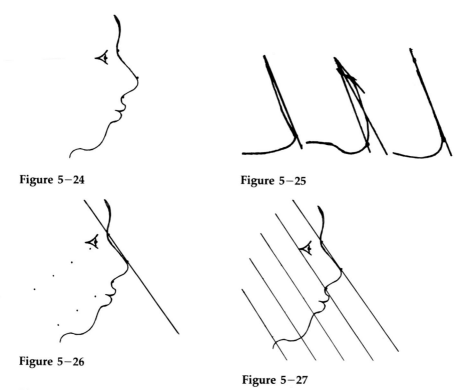

Figure 5—24

Figure 5—25

Figure 5—26

Figure 5—27

Figure 5—24 Lynn analysis soft tissue points: (1) soft tissue nasion (STN), (2) pupil of the eye (PE), (3) nasal tip superior (NTS), and (4) nasolabial point (NLP).

Figure 5—25 Nasal plane (NP): This line is critical to the entire analysis, as it orients the Bio-Facial Matrix grid over the facial profile. It is easily constructed by a line from STN to NTS. Note: When the profile of the nose is convex, a *corrected* nasal plane is substituted. It in turn represents a line that bisects an angle formed from the STN-NTS line and a line from STN to the most anterior portion of the nose, NA. Thus, the line bisecting the angle NTS-STN-NA forms the CNP or corrected nasal plane.

Figure 5—26 Nasal plane (extended to form matrix).

Figure 5—27 Matrix value (MV): Individual to each case, the MV is the distance from the NP or CPN to a parallel line through NLP. This linear distance separates all other parallel and perpendicular matrix lines.

patient's facial proportions that individualizes the entire Bio-Facial Matrix grid for each patient. It serves as a measuring rod for the equidistant construction of the lines forming the squares of the grid. It also serves other important treatment-planning and appliance-selection functions. It is determined not arithmetically but geometrically and anatomically by simply drawing a perpendicular line from NP (or CNP in the case of a convex nasal profile) to the NLP. This distance is defined as MV and serves as the key to the entire analysis system. Remember that MV is first individualized according to the anatomical proportion of the individual patient. Second, it only represents a true *ratio* and as such has no absolute numerical value, since it is constructed on an image (preferably a projected image according to Lynn) tracing that may not be actual life-size. The length of the matrix value must be measured linearly in some conventional fashion but only to produce the remaining lines of the grid. The first line is an extended version of the NP (or CNP in convex nasal profile cases). The second matrix line is one drawn parallel to NP through NLP. These two parallel lines are separated by the distances represented by MV, ie, the distance specific and individualized to each patient. The three remaining parallel lines are drawn equidistant apart in succession according to the proportions of the MV.

The counterpart to these lines, and thereby the ones that result in the formation of the grid, are based on what Lynn refers to as the optic plane (OP, not to be confused with the optic plane of the Sassouni analysis). Lynn defines his optic plane as a line drawn perpendicular from NP or CNP through PE. This serves as the superior posterior border of the grid, just as the NP or CNP serves as the superior anterior border. Four more equidistant lines are drawn parallel to OP, again using the MV to ensure their proper separation. Once completed, the Bio-Facial Matrix grid is formed consisting of 16 squares of equal size with the OP and the NP (or CNP in convex nasal profile cases) serving as the superior borders.

Accessory Planes

Once the Bio-Facial Matrix grid has been constructed, Lynn employs five additional diagnostic planes drawn at various intersections of the Matrix grid lines to serve as additional diagnostic and treatment-planning frames of reference.

Esthetic plane (EP)   The grid will always assume the position of a diamondlike configuration over the tracing of the facial profile. The superiormost point of the diamond would be at STN, which is the intersection of the OP with the NP, or the CNP if the nasal profile is convex. In this configuration the Bio-Facial Matrix grid may also be seen to have its

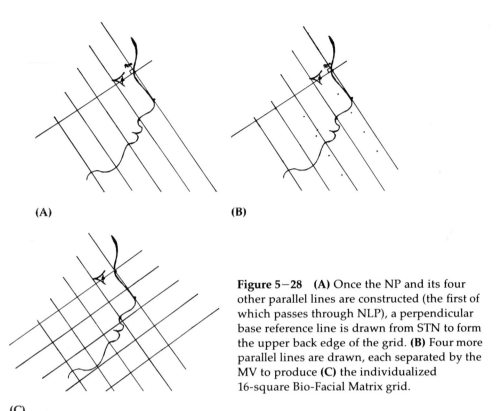

(A)   **(B)**

(C)

Figure 5−28   (A) Once the NP and its four other parallel lines are constructed (the first of which passes through NLP), a perpendicular base reference line is drawn from STN to form the upper back edge of the grid. **(B)** Four more parallel lines are drawn, each separated by the MV to produce **(C)** the individualized 16-square Bio-Facial Matrix grid.

three other corners at anterior, inferior, and posterior locations relative to the superior corner at STN. Lynn's EP is constructed from the first intersection of the planes to the right of the most superior STN and inferior points (or corners) of the grid. This straight line, starting at the intersection of the NP (or CNP) with the first grid line parallel to the OP, is drawn vertically so as to exactly bisect the first square to the right (and inferior) to the uppermost square of the grid. As a result, it must equally bisect the two grid squares directly beneath it. The EP passes directly through the first intersections of all the grid lines to the right of the midline (or superior and inferior points) of the Matrix grid. The EP is used to analyze the position of the NLP (which is a direct reflection of the location of the maxillary apical base as represented by the location of A-point).

Lip juncture plane (LJP)   The most anterior and posterior intersections (corners) of the Bio-Facial Matrix grid are connected by a horizontal straight line that Lynn uses to serve as the LJP. This plane represents the ideal vertical location, for that particular patient, of the juncture of the upper and lower lips when in a relaxed sealed state. The LJP separates the Bio-Facial Matrix into two equal triangles. It is geometrically perpendicular to the EP.

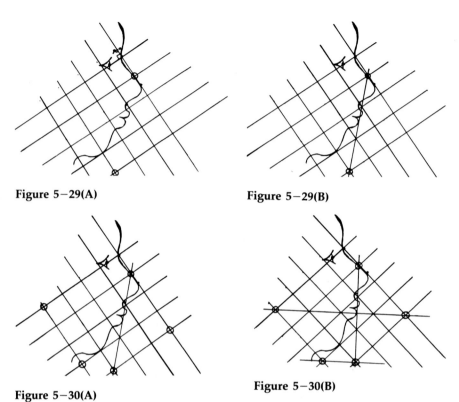

Figure 5−29(A)

Figure 5−29(B)

Figure 5−30(A)

Figure 5−30(B)

Figure 5−29   **(A)** Points on grid that locate the Lynn Bio-Facial Matrix esthetic line. **(B)** Constructed esthetic plane (EP).

Figure 5−30   **(A)** Points on grid that locate the lip juncture plane (LJP) and chin tissue plane (CTP). **(B)** LJP and CTP.

Chin tissue plane (CTP)   The bottommost square of the grid is bisected horizontally by a plane connecting the first two intersections of the grid lines superior to the most inferior point (corner) of the Matrix grid. This is the CTP and serves as a base reference line for the ideal location of the soft tissue inferior border of the chin. This little reference line is intimately related to the AFH and the vertical dimension of occlusion. Geometrically, it is parallel to the LJP.

Auxiliary esthetic planes (AEPs)   One of the important purposes of the EP is to serve as a basis for constructing the two AEPs that Lynn uses for evaluation and positioning of components of the soft tissue profile, one anterior and one posterior to the main EP. They are usually drawn in hashmarks for easier visualization. These AEPs are drawn parallel to the EP and equidistant anterior and posterior to it by a distance equal to *one third* the MV. The posterior AEP is used as a guide to the ideal location of

(1) the posterior border of the lip juncture anteroposteriorly on the horizontal plane (ideally, it should also align vertically with the grid bisecting LJP); and (2) the MC. The anterior AEP is used as a reference line for the ideal positioning of (1) the anterior borders of *both* upper and lower lips, and (2) the anterior border of the chin or soft tissue pogonion.

Ideal profile (IP)   It may now be seen that once the Bio-Facial Matrix has been completed, including the accessory planes, with knowledge of where the ideal locations of soft tissue landmarks of the profile should be, per the dictates of the Matrix itself, the intrepid hand of the clinician may then draw the IP, which is proportional to and dependent on (via the MV) the patient's anatomical proportions. This "constructed" ideal profile not only serves as a treatment goal, but it also offers an insight as to how hard the clinician will have to work to attain it. This is a product of the relationship of the IP to the pretreatment profile as interpreted by the ratios generated by the geometry of the Bio-Facial Matrix and Dr Lynn's vast clinical experience. *Zones* are created by the Matrix that offer insights and guidance to the treatment-planning techniques that will be called upon to deliver the case.

Lynn Bio-Facial Matrix Treatment Zones

In the effort to use the Bio-Facial Matrix as an aid in treatment planning, Lynn has divided the Matrix grid into four general treatment zones. These horizontal zones are layered on top of one another from the level of approximately the NLP down to the level of soft tissue menton on the Matrix-generated IP. Each zone has been designated by Lynn with a semiarbitrary percentage value derived from extensive clinical observation. These values, which give each zone its name, are 15%, 25%, 35%, and 45%. The 15% zone (representing the maxilla and upper lip) is where the least amount of physical change is effected via common orthodontic/orthopedic appliance mechanics. Conversely, the bottom zone, or 45% zone (representing soft tissue menton and pogonion), is where the greatest change is possible with modern appliance mechanics. It must be remembered that the pretreatment profile and the ideal Matrix (MV) generated profile are adjacent to one another on the completed tracing sheet. The various portions of the two profiles pass through each of the four horizontal zones (or layers) of assigned treatment potential.

These zones represent the areas that are amenable to appliance-mediated changes (be they functional, fixed, or combined) and are limited to the values assigned to the specific zones. The values are estimated as the aforementioned percentages of the MV for its respective zone. In other words, the amount of dimensional change possible in the anatomy for the 15% zone, by appliance mechanics alone of any sort, is estimated by Lynn to be limited to only 15% of the distance represented by the

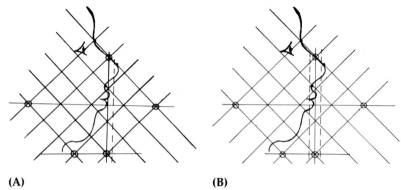

(A)   **(B)**

Figure 5−31 **(A)** Anterior auxiliary esthetic plane (AEP). **(B)** Posterior auxiliary esthetic plane.

MV. As stated previously, these percentage values of predicted possible therapeutic change by appliances alone for each of the four zones are not precise values, yet neither are they carelessly arbitrary. They represent reasonably accurate guidelines of treatment potential determined empirically by Lynn after study and evaluation of several thousand cases. Should changes greater than the estimates of the amount of change possible by the use of appliances alone be required to attain the ideal Matrix-drawn profile, either surgical intervention will be necessary, or the patient and clinician may have to simply settle for a compromised result.

The 15% zone This topmost zone includes the maxilla, premaxilla, ANS, the maxillary alveolar process, dentition, and ULP. Lynn estimates that the change possible here by conventional therapeutics (nonsurgical) is limited to 15% of the MV.

The 25% zone This zone, next to the top zone, includes the mandibular alveolus, mandibular dentition, and lower lip. The possible change for this area is estimated to be 25% of the MV.

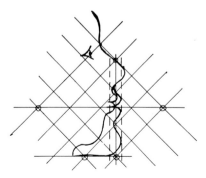

Figure 5−32 Freehand constructed individualized (by the MV) "ideal" profile.

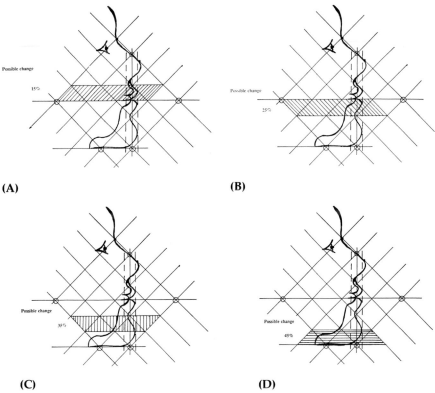

(A)

(B)

(C)

(D)

Figure 5−33   **(A)** 15% zone. **(B)** 25% zone. **(C)** 35% zone. **(D)** 45% zone.

The 35% zone   This zone includes the mandible and, therefore, its anterior limiting apical base landmark, B-point, and the MC of the soft tissue profile. The nonsurgical, appliance-mediated therapeutic change estimated for this zone is 35% of the MV.

The 45% zone   This bottommost zone represents the inferior border of the ramus and the soft tissue chin profile. Change possible here is greatest at 45% of the MV, because of the full scale changes in the position of the entire mandible in a downward and forward direction made possible by appliances such as the Bionator.

If changes required to achieve the ideal profile according to dictates of the Bio-Facial Matrix are within the limits of values calculated for each of the zones, then no compromises must be made in the treatment result, nor will surgical intervention be necessary. However, if the *facial changes* needed in the respective zones are substantially greater than the Matrix zone values, the decision must be made to either accept a compromised or less than ideal result, or to consider surgical intervention to augment the appliance mechanics necessary to deliver the case. In this light it may

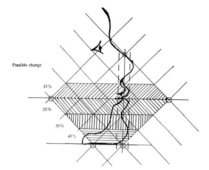

Figure 5–34 Completed Lynn Bio-Facial Matrix analysis.

be seen why the Bio-Facial Matrix method of facial analysis may be used to indicate when a rhinoplasty might be indicated to achieve the ideal profile. "Progress tracings" may also be used as an important and exciting patient motivational element during the course of treatment to show the patients the progress they are making and the changes the appliances are effecting during treatment.

Lynn strongly feels that the Bio-Facial Matrix adds another dimension to the modern orthodontic diagnosis and treatment-planning process. Realizing the therapeutic prowess represented by the orthopedically oriented functional appliances and active plates, and their abilities not only to change dental relationships but also to correct soft tissue profile deficiencies and neuromuscular imbalances as well, he feels (and justifiably so) that modern treatment may now more than ever be directed toward considering facial beauty as one of the most important criteria of successful treatment. But beauty *is* truly more than skin deep; it's bone deep. He has found that patients who have been treated to the ideal standards of the individualized Bio-Facial Matrix facial profile are observed to very seldom exhibit neuromuscular or TMJ pain, dysfunction, or degenerative arthritis. Lynn does not intend his facial analysis system to obviate the use of roentgenocephalometric analysis; rather it should be used as an important adjunct to comprehensive diagnosis. He also contends the treatment planning this method of analysis will necessarily generate will put proper attention to producing facial balance and beauty. A strong adherent to the philosophies of Moss, which theorize that control of facial dimensions rests with the functional operation of the soft tissues, Lynn summed up his feelings for the importance of considering the soft tissue (and neuromuscular) balance first over hard tissue positioning when he stated, "This analysis focuses on this important fact by directing dimensions and treatment-planning goals toward the tissues that actually control the biological changes we are ultimately trying to accomplish."[293]

FINAL STANZA

Thus our long pilgrimage through cephalometrics seems to have come full cycle. We have seen how it started in the days of the "mad Dutchman" with efforts at producing plaster reproductions of the facial profile, and sprouted early controversies over issues such as which way to trim something as seemingly mundane as the art bases of study models. We have seen how the early craniometricians studied and measured the skull and living face from every possible aspect in an effort to understand its deepest of mysteries. The sudden appearance of roentgenocephalometrics on the scene took the discipline by storm, and early investigators scrambled in a self-conscious effort to place the newfound science under control. Intimidated by their lack of knowledge of the subject, many investigators paid intellectual homage to the science of cephalometric x-ray interpretation by engaging in the most profuse and detailed study of its apparently innumerable components. We have seen how a movement arose which fantasized that there was some magical key, some secret formula, some concealed code that lay hidden among the lacy images of the cephalometric radiograph, only waiting for some scholarly champion to deliver it from the dungeons of intellectual darkness.

There were those who believed mathematical ratios held the answer. Others thought the true path lay in the proper employment of geometry. Some merely recorded nameless tables of nondescriptive numbers. For a time the obsession with exacting detail became paramount. Angulations of teeth were considered to within a fraction of a degree. The profession's concern over achieving combinations of precise positions of anterior teeth assumed heroic proportions as orthodontics wrestled with an inability to change jawbone size, location, or jaw-to-jaw relationships. Since the orthodontic therapeutic technique of the times was limited and its scope of vision was narrowed, the interpretation of the message of roentgenocephalometrics became equally distorted and narrowed to conform to that vision.

But then came the "bone movers" and the science of cephalometrics moved also, this time toward greater ranges of possibilities of treatment goals and with a vision encompassing a broader horizon. There were many false paths and, on occasion, scientific sins of omission in cephalometric's meandering and groping journey through the decades. Sometimes when the profession looked at cephalometrics, it saw only what it was told it should see. Surprisingly, even though the spectrum of its vision has gradually been broadened, some of the most important things as yet remain unseen, or at least uninterpreted. The most important of these, in a macabre sort of scientific irony, is that which ultimately governs the whole operation of the functional occlusal mechanism, the condyle/fossa relationship of the TMJs.

Not once in the history of roentgenocephalometric analysis has a system been developed that relates the significance and meaning of this most important of structural entities to the anatomical relationships of the components farther forward in the maxillofacial complex. And the hard tissue joint anatomy of this area is so simple! Yet, in spite of the slow and methodical manner in which it accumulated its findings, and in spite of the occasional faltering steps it has taken during its long journey in search of some form of mythical diagnostic nirvana, the discipline of roentgenocephalometrics has made great contributions to the orthodontic profession. The vision and the demands of the diagnostician have taken the science to the point where now cephalometric facially oriented analysis systems have been developed that are not even predicated upon the existence of a radiograph at all, but merely a facial profile photograph! Even the wonders of our technological age, the digital computers, have been enlisted to expedite and augment the process of deriving diagnostic and treatment-planning information from the science of cephalometrics. Nowadays the entire field of cephalometric analysis and interpretation can be organized, serialized, digitized, and even color-coded for the observer's convenience. All this has transpired in a sincere and honest effort to help the clinician help his patient. Old Van Loon would have been proud!

NOTE

It must be remembered that everything that we have discussed is qualified by one gigantic and overriding premise. The science of cephalometrics as we have examined it here presumes that the condyles are properly positioned within the TMJs prior to the initiation of therapeutics for correction of malocclusion. However, if they are not in proper relation in the pretreatment state, the correction of condylar malrelationships in both resting and full-occlusion positions takes precedence over any and all other preexisting conditions of the malocclusion. Proper treatment *must* include the necessary repositioning of these condyles to their correct locations within the TMJs, and this endeavor must be considered as the paramount treatment goal in the ultimate resolution of the case.

SECTION I
References

1. Van der Linden FPGM: A study of roentgenocephalometric bony landmarks. *Am J Orthod* 1971;59:111–125.
2. Yen PKJ: Identification of landmarks in cephalometric radiographs. *Angle Orthod* 1960;30:35–41.
3. Baumrind S, Frantz RC: The reliability of head film measurements. Pt I. *Am J Orthod* 1971a;60:111–127.
4. Rosenstein SW: A longitudinal study of anteroposterior growth of the mandibular symphysis. *Angle Orthod* 1964;34:153–167.
5. Hunter WS: Elementary principles of cephalometrics, in Enlow DH (ed): *The Human Face*. New York, Harper & Row, Hoeber Medical Division, 1968, pp 261–283.
6. Holdaway RA: The VTO procedure, in Schulhof RJ, Zierenberg RH, Walters RD: The mandibular dental arch. Pt II. Effects of lower incisor position on the soft tissue profile. *Angle Orthod* 1978;48:75–79.
7. Krogman WM: Craniometry and cephalometry as research tools in growth of the head and face. *Am J Orthod* 1951a;37:406–414.
8. Brown M: Eight methods of analyzing a cephalogram to establish anteroposterior skeletal discrepancy. *Br J Orthodont* 1981;8:139–146.
9. Van Loon JAW: A new method for indicating normal and abnormal relations of the teeth to the facial lines. *Dent Cosmos* 1915;57:973–983, 1093–1101, 1229–1235.
10. Angle EH: *Treatment of Malocclusion of the Teeth*, ed 7. Philadelphia, SS White Co, 1907.
11. Schwarz R: A new cephalometric method and apparatus and its application to orthodontia. *Int J Orthod Oral Surg* 1925;11:910–928, 989–1017.
12. Schwarz R: Cephalometric methods and orthodontia. *Int J Orthod Oral Surg* 1926;12:1078–1101.
13. Schwarz R: Labial deformities due to malocclusion. *Int J Orthod Oral Surg* 1930;16:808–819.
14. Schwarz R: Individual measurements of the face and jaws before and during orthodontic treatment. *Int J Orthod* 1933;19:22–54.
15. Simon P: *Fundamental Principles of a Systematic Diagnosis of Dental Anomalies*. Berlin, Hermann Meusser, 1922, translated by Lischer BC, Boston, Stratford Co, 1926.
16. Simon P: The orbital-canine law. *Int J Orthod Oral Surg* 1928;14:150–153.
17. Dewey M: The constancy of cusp position as related to facial form. *Int J Orthod Oral Surg* 1930;16:180–187.

18. Hellman M: A study of some etiological factors of malocclusion. *Dent Cosmos* 1914;56:1017−1032.

19. Hellman M: A further study of some etiological factors of malocclusion. *Dent Cosmos* 1916;58:189−201.

20. Hellman M: Nutrition, growth and dentition. *Dent Cosmos* 1923;65:34−49.

21. Hellman M: The process of dentition and its effects on occlusion. *Dent Cosmos* 1923;65:1329−1344.

22. Hellman M: Failures in orthodontic treatment. *Int J Orthod Oral Surg* 1936;22:343−360.

23. Hellman M: Fundamental principles and expedient compromises in orthodontic procedures. *Am J Orthod Oral Surg* 1944;30:429−436.

24. Hellman M: A preliminary study in development as it affects the human face. *Dent Cosmos* 1927;69:250−269.

25. Hellman M: Changes in the human face brought about by development. *Int J Orthod Oral Surg* 1927;13:475−516.

26. Hellman M: The orbital plane. *Int J Orthod Oral Surg* 1930;16:151−179.

27. Hellman M: Physiologic treatment. *Dent Cosmos* 1930;72:578−595.

28. Hellman M: An introduction to growth of the human face from infancy to adulthood. *Int J Orthod Oral Surg* 1932;18:777−798.

29. Hellman M: Morphology of the face, jaws, and dentition in Class III malocclusions of the teeth. *J Am Dent Assoc* 1931;18:2150−2173.

30. Hellman M: The face in its developmental career. *Dent Cosmos* 1935;77:685−699.

31. Pacini AJ: Roentgen ray anthropometry of the skull. *J Radiol* 1922;3:230−238, 322−331, 418−426.

32. Simpson CO: A procedure for obtaining radiographic images of the facial profile in the sagittal plane. *Int J Orthod Oral Surg* 1929;15:79−85.

33. Dewey MN, Riesner S: A radiographic study of facial deformity. *Int J Orthod Oral Surg* 1928;14:261−267.

34. Hofrath H: Die Bedeutung der Roentgenfernund Abstandsaufnahme fur Diagnostik der Kieferanomalien. *Fortschritte der Orthodontik* 1931;1:232.

35. Broadbent BH: A new x-ray technique and its application to orthodontia. *Angle Orthod* 1931;1:45−66.

36. Gregory WK: *Our Face from Fish to Man.* New York, GP Putnams' Sons, 1929.

37. Kieth A, Campion G: A contribution to the mechanism of growth of the human face. *Int J Orthod Oral Surg* 1922;8:607−633.

38. Krogman WM: The problem of growth changes in the face and skull as viewed from a comparative study of anthropoids and man. *Dent Cosmos* 1930;72:624−630.

39. Broadbent BH: The face of the normal child. *Angle Orthod* 1937;7:183−208.

40. Brodie AG, Downs WB, Goldstein A, Meyer E: Cephalometric appraisal of orthodontic results. *Angle Orthod* 1938;8:261−352.

41. Margolis HI: Standardized x-ray cephalographics. *Int J Orthod Oral Surg* 1940;26:725−740.

42. Higley LB: Lateral head roentgenograms and their relation to the orthodontic problem. *Am J Orthod Oral Surg* 1940;26:768−778.

43. Tweed CH: The application of the principles of the edgewise arch in the treatment of malocclusion. I, II. *Angle Orthod* 1941;11:5−69.

44. Tweed CH: A philosophy of orthodontic treatment. *Am J Orthod* 1945;31: 74–103.

45. Tweed CH: The Frankfort-mandibular plane angle in orthodontic diagnosis, classification, treatment planning and prognosis. *Am J Orthod Oral Surg* 1946;32:175–230.

46. Tweed CH: The Frankfort-mandibular incisors angle (FMIA) in orthodontic diagnosis, treatment planning and prognosis. *Angle Orthod* 1954;24:121–169.

47. Margolis HI: Basic facial pattern and its application in clinical orthodontics. *Am J Orthod Oral Surg* 1947;33:631–641.

48. Noyes HJ, Rushing CH, Sims HA: The axial inclination of the human central incisor teeth. *Angle Orthod* 1943;13:60–61.

49. Speidel Tom, Stoner MM: Variations of mandibular incisor axis in adult "normal" occlusion. *Am J Orthod Oral Surg* 1944;30:342–356.

50. Higley LB: Cephalometric diagnosis and its implication in treatment. *J Am Dent Assoc* 1945;32:3–15.

51. Mayne W: *A Study of the Skeletal Pattern of the Human Face*, thesis. Northwestern University, 1946.

52. Downs WB: Variation in facial relationships: their significance in treatment and prognosis. *Am J Orthod* 1948;34:812–840.

53. Thompson JR: The rest position of the mandible and its significance to dental science. *J Am Dent Assoc* 1946;33:151–180.

54. Thompson JR: Cephalometric investigations of the opening movements of the mandible. *Angle Orthod* 1948;18:30–31.

55. Thompson JR: Rest position of the mandible and its application to analysis and correction of malocclusion. *Angle Orthod* 1949;19:162–187.

56. Thompson JR, Craddock FW: Functional analysis of occlusion. *J Am Dent Assoc* 1949;39:404–406.

57. Thompson JR: Oral and environmental factors as etiological factors in malocclusion of the teeth. *Am J Orthod* 1949;35:33–53.

58. Riedel RA: *A Cephalometric Roentgenographic Study of the Relation of the Maxilla and Associated Parts of the Cranial Base in Normal and Malocclusion of the Teeth*, thesis. Northwestern University, 1948.

59. Luzi V: CV value in analysis of sagittal malocclusions. *Am J Orthod* 1982;81: 478.

60. Graber TM: New horizons in case analysis; clinical cephalometrics. *Am J Orthod* 1952;38:603–624.

61. Donovan RW: A radiographic cephalometric consideration of facial growth during orthodontic treatment. *Am J Orthod* 1953;39:341–357.

62. Buckley DE: *A Cephalometric Roentgenographic Study of the Facial Skeleton in Class II, Division 1 Malocclusion*, thesis. Northwestern University, 1948.

63. Freeman RS: *A Radiographic Method of Analysis of the Relation of the Structures of the Lower Face to Each Other and to the Occlusal Plane of the Teeth*, thesis. Northwestern University, 1950.

64. Rasmusson DF: *A Radiographic Analysis of the Structures of the Lower Face to the Mandibular Plane*, thesis. Northwestern University, 1950.

65. Carlson SD: *A Cephalometric Radiographic Study of the Change in Relation of Mandible to Maxilla in Orthodontic Treatment*, thesis. Northwestern University, 1951.

66. Williams JE: *A Radiographic Cephalometric Study of the Labiolingual Axial*

Inclination of the Central Incisors in Relation to the Mandible and Maxilla of Excellent Dentitions, thesis. Northwestern University, 1951.

67. Brown J: Specialization, a warning. *J Periodontol* 1950;21:97.

68. Salzmann JA: Resume of the workshop and limitations of the technique. *Am J Orthod* 1958;44:901–905.

69. Salzmann JA: The research workshop on cephalometrics. *Am J Orthod* 1960; 46:834–847.

70. Ricketts RM: A foundation for cephalometric communication. *Am J Orthod* 1960;46:330–357.

71. Ricketts RM: Planning treatment on the basis of facial pattern and an estimate of its growth. *Angle Orthod* 1957;27:14–37.

72. Ricketts RM: The influence of orthodontic treatment on facial growth and development. *Angle Orthod* 1960;30:103–133.

73. Ricketts RM: Cephalometric analysis and synthesis. *Angle Orthod* 1961;31: 141–156.

74. Ricketts RM: The evolution of diagnosis to computerized cephalometrics. *Am J Orthod* 1969;55:795–803.

75. Ricketts RM: *Introducing Computerized Cephalometrics*. Denver, CO, Rocky Mountain Communications, March 1969.

76. Ricketts RM, Bench R, Hilgers JJ, Schulhof R: An overview of computerized cephalometrics. *Am J Orthod* 1972;61:1–28.

77. Ricketts RM: A principle of archial growth of the mandible. *Angle Orthod* 1972;42:368–386.

78. Ricketts RM: *The Application of Computers to Orthodontics—Diagnosis, Prognosis and Treatment Planning*. Trans. 3rd IOC, Crosby Lockwood Staples, Great Britain, 1975.

79. Sassouni V: A roentgenographic cephalometric analysis of cephalo-facial-dental relationships. *Am J Orthod* 1955;41:735–764.

80. Sassouni V: Diagnosis and treatment planning via roentgenographic cephalometry. *Am J Orthod* 1958;44:433–463.

81. McNamara JA: A method of cephalometric evaluation. *Am J Orthod* 1984;86: 449–469.

82. McNamara JA: The electromyography of the mandibular postural position in the rhesus monkey (*Macaca mulatta*). *J Dent Res* 1974;53:949.

83. McNamara JA: An electromyographic study of mastication in the rhesus monkey. (*Macaca mulatta*). *Arch Oral Biol* 1974;19:821–823.

84. McNamara JA, Graber LW: Mandibular growth in the rhesus monkey (*Macaca mulatta*). *Am J Phys Anthrop* 1975;42:15–24.

85. McNamara JA: An experimental study of increased vertical dimension in the growing face. *Am J Orthod* 1977;71:382–395.

86. McNamara JA, Carlson DS: Quantitative analysis of temporomandibular joint adaptations to protrusive function. *Am J Orthod* 1979;76:593–611.

87. McNamara JA: Functional determinants of craniofacial size and shape. *Eur J Orthod* 1980;2:131–159.

88. McNamara JA: Components of Class II malocclusions in children 8–10 years of age. *Angle Orthod* 1981;51:177–202.

89. McNamara JA, Huge SA: The functional regulator (FR-3) of Frankel. *Am J Orthod*, in press 1981.

90. McNamara JA: Influence of respiratory pattern on craniofacial growth. *Angle Orthod* 1981;51:269–300.

91. McNamara JA: The Frankel appliance. I. Biological basis and appliance design. *J Clin Orthod* 1982;16:320–337.

92. McNamara JA: The Frankel appliance. II. Clinical management. *J Clin Orthod* 1982;16:390–407.

93. Bjork, A: Facial growth in man, studied with the aid of metallic implants. *Acta Odontal Scand* 1955;13:9–34.

94. Bjork, A: Facial growth in bilateral Rypoplasia of the mandibular condyle: A radiographic cephalometric study of a case using metallic implants, in Kraus BS and Reidel RA (eds): *Vistas in Orthodontics*. Philadelphia, Lea and Febiger, 1962, pp 347–358.

95. Bjork, A: Variations in the growth patterns of the human mandible: Longitudinal radiographic study by the implant method. *J Dent Res* 1963;42: 400–411.

96. Bjork, A: Sutural growth of the upper face studied by the implant method. *Acta Odontal Scand* 1966;24:109–127.

97. Bjork, A: The use of metallic implants in the study of facial growth in children. *Am J Phys Anthrop* 1968;29:243–254.

98. Bjork, A: The face in profile; an anthropological x-ray investigation on Swedish children and conscripts. *Svensk Tandl Tidskr* 1947;40:supp 5b.

99. Bjork, A, Skieller V: Facial development and tooth eruption: An implant study at the age of puberty. *Am J Orthod* 1972;62:339–382.

100. Bimler HP: Bimler therapy. Pt I. Bimler cephalometric analysis. *J Clin Orthod* 1985;19:501–523.

101. Bimler HP: A roentgenoscopic method of analyzing the facial correlations. *Trans Eur Orthod Soc* 1957;241–253.

102. Bimler HP: Facial pattern formula. *Trans Eur Orthod Soc* 1960;224–236.

103. Bimler HP: Stomatopedics in theory and practice. *Int J Orthod* 1965;2:5–20.

104. Bimler HP: The Bimler appliance, in Graber TM, Neumann B (eds): *Removable Orthodontic Appliances*, Philadelphia, WB Saunders Co, 1977, pp 337–500.

105. Baume LJ: Principles of craniofacial development revealed by experimental biology. *Am J Orthod* 1961;47:881–901.

106. Torrey TW: *Morphogenesis of the Vertebrates*. New York, John Wiley and Sons, 1962, pp 212–257.

107. Dodson EO: *Evolution: Process and Product*. New York, Reinhold Publishing Co, 1960, pp 155–166.

108. Baume LJ: Tooth and investing bone: A developmental entity. *Oral Surg Oral Med Oral Path* 1956;9:736–741.

109. Glucksmann A: The role of mechanical stresses in bone formation in vitro. *J Anat* 1942;76:231–239.

110. Blount WP, Zeier F: Control of bone length. *JAMA* 1952;148:451–457.

111. Zuckermann S: Age changes in the basiocranial of the human skull. *Am J Phys Anthro* 1955;13:521–539.

112. Baume LJ, Haupl K, Stellmach R: Growth and transformation of the temporomandibular joint in an orthopedically treated case of Pierre Robin's syndrome. *Am J Orthod* 1959;45:901–916.

113. Grant JCB, Basmajian JV: *Grant's Method of Anatomy*. Baltimore, Williams and Wilkins Co, 1965, pp 718–736.

114. Krogman WM, Sassouni V: *A Syllabus on Roentgenographic Cephalometry*. Philadelphia, University of Pittsburgh, 1957.

115. Elman ES: Studies on the relationship of the lower six-year molar to the mandible. *Angle Orthod* 1940;10:24−32.

116. Baldridge JP: A study of the relation of the maxillary first permanent molars to the face in Class I and Class II malocclusion. *Angle Orthod* 1941;11: 100−109.

117. Shoenwelter RF: The relation of the upper and lower first permanent molars to the face in Class III malocclusions. *Angle Orthod* 1948;18:16−19.

118. Staph WC: A cephalometric roentgenographic appraisal of the facial pattern in Class II malocclusions. *Angle Orthod* 1948;18:20−23.

119. Gilmore WA: Morphology of the adult mandible in Class II, division 1 malocclusions and excellent occlusions. *Angle Orthod* 1950;20:137−146.

120. Bjork A: Some biological aspects of prognathism and occlusion of the teeth. *Acta Odontal Scand* 1950;8:1−40.

121. Bjork A: Cranial base development. *Am J Orthod* 1955;41:198−225.

122. Coben SE: The integration of facial skeletal variants. *Am J Orthod* 1955;41: 407−434.

123. Ingervall B, Thilander B: The human spheno-occipital synchrondrosis. I. The time of closure appraised macroscopically. *Acta Odontal Scand* 1972;30: 349−356.

124. Ford EH: Growth of the human cranial base. *Am J Orthod* 1958;44:498−506.

125. Renfroe EW: A study of facial patterns associated with Class I, Class II, division 1 and Class II, division 2 malocclusions. *Angle Orthod* 1948;18: 12−15.

126. Moss ML: Correlation of cranial base angulation with cephalic malformations and growth disharmonies of dental interest. *NY State Dent J* 1955;24:452−454.

127. Hopkin GB, Houston WJB, James GA: The cranial base as an etiological factor in malocclusion. *Angle Orthod* 1968;38:250−255.

128. Brodie AG: The behavior of the cranial base and its components as revealed by serial cephalometric roentgenograms. *Angle Orthod* 1955;25:148−160.

129. Lewis AB, Roche AF: Elongation of the cranial base in girls during pubescence. *Angle Orthod* 1972;42:358−367.

130. Singh IJ, Savara BS: Norms of size and annual increments of seven anatomical measures of maxillae in boys from three to sixteen years of age. *Angle Orthod* 1968;38:104−120.

131. Savara BS, Singh IJ: Norms of size and annual increments of seven anatomical measures of maxillae in girls from three to sixteen years of age. *Angle Orthod* 1966;36:312−324.

132. Massler M, Schour I: The growth pattern of the cranial vault in the albino rat as measured by vital staining with alizarine red "S." *Anat Rec* 1941;110: 83−101.

133. Enlow DH, Bairg S: Growth and remodeling of the human maxilla. *Am J Orthod* 1965;51:446−464.

134. Brodie AG: Late growth changes in the human face. *Angle Orthod* 1953;23: 146−157.

135. Mills CM, Holman G, Graber TM: Heavy intermittant cervical traction in Class II treatment: A longitudinal cephalometric assessment. *Am J Orthod* 1978;74:361−379.

136. Harris JE: A cephalometric analysis of mandibular growth rate. *Am J Orthod* 1962;48:161−174.

137. Humphry G: The growth of the jaws. *Tr Cambridge Phil Soc* 1864.

138. Brash JC: *The Growth of the Jaws and Palate.* London, Dental Board of the United Kingdom, 1924, pp 23—66.
139. Brodie AG: On the growth pattern of the human head from the third month to the eighth year of life. *Am J Anat* 1941;68:209—262.
140. Sicher H: The growth of the mandible. *Am J Orthod* 1947;33:30—35.
141. Sicher H: *Oral Anatomy,* ed 2. St Louis, CV Mosby Co, 1952.
142. Enlow DH, Harris DB: A study of the postnatal growth of the human mandible. *Am J Orthod* 1964;50:25—50.
143. Horowitz SL, Thompson RH: Variations of the craniofacial skeleton in post-adolescent males and females. *Angle Orthod* 1964;34:97—102.
144. Enlow WH, McNamara J: Varieties of *in vivo* tooth movements. *Angle Orthod* 1973b;43:216—217.
145. Wylie WL: The relationship between ramus height, dental height, and overbite. *Am J Orthod Oral Surg* 1947;32:57—67.
146. Johnson EL: The Frankfort-mandibular plane angle and the facial pattern. *Am J Orthod* 1950;36:516—533.
147. Richardson A: A cephalometric investigation of skeletal factors in anterior open bite and/or deep bite. *Trans Eur Orthod Soc* 1967;159—171.
148. Creekmore TD: Inhibition or stimulation of the vertical growth of the facial complex, its significance to treatment. *Angle Orthod* 1967;37:285—297.
149. Schudy FF: The rotation of the mandible resulting from growth: Its implications in orthodontic treatment. *Angle Orthod* 1965;35:36—53.
150. Schudy FF: Control of vertical overbite in clinical orthodontics. *Angle Orthod* 1968;38:19—39.
151. Bjork A: Prediction of mandibular growth rotation. *Am J Orthod* 1969;55: 585—599.
152. Odegaard J: Mandibular rotation studied with the aid of metal implants. *Am J Orthod* 1970;58:448—454.
153. Isaacson JR, Isaacson RJ, Speidel TM, Worms FW: Extreme variation in vertical facial growth and associated variations in skeletal and dental relations. *Angle Orthod* 1971;41:219—229.
154. Moss ML: Embryology, growth and malformation of the temporomandibular joint, in Schwarz L (ed): *Disorders of the Temporomandibular Joint.* Philadelphia, WB Saunders Co, 1959.
155. Moss ML: A functional analysis of human mandibular growth. *J Prosthet Dent* 1960;10:1149—1160.
156. Moss ML: Extrinsic determination of sutural area morphology. *Acta Anat* 1961;44:263—272.
157. Moss ML: The functional matrix, in Kraus BS and Reidel R (eds): *Vistas in Orthodontics.* Philadelphia, Lea and Febiger, 1962.
158. Moss ML: The vertical growth of the human face. *Am J Orthod* 1964;50: 354—376.
159. Moss ML: The primacy of functional matrices in orofacial growth. *Practitioner* 1968;19:65—73.
160. Moss ML, Greenberg S: Functional cranial analysis of the human maxillary bone. I. Basal bone. *Angle Orthod* 1967;37:151—164.
161. Moss ML, Rankow R: The role of the functional matrix in mandibular growth. *Angle Orthod* 1968;38:95—103.
162. Moss ML, Simon M: Growth of the human mandibular angular process: A functional cranial analysis. *Am J Phys Anthropol* 1968;28:127—138.

163. Moss ML, Salentijn L: The primary role of functional matrices in facial growth. *Am J Orthod* 1969a;55:566–577.

164. Moss ML: Neurotropic processes in orofacial growth. *J Dent Res* 1971;50: 1492–1494.

165. Moss ML: Twenty years of functional cranial analysis. *Am J Orthod* 1972c;61: 479–485.

166. Bosma JF: Oral and pharyngeal development and function. *J Dent Res* 1963; 42:375–380.

167. Bosma JF: Maturation and function of the oral and pharyngeal region. *Am J Orthod* 1963;49:94–100.

168. Latham RA: The sella point and postnatal growth of the human cranial base. *Am J Orthod* 1972a;61:156–162.

169. McNiel RW: *A Roentgenocephalometric Study of the Nasopharyngeal and Cranial Base Growth in Cleft Palate Children*, thesis. University of Pennsylvania, 1962.

170. Baume LJ: A biologist looks at sella point. *Trans Eur Orthod Soc* 1957; 150–159.

171. Bergerson EO: A comparative study of cephalometric superimposition. *Angle Orthod* 1961;31:216–299.

172. Steuer I: The cranial base for superimposition of lateral cephalometric radiographs. *Am J Orthod* 1972;10:493–500.

173. Melson B: Time of closure of the spheno-occipital synchrondrosis determined on dried skulls: A radiographic cephalometric study. *Acta Odontal Scand* 1969;27:73–90.

174. Prichard JJ, Scott JH, Girgis FG: The structure and development of cranial and facial sutures. *J Anat* 1956;90:73–86.

175. Scott JH: Growth at facial sutures. *Am J Orthod* 1956;42:381–387.

176. Brodie AG: Behavior of normal and abnormal growth patterns. *Am J Orthod Oral Surg* 1941a;27:633–647.

177. Brodie AG: Some recent observations on the growth of the face and their implications to the orthodontist. *Am J Orthod Oral Surg* 1940;26:741–757.

178. Brodie AG: Facial patterns: A theme and variations. *Angle Orthod* 1946;16: 75–87.

179. Sved, Alexander: A critical review of cephalometrics. *Am J Orthod* 1954;40: 567–590.

180. DeCoster L: Hereditary potentiality versus ambient factors. *Trans Eur Orthod Soc* 1951;227–234.

181. DeCoster L: The familial line, studied by a new line of reference. *Trans Eur Orthod Soc* 1952;50–55.

182. DeCoster L: A new line of reference for the study of lateral facial teleradiographs. *Am J Orthod* 1953;39:304.

183. Scott JH: The growth of the human face. *Proc Roy Soc Med* 1954;47:91–100.

184. Richardson A: An investigation into the reproducability of some points, planes and lines used in cephalometric analysis. *Am J Orthod* 1966;52: 637–651.

185. Moore, AW: Observations on facial growth and its clinical significance. *Am J Orthod* 1959;45:399–423.

186. Ricketts RM, Schulhof RJ, Bagha L: Orientation: Sella-nasion or Frankfort horizontal. *Am J Orthod* 1976;69:648–654.

187. Waldo CM: A practical approach to the problem of orthodontics. *Am J Orthod* 1953;39:322–339.

188. Koski K: The norm concept in dental orthopedics. *Angle Orthod* 1955;25: 113—117.
189. Hixon HE: The norm concept and cephalometrics. *Am J Orthod* 1958;42: 898—906.
190. Hixon HE: Cephalometrics: A perspective. *Angle Orthod* 1972;42:200—211.
191. Graber TM: Problems and limitations of cephalometric analysis in orthodontics. *J Am Dent Assoc* 1956;53:439—454.
192. Kraus BS, Wise WJ, Frei RH: Heredity and the craniofacial complex. *Am J Orthod* 1959;45:172—217.
193. Horowitz SL, Osborne RH, DeGeorge FV: A cephalometric study of craniofacial variation in adult twins. *Angle Orthod* 1960;30:1—5.
194. Schulhof RJ, Nakamurg S, Williamson WV: Prediction of abnormal growth in Class III malocclusions. *Am J Orthod* 1977;71:421—430.
195. Greenberg LZ, Johnston LE: Computerized prediction: The accuracy of a contemporary long-range forecast. *Am J Orthod* 1975;67:243—252.
196. Schulhof RJ, Bagha L: A statistical evaluation of the Ricketts and Johnston growth forecasting methods. *Am J Orthod* 1975;67:258—275.
197. Lande MS: Growth behavior of the human bony profile as revealed by cephalometric roentgenology. *Angle Orthod* 1952;22:78—80.
198. Bjork A, Palling M: Adolescent age changes in sagittal jaw relation, alveolar prognathy and incisal inclination. *Acta Odontal Scand* 1955;12:201—232.
199. Harvold E: Some biologic aspects of orthodontic treatment in the transitional dentition. *Am J Orthod* 1963;49:1—14.
200. Jones BH, Meredith HV: Vertical change in osseous and odontic portions of human face height between the ages of 5 and 15 years. *Am J Orthod* 1966;52: 902—921.
201. Hixon EH: Prediction and facial growth. *Trans Eur Orthod Soc* 1968;127—139.
202. Johnston LE: A statistical evaluation of cephalometric prediction. *Angle Orthod* 1968;38:284—304.
203. Balbach DR: A cephalometric relationship between the morphology of the mandible and its future occlusal position. *Angle Orthod* 1969;39:29—41.
204. Hirschfeld WJ, Moyers RE: Prediction of craniofacial growth: The state of the art. *Am J Orthod* 1971;60:435—444.
205. Schwarz AM, Gratzinger M: *Removable Orthodontic Appliances*. Philadelphia, WB Saunders Co, 1966.
206. Graber TM: Orthodontics, Principles and Practices. Philadelphia, WB Saunders Co, 1961.
207. Salzmann JA: *Practice of Orthodontics*. Philadelphia, JB Lippincott Co, 1966.
208. Ricketts RM, et al: *Orthodontic Diagnosis and Planning*. Denver, Rocky Mountain/Orthodontics, 1982.
209. Jacobson A: The "Wits" appraisal of jaw disharmony. *Am J Orthod* 1975;67: 125—134.
210. Jacobson A: Application of the "Wits" appraisal. *Am J Orthod* 1976;70: 179—189.
211. Jacobson A, Caufield PW: *Introduction to Radiographic Cephalometry*. Philadelphia, Lea & Febiger, 1985, pp 63—71.
212. Hellman M: Racial characteristics in human dentition. *Proc Am Philos Soc* 1929;67:157—174.
213. Vorhies JM, Adams JW: Polygonic interpretations of cephalometric findings. *Angle Orthod* 1951;21:194—197.

214. Wylie WL, Johnson EL: Rapid evaluation of facial dysplasia in the vertical plane. *Angle Orthod* 1952;22:165−182.
215. Steiner CC: Cephalometrics for you and me. *Am J Orthod* 1953;39:729−755.
216. Steiner CC: Cephalometrics in clinical practice. *Angle Orthod* 1959;29:8−29.
217. Steiner CC: The use of cephalometrics as an aid to planning and assessing orthodontic treatment. *Am J Orthod* 1960;46:721−735.
218. Wylie WL: The assessment of anteroposterior dysplasia. *Angle Orthod* 1947; 17:97−109.
219. McWilliam JS, Welander U: The effect of image quality on identification of cephalometric landmarks. *Angle Orthod* 1978;48:49−56.
220. Jarabak JR, Fizzell JA: *Technique and Treatment with Light Wire Appliances.* St Louis, CV Mosby Co, 1963, p 146.
221. Steyn CL, et al: Calculation of the position of the axis of rotation when single-rooted teeth are orthodontically tipped. *Br J Orthod* 1978;5:153−156.
222. Davidian EJ: Use of a computer to study force distribution on the root of the maxillary central incisor. *Am J Orthod* 1971;59:581−588.
223. Christiansen RL, Burstone CJ: Centers of rotation within the periodontal space. *Am J Orthod* 1969;55:353−369.
224. Jacobson RL, Jacobson A: Point A revisited. *Am J Orthod* 1980;77:92−96.
225. Ricketts RM, et al: *Orthodontic Diagnosis and Planning.* Denver, Rocky Mountain Orthodontics, 1982, pp 283−288.
226. Welchons AM, Krickenberger WR, Pearson HR: *Plane Geometry.* Boston, Ginn and Co, 1958.
227. Sassouni V: A roentgenocephalometric analysis of cephalofaciodental relationships. *Am J Orthod* 1955;41:735−764.
228. Beistle R: Sassouni Plus lecture, presented at University of Notre Dame, Sept 15, 1986.
229. Sassouni V: Diagnosis and treatment planning via roentgenographic cephalometry. *Am J Orthod* 1958;44:433−463.
230. Sassouni V: *Clinical Cephalometry.* Philadelphia Center for Research in Child Growth, Philadelphia, 1959.
231. Sassouni V: *The Face in Five Dimensions,* ed 1. Philadelphia Center for Research in Child Growth, Philadelphia, 1960.
232. Sassouni V: *The Face in Five Dimensions,* ed 2. University of West Virginia Publication, Morgantown, West Virginia, 1962.
233. Sassouni V, Nanda S: Analysis of dentofacial vertical proportions. *Am J Orthod* 1964;50:801−823.
234. Sassouni V, Nanda S: Planes of reference in roentgenographic cephalometry. *Angle Orthod* 1965;35:311−319.
235. Sassouni V: A classification of skeletal facial types. *Am J Orthod* 1969;55: 109−123.
236. Sassouni V: The Class II syndrome: Differential diagnosis and treatment. *Angle Orthod* 1970;40:334−341.
237. Sassouni V, Forrest E: *Orthodontics in Dental Practice.* St Louis, CV Mosby Co, 1971.
238. Sassouni V: *A Syllabus in Cephalometric Analysis (Archial),* School of Dentistry. University of Pittsburgh, Pittsburgh, PA, course material, 1959.
239. Beistle R: Personal communication, December 1986.
240. McNamara JA: *Integrated Treatment of the Orthodontic Patient: Diagnosis Treat-*

ment Planning and Clinical Management. University of Michigan, Ann Arbor, MI, 1986.

241. Broadbent BH Sr, Broadbent BH Jr, Golden WH: *Bolton Standards of Dentofacial Development and Growth.* St Louis, CV Mosby Co, 1975.

242. Scheideman GB, Bell WH, Legan HL, Finn RA, Reisch JS: Cephalometric analysis of dentofacial normals. *Am J Orthod* 1980;78:404−420.

243. Harvold EP: *The Activator in Interceptive Orthodontics.* St Louis, CV Mosby Co, 1974.

244. Woodside DG: Cephalometric roentgenography, in Clark J (ed): *Clinical Dentistry.* Philadelphia, WB Saunders Co, 1975, vol 2.

245. Ricketts RM: Perspectives in the clinical application of cephalometrics. *Angle Orthod* 1981;51:105−115.

246. Bimler HP: *The Bimler Cephalometric Analysis.* Great Falls, MT, V Nord, 1969.

247. Bimler HP: Possibilities and limitations of treatment in Class II cases. *Trans Eur Orthod Soc* 1956;55−67.

248. Bimler HP: Personal communication, September 1985.

249. Friel S: Further investigations concerning muscles and their relation to growth of the jaws. *Int J Orthod* 1929;15:1078−1086.

250. Campion GG: Orthodontics: A study in six dimensions. *D Record* 1920;40: 345−353.

251. Campion GG, Campion DH: Facial measurements in diagnosis. *Int J Orthod* 1932;18:1170−1180.

252. Goldstein MS, Stanton FL: Facial growth in relation to dental occlusion. *Int J Orthod* 1937;23:859−892.

253. Pelton WJ, Elasser WA: Studies of dentofacial morphology. IV. Profile changes among 6829 white individuals according to age and sex. *Angle Orthod* 1955;25:199−207.

254. Krogman WM: The problem of timing in facial growth with special reference to the period of the changing dentition. *Am J Orthod* 1951;37:253−276.

255. Coben SE: The integration of facial skeletal variants: A serial cephalometric roentgenographic analysis of craniofacial form and growth. *Am J Orthod* 1955;41:407−434.

256. Meredith HV, Knott VB, Hixon HE: Relation of the nasal and subnasal components of facial height in childhood. *Am J Orthod* 1958;44:285−294.

257. Gresham H: A cephalometric comparison of some skeletal and denture pattern components in two groups of children with acceptable occlusions. *Angle Orthod* 1963;33:114−119.

258. Bergersen EO: The direction of facial growth from infancy to adulthood. *Angle Orthod* 1966;36:18−43.

259. Schudy FF: Vertical growth vs. anteroposterior growth as related to function and treatment. *Angle Orthod* 1964;34:75−93.

260. Riedel RA: Esthetics and its relation to orthodontic therapy. *Angle Orthod* 1950;20:168−178.

261. Burstone CJ: The integumental profile. *Am J Orthod* 1958;44:1−25.

262. Bjork A: The significance of growth changes in facial patterns and their relationship to changes in occlusion. *D Record* 1951;71:197−208.

263. Subtelny JD: A longitudinal study of soft tissue facial structures and their profile characteristics defined in relation to underlying skeletal structures. *Am J Orthod* 1959;45:481−507.

264. Liddle DW: Second molar extraction in orthodontic treatment. *Am J Orthod* 1977;72:599–616.

265. Yerkes I: Are you doing all you can for your patients? lecture, handout materials, Minneapolis, May 1983.

266. Enlow DH: *Handbook of Facial Growth*, ed 1. Philadelphia, WB Saunders Co, 1975.

267. Gottlieb EL: A new look at Class II malocclusion. *J Clin Orthod* 1982;16: 571–572.

268. Moyers RE, et al: Differential diagnosis of Class II malocclusions. *Am J Orthod* 1980;78:477–494.

269. Witzig J: Lecture notes, Minneapolis, August 1984.

270. Bean M: The Facial Seminar, Des Moines, April 1983.

271. Bowbeer GRN: Five keys to facial beauty and TMJ health. *The Functional Orthodontist* 1985;2:12–29.

272. Riedel RA: An analysis of dentofacial relationships. *Am J Orthod* 1957;43: 103–119.

273. Peck H, Peck S: A concept of facial esthetics. *Angle Orthod* 1970;40:284–317.

274. Bowbeer GRN: Saving the face and the TMJ. I. *The Functional Orthodontist* 1985;2:32–44.

275. Jervinen S: Relation of the SNA angle to the saddle angle. *Am J Orthod* 1980;79:670–673.

276. Bowbeer GRN: Saving the face and the TMJ. II. *The Functional Orthodontist* 1986;3:9–24.

277. Bowbeer GRN: Saving the face and the TMJ. III. *The Functional Orthodontist* 1986;3:6–18.

278. Chambers J, Mullich S, Smith DD: How to choose the right forecasting technique. *Harvard Business Review* 1971;49:45–74.

279. Chambers J, Mullich S, Smith DD: *An Executive's Guide to Forecasting*. New York, John Wiley & Sons, 1973.

280. Smith DD, Schrieber N: *Corporate Simulation Models*. Institute of Management Science, University of Washington Press, 1970.

281. Smith DD, Smith NK: *SST—Searching for Structure Technique*. Pittsburgh, On-Line Systems Inc, 1972.

282. Burstone CJ, Park YC: Soft tissue profile—Fallacies of hard tissue standards in treatment planning. *Am J Orthod* 1986;90:52–62.

283. Looi L, Mills J: The effects of two contrasting forms of orthodontic treatment on the facial profile. *Am J Orthod* 1986;89:507–517.

284. Van der Linden FPG: *Facial Growth and Facial Orthopedics*. Kingston-upon-Thames, Surrey, UK, Quintessence Ltd, 1980.

285. McNamara JA: *Neuromuscular and Skeletal Adaptations to Altered Orofacial Function*, thesis. University of Michigan, Ann Arbor, 1972.

286. Subtelny JD: A longitudinal study of soft tissue facial structures and their profile characteristics, defined in relation to underlying skeletal structures. *Am J Orthod* 1959;45:481–507.

287. Kiser JVL: *A Serial Radiographic Cephalometric Study on the Growth of the Soft and Hard Tissues of the Nose in the Midsagittal Plane*, thesis. Northwestern University Dental School, 1960.

288. Subtelny JD: The soft tissue profile, growth and treatment changes. *Angle Orthod* 1961;31:105–122.

289. Bowker WD, Meredith HV: A metric analysis of the facial profile. *Angle Orthod* 1959;29:149–160.
290. Davenport GB: Postnatal development of the human outer nose. *Proc Am Philos Soc* 1969;80:175–356.
291. Posen JM: A longitudinal study of the growth of the nose. *Am J Orthod* 1967;53:746–756.
292. Chaconas SJ: A statistical evaluation of nasal growth. *Am J Orthod* 1969;56:403–414.
293. Lynn JM: Bio-facial matrix—Soft tissue analysis. *The Functional Orthodontist* 1986;4:24–32.

Section II
Sequential Treatment

"The old order changeth, yielding place to new,
And God fulfills himself in many ways,
Lest one good custom should corrupt the world."
(Dying King Arthur to Sir Bedivere)
Morte d'Arthur, from "Idylls of the King"
Alfred Lord Tennyson 1809—1892

CHAPTER 6
Sequential Treatment

PREFERRED EARLY TREATMENT: URGENCY CASES

It would be presumptuous for one clinician to tell others how to treat their own patients. Only the respective treating clinicians have that particular privilege, for it is the individual practitioner that is in the best position to judge what it best for the patients for whom he is responsible. However, in the application of FJO there are certain principles of basic appliance or active plate usage combinations that, though not immutable, are generally accepted as being the most efficient and logical methods of approach to representative cases.

We saw in Volume 1 concerning the Bionator, Sagittal, Transverse, and Straight Wire appliances the techniques of *how* to utilize these devices. And, considering their use individually in isolated examples, we have even alluded to the question of *why* we use them—to obtain proper arch form and, ultimately, to correct interarch alignment. What we will not attempt to address are the questions which follow naturally on the heels of the first two: *When* do we use these appliances? Under what conditions should each appliance be used? When more than one series of appliances is needed to complete a given case, we hope to make clear in what order they should be used. The answers lie in proper diagnosis, which in turn implies clinical examinatory model analysis and, of course, the use of cephalometrics. When one has complete knowledge of what the individual appliances are capable of doing (ie, what they were originally designed for), and once it has been determined what the *needs* of the patient are, these needs themselves will dictate which appliances are required for treatment. Should the patient's needs demand more than one type of appliance, the order of their use is determined by the observance of some simple guidelines, which we shall consider, in a coordinated plan of sequential treatment.

We shall consider some of the treatment-planning philosophies developed by experienced and competent clinicians. Consideration of such experience can help us manage maxillofacial orthopedic appliances so as to obtain the maximum efficiency and benefit from their use. It is not possible to address every conceivable type of malocclusion in this review. However, the functional appliance/active plate methodology never claimed to be able to treat to perfection every type of malocclusion, but it can certainly treat most of them, especially the most common varieties. Yet when the treating clinician is able to augment his removable appliance therapy with even the most basic principles of Straight Wire® technique, he will find that there will be few cases presented in daily practice that will require additional or more sophisticated techniques. One will find in this premise an ideal enactment of what has been termed "Sutton's law": "Common things happen commonly, and rare things happen rarely." And for most of the common malocclusions seen in orthodontics, these most common treatments usually suffice. This review, then, explores the more commonly accepted approaches to orthodontics, utilizing the FJO philosophy.

The question often arises as to when to begin treatment. Many factors come into play here, and each case must be considered individually. Certain times are better for treatment than others, relative to the age of the patient, but certain conditions command immediate intervention, at least as much as is practical. The Class I crowded case in the mixed dentition, the Class II, Division 1, and Division 2 mixed dentition cases automatically imply the patient to be at least 7 to 8 years old, since these are the times the upper and lower permanent centrals, laterals, and first permanent molars appear in the mouth. Many practitioners prefer to wait with such cases until the first permanent bicuspids are very near or just starting to erupt. By this time patients are usually old enough to understand what is expected of them and why their orthodontic treatment is so important.

Patients are usually quite well motivated in the age range of 10 to 12, and the "bioplastic" aspects of the facial bones are usually excellent. Mid-teen patients generally require more stringent supervision and a little longer treatment time. Mid- to late-teenage males are often the most difficult to manage and motivate, though many are self-motivated to the point where the disciplines of protracted treatment are not a hindrance to excellent treatment results. It must be remembered that the child and the parents must desire extended, and often expensive, orthodontic treatment before it is presented by the doctor. It must be stressed prior to the "orthodontic workup" as well as during the treatment conference that the orthodontic program involving removable appliances is a three-way team effort requiring the participation of not only the patient and the doctor, but the parents as well—not only for the financial responsibility but also for supervising appliance wearing, screw turning, and other incidental aspects of the treatment plan. Should there be lack of motivation in either the child or parent, it may be wise to postpone treatment until they are in complete agreement with the doctor about the importance of the treatment.

Certain types of malocclusions mandate that the treating clinician strongly urge the parents to authorize treatment as soon as the conditions are diagnosed. These types are (1) anterior crossbites, (2) posterior crossbites, and (3) anterior open bites as a result of thumb- or finger-sucking habits in conjunction with tongue-thrust habits. Regardless of the course of growth of the rest of the maxillofacial complex, when any of these conditions exist they will seldom, if ever, correct themselves, and usually without treatment they will only get worse. The rest of the dentition, or even the TMJs, may also suffer severe consequences later in life.

These three conditions, aside from all worsening with time, have one other trait in common: Not a single one is fully diagnosable from a cephalometric radiograph! Each one is diagnosed from direct and simple clinical observation. It is true that, with respect to a tongue thrust or deviant swallowing habit, in late mixed and early adult dentitions if the flared forward angulations of the anteriors exhibit a low interincisal angle (120-degree range or less), it is a tip-off that some lateral expansion may be necessary, especially if all contacts are closed, or, if crowding is present, some first molar distalization techniques may be required—with or without arch development laterally—yet the main (initial) diagnosis of tongue thrust is still determined clinically. The importance of direct observation of the patient and accurate model analysis become obvious.

ANTERIOR CROSSBITE

The simple anterior lingual crossbite of a single tooth, such as an upper central or lateral incisor, is one of the easiest conditions to correct with a removable appliance. It is easiest to treat at a time when the offending tooth is just erupting to the level of the occlusal plane. As an upper incisor approaches the lower incisors and displays an eruption path indicative of a lingual crossbite, a simple removable acrylic plate may be constructed on an accurate set of plaster casts with the aid of a simple construction bite in habitual occlusion no more than 1 mm thick. The occlusal coverings of acrylic help hold the bite open so that the upper tooth may freely pass from its position lingual to the lower incisors, to its correct labial relationship without its path of movement labially being inhibited by lower teeth. A simple finger spring, preferably with a double helical loop, is used as a force system to push the tooth forward into its proper overjet position. A labial bow may or may not be added, depending on individual preference. The same is true of the use of a small expansion screw instead of the finger spring.

Adams clasps are used on the first permanent molars, and ball clasps are also added to the embrasure area between the deciduous first and second molars to aid retention. The finger spring is activated by the doctor about once per week to apply gentle pressure to the tooth until the desired movement is effectuated. Advancing the contact portion of the wire spring about 1 mm per adjustment is usually adequate. Once the tooth is in its proper position and there exists some overbite beyond the level of the incisal edges of the lower teeth, the forces of occlusion will easily hold the tooth in place and retention is not necessary. Since such cases as this occur at the 6- to 8-year-old stage, patient motivation is usually easy to effect, because children of that age are eager to please, thrive on attention, and adapt to wearing an appliance as simple as the one described almost overnight.

If caught in an erupting stage, and if space is present for it, moving such a tooth seldom takes longer than 4 to 6 weeks. Left untreated, the condition soon worsens and requires more extensive and lengthy treatment, as well as thicker construction bites, as the tooth deepens its overbite behind the lowers. (This requires thicker acrylic pads on the appliance to open the bite farther to clear the incisal edge of the upper as it is moved labially past the lowers.) This entire process, however, is predicated upon the absence of crowding and the presence of adequate

---

Figure 6–1 Anterior crossbite (single tooth). Anterior crossbites in the mixed dentition should be considered as "urgency cases" and treated as early as possible. This 7-year-old boy exhibits a pretreatment state of anterior lingual crossbite of the maxillary left central incisor **(A)–(C)** and a slight loss of maxillary arch width also. The anterior crossbite and slight maxillary constriction results in a midline shift to the left **(B)**. Treatment consisted of a simple Schwarz plate with occlusal acrylic coverings to open the bite enough to clear the anteriors **(D)** as the tooth is advanced by a simple, double-helical finger spring. The tooth was advanced to correct position **(E)–(F)** in one month. The spring was adjusted to apply firm but gentle pressure to the tooth at weekly intervals. Lateral development of the maxillary arch by standard Schwarz plate technique took several more months.

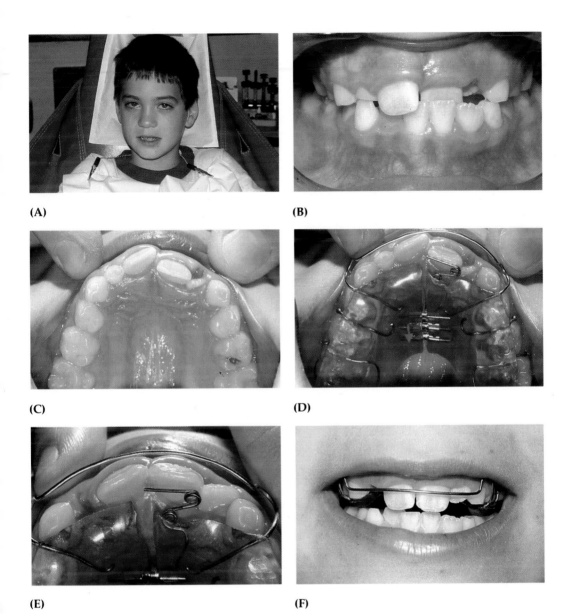

(A)

(B)

(C)

(D)

(E)

(F)

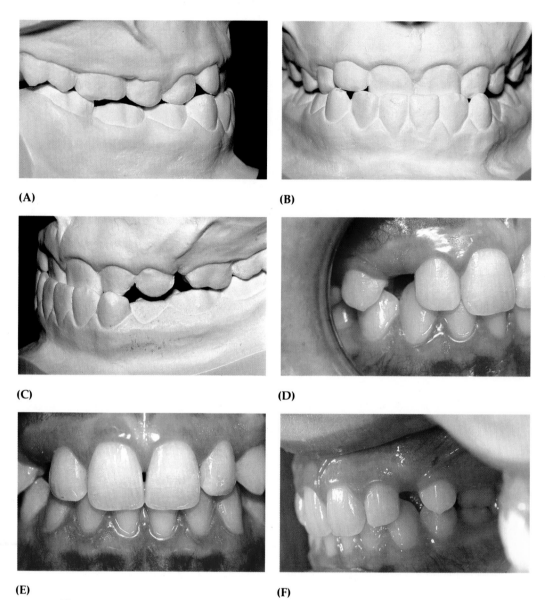

(A)

(B)

(C)

(D)

(E)   (F)

Figure 6–2 Anterior crossbite (multiple teeth). In more severe examples of anterior crossbites involving multiple teeth, as in pseudo-Class III situations, instead of using multiple finger springs or lap springs, the clinician may opt for the increased tooth-moving power of the Sagittal II. In this example the four maxillary anterior permanent incisors are locked in lingual crossbite **(A)–(C)**. After 4 months of treatment with a Sagittal II (using retained second molars as anchorage), note the advancement of teeth **(D)–(F)**. Also note how the extra arch length represented by such advancement helps eliminate the shortage of arch length from a pretreatment state **(G)** to a much less crowded arch **(H)**. With the

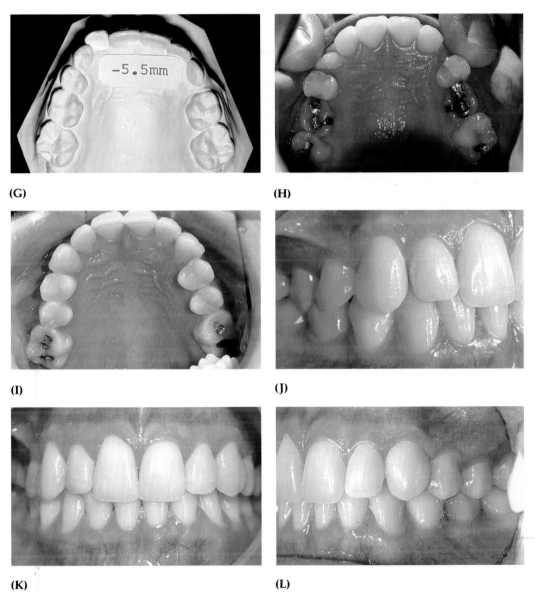

(G)

(H)

(I)

(J)

(K)

(L)

exfoliation of the remaining deciduous teeth, enough space was gained to permit cuspids to erupt. Additional space was also gained by insertion of a Bionator I immediately upon completion of Sagittal II phase of treatment, to increase vertical and widen the arches slightly via adjustment of the midline screw and Coffin spring **(I)−(L)**. This helped eliminate the arch width deficiencies represented by the −5.5-mm shortage across the bicuspids, according to the Schwarz analysis.

space for the lingually positioned tooth. This is usually the case in very early mixed dentition situations, because the upper cuspids have not erupted yet and diastemata are commonly present between the upper centrals or laterals. In the event all contacts are closed and insufficient space exists for the labial movement of the tooth in crossbite, an entirely different situation exists, which requires far more sophisticated diagnostic procedures and treatment methods. This will be discussed in the section on Class I crowded cases.

POSTERIOR CROSSBITE

Posterior crossbites may occur in children whose first permanent molars have not erupted, but the very young age of patients with only their deciduous teeth present usually precludes treatment with removable appliances. But once the first permanent molars have erupted and exist in crossbite, treatment may be initiated. Left untreated, the condition will only worsen and deform the growing face and disrupt facial symmetry. Posterior crossbite of molars often leads to TMJ problems, especially if the crossbite is fully bilateral, because it is difficult for the patient to execute lateral excursive movements during function without incurring balancing side interferences which are universally hard on supporting musculature and connective tissues of the joint.

In the mixed dentition stage the child is young enough that adapting to the wearing of a removable plate offers little problems. The bioplasticity of the palate is extremely conducive to transverse development. The first task is to determine whether the crossbite is unilateral or bilateral. Patients will often accommodate a slightly narrower than appropriate upper arch by shifting the mandible to one side or another in order to obtain more compatible interdigitation of the posterior teeth upon full occlusion. They usually shift to the most constricted side, which exhibits the greatest loss of vertical. This often makes a bilateral crossbite appear like a unilateral crossbite. Checking the toothy and soft tissue or frenum midlines will divulge whether the patient is shifting the mandible upon closure. This is usually what happens; a true unilateral posterior crossbite is a rather rare occurrence and is less frequently seen in clinical situations.

Use of the symmetroscope, as previously discussed,[1] is extremely valuable here. The bilateral crossbite, disguising itself as a unilateral crossbite due to mandibular shift, will exhibit a symmetrical loss of arch width in the posterior segments of the upper arch as divulged by the symmetroscope. A true unilateral crossbite will appear as an obviously asymmetric collapse inward of one of the two maxillary posterior segments.

For bilateral crossbites in the mixed dentition, two excellent choices exist as to appliances which may be selected from the removable active plate category: the Schwarz plate and the Transverse appliance. The determining factor as to which is selected for mixed dentition treatment is the status of the lower arch. If slight crowding exists in the lower dentition, the simple Schwarz plate is the appliance of choice. Since the Schwarz plate has no occlusal acrylic covering the biting surfaces of the upper teeth, the teeth are exposed and may make contact with the lowers. As the plate is expanded, the inclined plane action of the upper teeth on the lower teeth has a tendency to "drag" the lowers with them as they gradually expand laterally during constant function. This occasionally is all that is needed to relieve slight crowding on lowers housed and crowded under a slightly narrow upper arch. Since the mandible shifts to a favored side during function, the bilateral expansion of the narrow upper arch will allow the mandible to "seek its own level" upon closure as treatment progresses. This will bring the mandible back to its correct, unmitigated "straight line" arc of closure and also allow the forces of function-initiated expansion of the lower arch to progress in a symmetrical fashion. However, major amounts of lower arch constriction generally require treatment with appliances designed for such lateral development corrections, since the "dragging" effect of the bilaterally expanding upper arch is only capable of limited, lower lateral development. Reduction of expansion screw activation to one turn per week also aids in the dragging effect of the uppers on the lowers, because the inclined plane action during function of the upper teeth requires time to take effect on the lowers.

If the lower arch is uncrowded and has proper arch form, the appliance of choice for laterally developing the upper is the Transverse, with its acrylic pads covering the occlusal surfaces of the upper posterior teeth. As it is expanded, the acrylic, which is kept relatively flat at its contact with the lowers, protects the lower teeth from the expanding effect of the laterally moving upper teeth and the inclined planes of their cusps. Thus, the lowers remain undisturbed while the uppers are expanded laterally to their proper arch width. In young children with small mouths, these acrylic occlusal coverings need only be 1 to 2 mm thick to maximize comfort and aid in the patient's ability to adapt to the appliance. Either appliance may be used in conjunction with a labial bow, depending on any need for anterior lingual crown movement.

Sometimes a combination of appliances is needed to treat a bilateral posterior crossbite with one side more constricted than the other, thus imitating a unilateral crossbite. This is determined by analysis of the upper cast by means of the symmetroscope.

If the midline of the symmetroscope (orthodontic cross) is placed over the midpalatal raphe, an asymmetrically constricted arch will reveal the side of greatest constriction closer to the midline. In such a case, it would be best to start with a Nord crossbite appliance to push the more constricted side laterally until the first molars are equidistant from the

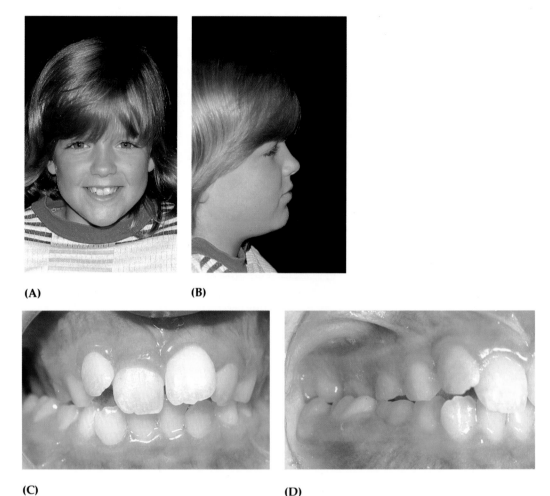

(A)   **(B)**

(C)   **(D)**

Figure 6–3 Posterior crossbite. This patient presented with a bilateral posterior crossbite in the mixed dentition **(A)**−**(D)** and severe crowding of the maxillary arch **(E)** represented by a deficiency of −9.1 mm according to the Schwarz index at the bicuspids. Treatment consisted of first removing the second molars in order to allow thirds to erupt. This would aid in the relief of crowding and in long-term stability of the case. A maxillary Transverse appliance was used for 12 months to develop the maxillary arch laterally **(F)**−**(H)**. Active treatment lasted

midline. Then the holding wing of acrylic on the Nord that acts as anchorage extending to the lingual surfaces of the lower teeth may be trimmed off, along with any excess acrylic in the nasopalatine area that may act as an interference, making a Transverse appliance out of the plate. If lower crowding exists, one may opt to make a whole new Schwarz appliance.

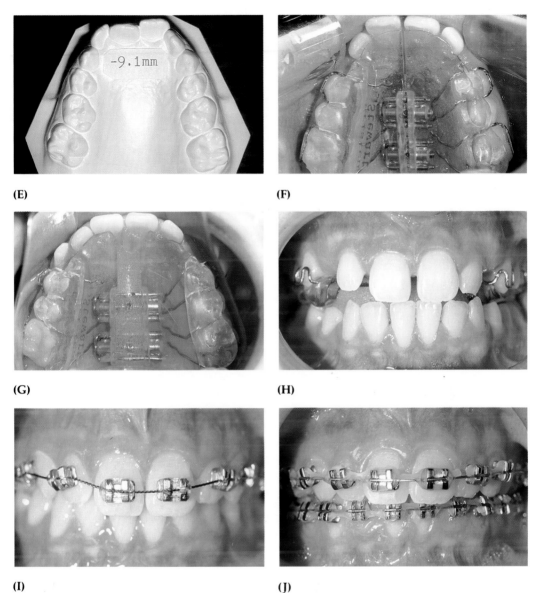

(E)   **(F)**

(G)   **(H)**

(I)   **(J)**

approximately 4 to 5 months, at which time screw activation was stopped and the midline space was filled in with acrylic **(G)** to let the appliance act as its own retainer for 6 to 7 months, to allow the midpalatal suture to fully "fill in" and allow the case to stabilize. As the cuspids erupted **(G)**, an upper Sagittal I appliance was inserted (upper seconds are already removed), and after 5 months of additional active plate treatment, the Sagittal I delivered the cuspids nicely. This was followed by 5 more months of standard Straight Wire treatment to level,

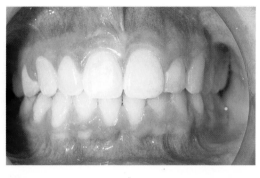

(K)

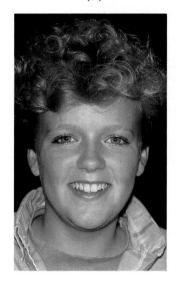

(L)

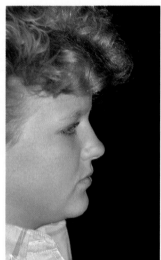

(M)

align, and rotate teeth **(I)**−**(J)**. Final case **(K)** was retained with Tru-tains, 6 months active (24 hours per day), 6 months passive (night only). Note final full facial contours and profile **(L),(M)**.

In the unlikely event a patient exhibits a unilateral posterior cross-bite where the toothy and frenum midlines are in perfect alignment vertically, a true unilateral situation exists. The previously discussed Nord plate serves adequately to correct this situation. The importance of treating posterior crossbite at an early age cannot be overly stressed. Lateral development is far more easy to accomplish and maintain at ages up to 11−12 years old. From then to adulthood the chances of relapse to some degree steadily increase. Past this age many clinicians feel that actual bony expansion becomes more difficult to achieve, and more buccal tipping of teeth is likely to occur. Moving the apical bases laterally is greatly enhanced by the bioplasticity of prepubertal bone. The post-pubertal adult dentition is more prone to keeping its apical base size relatively constant and to permitting tooth movement only about the apical bases. When the apices are relatively close to their correct position in the apical bases, simple tipping is all that would be required. Early correction of posterior crossbites does not guarantee the patient will not need further treatment once the transition from early mixed to young adult dentition is complete, but it at least allows for the possibility while protecting the facial bones from the inhibiting aspects of this type of malocclusion so that Nature may have a free hand in expressing itself in the growth and development of the face and jaws.

ANTERIOR OR LATERAL OPEN BITES AND THE TONGUE THRUST

The tongue-thrust patient has always been a stepchild of the dental profession. Everybody acknowledges the problem, but nobody as yet has developed a clear-cut, simple way to handle it. Even its role in the etiology of malocclusion is seriously debated. Innumerable types of tongue-thrust appliances of every conceivable type have been utilized over the years in an effort to retrain or irritate the tongue into staying out of the lingual gingival crest area of the premaxilla. They range from simple palatal arch wires to sharpened barbed devices that might have been designed by a weapons manufacturer! And once the bands and arch wires have been removed, many a beautiful orthodontic result has been spoiled by a return of the premaxilla to its pretreatment "gothic arch" shape, with flaring maxillary anterior teeth, and improper, untreated tongue posture and associated muscle function.

Speech therapists often throw up their hands in despair when confronted with the problem of endogenous tongue thrust, and many declare such a condition as untreatable strictly from a speech therapy standpoint. Myofunctional therapists approach some degree of success with carefully designed and monitored programs of myofunctional ther-apy, but they also are the first to admit that in such cases a teamwork approach involving the services of all the appropriate disciplines, es-pecially orthodontics, is needed. However, one thing dentists, orthodon-tists, myofunctional therapists, and speech therapists all agree on is to attack the problem *early*. Left untreated, endogenous anterior or lateral tongue thrust, anterior displaced tongue posture (rest), and associated muscle imbalances can do great damage to the growing, developing jaws. Just about every conceivable type of anterior open bite is possible as a result of an untreated tongue posture imbalance and accompanying swallowing tongue thrust. The irony of the whole situation is that every infant is born skeletally Class II, closed bite with a near vaultless palate and, by the necessity of this anatomical circumstance, an anterior tongue-thrusting-type swallow reflex.

This thrusting-type swallow reflex may persist until the age of 7 or 8 before the child outgrows it on his own and goes on to develop a more correct adult swallowing reflex. Some studies claim there may be anywhere from 20 to 50% of the adolescent and adult population with some form of "retained" improper or imbalanced muscle activity during swallowing,[2-4] although these remaining thrusts or imbalances are not major. Some even feel that the thrust itself is merely an unrecognized variation of a normal swallowing pattern.[5-6] Some feel the thrust itself is of no etiological consequence, since its total time of activity is so short.[7, 8] Instead they point to resting tongue posture and other forms of associated muscle imbalance, which we do not yet fully understand, as the culprits responsible for the anterior open bite and gothic-arch-type malocclusions. However, the infantile thrusting-type swallowing reflex is usually replaced by the adult swallowing pattern about the age of 4 or 5 years. If it is retained beyond this age an ever-increasing likelihood arises that the endogenous thrust will remain along with some sort of imbalance and improper resting tongue posture to cause in turn some sort of orthodontic or orthopedic problem.

The most common sequelae of imbalanced tongue posture and a retained tongue-thrusting or infantile swallowing reflex is the anterior open bite with the characteristic forward flaring of the maxillary anteriors. These teeth may also be unerupted to a certain degree, especially if the child has a concomitant thumb- or finger-sucking habit. A retruded mandible, posterior crossbite, labially or lingually inclined lower anteriors, and incompetent lip seal may also accompany the anterior tongue-thrusting condition either singly or in any number of combinations.

At the age the child should be progressing from the infantile swallowing reflex to the adult pattern of posture and swallowing action, the bioplasticity of the developing maxillofacial complex, with its eagerly erupting adult dentition, is extremely susceptible to the guiding influences of the ever-present surrounding and enveloping muscle activity. If the muscle activity is improper, especially the activity of a muscle as overwhelmingly powerful as the tongue, the battle between developing bone and developing muscle soon shifts in favor of the muscle, as it always will, and the bone must misshape itself as a result of being forced to allow the errant muscle to have its way. The teeth then, the innocent victims of this combat since they are merely passengers in the highly bioplastic alveolar bone, must display the effects of improper muscle function by erupting into improper dental relationships. Even the speech patterns are affected by retained tongue thrusting. Children who suffer from this condition often exhibit what speech therapists call "frontal lisping." The sibilant s sound is replaced by the th sound. Words like swell or yes are pronounced as thwell or yeth.

By the age of 8 or 9 the problems heralded by the anterior thrust and its resultant effects have usually become obvious, and interceptive treatment becomes necessary. It also works out, fortunately, to be a good age to begin treatment from a psychological aspect, since children of that age, as we have said, thrive on attention and are eager to please. This is especially true of the child who has both tongue-thrusting and thumb- or finger-sucking habits. They are aware of their own problems, since they have no doubt been incessantly reprimanded by well-meaning and concerned parents about the latter and are often frustrated at their own inability to help themselves. Treating them with an orthopedic appliance that they know will not only correct their disfiguring malocclusion but also help them eliminate their other unwanted habits is something that they can easily understand. Hence patient compliance with appliance wearing is seldom a problem.

After assessing the patient's individual needs, a certain group of requirements for treatment commonly appear. Both orthopedic and orthodontic correction is required for the flared forward and gothic-arch-shaped upper premaxilla, and orthopedic or orthodontic correction of the mandible may or may not also be required. Adult dentition arch width must be checked first; if grossly inadequate, it should be developed to Pont's or Schwarz's individualized facially corrected widths with maxillary Schwarz and mandibular Jackson or Schwarz appliances. Mixed or primary dentition arch widths may have to be developed to only a *slightly* lesser width than the indexed ideal values according to the age of the patient. Of course, with any patient, ideal arch width values should be mitigated by facial type. Once proper arch width is gained, the tongue has more room in which to move around during retraining with other appliances.

The initial cause of the problems, improper tongue resting posture and swallowing function, as well as perioral musculature abnormalities, must also be addressed. These requirements are a glaring mandate for enlisting the services of the one family of muscle-readapting appliances ideal for such conditions, the Bionators. If the mandibular length and vertical dimension of occlusion are both adequate, the appliance of choice is the Bionator II. The acrylic pads between the occlusal surfaces of the opposing teeth in the posterior segments hold the vertical constant while allowing the induced muscle forces of the perioral musculature and upper lip to exert their normal pressure on the anterior teeth and premaxillary area.[9,10] This is partly responsible for the maxillary anterior teeth moving down into their proper anterior relationship. The lower anterior cap may be used if the level of eruption of the lower incisors is adequate. If extra eruption is needed in the lower incisor area, the appliance is constructed without the acrylic incisal cap. Since maximum premaxillary correction and retraction is desired, the labial guide bow is adjusted so that it contacts the maxillary anterior teeth immediately upon insertion of the appliance at the beginning of treatment. As the anteriors retract, the labial guide bow must be adjusted periodically so as to maintain proper contact.

The lingual wire may play an extremely important role here, too. Normally not used as a standard component to Bionator II construction, the lingual wire may be added in a slightly modified fashion and utilized for tongue retraining purposes. In standard Bionators, if a lingual retention wire is used at all, as in follow-up treatment after active plate usage, such as Sagittal II appliances pushing upper anteriors forward for more favorable angulations, it is fabricated such that it follows as nearly as possible a perfect arch form up behind the cingula of the four upper anterior teeth when the appliance is in full contact in the mouth. For tongue retraining purposes the lingual wire of the Bionator II is fashioned in an entirely different manner. It is arched across the top of the lower incisor area so that it may be cut at its midpoint and bent back at the tips just enough to cause a mild irritation to a forward-thrusting tongue during swallowing. Other types of tongue-restraint wire grids or simple loops may be fashioned also.

The use of tongue-restraining wires, combined with the restricting effect of the acrylic wings of the appliance, which prevent the tongue from widening out over the occlusal surfaces of the posterior teeth, and coupled with the action of the Coffin spring in the vault area, forces the tongue to seal itself properly against the soft and hard palates during swallowing. The labial bow forces the lips to work harder in an effort to seal against one another during the swallow reflex, thus aiding in the correction of improper function in this area. This helps rebalance hypertonic and hypotonic perioral musculature, which often accompanies the tongue-thrust condition.

A superactive mentalis or "peach stone" chin button upon swallowing is the classic example of a muscle function pattern that would contribute to the labial flaring of the maxillary anterior teeth. The constricting mentalis forces the lower lip up under the lingual surfaces of the protruding upper incisors, intensifying the forces that result in the protrusion of the teeth. In a correct swallowing reflex, the lips and perioral musculature should remain essentially flaccid. The beauty of the Bionator II approach to the malocclusion—tongue-thrust problem is that it offers a medium for not only treating the result of the problem, the protrusive premaxilla and anterior open bite, but also the cause of the problem—improper muscle function in the form of improper resting tongue posture in conjunction with the lingering infantile tongue-thrusting swallow reflex.

Both patient and doctor are often pleasantly surprised with the speed at which dramatic results in the reduction of the anterior open bite occur. It is common to see such purely dental open bite malocclusions greatly reduced to nearly normal overbite/overjet relationships in as short as 6 to 8 months! Treatable skeletal open bites take longer. But

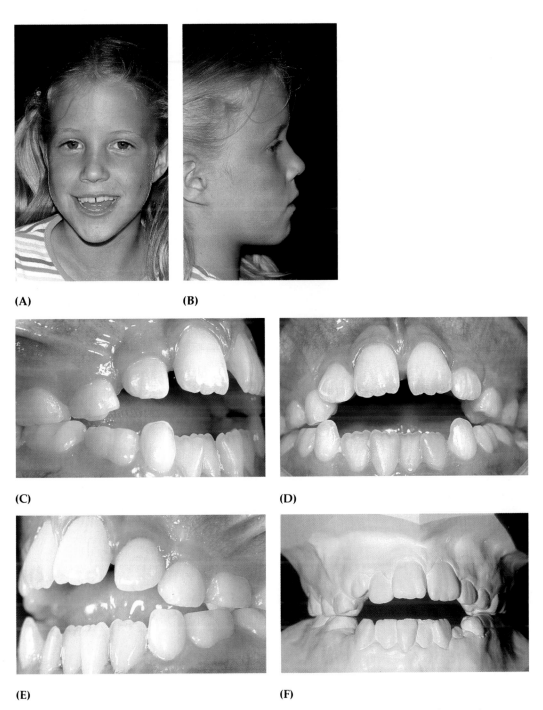

(A)   (B)

(C)   (D)

(E)   (F)

Figure 6−4 Anterior open bite: this patient exhibited an anterior open bite with severe crowding, an upper midline shifted to the left 3.5 mm, all of which was

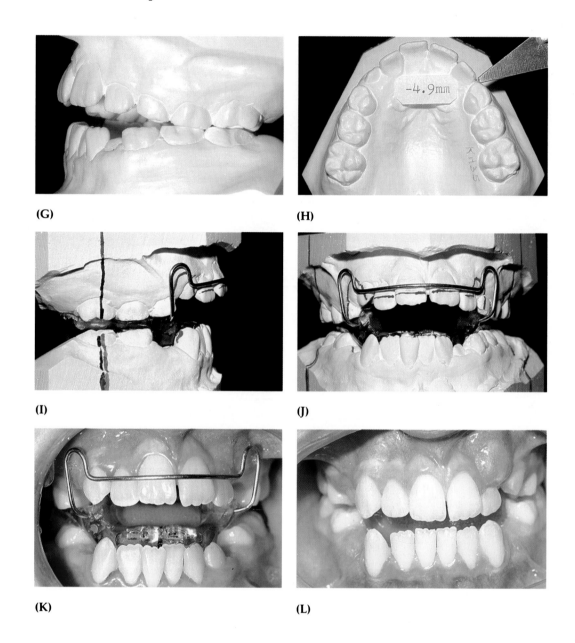

(G)

(H)

(I)

(J)

(K)

(L)

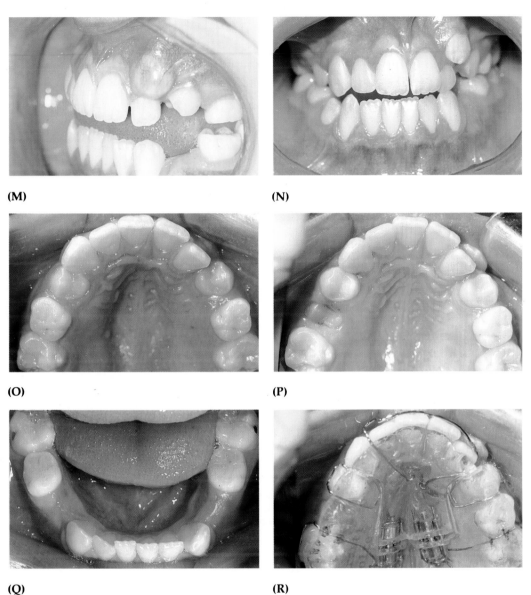

(M)

(N)

(O)

(P)

(Q)

(R)

compounded by a thumb-sucking habit at age 7 years 11 months **(A)**−**(G)**. The maxillary arch also exhibits an arch width loss of −4.9 mm according to the Schwarz index at the deciduous first molar area **(H)**. Treatment began at age 9 years 5 months with the removal of all four second molars. The following month appliance treatment began by inserting a Bionator II for 8 months **(I)**−**(K)** to close down the anterior open bite. Note bulge in gingiva that represents the location of unerupted maxillary left cuspid **(L), (M)**. As cuspid erupts **(N)**, the extent of A-P crowding is evident. Note how maxillary first bicuspid is crowded forward

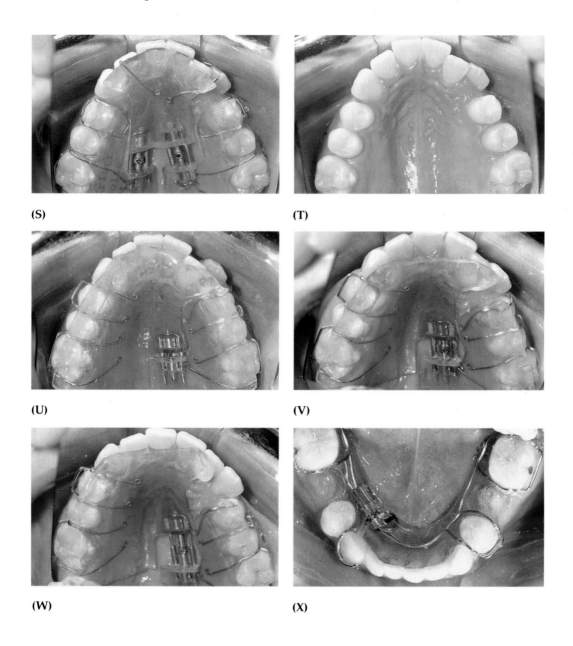

(S)

(T)

(U)

(V)

(W)

(X)

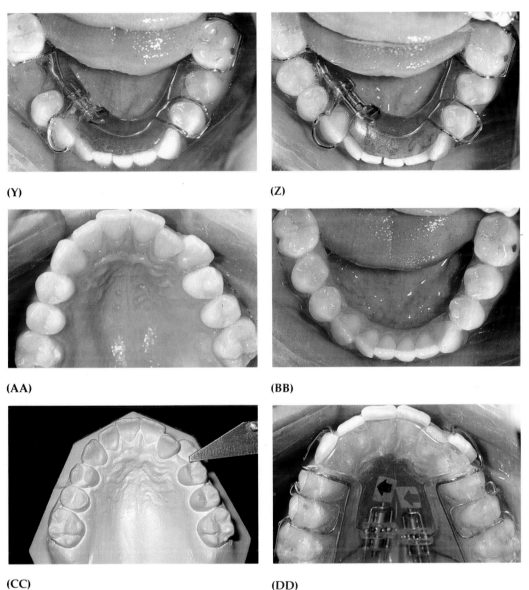

(Y)

(Z)

(AA)

(BB)

(CC)

(DD)

against the lateral, completely blocking out the cuspid as it erupts **(O)**, **(P)**. Lower arch exhibits exfoliated deciduous first molars and fully erupted lower cuspids **(Q)**. At this point an upper Sagittal I was inserted with screws offset to aid in midline correction **(R)**−**(T)** for 6 months. A second unilateral Sagittal was used **(U)**−**(W)** to complete the distalization of the upper left posterior quadrant to make room for the cuspid. Lower-right quadrant was distalized also with unilateral mandibular Sagittal I **(X)**−**(Z)**. This second stint with both upper and lower Sagittals took 8 more months to produce arches in **(AA)**, **(BB)**. Note there is still not enough room **(CC)** for the proper uncrowded eruption of the maxillary

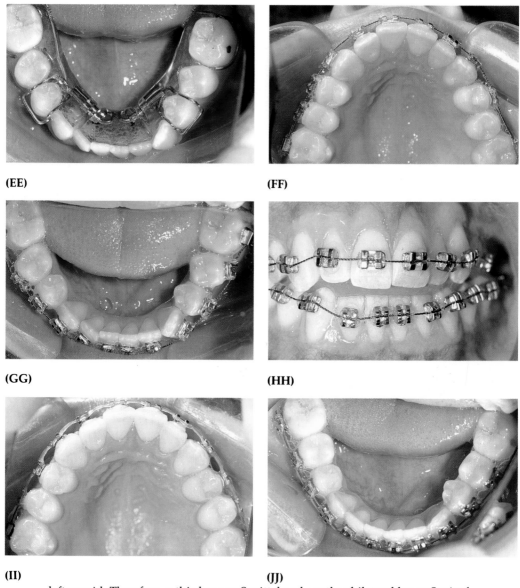

(EE)

(FF)

(GG)

(HH)

(II)

(JJ)

left cuspid. Therefore, a third upper Sagittal and another bilateral lower Sagittal were inserted **(DD), (EE)**, and remaining A-P crowding was relieved. Straight Wire appliance on upper and lower arches was used for 8 months **(FF)−(KK)** to finish case to completion **(LL)−(PP)**. Retention was accomplished with Tru-tains used for 10 months. Final photos are 1 year after completion.

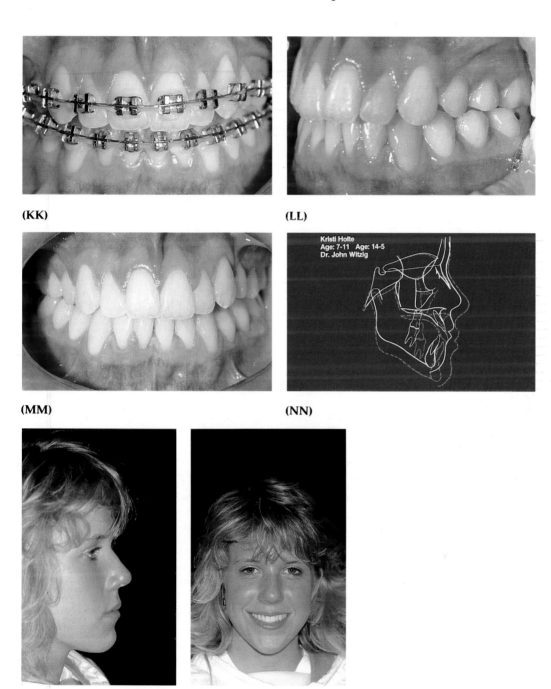

(KK)

(LL)

(MM)

(NN)

Kristi Holte
Age: 7-11   Age: 14-5
Dr. John Witzig

(OO)

(PP)

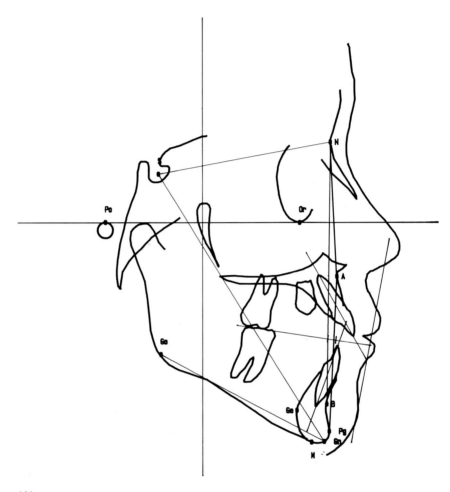

(A)

again, this initially rapid change is because the case is treated early and the Bionator merely takes advantage of unlocking and utilizing the nat urally occurring forces of growth that are universally present and merely waiting for a little help to manifest themselves. Once the lopsided effect of the muscle-bound tongue is negated and redirected, other naturally occurring muscle forces may be brought into play along with naturally occurring eruptive forces that help the maxillofacial complex correct itself and develop normally once again. The Bionator moves bone and teeth together and helps retrain muscles, a multidisciplined approach to a multifaceted problem.

There is a caveat associated with treating this condition, however, about which the parents of the patient must be informed—ongoing treatment. Essentially, the concept of ongoing treatment provides that

MODIFIED STEINER ANALYSIS

SKELETAL

MEASUREMENT	NORM	ACTUAL	COMMENT
SNA	80.0° to 84.0°	82.5°	
SNB	78.0° to 82.0°	78.8°	
ANB	0.0° to 4.0°	3.7°	SKELETAL CLASS I
WITS	-2.0mm to 2.0mm	-3.2mm	SKELETAL CLASS III
UPPER FACIAL HEIGHT	50.0%	40.8%	
LOWER FACIAL HEIGHT	50.0%	59.2%	
Go-Gn to SN	28.0° to 36.0°	37.9°	SKELETALLY OPEN
Y-Axis to SN	63.0° to 69.0°	68.0°	
			Normal skeletal bite.
OCCL to SN	14.0° to 15.0°	18.8°	ANY CHANGE IN POSTERIOR VERTICAL SUPPORT WILL HAVE A THREE-FOLD PROPORTIONAL CHANGE IN ANTERIOR VERTICAL
Pg to NB	1.5mm to 3.5mm	1.2mm	$NOT MUCH BONE STRUCTURE FOR MOVING MANDIBULAR TEETH ANTERIORLY

DENTAL

MEASUREMENT	NORM	ACTUAL	COMMENT
UP1 to NA DIST	4.0mm	5.9mm	
UP1 to NA ANG	20.0° to 24.0°	27.1°	BUCCOVERSION
LOW1 to NB DIST	4.0mm	4.9mm	
LOW1 to NB ANG	23.0° to 27.0°	19.5°	LINGUOVERSION
LOW1 TO UP1	120.0° to140.0°	129.7°	
A-Pg to LOW1	-2.0mm to 3.0mm	2.8mm	
6+6 to PTV	10.0mm	15.5mm	

SOFT TISSUE

MEASUREMENT	NORM	ACTUAL	COMMENT
UPPER LIP	0.0mm to 2.0mm	2.2mm	
LOWER LIP	0.0mm to 2.0mm	2.0mm	

Figure 6–5   Pretreatment Steiner **(A)** and Bimler **(B)** and posttreatment Steiner **(C)** and Bimler **(D)** cephalometric analysis of patient in Figure 6–4. Note change in angulation of upper centrals to NA line (Steiner) from 27.1 to 22.3 degrees and the change in the interincisal angle from 129.7 to 138.2 degrees. Also note the change in the Bimler Factor 4 from −5.2 to −2.0 degrees. All these changes are helpful in correcting anterior open bite cases.

REFERENCE I.D. GRID

ANTERIOR PROFILE ANGLE	BASIC ANGULAR RELATION	SUBORBITAL FACIAL INDEX	FACIAL FORMULA
Class I 0-10°	Upper Basic Angle	Dolico —	
Class II >15°	DLM DLM	Meso — Prosopic	
Class III <0°	Lower Basic Angle	Lepto —	

BONY OVERJET		TEMPORAL POSITION	GNATHIC INDEX
A-B Distance (Projected)	Factor Ⓐ (+) (±) (−)	T-TM Distance	
Class III (−)		Short 20-24 Class III	
Mean -4 to 8 mm*	Factor Ⓑ	Med. 28-32 Normal	
Class II (+)	(+) (±) (−)	Long 36-40 Class II	

INTERINCISOR ANGLE		STRESS AXIS	ANGLE CLASS	DENTAL FORMULA
BIPRO <120	Upper Bicuspid Inclination	Per	I	
DIV 1 120-140	P.O.R.	Post	II	
DIV 2 >140	P.O.R. Lower Bicuspid Inclination	Pre	III	

* − 0 to 8mm is The American interpretation
− 4 to 8mm is The True Bimler interpretation

PATIENT'S I.D. GRID

			FACIAL FORMULA
4.7	L/L	LEPTO	
	−5.2/		
			GNATHIC INDEX
4	8.5	22.9	
			DENTAL FORMULA
129.7	P/P	PRE/I	

(B)

Accurad-200™

Now that TMJ evaluation and health are the **Standard of Care** for dental procedures, it is essential to have an accurate, easy-to-use unit for TMJ radiographs. Evaluate condylar positioning **before** and **after** treatment.

The Accurad-200 conveniently attaches to standard dental x-ray machines and delivers clear, accurate, repeatable joint films. Shoot up to 6 views on a single 5 x 7 sheet of film. (See: **Radiograph Duplicator** for getting your x-rays ready quickly to send off to the insurance company: Speed up payments without risking your x-ray originals.)

Complete Accurad-200 Kit Includes:
Headholder, Cassette w/intensifying screen, 50 sheets Film, Film Record Envelopes, installation and operation Reference Chart.

Price: $995.

Choice of payment options:
A) $100 deposit; Balance due 30 days after shipment.
B) 1/3 deposit; 1/3 due 30 days after shipment; 1/3 due 60 days after shipment.

[Make deposits via VISA, MasterCard, or check made out to eop.]

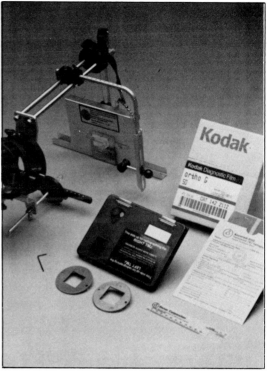

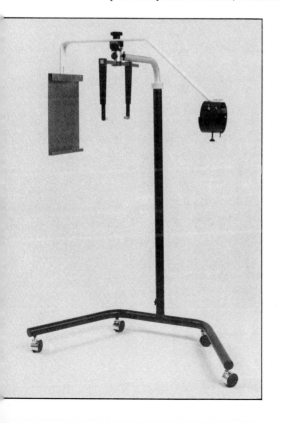

Versa-Tech™

Another precision attachment which allows expansion of radiographic applications with standard dental X-ray units. The Versa-Tech delivers Submental Vertex radiographs from which easy measurements are derived, which then permit 'corrected' transcranial TMJ X-rays to be taken (See: **T.C.D.** on back). The AP View shows the form and size of the condyle and permits viewing of cortical bone characteristics such as fractures, cysts, and other erosions. The AP View also displays the form and size of the mandibular neck.

Other radiographs necessary for routine Orthodontics and Full-mouth Reconstruction provided by the Versa-Tech are: Waters, Reverse Townes, Innercanthus, and Transmaxillary Views. These projections show condylar size, shape, and surface, to assist in locating pathologies and examining fractures. Uses standard 8 x 10 Cassette.

The Versa-Tech comes on a convenient Rolling Stand. $780.00.

Requires a $100 order-initiation deposit via VISA, MasterCard, or Check.

T.C.D.™

Transcranial Correction Device easily and quickly attaches to Accurad-200 or Accurad-100 and, from measurements derived from the submental vertex radiograph provided by the Versa-Tech, adjusts patient head position to facilitate taking of 'corrected' transcranial TMJ X-rays (down the long axis of the condyle).

Price includes Manual and Instructional Video. When ordering, be certain to indicate which Accurad model (200 or 100) the T.C.D. is to fit. $129.95

*Get paid **faster**—*without having to worry about your radiograph originals!

X-ray Duplicator

Scientifically designed for perfect x-ray duplication. Special dual-diffusion reflecting system delivers even illumination. Fluorescent BLB Light will light instantly, thereby avoiding loss of exposure time. Built-in safelight allows proper film positioning.

Compact for easy storage. Accommodates all intra-oral, extra-oral, 8 x 10, 5 x 7, 5 x 12, and 6 x 12 films. Complete and send your insurance claims fast!

Reg. price, $259   Special: $214

X-ray Duplicating Film: 5 x 7, 50/pkg., $25
8 x 10, 100/pkg., $88

X-ray Tracing Paper

Premier-quality tracing paper which is nearly transparent and has a smooth, matte finish for extra-clear, detailed X-ray tracing. For tracing all types of radiographs: Cephs, TMJs, Sub-mental Vertex, etc.

Uniformly cut in 8 x 10 sheets. 100 sheets/pkg.
$19.60/pkg.   3 or more pkgs., $17.90/pkg.

Cephalometric Protractor with Tooth Templates

Special combination tool for improved accuracy and speed in Ceph tracing and analysis.
$18.45 ea.   3 or more, $16.60 ea.

Deluxe X-ray Tracing-Viewing Lightbox

New viewbox features advancements designed to speed up and improve X-ray tracing and analysis: "Double-brite" twin-bulb illumination eliminates dead spots, and the more-rigid tracing surface minimizes distortion during tracing. Conveniently fits in attaché case for easy transport to satellite offices and to X-ray training courses.

Special: $89

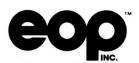

eop™
INC.

MODIFIED BIMLER ANALYSIS

MEASUREMENT	NORM	ACTUAL	COMMENT

FACTOR 1:
  UPPER PROFILE ANGLE N TO A   -1.0° to 1.0°   3.4° PROGNATHIC

FACTOR 2:
  LOWER PROFILE ANGLE AB TO VERT   4.9°

  ANTERIOR PROFILE ANGLE (F1+F2)   0.0° to 10.0°   8.3° SKELETAL CLASS I

FACTOR 3:
  MANDIBULAR INCLINATION   29.0°

FACTOR 4:
  MAXILLARY INCLINATION ANS-PNS   -3.0° to 3.0°   -2.0°

  LOWER BASIC ANGLE (F3-F4)   15.0° to 30.0°   31.0° VERTICAL GROWTH (LEPTO)

  ALVEOLAR HEIGHT   6.9mm

FACTOR 5:
  CLIVUS INCLINATION   60.0° to 70.0°   70.7° STEEP POSTERIOR CRANIAL BASE

  UPPER BASIC ANGLE (F5+F4)   60.0° to 70.0°   68.8° MESO PROSOPIC

  FACIAL HARMONY   M/L   OPEN VERTICAL: D/L

  SUBORBITAL FACIAL INDEX (A1M/AC) 1.00 to 1.05   1.21   LONG FACE

FACTOR 6:
  STRESS AXIS   113.3mm CLASS III (PRE)

FACTOR 7:
  N-S INCLINATION   9.2°

FACTOR 8:
  MANDIBULAR FLEXION   -5.0° to 5.0°   7.6° HYPERFLEXION - UNDER-
                                                                DEVELOPMENT OF MIDDLE FACE;
                                                                FAVORABLE IN CLASS III
                                                                CASES; IT WILL BE REDUCED
                                                                iN BITE OPENING IN TREATMENT

LINEAR MEASUREMENTS
  MAXILLA LENGTH (AT)   53.5mm
  TEMPORAL POSITION (T-TM)   23.0mm to 32.0mm   27.2mm MEDIUM
  OVERJET OF BONY BASES (A1-B1)   3.9mm
  MANDIBULAR LENGTH (B1-TM)   76.8mm
  MANDIBULAR DIAGONAL   123.0mm
  MANDIBULAR HEIGHT   97.3mm
  HORIZONTAL TOTAL   80.7mm

ANGLES
  UPPER INCISAL ANGLE   115.7°
  LOWER INCISAL ANGLE   106.1°
  INTERINCISAL ANGLE   120.0° to 140.0°   138.2°
  GONIAL ANGLE   105.0° to 120.0°   126.6° LEPTOGNATHIC
  IMPA   77.1°

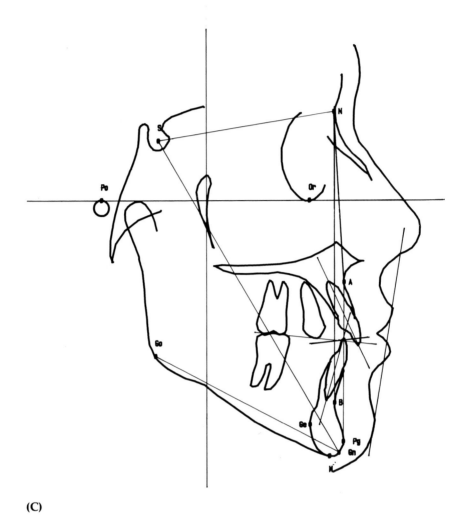

(C)

MODIFIED STEINER ANALYSIS

SKELETAL

MEASUREMENT	NORM	ACTUAL	COMMENT
SNA	80.0° to 84.0°	84.2°	PROGNATHIC MAXILLA
SNB	78.0° to 82.0°	80.8°	
ANB	0.0° to 4.0°	3.4°	SKELETAL CLASS I
WITS	-2.0mm to 2.0mm	-0.6mm	SKELETAL CLASS I
UPPER FACIAL HEIGHT	45.0%	43.4%	
LOWER FACIAL HEIGHT	55.0%	56.6%	
Go-Gn to SN	28.0° to 36.0°	36.5°	SKELETALLY OPEN
Y-Axis to SN	63.0° to 69.0°	68.6°	
			Normal skeletal bite.
OCCL to SN	14.0° to 15.0°	14.9°	
Pg to NB	1.5mm to 3.5mm	3.5mm	

DENTAL

MEASUREMENT	NORM	ACTUAL	COMMENT
UP1 to NA DIST	4.0mm	5.2mm	
UP1 to NA ANG	20.0° to 24.0°	22.3°	
LOW1 to NB DIST	4.0mm	5.0mm	
LOW1 to NB ANG	23.0° to 27.0°	16.1°	LINGUOVERSION
LOW1 TO UP1	120.0° to140.0°	138.2°	
A-Pg to LOW1	-2.0mm to 3.0mm	1.3mm	
6+6 to PTV	18.0mm	19.5mm	

SOFT TISSUE

MEASUREMENT	NORM	ACTUAL	COMMENT
UPPER LIP	0.0mm to 2.0mm	0.1mm	
LOWER LIP	0.0mm to 2.0mm	1.6mm	

REFERENCE I.D. GRID

ANTERIOR PROFILE ANGLE	BASIC ANGULAR RELATION	SUBORBITAL FACIAL INDEX		FACIAL FORMULA
Class I 0-10° Class II >15° Class III <0°	Upper Basic Angle DLM Lower Basic Angle	Dolico —— Meso —— Prosopic Lepto ——		
BONY OVERJET		**TEMPORAL POSITION**		**GNATHIC INDEX**
A-B Distance (Projected) Class III (−) Mean -4 to 8 mm* Class II (+)	Factor Ⓐ (+) (±) (−) Factor Ⓑ (+) (±) (−)	T-TM Distance Short 20-24 Class III Med. 28-32 Normal Long 36-40 Class II		
INTERINCISOR ANGLE		**STRESS AXIS**	**ANGLE CLASS**	**DENTAL FORMULA**
BIPRO <120 DIV 1 120-140 DIV 2 >140	Upper Bicuspid Inclination P.O.R. Lower Bicuspid Inclination	Per Post Pre	I II III	

* − 0 to 8mm is The American interpretation
− 4 to 8mm is The True Bimler interpretation

PATIENT'S I.D. GRID

FACIAL FORMULA				GNATHIC INDEX				DENTAL FORMULA		
4.9	M/L	MESO		3.9	-2/ 7.6	27.2		138.2	P/P	PRE/II

(D)

MODIFIED BIMLER ANALYSIS

MEASUREMENT	NORM	ACTUAL	COMMENT
FACTOR 1:			
UPPER PROFILE ANGLE N TO A	-1.0° to 1.0°	2.8°	PROGNATHIC
FACTOR 2:			
LOWER PROFILE ANGLE AB TO VERT		4.7°	
ANTERIOR PROFILE ANGLE (F1+F2)	0.0° to 10.0°	7.5°	SKELETAL CLASS I
FACTOR 3:			
MANDIBULAR INCLINATION		30.6°	
FACTOR 4:			
MAXILLARY INCLINATION ANS-PNS	-3.0° to 3.0°	-5.2°	NASAL FLOOR CONTRIBUTES TO OPEN BITE
LOWER BASIC ANGLE (F3-F4)	15.0° to 30.0°	35.8°	VERTICAL GROWTH (LEPTO)
ALVEOLAR HEIGHT		2.3mm	
FACTOR 5:			
CLIVUS INCLINATION	60.0° to 70.0°	75.3°	STEEP POSTERIOR CRANIAL BASE
UPPER BASIC ANGLE (F5+F4)	60.0° to 70.0°	70.1°	LEPTO PROSOPIC
FACIAL HARMONY		L/L	NEUTRAL (L/L, M/M, D/D)
SUBORBITAL FACIAL INDEX (A1M/AC)	1.00 to 1.05	1.12	LONG FACE
FACTOR 6:			
STRESS AXIS		119.2mm	CLASS III (PRE)
FACTOR 7:			
N-S INCLINATION		10.3°	
FACTOR 8:			
MANDIBULAR FLEXION	-5.0° to 5.0°	8.5°	HYPERFLEXION - UNDER-DEVELOPMENT OF MIDDLE FACE; FAVORABLE IN CLASS III CASES; IT WILL BE REDUCED IN BITE OPENING IN TREATMENT

LINEAR MEASUREMENTS			
MAXILLA LENGTH (AT)		52.2mm	
TEMPORAL POSITION (T-TM)	23.0mm to 32.0mm	22.9mm	EXTREMELY SHORT (CLASS III)
OVERJET OF BONY BASES (A1-B1)		4.0mm	
MANDIBULAR LENGTH (B1-TM)		71.1mm	
MANDIBULAR DIAGONAL		109.6mm	
MANDIBULAR HEIGHT		83.5mm	
HORIZONTAL TOTAL		75.1mm	

ANGLES			
UPPER INCISAL ANGLE		119.9°	
LOWER INCISAL ANGLE		110.4°	
INTERINCISAL ANGLE	120.0° to 140.0°	129.7°	
GONIAL ANGLE	105.0° to 120.0°	129.2°	LEPTOGNATHIC
IMPA		79.7°	

when interceptive orthodontics is instituted in the early mixed dentition, it is no guarantee that additional treatment may not be required later on in the development of the patient once all of the deciduous teeth have exfoliated and all of the adult dentition has erupted. Usually, however, if additional therapy is required, it often is, to much less of an extent, due to initial "groundwork laid" in the mixed dentition by the interceptive treatment than if the case were treated all at once in the early teens.

Ironically, orthodontics up until now has been one of the few components of the health care delivery system that has a penchant for allowing the patient to progress to the worst possible state before initiating a corrective form of treatment! This was no doubt due to the restrictions of fixed appliance usage. Fixed appliance technique was predicated upon a nearly complete set of adult teeth upon which to afix the individual bands. That placed the patient in the 12- to 14-year-old age bracket, a time when growth-disrupting myofunctional and occlusion-disrupting orthopedic imbalances had already gotten a good head start. An application of the principle of ongoing treatment is pertinent to treatment of anterior open bites. On occasion, after the bite has been corrected, a persistent tongue thrust will return (actually, it had never been corrected fully in the first place) to push anteriors labially once again, and posterior segments may even exhibit a slight tendency to relapse lingually. In such circumstances appliance therapy is reinitiated with longer periods of night-only wear during the retentive phase of treatment and a more concerned approach to myofunctional therapy.

MYOFUNCTIONAL CONSIDERATION

Many believe that improper muscle function is the chief etiological agent responsible for all malocclusion (aside from outright genetic defects like micrognathia or leptoid dysplasia). As stated previously, this relationship has long been observed and was first formally brought to the attention of the orthodontic community by Rogers.[11–14] Also observed was the fact that once muscle function became deviant and developed "bad behavior," it resisted return to normal activity.

It was also realized from the onset that myofunctional therapy would be difficult to carry out without the cooperation of the patient and parents involved and the systematic and faithful adherence to a prescribed daily exercise program. In no instance is the importance of muscle retraining made more evident than when an excellent orthodontic result is destroyed over a period of time after treatment by a returning myofunctional irregularity, such as persistent tongue thrust, improper resting tongue posture, mouth breathing, lip posture, and so on. It must be remembered that simplistically the teeth and alveolar bone occupy a neutral zone between the weight and pressures pushing them in (the perioral musculature) and the one big force pushing them out, the tongue. Great efforts are being made in the field of myofunctional therapy, yet it has received little attention from the bulk of the dental community.

Fortunately, there are several myofunctional aspects already built right into functional appliances such as the Bionator. It is not claimed that myofunctional therapy alone can correct or modify preexisting malocclusions; rather its goal is to produce a balanced teamwork effect between the muscles, bones, and teeth so that a totally normal and natural structural and functional environment may be maintained within the patient's stomatognathic system. But balanced muscle forces can never be obtained until the bones against which they exert their forces are of themselves in proper structural balance. Thus it may be seen that if any form of myofunctional therapy is to be instituted when true structural and myofunctional problems exist in the maxillofacial complex, it should be done in conjunction with structurally corrective orthodontic/ortho-pedic therapy.

A functional analysis should be a part of every orthodontic clinical workup. Examination procedures may be as extensive as the clinician's training and desires permit, but simple basic observation of the more pertinent areas of concern is not difficult. First, however, it must be clear as to what is normal. Since we know that an average individual swallows from 1500 to 2000 times per day,[15] this is obviously one of the most important myofunctional activities of the maxillofacial environment. All of the important external perioral musculature is involved directly or indirectly in the production of *incoming* forces to the teeth while the tongue must posture itself and develop a swallowing seal somewhere within the oral cavity in order to produce the main component of counter-balancing *outgoing* forces. It must also be remembered that the teeth occlude, or at least try to, at every instance of this reflexive swallowing activity and they do so with a considerable degree of force. Considering the enormous frequency of this act on a daily basis and the additive power generated by the muscles involved during each incident against intervening structures, it may readily be seen how the bioplastic alveolar processes and their passenger teeth may be biologically "drop forged" into whatever arch shape or position the surrounding muscles wish to place them.

Membrane-type bones are characteristically sensitive to pressures, and the alveolar processes are of membrane-type embryonic origins. Though true that some bracing effect is derived from the interdigitation of the teeth during the occlusion component of the swallow, an improper tongue posture in conjunction with a deviant form of muscle activity during such a repetitive event as swallowing will soon have its way. To repeat, in the battle between muscle and bone, bone loses, especially the "green" ever-growing, ever-changing extremely bioplastic alveolar bone of the young child or adolescent.[16−21]

Briefly, in a normal swallowing pattern the tip of the tongue seals itself in the rugae portion of the premaxilla slightly posterior to the nasopalatine area. The main muscular portion of the dorsal surface of the tongue rises, seals, and fills in the hard palate or vault while the posterior portion or base of the tongue tapers off through the soft palatal area at about a 45-degree angle. The masseter, temporalis, and medial pterygoid muscles constrict to pull the mandible closed, with the masseter and buccinator applying pressure inward against the alveolar processes and their teeth in the posterior segments. Anteriorly, the orbicularis oris exerts slight internal pressure against the anterior teeth and their alveolar processes. Note that the mentalis remains *passive*!

Thus it may be seen that during a normal swallow there are many muscular forces at work, all exerting pressure form the outside in, both anteriorly and posteriorly. There is also a singularly mighty counteracting force in the form of the tongue pressing upward in the vault area and slightly laterally, due to the tongue's thickness, in the posterior segments. But nowhere may there be seen, if the swallow is indeed normal, any appreciable source of force against the anterior teeth to drive them labially. Thus the anterior open bite of various varieties with their flared forward upper anteriors, or the less frequent posterior open bite, either unilaterally or bilaterally, are telltale signs of what must obviously be some sort of disturbance or imbalance of some form of a frequently occurring orofacial muscular pattern. (The evidence starts stacking up against tongue thrusts rather quickly when viewed in this light!)

It must also be remembered that the tongue can assume three roles in the malocclusion process. It can act as a force *for movement* of teeth and alveolar processes; it can act as a force for *inhibiting the movement* (eruption) of teeth and alveolar processes; or it can act as a *combination* of both. Though not the sole culprit in the development of malocclusions of the teeth and jaws, the tongue is such a muscle-bound member of the reflexive muscular team responsible for the swallowing action that it should receive a certain amount of attention during the functional analysis aspect of the clinical exam.

Obviously, the anterior open bite may be of several varieties if caused by improper tongue posture in conjunction with a tongue thrust during swallowing. The open bite may be *dental,* where the teeth are merely inhibited from completing their proper eruption by an intervening tongue. Or the open bite may be *skeletal,* where the teeth and their supportive alveolar processes have actually been moved or torqued labially by the moving forces of a forward-driving tongue. Both conditions may also be present concomitantly. The severity of the problem is paralleled by the intensity of the muscle imbalance. While the tongue is incorrectly posturing and thrusting forward, it is, by default, sacrificing some of the lateral bracing forces it should be providing against the lingual surfaces of the posterior segments.

As a result of this, it is easy to understand how the equilibrium of functional muscle forces is soon shifted in favor of the external forces pushing in, ie, the masseter and buccinator. In spite of a good cusp-fossa locking occlusion, the alveolar process of one or both sides of the upper and lower arches that absorb the brunt of this force soon surrender to the imbalance of functional forces, with the maxillary arch almost always the first to give way, and thus the unilateral or bilateral posterior crossbite ensues. The forces *"in"* versus the forces *"out"*—the battle is constant.

Another diagnostic observation to note is the activity of the "chin button" or mentalis muscle. In most cases of anterior dental (simple) open bite, anterior skeletal (complete) open bite, and bimaxillary protrusion, there is usually a constricture, improperly so, of the mentalis muscle upon swallowing. This pushes the base of the lower lip up under the protruding maxillary incisors. This helps obtain the needed, albeit improper, lip seal needed for swallowing, but it also reinforces the action of the tongue in helping to keep the anteriors torqued labially and aids in resisting the forces of the orbicularis and upper lip tissues in their natural attempt to drive the anteriors back lingually again. (Add a thumb- or finger-sucking problem to this milieu and it is a wonder why the anteriors are not pushed straight out parallel to the floor!)

Clinical observations pertinent to this area include the tonicity of the lips and their natural posture, ie, either flaccid (hypotonic) or active and muscular (hypertonic). During swallowing, do the lips tense unduly? Is there mentalis activity? Are there any other forms of facial muscle constricture during swallowing? Also note if the vault of the palate is high enough and wide enough to accommodate the wide dorsum of the tongue. A narrow vault often forces (or reinforces) the tongue to seal anteriorly, instead of palatally, during swallowing. This poses the classic etiological question: Does the narrow vault *cause* the tongue thrust, or does the tongue thrust cause the narrow vault? Either way, the two represent a true myofunctional/anatomic vicious cycle. Does the patient have an "adenoid face" or is he or she a mouth breather? Are there any speech defects present, such as a sibilant *s* lisp? Much of this information may be observed while patients are in their normal relaxed posture, unaware that such things are being observed. Directly observing the presence of a tongue thrust on a patient may require a bit of facile technique. Self-consciousness often alters this activity, even without the patient's effort. Gently parting the lips slightly often allows the clinician to observe the tongue as it thrusts between the teeth during repeated swallowing.

Oral muscle dysfunctions basically resolve themselves to one of two types of tonicity problems, too much or too little. The hypotonicity of lips during swallowing can contribute to the forcing of the tongue to create a seal improperly in the anterior area. Myofunctional therapists have devised many forms of facial muscle exercises, including having patients practice holding a pencil or tongue blade firmly between their lips while watching TV, for example. Performed on a daily basis for 10-minute intervals until the periods of control become longer and longer, some therapists believe that such exercises strengthen the orbicularis oris and improve its tonicity so as to make it easier for the patient to habitually obtain a proper lip seal without thinking about it. This better enables the patient to retrain the tongue to seal properly against the premaxillary area instead of thrusting to seal against the cervical area of the anterior teeth.

The same type of exercises are also recommended for mouth breathers. The correlation between mouth breathing and maxillofacial malocclusion has been well established by McNamara. Increasing muscle tonicity in the orbicularis oris is thought to increase the potential for permanent lip seal forcing the much more desirable nasal breathing. However, tonsil and adenoidal problems may also make a contribution here. Therapists augment these exercises by telling the patient why they are necessary and by admonishing the patient to make a persistent effort to avoid the untoward muscular activity. Remembering, or trying to remember, to make a conscious effort to keep lips together during relaxed breathing or keep the tip of the tongue at its proper place in the premaxilla during swallowing, is considered an important aspect of any myofunctional training program.

Lip exercises to increase the tonicity of improperly sealing lips are designed to help maintain anterior tooth alignment in protrusive cases. Increasing the strength of flaccid perioral musculature is one way of dealing with hypotonic problems. On the other hand, hypertonic problems, like anterior tongue posture, tongue thrust, or overactive mentalis or orbicularis oris, require a slightly different approach. The best way to deal with muscle hyperactivity is to retrain it to operate more desirably or to redirect it so its net effect in constructive and not destructive (ie, supportive and not deforming). This approach is taken by the rebalancing of orthopedic and orthodontic irregularities. Once teeth and bones are aligned correctly, these extra muscular forces may properly direct themselves so as to increase the stability and maintain the balance of the case. The bracing effect of muscle hypertonicity levels itself out in the properly formed maxillofacial complex such that the forces "in" and forces "out" isometrically counteract each other; even if they persist, they will do no harm.

Leveling out muscle imbalances is one of the main attributes of appliances like the Bionator. Not only does it perform active functions on the teeth and jaws by means of its own internal energy source, but it is also designed to counteract improper muscle function and to redirect, retrain, or stimulate the particular muscles involved to ensure their proper posture. In conjunction with a well-designed and faithfully implemented regimen of indicated myofunctional therapy, the Bionator gives the patient the best of what the total-patient-care-oriented FJO system of treatment has to offer.

It is not within the scope of this text to discuss the entire spectrum of such an involved and subjective science as myofunctional therapy and its relationship to malocclusions. However, when occasional difficulties do occur with recurrent or persistent tongue posturing and thrusting problems, patients may do some simple oral exercises while wearing their appliances during treatment to help retrain the tongue to seal itself correctly during swallowing.

One exercise, advocated by Dr J. W. Truitt, Jr, is as follows. Instruct the parent to assist the child in performing this exercise. For at least 10 minutes or more by the clock each day have the child place a sip of water in the mouth while wearing the appliance and making a determined effort to keep the tip of the tongue as close as possible to the loop of the Coffin spring in the vault of the palate. The patient should be instructed to swallow such that the base of the tongue must seal against the posterior palatal area. Continue this exercise faithfully on a daily basis until the case retains.

It must also be stressed that the parents maintain a patient and understanding attitude during treatment; their participation and supervision of the daily swallowing exercise activities is essential in the correction of persistent tongue-thrust problems. The child must never be made to feel that this condition is somehow his or her fault. Nor should the parents' frustration over the difficulty of the daily exercises or the stubbornness of the problem be reflected in their dealings with the child. Every effort should be made to make the experience positive.

As in any type of physical training program, a little bit done steadily and faithfully over a protracted period of time will do better than a lot done sporadically. Once the malocclusion has been reduced, the clinician may wish to have the child continue the exercises while wearing the appliance only at night for as long (3 to 12 months) as necessary to ensure retention of the case.

In ongoing treatment it must also be made clear to the parents that as the patient grows and matures, the maxillofacial development may need further assistance as the rest of the adult dentition erupts and the facial bones complete their growth. Should further treatment be needed in subsequent years, it will often be easier to accomplish and require less involved forms of therapy than if everything is left until then to be done all at once. Leaving improper muscle patterns, such as tongue thrusts, untreated until teenage years merely increases the chances of an unsuccessful outcome. It is far better to treat such conditions early and allow for the natural development to possibly preclude the need for further treatment later on.

Occasionally an upper Schwarz plate may be all that is needed to retract a protruding set of maxillary anteriors, especially if the problem is a result of thumb- or finger-sucking unaccompanied by an adaptive or secondary anterior tongue thrust. Such a thrust is merely a result of the tongue eagerly adapting to the gothic shape of the premaxilla. If the intramolar arch width is correct but the anterior part of the arch across the bicuspid area is too gothic in shape, the upper Fan appliance may be employed. As the labial bow shortens with the expansion screw activation of either appliance, it will retract the protruding incisors nicely. Of course, the lingual acrylic must be reduced to allow for the lingual movement of the teeth, and if the arch is excessively narrow the standard adjustments must be made on the acrylic adjacent to the palatal vault tissue to allow for proper expansion and separation of the two alveolar ridges. Active plate use implies adequate vertical. One thing all of these appliances have in common is that they often satisfy the nighttime sucking urge in children with thumb- and finger-sucking habits.

Even in these three types of "urgency" malocclusion situations, the anterior crossbite, the posterior crossbite, and the tongue-thrust−anterior open bite, there is a desirable sequencing of treatment. And that is the order in which they have been presented.

When more than one malocclusion is present, it is best to start with the anterior crossbite first because it is the simplest, quickest, and easiest way for the patient to become initiated into removable appliance usage. It also may unlock a mandible that is forced into an aberrant arc of closure in an attempt to accommodate the inclined plane action of the maloccluding anterior teeth. This is important if further treatment is to follow. If the case is too crowded anteriorly because of lateral collapse of the arch to permit simple correction of anterior crossbite first, it may be incorporated as part of concomitant lateral development by appropriate addition of finger springs to a transverse-type appliance of the proper variety.

The next most important, and far more prevalent, condition to receive consideration is the posterior crossbite. A general orthodontic rule of thumb is that lateral development should always precede any other form of development, be it horizontal or vertical, anterior or posterior. Many times an anterior or lateral tongue thrust will produce an anterior open bite situation accompanied by some sort of posterior crossbite. As the tongue pushes the anterior teeth and premaxilla forward, the pressure of the cheek muscles and buccal fat pads force the posterior alveolar processes inward lingually, especially in the maxilla. In certain Class II skeletal conditions of this nature, the upper posterior teeth may seem to occlude and interdigitate properly as far as lateral overjet with the lower molars is concerned. This occurs because the mandibular arch, which may be relatively wider than the upper arch, is retropositioned in order that its cusps may interdigitate on a more stable cusp-to-fossa basis with the wider, more posterior part of the upper arch. However, if the Class II mandible is advanced forward by the patient to the proposed "as if" position that could be effected by Bionator treatment, it would be observed that the upper arch is too narrow to allow proper posterior molar overjet to occur with the mandible in a corrected advanced position. Thus the telltale buccal-cusp-to-buccal-cusp apposition of the upper to lower posterior teeth with the mandible in this position mandates lateral development of the maxillary arch to proper widths prior to Bionator treatment. Proper model analysis with either the Ponts or Schwarz tables corrected to facial type will usually also reveal the "hidden" arch width discrepancy.

So, if the anterior open bite is to be reduced with a Bionator II and the mandible also happens to be in a skeletal Class II condition, the width of the upper arch should be checked *first* to see if a bilateral posterior crossbite does exist and is merely being disguised by the retruded condition of the mandible. If so, the case should be begun first with either a Schwarz or Transverse plate (depending again on the status of the amount of crowding present in the lower arch or if TMJ symptoms are already present), and once adequate arch width is obtained the transition may be made to the Bionator II; its work of retracting the premaxilla and anterior teeth having been already partially completed (and sometimes to an amazing degree) by the labial bow action of the particular active plate that preceded it.

Should the vertical *and* horizontal relationships of the lower jaw to the upper jaw be satisfactory, precluding the need for the mandibular advancing or vertical increasing aspects of the Bionator I, then the question is: Should the Bionator II or active plate be used to reduce the anterior open bite? The differential diagnosis here is the key to appliance selection; ie, is one dealing with a true endogenous (forceful) tongue thrust with accompanying anterior tongue posture or merely with concomitant adaptive thrust secondary to thumb-sucking, etc? If the anterior open bite is open to any appreciable extent and the clinician suspects any form of remaining endogenous tongue thrust is present, which it usually is in more severe open bite cases, the appliance of choice is the Bionator II because of its tongue-retraining aspects. However, if the case exhibits more innocuous labial flare and protrusion of the maxillary incisors, and less vertical movement or closure is required of the upper incisors and the thrust is only adaptive in nature (not a true thrust), an active plate may suffice. The reason is that when the upper incisors are retracted by the labial bow of the active plate, the bite closes down slightly anteriorly. But again the arch width should be checked first. If it is already wide enough, there is no need for Schwarz plate lateral development. Therefore one must still resort to the Bionator II.

If the anterior open bite is complicated by a skeletally Class II mandibular retrusion, several modifications in treatment approach must be made. The construction bite for the Bionator II may be taken with the mandible protruded in a more advanced position using the "as if" position and molar and cuspid (if permanent cuspids are present) alignment as a guide. This allows mandibular advancement and premaxillary reduction to take place simultaneously. But since the acrylic pads hold the vertical constant, there is *no* increase in vertical, but that is seldom needed in open bite cases. The question that often arises in the Class II anterior open bite case is, how far must the mandible be advanced during construction bite registration? If the clinician is uncertain as to what would constitute adequate mandibular advancement with respect to the registration of the construction bite, the problem can easily be solved by construction of an Orthopedic Corrector II. The construction bite may be registered in a moderately advanced position, and if more mandibular advancement is needed once treatment is in progress, the typical adjustments of side screws and acrylic reduction, this time both interproximally and on the underside of the acrylic pads, may be called upon to steadily advance the mandible to its correct position.

Thus, in these "urgent" cases of anterior crossbite, posterior crossbite, and anterior or lateral open bite in the growing child, the process of addressing the needs of the patient implies not only initiating treatment as early as possible, but also in the correct sequence—anterior crossbites first, followed by whatever other treatment is needed to correct the rest of the case. It may also be seen that one of the "needs" to be addressed by the clinician is whether tongue retraining is required for a particular case, since this is an important point of differential diagnosis and appliance selection. Early treatment of the above conditions coupled with ongoing treatment give the patient, the parents, and the treating practitioner the best possible chance of obtaining long-term successful results. Enumerating the individual needs of the patient is also applied to the larger, more generalized group of malocclusions in the late mixed, adolescent, and adult dentitions. Clearly, diagnosing these needs by clinical examination, cephalometric and study model analysis, and succinctly cataloging them is the key to appliance selection. Determining the sequence of their use in the adult dentition follows essentially the same set of basic guidelines as in the mixed dentition. However, in the more advanced dentitions these guidelines must be expanded to accommodate the larger number of combinations of malocclusions and adult dentition techniques available.

The adult Class I posterior crossbite is treated best by an upper Schwarz plate because Crozat appliances are totally *contraindicated* in these situations. If Crozats are used, they might not expand the palate perfectly symmetrically, and the side of the upper arch that "jumps" the cusp tips of the lower arch first will accelerate laterally quickly as the "unjumped" side digs in and acts as an anchor, due to the interdigitation and inclined plane action of the upper cusps with the lower fossae. In the rare event that the case is an actual unilateral posterior crossbite, the Nord appliance is used. Once properly developed and retained, the case may be finished as the previously discussed cases, if need be. In the adolescent or *early* adult (ie, teenage) dentitions the Rapid Palatal Expander may also be considered, since this appliance is best utilized for severe bilateral posterior crossbites in the late mixed and early adult dentitions. For the adult patient 20 years old or older, use of the Rapid Palatal Expander is accompanied by surgical intervention such as the Epker-Wolford procedure to mechanically free up the two halves of the palate prior to activation of the appliance.

The anterior open bite with a tongue thrust in the adult Class I dentition poses an increasingly unfavorable prognosis with the increased age of the patient. It is treated as described under "urgency" cases but with extra emphasis on the myofunctional therapy, such as the water-swallowing exercises previously described and increased periods of night-time appliance wear during the retentive phase. These cases are difficult to treat, and the patient must be made well aware of the compromised situation it presents to the clinician. By the time the case has reached full adulthood, the chances for a long-term successful elimination of the problem are greatly reduced. If cephalometric analysis indicates an individual with signs that approach the leptoid dysplasia type, resolution with functional appliances may well be impossible, and the case should be evaluated for possible surgery.

"Ohne Hast, aber ohn Rast."
"Without haste, but without rest."
Johann Wolfgang Von Goethe
German poet 1749—1832

CHAPTER 7

Appliance Sequencing in Conventional Treatment: Class I Malocclusions

The approach one takes to treating malocclusions in the mixed, adolescent, or adult dentition stages usually consists of first determining what the specific needs of the patient are, which is the cornerstone of determining, in turn, what the treatment goals for the case under consideration will be. When the clinician uses the FJO series of techniques, obtaining these goals often follows the structured pattern of first obtaining proper individual arch form followed by securing proper interarch form (ie, alignment in all three planes: horizontal, vertical, and lateral). In some instances merely producing the proper individual dental arch form will automatically secure the proper interarch form or orthopedic jaw-to-jaw relationships.

Conversely, in certain cases, obtaining the correct orthopedic relationships may automatically secure proper dental relationships. What is important to remember is that the FJO philosophy is dedicated to placing equal importance to treating both dental and skeletal relationships on an

422

equal basis in the goal of providing the best and most complete care possible for the patient. Proper appliance sequencing during treatment consists of nothing more than the most logical way of addressing one problem (either orthopedic or orthodontic) so that its correction may pave the way for the most efficient and expeditious treatment of the other problems. The following guidelines to treatment are offered for the consideration of the reader, not as an ironclad set of rules to be mindlessly obeyed, but a series of time-honored and generally accepted methods of approaching the various types of malocclusions the practitioner commonly confronts.

Individual modifications are always the prerogative of the treating clinician. When faced with specific treatment circumstances, especially of a more difficult nature, most practitioners will resort to that technique which they do best. Fortunately, there is often an august selection of appliances and modalities in the FJO philosophy to broadly appeal to the various clinical skills of the individual. It is these universal and temperate aspects of the technique that make it a humane system for both the patient and the doctor.

It is most logical that we begin our discussion of appliance sequencing with Class I type malocclusions, although this does not mean to imply that they are the easiest to treat. Although a case may exhibit an Angle Class I dental relationship with respect to interdigitation of certain upper and lower teeth and may be in skeletal Class I orthopedic harmony, these traits do not necessarily mean the case is not in dire need of orthopedic/orthodontic treatment. The aforementioned types of "urgency" malocclusions (anterior crossbite, posterior crossbite, and anterior/lateral open bite) may all exist in skeletal and dental Class I categories. (The anterior single- or multiple-tooth crossbite, by necessity, is nearly always at least Class I and sometimes may even be a "super-Class I" tending to a pseudo-Class III.) Yet, as we have seen, these require the most critical scrutiny in the early mixed dentition with treatment preferred as early as possible. But there are also more innocuous Class I situations that, though not as petulant as the urgency-type cases, still require orthodontic or orthopedic intervention. Here again the proper sequencing of appliances efficiently uses time and energy.

CLASS I MIXED DENTITION

In the mixed dentition the developing dental arches may be too narrow (arch width discrepancies), too short (arch length discrepancies), too long (protrusive permanent anteriors), too close to one another (insufficient vertical), or any combination of these. When more than one discrepancy is present, it is usually best to *develop laterally first*. Arch widening may then be followed, if needed, by arch lengthening procedures, followed, again if needed, by vertical increasing techniques. This entire sequence is nearly always performed by removable active plates, such as the Schwarz/Transverse, Sagittal, Jackson, and, occasionally, the Bionator if increased vertical is deemed vital at the time. Except for the special instance of the use of Brehm Utility Arches, traditional-style, fixed appliance therapy is seldom used in early mixed dentition cases, but is reserved for a time when the permanent dentition has fully erupted.

Class I mixed dentition treatment is predicated on the case actually being Class I. Recall that in the vast majority of cases in the mixed dentition the first permanent molars, in order to be correct, are not in their usual Angle Class I dental relationship but are vertically superimposed on one another with their mesial surfaces in line with the imaginary vertical line referred to as the "flush terminal plane."[22-25] This makes them appear as if they are in a half-Class II situation, because the lower first permanent molar is a little more distal to its final correct anatomic location due to the extra width mesiodistally of the lower deciduous second molar. Once exfoliated, this extra "E-space" will be eliminated as the lower first permanent molar drifts forward, slipping into a full Class I dental relationship with the upper in doing so.

The Class I skeletal designation may be determined cephalometrically by various means. The Wits analysis will show the AO and BO perpendiculars within 0 to +2 mm of one another. (The −1 to +2 mm designation for males is somewhat suspect here, as prepubescent males of 8−9 years of age do not usually show the effects of male hormones in bone growth.) A McNamara analysis will reveal the "effective" maxillary and mandibular lengths to be within about 20 mm of each other, with an ANS-ME LFH hovering somewhere around 60 mm. A-point should lie within ±2 mm, and Pog within −8 to +2 mm of the N-perpendicular. A Sassouni analysis will reveal A-point and B-point close to or right on the Basal Arc, and the mesial surface of the maxillary first molar should fall on the Midfacial Arc. But since both the maxilla and mandible may be retropositioned by the same amount, making the case appear Class I due to the relative alignments of A-point and B-point on the Basal Arc, it is very important that the Class I status of the case be determined by the locations of N, ANS, and Pog relative to the Anterior Arc. A Bimler analysis should reveal an Anterior Profile Angle (the arithmetic summation of Factors 1 and 2) in the positive range from 0 to 10 degrees, the Factor 8 near 0 to 8 degrees in a state of orthoflexion or near parallel to the C-vertical. Factor 7 length, the AT length, the T-TM length, and the diagonal length of the mandible should all fall proportionately close to the 7:5:3:11.5 Bimler ratio if the patient is of the mesoprosopic facial pattern type. The Factor 6, or Stress Axis, should be on or very near the

PER configuration if the case is sufficiently developed (apicale present) to permit its construction.

Beginning with arch width discrepancies first, a model analysis with an accent on anterior crowding will indicate the degree of correction necessary for lateral development with an upper Schwarz and lower Jackson appliance if anterior crowding is present in both arches. If crowding is slight and arch width loss symmetrical, an upper Schwarz may be all that is required, because the inclined plane action of upper cusps against lower cusps during function of the expanding uppers may be sufficient to "drag" the lowers with them laterally. However, this is considered by some as tenuous at best. Crossbites should be treated as described under "urgency" treatment. Once treatment is begun in the narrow-arch, crowded case, the labial bow of the upper Schwarz may be enlisted in conjunction with appropriate adjustment of lingual acrylic to assist in correcting the anterior rotations that give up much needed arch length. Final perfection of tooth position may be attained with Brehm Utility Arches, or the clinician may choose to wait until early permanent dentition stages when a full complement of teeth are present, so Straight Wire appliances may be employed.

Division 1 problems of maxillary anterior flaring in Class I crowded cases must also be approached with an eye for first determining if there is an arch width deficit, which there usually is. The maxillary Schwarz is again the appliance of choice, but this type of case calls for the use of the labial bow across the protruding maxillary teeth acting as an active force for retraction of flared upper anteriors as the appliance expands the narrow arch laterally. The mandibular Jackson appliance complements arch development on the lower. In such cases diastemata commonly exist between the maxillary anteriors in the pretreatment state, which will reduce somewhat as the teeth are retracted by the labial bow. Final reduction might have to wait until the natural "diastema-closing" forces are exhibited as the permanent cuspids erupt.

If both upper and lower arches are protrusive, in what may be termed a Division 3 situation, where the interincisal angle is 120 degrees or less, to retract the lower anteriors to a more upright position, the practitioner substitutes a lower Schwarz with a labial bow for the lower Jackson. Again, as with the upper, the lingual acrylic on the lower Schwarz must be reduced. Caution must be exercised here because such cases are commonly associated with anterior tongue thrusts. Any tendency to anterior open bite or clinically observed signs of a forward resting posture of the tongue or thrusting swallowing pattern should cause one to consider the use of the Bionator II as described under "urgency" treatment. If no arch width discrepancy exists, yet the upper anteriors are still protruded and require retraction, the case may be treated as if it were an anterior open bite and thus reduced with the Bionator II.

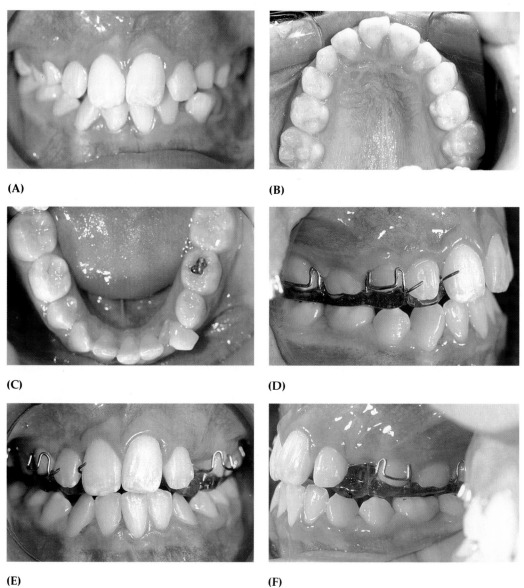

(A)   **(B)**

(C)   **(D)**

(E)   **(F)**

Figure 7−1   Class I crowded (early mixed dentition). In this example we see a Class I crowded case in the early mixed dentition that also exhibits an upper midline shift to the right of 6 mm **(A),(B)**. The patient also lost his lower right central incisor in a gym accident prior to initiation of orthodontic treatment **(C)**. To assist with midline correction in this case, only the upper left second molar is removed. The upper right second molar is retained to act as achorage for appliances that will shift the anterior teeth around the arch to the left. Upper

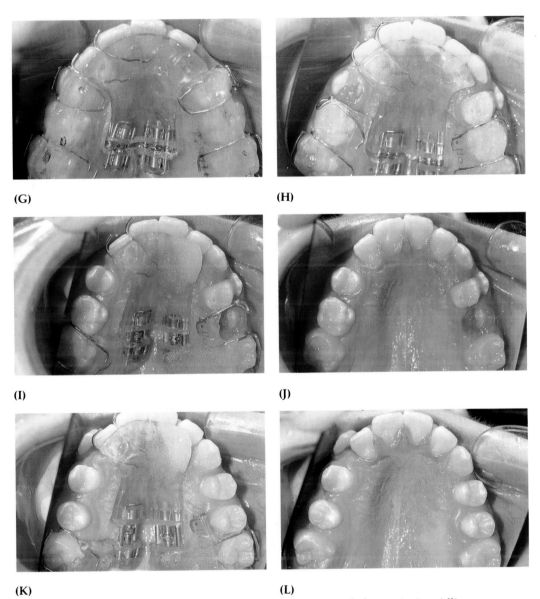

(G)   **(H)**

(I)   **(J)**

(K)   **(L)**

Sagittal appliance is inserted with expansion screws angled to assist in midline correction, and finger springs placed distal to upper right central and lateral **(D)–(G)**. After 8 months of treatment a second Sagittal appliance was constructed with acrylic relieved over areas where upper deciduous first molars exfoliate **(H)**. Treatment time with second upper Sagittal was 10 months, since once expanded **(I),(J)** the appliance was used (and repaired) as its own retainer **(K),(L)** to allow

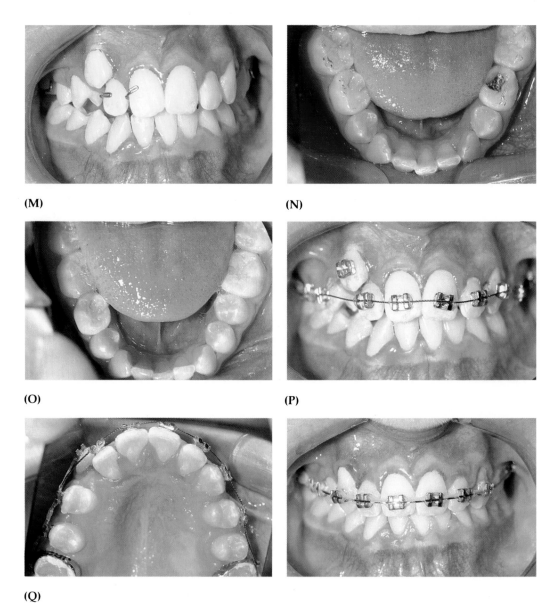

(M)   **(N)**

(O)   **(P)**

(Q)

time for remaining deciduous teeth to exfoliate and upper right cuspid to appear
(M). Exfoliation of deciduous second molars **(N),(O)** provides enough space for
permanent second bicuspid to erupt. Straight Wire appliance is applied to
maxillary arch, temporarily skipping cuspid **(P),(Q)** until it erupts enough to be
engaged by wire. Note how overcorrection depicted in earlier stages of treatment
is easily condensed as Straight Wire phase of treatment (8 months) is completed.

Division 2 problems in Class I cases of high interincisal angles of 140-degree range or more offer one of the few exceptions to the "develop laterally first" concept. A mere case of a high interincisal angle in a very early mixed dentition, just as the upper centrals are erupting, may be more apparent than real. But, as the case develops and it starts to exhibit the classic Division 2 positioning of the retroclined maxillary centrals with the labially flared and crowded laterals, treatment should be initiated first by a Sagittal II, designed to push the upper centrals labially to a more reduced interincisal angle relationship with the lowers. The purpose of this is to unlock what may be strained or even compressed TMJs. By the time a fully developed Division 2 anterior relationship has manifested itself, the mandibular development has probably been constrained to the point where the case has slipped from Class I to Class II. Either way, unlocking the joint and freeing the mandible from the "Division 2 trap" is paramount to the proper growth and development of the individual. Once corrected, the case may then be considered as all others; check for adequate arch width first, and if insufficient develop with a maxillary Schwarz and mandibular Jackson to proper arch form.

Another important point to bear in mind in Class I, Division 2, treatment in the mixed dentition is that though the Sagittal II is designed and adjusted to place nearly all of the expansion forces on the upper anterior area, this may not actually happen in the early mixed dentition. The Sagittal II depends for its action on the stout anchorage of the second molars. Yet at age 8 to 9 these teeth are so far up in the alveolar process that they offer little aid in resisting the distal component of the forces of the Sagittal II, and as a result it begins to assume the performance characteristics of the Sagittal I due to the "green" nature of the young and bioplastic arches, and some distalization, whether desired or not, will occur in spite of proper adjustments to keep the occlusion heavy on both the anterior and posterior portions of the plate. But this is an excellent trade-off for the benefit of obtaining proper maxillary anterior angulation. For what slight excess space might be created in the posterior segments will readily "slam shut" once the enormous forward thrust of the second molars comes into play during their eruption. In the meantime the worst that can happen is the patient will be given a short-term iatrogenic pseudo-Class III occlusion in the molar area. But, far more important benefits are reaped as the upper centrals are proclined properly and the TMJ and entire mandible are decompressed and allowed to freely develop normally. As always, Division 2 development requires retention.

If patient cooperation with appliance wear is suspect, or for a variety of other reasons, the Brehm Utility Arch is an alternative to the Sagittal II in Class I, Division 2, mixed dentition situations. Beginning with the .14 or .16 round arch wires, the teeth may be nicely aligned in the relatively short time of 2 to 3 months, at which time the rectangular .16 × .16

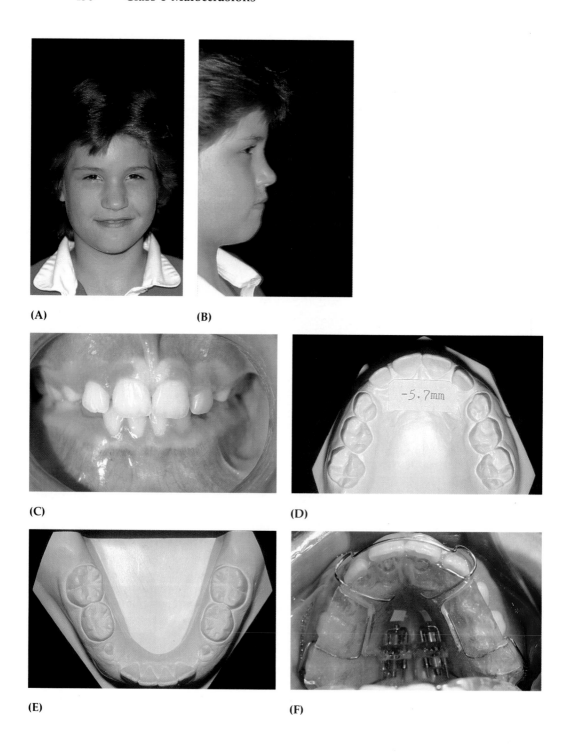

(A)

(B)

(C)

(D)

(E)

(F)

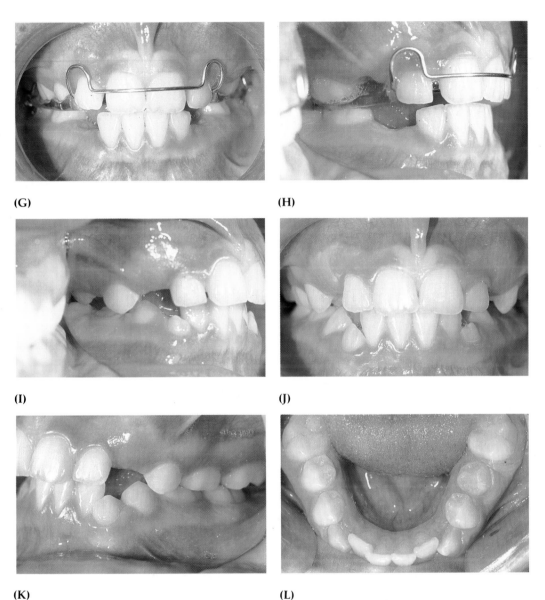

(G)   **(H)**

(I)   **(J)**

(K)   **(L)**

Figure 7−2 Class I crowded (early mixed dentition). At the early mixed
dentition stage, this patient presented with severe crowding, −5.7-mm arch
width loss at the ''D's'' according to the Schwarz analysis **(A)−(E)**, and enough
forward drift of the posterior quadrants to ensure the unerupted cuspids will be
crowded out once they appear. Treatment began with removal of all four second
molars prior to distalization procedures with upper Sagittal I appliance with a
labial bow wire tucked in distally to the maxillary permanent laterals **(F)−(H)**.
After 7 months of treatment note space created for unerupted upper cuspids

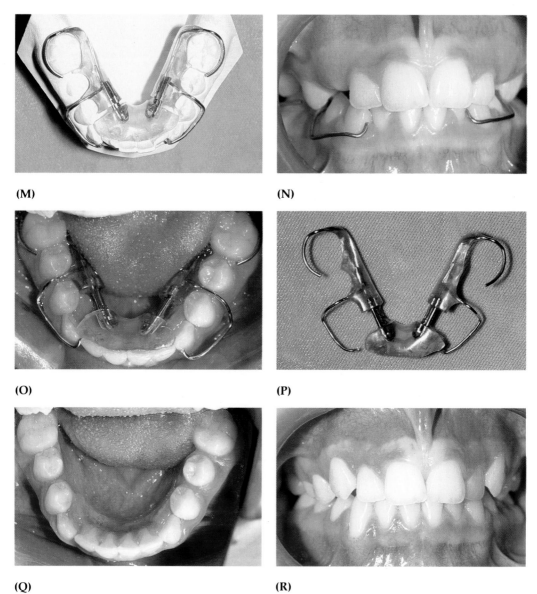

(M)   (N)

(O)   (P)

(Q)   (R)

(I)−(K). Mandibular crowding, which was due to forward migration of posterior quadrants, was corrected in 3 months by lower Sagittal I appliance technique employing cuspid retraction springs (L)−(Q). Final perfection of upper arch was attained in 7 months with Straight Wire technique (R)−(T). Final case retains skeletal Class I status (U)−(W).

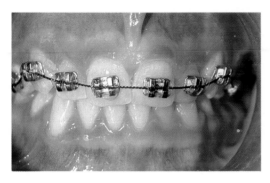

(S)

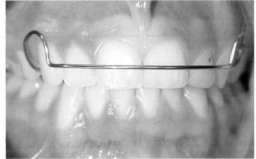

(T)

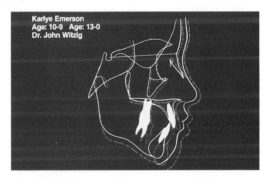

(U)

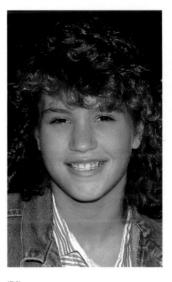

(V)

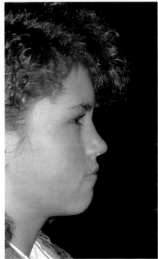

(W)

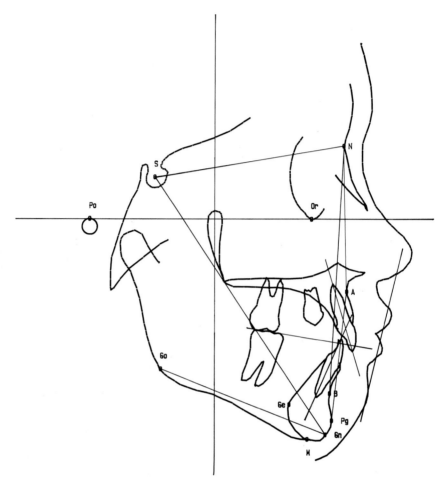

(A)

MODIFIED STEINER ANALYSIS

SKELETAL

MEASUREMENT	NORM	ACTUAL	COMMENT
SNA	80.0° to 84.0°	82.1°	
SNB	78.0° to 82.0°	77.5°	RETROGNATHIC MANDIBLE
ANB	0.0° to 4.0°	4.5°	SKELETAL CLASS II
WITS	-2.0mm to 2.0mm	0.2mm	SKELETAL CLASS I
UPPER FACIAL HEIGHT	50.0%	42.0%	
LOWER FACIAL HEIGHT	50.0%	58.0%	
Go-Gn to SN	28.0° to 36.0°	30.4°	
Y-Axis to SN	63.0° to 69.0°	64.9°	
			Normal skeletal bite.
OCCL to SN	14.0° to 15.0°	18.6°	ANY CHANGE IN POSTERIOR VERTICAL SUPPORT WILL HAVE A THREE-FOLD PROPORTIONAL CHANGE IN ANTERIOR VERTICAL
Pg to NB	1.5mm to 3.5mm	1.5mm	NOT MUCH BONE STRUCTURE FOR MOVING MANDIBULAR TEETH ANTERIORLY

DENTAL

MEASUREMENT	NORM	ACTUAL	COMMENT
UP1 to NA DIST	4.0mm	3.3mm	
UP1 to NA ANG	20.0° to 24.0°	15.9°	LINGUOVERSION
LOW1 to NB DIST	4.0mm	4.4mm	
LOW1 to NB ANG	23.0° to 27.0°	21.0°	LINGUOVERSION
LOW1 TO UP1	120.0° to 140.0°	138.5°	
A-Pg to LOW1	-2.0mm to 3.0mm	1.2mm	
6+6 to PTV	14.0mm	14.1mm	

SOFT TISSUE

MEASUREMENT	NORM	ACTUAL	COMMENT
UPPER LIP	0.0mm to 2.0mm	1.8mm	
LOWER LIP	0.0mm to 2.0mm	1.0mm	

Figure 7–3   Pretreatment Steiner **(A)** and Functional Orthopedic **(B)** and post-treatment Steiner **(C)** and Functional Orthopedic **(D)** cephalometric analysis of patient in Figure 7–2. Note that both skeletal and dental Class I status is retained throughout treatment. The main body of cephalometric changes are due to growth.

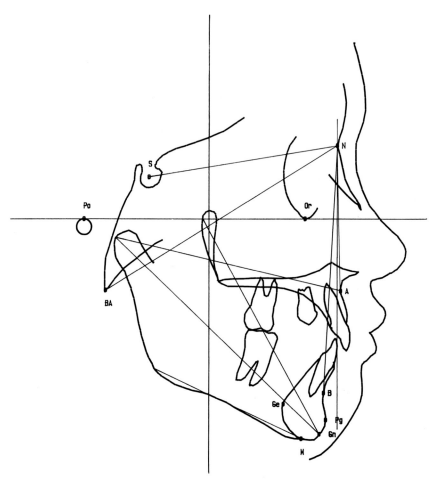

(B)

FUNCTIONAL ORTHOPEDIC ANALYSIS

MEASUREMENT	NORM	ACTUAL	COMMENT
A. RELATING THE MAXILLA TO THE CRANIAL BASE			
A Pt to N Perp	-2.0mm to 2.0mm	1.2mm	
B. RELATING THE MANDIBLE TO THE MAXILLA			
Eff. MAXILLA Lgth	***	90.4mm	
Eff. MANDIBLE Lgth	113.0mm to118.0mm	109.4mm	SHORT MANDIBLE
Diff=MAX-MAND Lgth	***	20.2mm	
Lower Facial Ht[Vert Dim]	63.5mm to 67.7mm	67.1mm	
C. RELATING THE UPPER INCISOR TO THE MAXILLA			
Up1 to A Perp	4.0mm to 6.0mm	3.7mm	
D. RELATING THE LOWER INCISOR TO THE MANDIBLE			
Low1 to A-Pg Line	1.0mm to 3.0mm	1.2mm	
E. MANDIBULAR POSITION			
Pg to N Perp	-5.4mm to -1.6mm	-4.5mm	
F. OTHER USEFUL CEPHALOMETRIC MEASUREMENTS			
SNA	80.0° to 84.0°	82.1°	
SNB	78.0° to 82.0°	77.5°	RETROGNATHIC MANDIBLE
ANB	0.0° to 4.0°	4.5°	SKELETAL CLASS II
Interincisal Angle	120.0° to140.0°	138.5°	
Mandibular Plane Angle	20.0° to 30.0°	21.2°	
Facial Axis (Ricketts)	86.5° to 93.5°	92.1°	
WITS	-2.0mm to 2.0mm	0.2mm	SKELETAL CLASS I

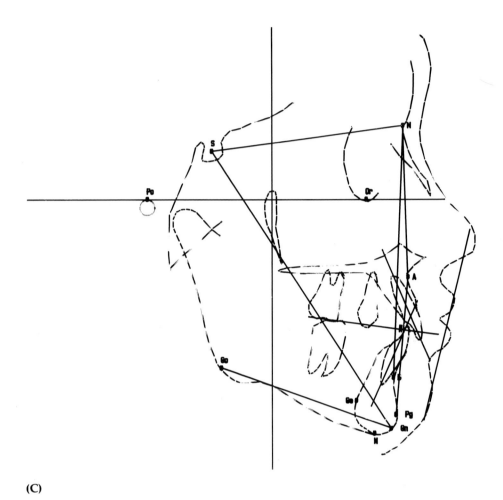

(C)

MODIFIED STEINER ANALYSIS

SKELETAL

MEASUREMENT	NORM	ACTUAL	COMMENT
SNA	80.0° to 84.0°	84.4°	PROGNATHIC MAXILLA
SNB	78.0° to 82.0°	80.2°	
ANB	0.0° to 4.0°	4.3°	SKELETAL CLASS II
WITS	-2.0mm to 2.0mm	0.7mm	SKELETAL CLASS I
UPPER FACIAL HEIGHT	50.0%	41.8%	
LOWER FACIAL HEIGHT	50.0%	58.2%	
Go-Gn to SN	28.0° to 36.0°	26.7°	TENDENCY FOR INSUFFICIENT VERTICAL DEVELOPMENT
Y-Axis to SN	63.0° to 69.0°	63.9°	
			Normal skeletal bite.
OCCL to SN	14.0° to 15.0°	15.1°	ANY CHANGE IN POSTERIOR VERTICAL SUPPORT WILL HAVE A THREE-FOLD PROPORTIONAL CHANGE IN ANTERIOR VERTICAL
Pg to NB	1.5mm to 3.5mm	1.6mm	

DENTAL

MEASUREMENT	NORM	ACTUAL	COMMENT
UP1 to NA DIST	4.0mm	4.8mm	
UP1 to NA ANG	20.0° to 24.0°	21.8°	
LOW1 to NB DIST	4.0mm	5.9mm	
LOW1 to NB ANG	23.0° to 27.0°	22.2°	LINGUOVERSION
LOW1 TO UP1	120.0° to140.0°	131.8°	
A-Pg to LOW1	-2.0mm to 3.0mm	2.6mm	
6+6 to PTV	16.0mm	14.3mm	BE SURE ENOUGH TUBEROSITY EXISTS TO DISTALLIZE MOLARS IF NECESSARY

SOFT TISSUE

MEASUREMENT	NORM	ACTUAL	COMMENT
UPPER LIP	0.0mm to 2.0mm	0.4mm	
LOWER LIP	0.0mm to 2.0mm	2.4mm	

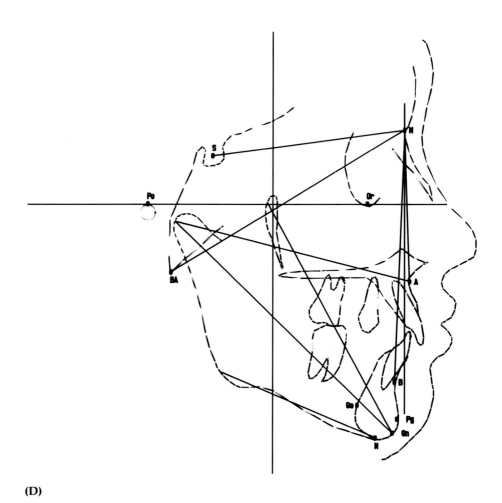

(D)

FUNCTIONAL ORTHOPEDIC ANALYSIS

MEASUREMENT	NORM	ACTUAL	COMMENT

A. RELATING THE MAXILLA TO THE CRANIAL BASE

A Pt to N Perp	-1.0mm to 3.0mm	1.9mm	

B. RELATING THE MANDIBLE TO THE MAXILLA

Eff. MAXILLA Lgth	***	94.1mm	
Eff. MANDIBLE Lgth	119.2mm to124.2mm	116.8mm	SHORT MANDIBLE
Diff=MAX-MAND Lgth	***	24.6mm	
Lower Facial Ht[Vert Dim]	66.2mm to 70.9mm	70.5mm	

C. RELATING THE UPPER INCISOR TO THE MAXILLA

Up1 to A Perp	4.0mm to 6.0mm	5.5mm	

D. RELATING THE LOWER INCISOR TO THE MANDIBLE

Low1 to A-Pg Line	1.0mm to 3.0mm	2.6mm	

E. MANDIBULAR POSITION

Pg to N Perp	-4.6mm to -0.4mm	-3.0mm	

F. OTHER USEFUL CEPHALOMETRIC MEASUREMENTS

SNA	80.0° to 84.0°	84.4°	PROGNATHIC MAXILLA
SNB	78.0° to 82.0°	80.2°	
ANB	0.0° to 4.0°	4.3°	SKELETAL CLASS II
Interincisal Angle	120.0° to140.0°	131.8°	
Mandibular Plane Angle	20.0° to 30.0°	19.2°	LOW VERTICAL DIMENSION
Facial Axis (Ricketts)	86.5° to 93.5°	91.7°	
WITS	-2.0mm to 2.0mm	0.7mm	SKELETAL CLASS I

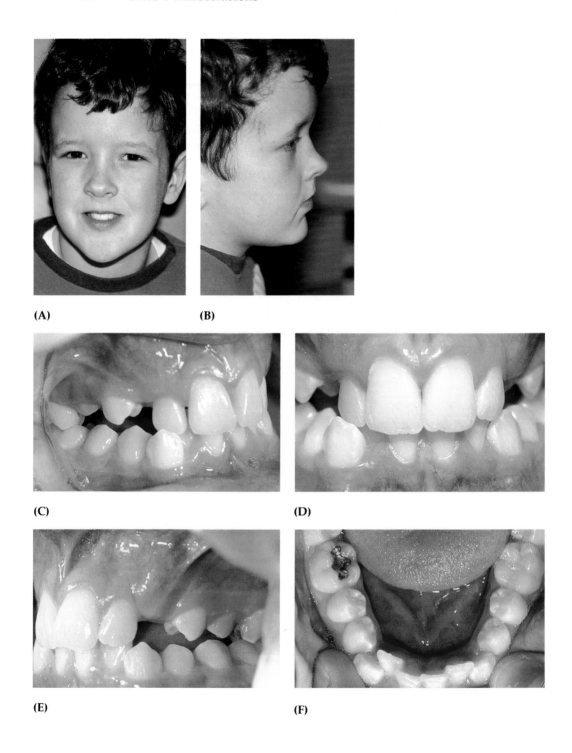

(A)

(B)

(C)

(D)

(E)

(F)

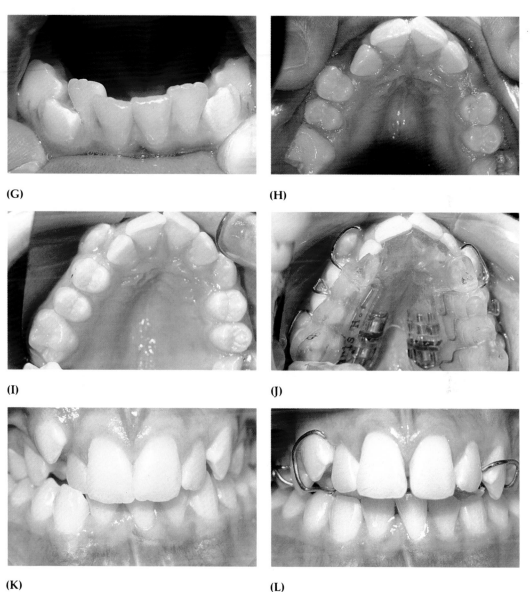

(G) (H) (I) (J) (K) (L)

Figure 7–4 Class I crowded (late mixed dentition). This patient consulted a clinician who wanted four bicuspids removed as part of the treatment plan. The patient's mother had a history of prior treatment involving removal of four bicuspids and conventional fixed appliances when she was a teenager. She was displeased with the outcome of the treatment. Therefore, she obtained a second opinion at Dr Witzig's office. The patient exhibited severe crowding in the late mixed dentition (all deciduous teeth had been lost just prior to time when photographs were taken) **(A)–(G)**. Treatment began with removal of all four second molars (thirds allowed to erupt). Upper Sagittal I appliance used for 7 months (not pictured). Note that early in the treatment the upper cuspids erupt and are blocked out labially, with the upper right cuspid being the worst of the two by far **(H), (I)**. Then a second Sagittal I appliance was constructed and

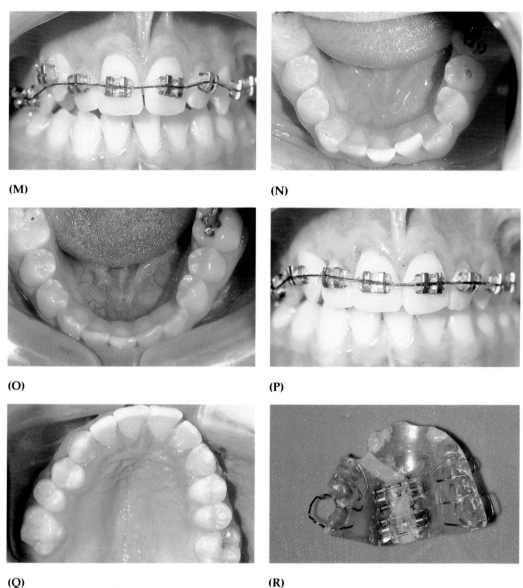

(M)

(N)

(O)

(P)

(Q)

(R)

inserted **(J)**−**(L)**. The second Sagittal was also used for 7 to 8 months (3 to 4 months to open screws, then 3 to 4 more months to act as its own retainer to allow things to stabilize). Straight Wire appliance was then used for 7 months **(M)**. No appliances were used on the mandibular arch. Spontaneous correction of crowding in the lower arch occurred in a most dramatic fashion merely from the removal of the lower second molars **(N)**, **(O)**. At the completion of Straight Wire phase of treatment **(P)**, the arch form became unsatisfactory due to slight lateral collapse of the arch in an asymmetric fashion that resulted in a near posterior crossbite **(Q)**. Therefore, a combination Transverse-Sagittal appliance with offset screws **(R)** was designed and used for 6 months to obtain final case results **(S)**−**(X)**.

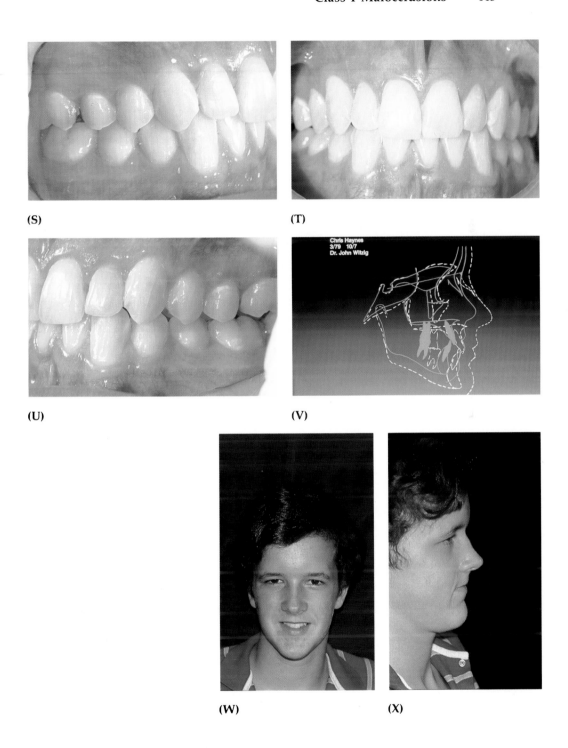

(S)

(T)

(U)

(V)

(W)

(X)

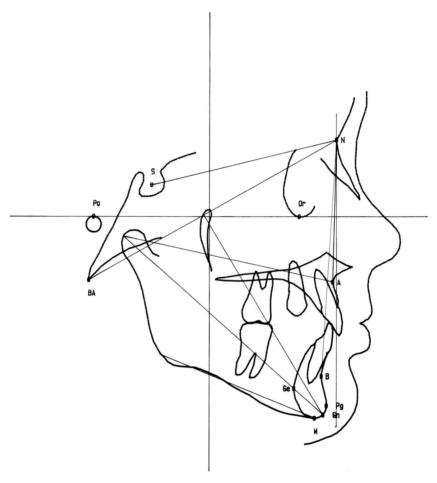

(A)

FUNCTIONAL ORTHOPEDIC ANALYSIS

MEASUREMENT	NORM	ACTUAL	COMMENT
A. RELATING THE MAXILLA TO THE CRANIAL BASE			
A Pt to N Perp	-2.0mm to 2.0mm	-1.5mm	
B. RELATING THE MANDIBLE TO THE MAXILLA			
Eff. MAXILLA Lgth	***	83.4mm	
Eff. MANDIBLE Lgth	101.6mm to106.6mm	103.3mm	
Diff=MAX-MAND Lgth	***	18.4mm	
Lower Facial Ht[Vert Dim]	58.5mm to 61.9mm	59.3mm	
C. RELATING THE UPPER INCISOR TO THE MAXILLA			
Up1 to A Perp	4.0mm to 6.0mm	3.9mm	
D. RELATING THE LOWER INCISOR TO THE MANDIBLE			
Low1 to A-Pg Line	1.0mm to 3.0mm	1.1mm	
E. MANDIBULAR POSITION			
Pg to N Perp	-5.4mm to -1.6mm	-3.8mm	
F. OTHER USEFUL CEPHALOMETRIC MEASUREMENTS			
SNA	80.0° to 84.0°	75.1°	RETROGNATHIC MAXILLA
SNB	78.0° to 82.0°	72.9°	RETROGNATHIC MANDIBLE
ANB	0.0° to 4.0°	2.2°	SKELETAL CLASS I
Interincisal Angle	120.0° to140.0°	141.2°	
Mandibular Plane Angle	20.0° to 30.0°	19.8°	LOW VERTICAL DIMENSION
Facial Axis (Ricketts)	86.5° to 93.5°	87.1°	
WITS	-2.0mm to 2.0mm	1.9mm	SKELETAL CLASS I

Figure 7-5   Pretreatment **(A)** and posttreatment **(B)** Functional Orthopedic cephalometric analysis of patient in Figure 7-4. Note how maxillomandibular differential increases nicely due to male growth spurt and enlargement of pogonion.

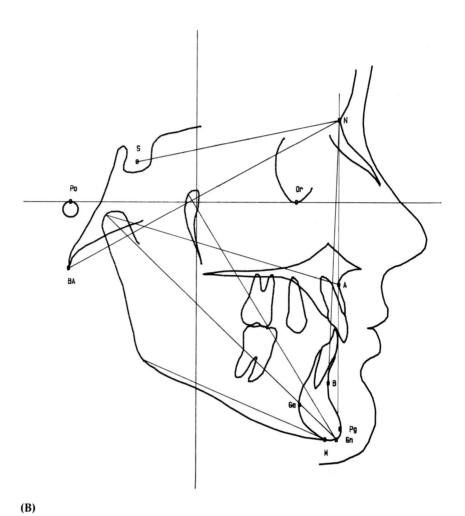

(B)

FUNCTIONAL ORTHOPEDIC ANALYSIS

MEASUREMENT	NORM	ACTUAL	COMMENT
A. RELATING THE MAXILLA TO THE CRANIAL BASE			
A Pt to N Perp	-1.0mm to 3.0mm	0.0mm	
B. RELATING THE MANDIBLE TO THE MAXILLA			
Eff. MAXILLA Lgth	***	94.6mm	
Eff. MANDIBLE Lgth	119.9mm to124.9mm	124.0mm	
Diff=MAX-MAND Lgth	***	29.4mm	
Lower Facial Ht[Vert Dim]	66.5mm to 71.3mm	66.3mm	SHORT VERTICAL DIMENSION
C. RELATING THE UPPER INCISOR TO THE MAXILLA			
Up1 to A Perp	4.0mm to 6.0mm	3.6mm	
D. RELATING THE LOWER INCISOR TO THE MANDIBLE			
Low1 to A-Pg Line	1.0mm to 3.0mm	-0.5mm	
E. MANDIBULAR POSITION			
Pg to N Perp	-3.5mm to 1.5mm	0.8mm	
F. OTHER USEFUL CEPHALOMETRIC MEASUREMENTS			
SNA	80.0° to 84.0°	78.5°	RETROGNATHIC MAXILLA
SNB	78.0° to 82.0°	76.2°	RETROGNATHIC MANDIBLE
ANB	0.0° to 4.0°	2.3°	SKELETAL CLASS I
Interincisal Angle	120.0° to140.0°	143.3°	
Mandibular Plane Angle	20.0° to 30.0°	21.8°	
Facial Axis (Ricketts)	86.5° to 93.5°	86.2°	CLOSED BITE TENDENCIES
WITS	-2.0mm to 2.0mm	-0.3mm	SKELETAL CLASS I

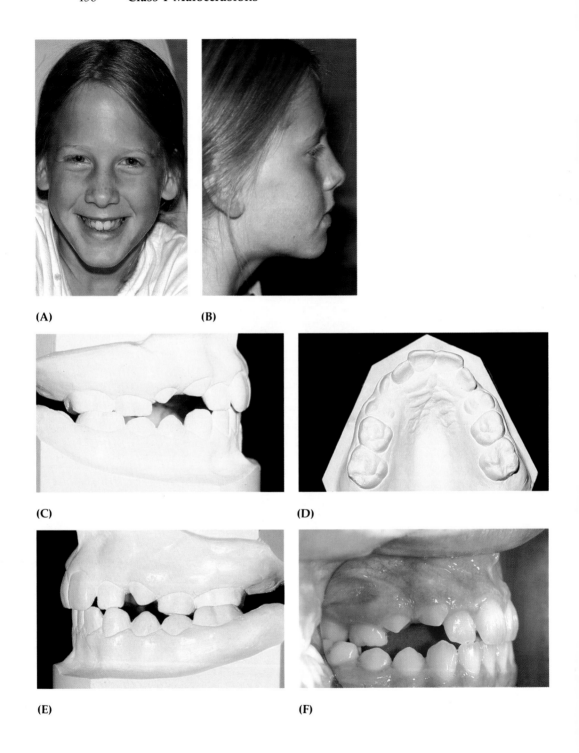

(A)

(B)

(C)

(D)

(E)

(F)

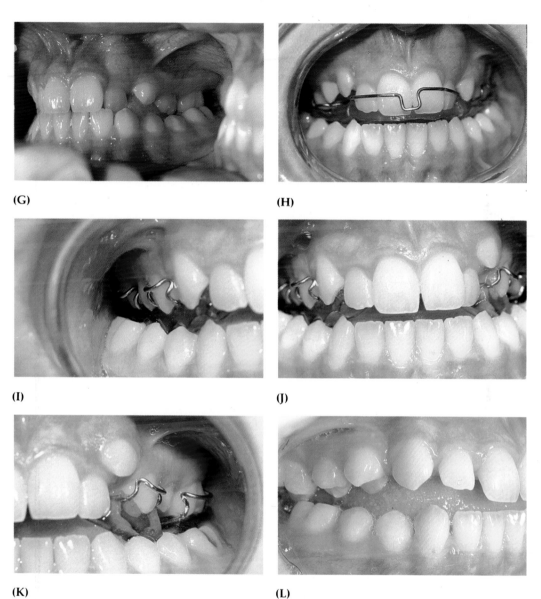

(G)

(H)

(I)

(J)

(K)

(L)

Figure 7−6   Class I crowded, posterior crossbite. This patient exhibited a pre-treatment state of Class I crowding with a bilateral posterior maxillary crossbite **(A)−(G)**. Since the case is skeletally Class I and upper anterior incisors are near labial limits of normality, any AP arch collapse is corrected via distalization techniques. Treatment began with removal of all four second molars to permit distalization of the upper posterior quadrants with maxillary Sagittal I **(H)** with a labial bow. The loop in the labial bow was used to tip the crowns of the two upper centrals inward slightly. After 4 months of Sagittal I treatment, an upper

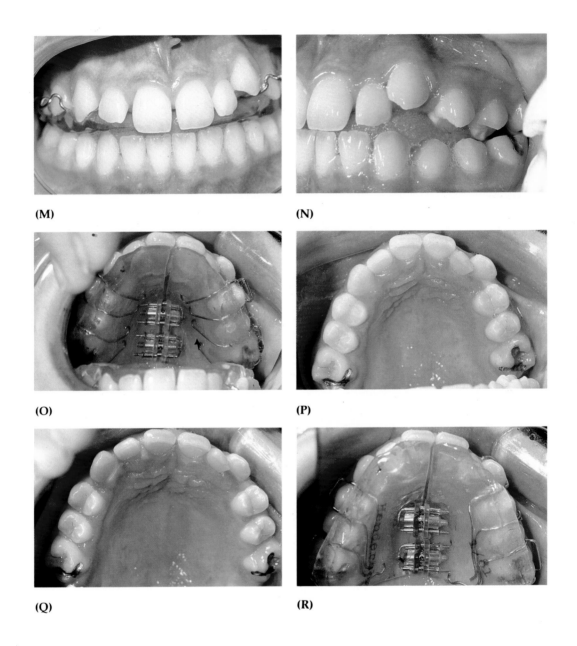

(M)

(N)

(O)

(P)

(Q)

(R)

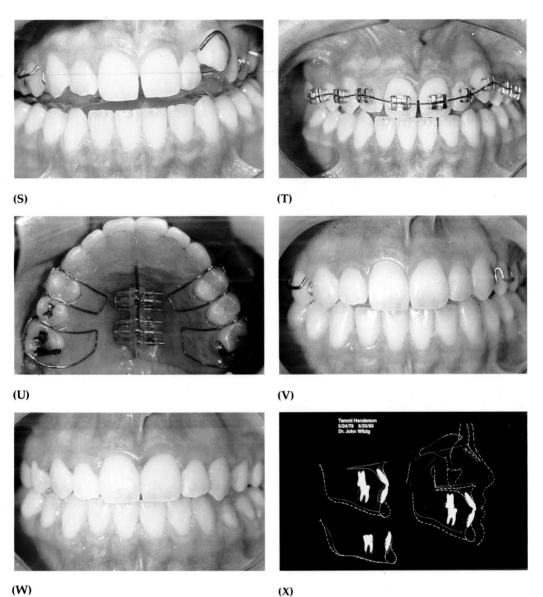

(S)

(T)

(U)

(V)

(W)

(X)

Transverse appliance was inserted **(I)**−**(N)** and used for 9 months. Following this, a second Transverse appliance was used for 9 more months, both actively and passively **(O)**, **(P)**. Note overcorrection imparted in anticipation of impending relapse **(Q)**. A third Transverse appliance was inserted **(R)** with a "C" clasp to tease cuspid into place **(S)**. Straight Wire appliance was used in upper arch only for 8 months **(T)**, followed by a Transverse Hawley to both retain and regain slight arch width loss incurred during Straight Wire phase of treatment **(U)**−**(W)**. Since case was skeletally Class I, most cephalometric changes of a skeletal nature were due to growth **(X)**−**(Z)**.

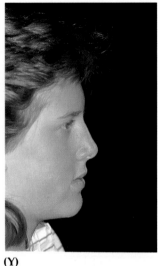

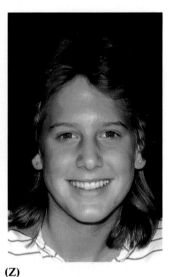

(Y)   **(Z)**

standard or preformed Brehm Utility Arches may be employed for final anterior positioning per routine Utility Arch technique. The advantage of the Brehm Utility Arch over the Sagittal II (other than the fact that the patient can't remove it) is its ability to distally rotate molars if need be, which can gain up to 2 mm additional arch length per quadrant.

Class I mixed dentition vertical deficiencies are ubiquitous through-out the spectrum of early childhood and usually offer no serious concern at the 7–8 year range. As the child progresses, the permanent molars continue to erupt and open the vertical, with alveolar process bone height also increasing. A Class I Bionator, solely for the purpose of increasing the vertical and constructed on a neutral or only slightly advanced construction bite, is an appliance that does not have to be called upon very often at this stage of development. However, if after an adequate period of observation it is evident that a glaring deficiency in vertical dimension is persistent or if the patient has a history of TMJ-type headaches or myofacial involvement, serious consideration should be given to opening the bite with interceptive Bionator therapy. But again, start with assessing arch width first. If inadequate, the mere widening of the arches will open the vertical slightly, which may be all that is needed to relieve the tension on the masticatory mechanism and decompress the TMJs in the case until natural growth may once again proceed at its normal rate. If not, once properly prepared, the arches are ready to be fit with the Bionator.

Class I severely closed bite cases in the mixed dentition are rare. But as with the Division 2, since the inclined plane action of the lower incisors against the cingula of the lingual surfaces of the uppers in a skeletal deep bite causes neuromuscular reflexive displacement of the mandible (NRDM) distally, such a malocclusion cannot only compress the developing joint but also can force the case out of a dental Class I back to a dental and even skeletal Class II. The older the child gets, the more serious becomes the problem of an inadequate amount of vertical. By 9 years of age the McNamara analysis tells us we should be seeing something around the 60-mm ANS-Me LFH measurement. But symptoms also have to be considered along with the numbers. In some cases the anamnesis may be more important than the cephalometrics. Growing up may be difficult, but it shouldn't be painful. When the child's body talks in the form of chronic headaches or myofacial discomfort, it is the duty of parents and professionals to listen.

CLASS I PERMANENT DENTITION

Class I malocclusions in the adult dentition may fall into the same categories as that of the mixed dentition. The only difference is that the deciduous teeth have all been replaced by permanent teeth. However, now that all the permanent teeth are present, there are several added techniques that may be utilized during treatment that were unavailable in the mixed dentition stages, namely the Straight Wire appliance and the Crozat.

If left untreated, the "urgency" cases that should have been treated in the mixed dentition stage may still be in both skeletal and dental Class I but with crossbites or anterior open bites that have worsened. The Class I crowded case may also exist that has adequate arch width and correct skeletal orthopedic alignment requiring only the purely orthodontic "straightening" of teeth. Thus we see that even though a Class I skeletal or dental situation may exist due to such things as vertical problems, posterior crossbites, and anterior open bites, both orthopedic and orthodontic techniques might still have to be called upon to correct the situation.

An important point to remember when treating bilateral maxillary posterior crossbites in the late mixed and early adult dentitions is the posttreatment increased prominence of the huge mesiolingual cusps of the upper molars. This is a result of the fact that often the upper molars will tip buccally somewhat as the arches are developed laterally. This is especially true in the late teenage or early adult patients or if the maxillary arch must be widened a relatively great distance. Occlusal function aids in uprighting these teeth, but often this may not be enough. The result is that upon seeming completion of the case, the increased prominence of these upper molar mesiolingual cusps causes *balancing side interferences* to be struck with the buccal cusps of the lower molars (especially the last molars in the arch), which is widely conceded to be universally hard on

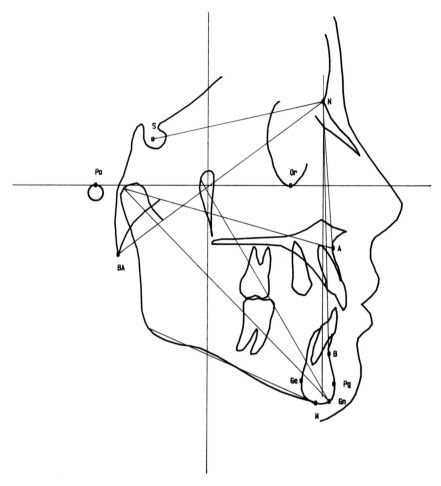

(A)

FUNCTIONAL ORTHOPEDIC ANALYSIS

MEASUREMENT	NORM	ACTUAL	COMMENT
A. RELATING THE MAXILLA TO THE CRANIAL BASE			
A Pt to N Perp	-2.0mm to 2.0mm	4.1mm	OVERDEVELOPED PRE-MAXILLA
B. RELATING THE MANDIBLE TO THE MAXILLA			
Eff. MAXILLA Lgth	***	84.9mm	EFFECTIVE MAXILLA LENGTH AFTER ADJUSTMENT FOR 'A' PT. LOCATION: 80.8
Eff. MANDIBLE Lgth	97.3mm to 102.3mm	113.9mm	LONG MANDIBLE
Diff=MAX-MAND Lgth	***	33.2mm	
Lower Facial Ht[Vert Dim]	56.6mm to 59.6mm	66.1mm	LONG VERTICAL DIMENSION
C. RELATING THE UPPER INCISOR TO THE MAXILLA			
Up1 to A Perp	4.0mm to 6.0mm	5.2mm	
D. RELATING THE LOWER INCISOR TO THE MANDIBLE			
Low1 to A-Pg Line	1.0mm to 3.0mm	1.4mm	
E. MANDIBULAR POSITION			
Pg to N Perp	-5.4mm to -1.6mm	4.6mm	POSSIBLE PROTRUSION
F. OTHER USEFUL CEPHALOMETRIC MEASUREMENTS			
SNA	80.0° to 84.0°	81.9°	
SNB	78.0° to 82.0°	79.2°	
ANB	0.0° to 4.0°	2.6°	SKELETAL CLASS I
Interincisal Angle	120.0° to 140.0°	137.0°	
Mandibular Plane Angle	20.0° to 30.0°	21.4°	
Facial Axis (Ricketts)	86.5° to 93.5°	95.2°	OPEN BITE TENDENCIES
WITS	-2.0mm to 2.0mm	-3.3mm	SKELETAL CLASS III

***See Instructions RE: Reliability of analysis with uncertain Porion location.

Figure 7−7 Pretreatment **(A)** and posttreatment **(B)** Functional Orthopedic cephalometric analysis of the patient in Figure 7−6. Note that the pretreatment status of the upper anteriors indicates that they are almost at the outer limits of the range of normality; therefore, any relief of arch crowding cannot employ Sagittal II techniques but must rely on Sagittal I (distalization) techniques, lateral development techniques, or in this case a combination of both. Note how well face tolerates "extra" cephalometric protrusion due to mandibular and pogonial growth.

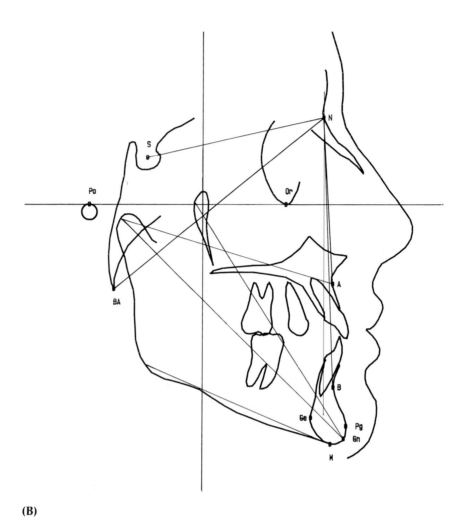

(B)

FUNCTIONAL ORTHOPEDIC ANALYSIS

MEASUREMENT	NORM	ACTUAL	COMMENT
A. RELATING THE MAXILLA TO THE CRANIAL BASE			
A Pt to N Perp	-1.0mm to 3.0mm	3.6mm	OVERDEVELOPED PRE-MAXILLA
B. RELATING THE MANDIBLE TO THE MAXILLA			
Eff. MAXILLA Lgth	***	86.2mm	EFFECTIVE MAXILLA LENGTH AFTER ADJUSTMENT FOR 'A' PT. LOCATION: 82.6
Eff. MANDIBLE Lgth	100.2mm to105.2mm	120.4mm	LONG MANDIBLE
Diff=MAX-MAND Lgth	***	37.9mm	
Lower Facial Ht[Vert Dim]	57.9mm to 61.2mm	71.6mm	LONG VERTICAL DIMENSION
C. RELATING THE UPPER INCISOR TO THE MAXILLA			
Up1 to A Perp	4.0mm to 6.0mm	6.2mm	
D. RELATING THE LOWER INCISOR TO THE MANDIBLE			
Low1 to A-Pg Line	1.0mm to 3.0mm	1.2mm	
E. MANDIBULAR POSITION			
Pg to N Perp	-3.1mm to 2.1mm	8.9mm	POSSIBLE PROTRUSION
F. OTHER USEFUL CEPHALOMETRIC MEASUREMENTS			
SNA	80.0° to 84.0°	80.8°	
SNB	78.0° to 82.0°	79.7°	
ANB	0.0° to 4.0°	1.1°	SKELETAL CLASS I
Interincisal Angle	120.0° to140.0°	130.9°	
Mandibular Plane Angle	20.0° to 30.0°	19.9°	LOW VERTICAL DIMENSION
Facial Axis (Ricketts)	86.5° to 93.5°	95.5°	OPEN BITE TENDENCIES
WITS	-2.0mm to 2.0mm	-1.6mm	SKELETAL CLASS I

TMJs and associated musculature whenever the patient executes a lateral protrusive movement of the mandible. In such situations, the patient complains of "tightness," soreness, or myofacial discomfort of the facial area in the absence of any actual TMJ reciprocal clicking or other evidence of the classic NRDM/SPDC phenomenon. Here anterior interference is not the problem. Rather *posterior* interferences in lateral excursive movements on the balancing side are the culprits. This will occur in spite of perfect skeletal Class I mandibular positioning with the condyles perfectly on the discs in full occlusion, and as such it represents a condition of a true form of primarily muscular trauma during function.

Simple equilibration to free the lingual slopes of the upper molars from interfering with the buccal cusps of the lower molars during both lateral and lateral-protrusive movements of the mandible almost instantly brings noticeable relief to the patients as they execute these movements. This places the occlusion back on the "cuspid protected track" again (or at least reemploys group function of other teeth in the front of the arch), which greatly helps the TMJs and their associated muscles of mastication. Therefore, whenever lateral development of a maxillary arch is employed, the occlusion should be checked at the completion of treatment to determine if posterior *balancing side interferences* exist; if so, steps should be taken to judiciously eliminate them.

Cephalometrically, the Class I skeletal relationship is verifiable by the same means as that used for the mixed dentition, with some modifications. The Wits would reveal the AO and BO perpendiculars to be within 0 to +2 mm of each other for females and −1 to +2 mm of each other for males. (The extra tolerance of the −1 boundary is due to the fact that the secondary characteristics of male hormones may have started to take effect in adolescent males, giving them the more protrusive mandible often associated with the masculine profile.) If the vertical is near normal, the Steiner will reveal an ANB angle of around 2 degrees. However, this may be suspect due to the location of N, ie, the linear length of the S-N line or Bimler Factor 7. A Sassouni analysis would show A-point and B-point close to or on the Basal Arc, with the mesial surface of the maxillary first permanent molar touching the Midfacial Arc. N, ANS, and Pog should fall on the Anterior Arc. Gonion will fall on the Posterior Arc at age 12 and progressively farther past it posteriorly according to the increased age of the patient.

The numerical values of the measurements used in the McNamara will differ from that for the mixed dentition. Depending on the age of the patient and how close he is to complete adult growth, the effective lengths of the maxilla versus the mandible should be approaching the adult difference of 27 mm in females and 30 mm in males. The ANS-Me LFH also would be approaching the adult norms of 66 mm and 70 mm for females and males, respectively. And the purely orthopedically oriented Bimler analysis will again reveal the Anterior Profile Angle of a positive

0–10 degrees, the Factor 7 length, AT length, T-TM distance, and diagonal length of the mandible (DLM) should correspond to the 7:5:3:11:5 ratio if the patient is of the mesoprosopic facial type, and Factor 8 would be near 0 degrees or slightly positive in a neutral state of orthoflexion. Because we are in the adult dentition, we may also use the Factor 6 Stress Axis analysis, and it should show a PER designation. (Factor 6 line travels through the apex of the root of the upper first bicuspid.)

The simplest type of case in the Class I permanent dentition category would be the one where there is excellent orthopedic harmony to the maxillofacial complex, exhibiting a normal skeletal Class I with the molars and cuspids in an Angle Class I, but in which several of the teeth in the arch may be rotated or tipped in one fashion or another so as to require some modicum of orthodontic correction, usually for esthetic purposes. This type of case is often of adequate arch width being on or within 5 mm of Ponts or Schwarz corrected indices for lateral development, with good arch form and near normal interincisal angle. This is a purely orthodontic case that does not require changes in the position or shape of supportive bone but merely the position of teeth within the bone in which they are being carried. And when it comes to such pure type of orthodontic tooth movement, ie, the need to level, align, and rotate teeth, nothing available appliancewise comes even close to the efficient and expedient performance of the Straight Wire appliance. Since little actual movement of teeth will be required, the treatment time may be relatively short, somewhere in the 6–8 month category. Active retention with spring retainers with Hawley palates or vacuum-formed Tru-tains may take place for 6–12 months after fixed appliance removal followed by 6 months of passive retention (night wear only).

Major rotations corrected with the use of rotation wedges have their stability increased by use of the modified Edwards technique of transeptal fibrotomy and slight overcorrection with the wedges under the arch wire. The molars may be banded as in conventional Straight Wire therapy, or they may merely be secured with bonded molar brackets as are the other teeth. Nitinol or the standard series of twisted round wires may be gone through in such a case, ending with the torquing effects of the finishing rectangular .018 x .025 wire. The older the patient the longer the treatment, and periods of active retention should last. But this simple treatment is entirely predicated upon having adequate space in which to move, tip, or rotate these teeth. Tight contacts or a more severe level of dental crowding all the way around the arch present an entirely different orthodontic situation.

For the Class I crowded case the rotations of the anterior teeth have given up arch length, and the thrust of the erupting second molars have jammed all the teeth in front of them forward, collapsing the arch and increasing the degree of rotation of the anteriors and tilting of cuspids and bicuspids mesially. Here the analysis of arch form is critical, and the

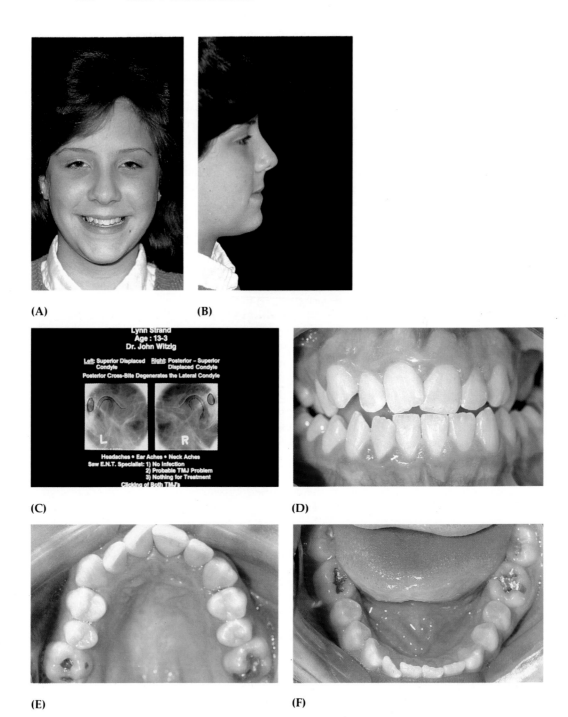

(A)

(B)

(C)

(D)

(E)

(F)

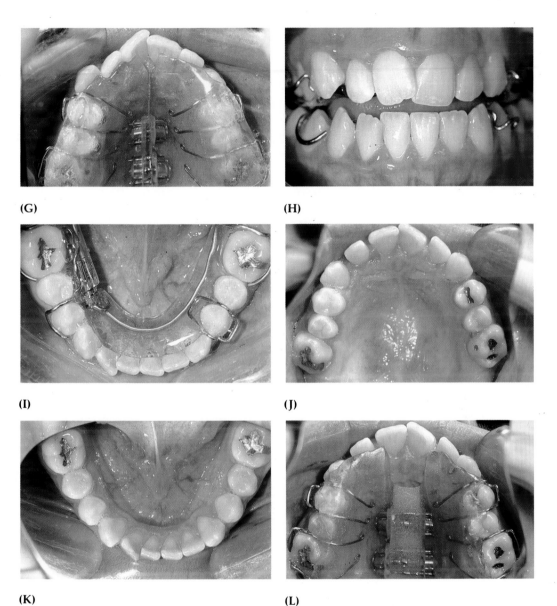

(G)

(H)

(I)

(J)

(K)

(L)

Figure 7−8   Class I crowded posterior crossbite (adult dentition).
This 13-year-old patient and her parents were told by a dental office that she
would need surgery on the maxilla followed by "braces" after surgery. The
patient's parents thought surgery was too drastic an approach and obtained a
second opinion at Dr Witzig's office. The patient exhibited not only a Class I
crowded malocclusion with an accompanying bilateral posterior crossbite, but
also suffered from TMJ-type pain and related headaches as well as reciprocal
clicking in both TMJs **(A)−(F)**. All four second molars were removed, and an
upper Transverse appliance and a lower unilateral Sagittal I were inserted
(G)−(I). After 8 months (4 active, 4 passive), lateral development of maxilla is

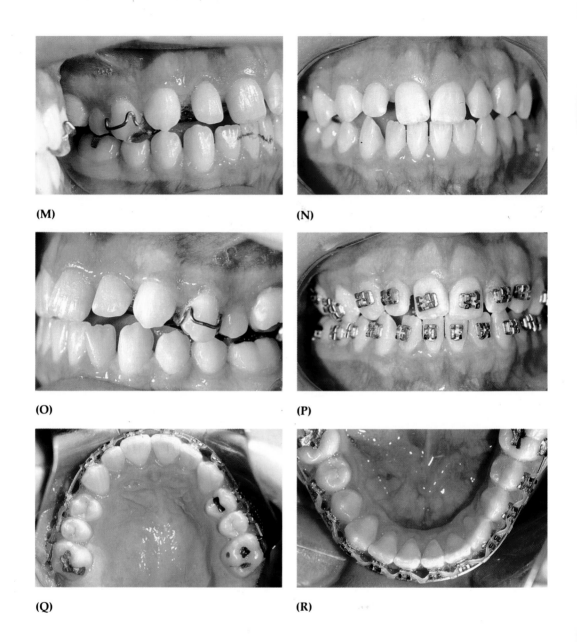

(M)

(N)

(O)

(P)

(Q)

(R)

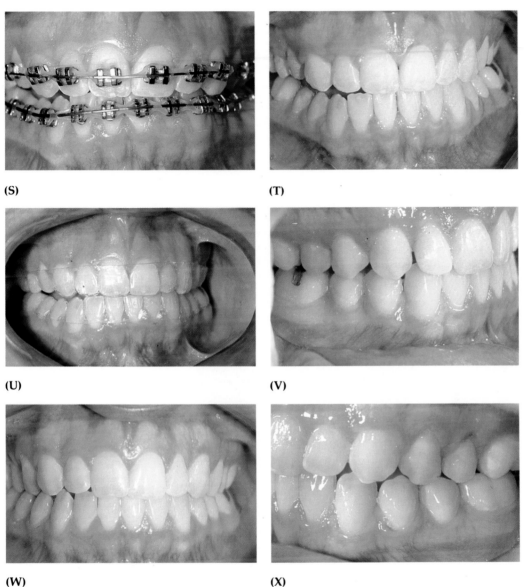

(S) (T)

(U) (V)

(W) (X)

evident, (J)−(K). For a portion of the 8-month period, the space in the middle of the Transverse was filled in with acrylic to act as its own retainer for a short while (passive phase) (L) to allow things to stabilize somewhat prior to construction and insertion of a second Transverse appliance (M)−(O). Slight overcorrection is evident. The second Transverse was used in a similar manner to the first for about 8 months. Straight Wire appliance technique was then used for 8 months (P)−(S). Note that although occlusion is not perfect when Straight Wire appliance is removed (T) and Tru-tain retainers (U) are inserted, the case nevertheless "settled in" very nicely (V)−(AA) for a good final result.

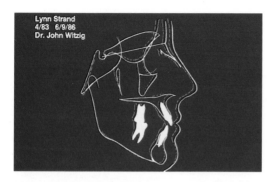

Lynn Strand
4/83 6/9/86
Dr. John Witzig

(Y)

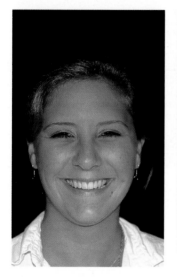

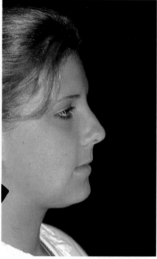

(Z)   **(AA)**

value of the Pont or Schwarz indices becomes obvious. If the case is within 5 mm of corrected Pont or Schwarz, merely applying the Straight Wire appliance may be all that is needed to correct the case. Remember that when the arch wires are inserted, usually the twisted variety first, they are flared widely in a lateral direction (or straight non-arch-formed twisted wire is used), which has a tendency when ligated to the brackets to not only level, align, and rotate but also to slightly flare the arch outward facially in all directions, especially to the labial. This greatly aids in correcting such crowding, since the end result is a generally larger all around arch.

If the patient is young enough so that the thirds have not developed roots yet, extraction of the second molars may also help here. (It should be seriously considered as a convenience to preclude the necessity for difficult third molar surgery for the patient anyway.) If this is not enough to correct the case and if no lateral development is indicated, and if the anteriors are already torqued far enough forward, then the correction cannot be accomplished unless the second molars are extracted and the case first treated with a Sagittal I to distalize the posterior segments enough so that the arch length becomes great enough that the teeth may then be freely rotated and aligned properly by the Straight Wire appliance without the inhibiting effects of the second molars of the severely crowded arch preventing individual tooth rotation.

Without second molar extraction and posterior quadrant distalization, even if the Straight Wire appliance could flare the anteriors far enough forward to correct the rotations, the interincisal angle would become so great that once the brackets were removed, because of the combined pressure of the perioral musculature in the front and pressure from the forward thrusting second molars from the rear, relapse and recollapse of the arch anteriorly could not help but remain imminent. Nature will not tolerate overexpansion anteriorly any more than it will tolerate overexpansion past Schwarz or Pont indices laterally in the posterior area. What the latter form of treatment attempts to do is simply the reverse of how the case got that way in the first place. Being Class I, both structurally and dentally, the powerful erupting second molars push the posterior segments forward. Yet the tongue is powerful enough to resist collapse lingually, and the perioral musculature is strong enough anteriorly to prevent protrusion of the anteriors. Bimler refers to this inward force of the lips and musculature against the anterior teeth as the "perioral tension brace." As a result of the forces of posterior quadrants pushing forward meeting forces of the perioral tension brace pushing inward, labially blocked out cuspids and even some anterior jumbling of teeth ensue. To treat, merely reverse the process, first eliminating the offending etiological agent, the second molar, distalize the improperly advanced posterior segments back to their normally correct anatomical location (obtained once adequate arch length exists as determined by a Carey analysis), *then* level, align, and rotate with the Straight Wire appliance in the conventional manner. Treatment time is shortened, and retention is much less of a problem with the employment of second molar removal techniques where age and dental status of the patient permit.

But using the Sagittal first depends on the existence of proper arch width. If the arch width discrepancy is over the 5-mm limit of tolerance for Straight Wire only and is combined with more severe anterior crowding and rotation, one should develop the arches *laterally first* with the upper Schwarz and lower Jackson for a case still in the late mixed dentition or, if more individual control of specific teeth in the adult dentition arch is desired, upper and lower Crozat appliances may be

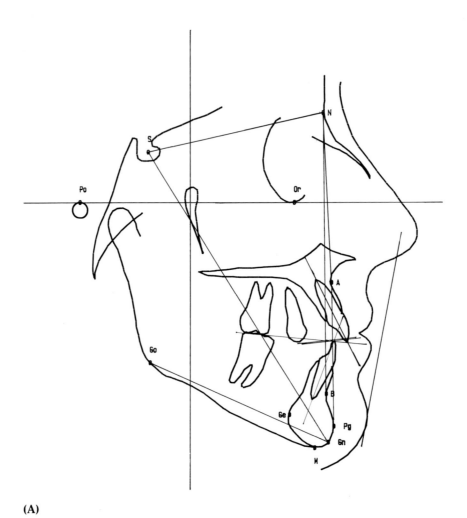

(A)

MODIFIED STEINER ANALYSIS

SKELETAL

MEASUREMENT	NORM	ACTUAL	COMMENT
SNA	80.0° to 84.0°	80.6°	
SNB	78.0° to 82.0°	78.3°	
ANB	0.0° to 4.0°	2.3°	SKELETAL CLASS I
WITS	-2.0mm to 2.0mm	-1.7mm	SKELETAL CLASS I
UPPER FACIAL HEIGHT	50.0%	44.0%	
LOWER FACIAL HEIGHT	50.0%	56.0%	
Go-Gn to SN	28.0° to 36.0°	35.9°	
Y-Axis to SN	63.0° to 69.0°	69.8°	CLOCKWISE GROWER
			Normal skeletal bite.
OCCL to SN	14.0° to 15.0°	17.6°	ANY CHANGE IN POSTERIOR VERTICAL SUPPORT WILL HAVE A THREE-FOLD PROPORTIONAL CHANGE IN ANTERIOR VERTICAL
Pg to NB	1.5mm to 3.5mm	2.9mm	

DENTAL

MEASUREMENT	NORM	ACTUAL	COMMENT
UP1 to NA DIST	4.0mm	5.6mm	
UP1 to NA ANG	20.0° to 24.0°	24.1°	BUCCOVERSION
LOW1 to NB DIST	4.0mm	3.9mm	
LOW1 to NB ANG	23.0° to 27.0°	21.5°	LINGUOVERSION
LOW1 TO UP1	120.0° to140.0°	132.1°	
A-Pg to LOW1	-2.0mm to 3.0mm	1.2mm	
6+6 to PTV	16.0mm	19.7mm	

SOFT TISSUE

MEASUREMENT	NORM	ACTUAL	COMMENT
UPPER LIP	0.0mm to 2.0mm	5.5mm	
LOWER LIP	0.0mm to 2.0mm	3.3mm	

Figure 7–9 Pretreatment **(A)** and posttreatment **(B)** Steiner cephalometric analysis of patient in Figure 7–8. Note how the Class I status is retained throughout the case.

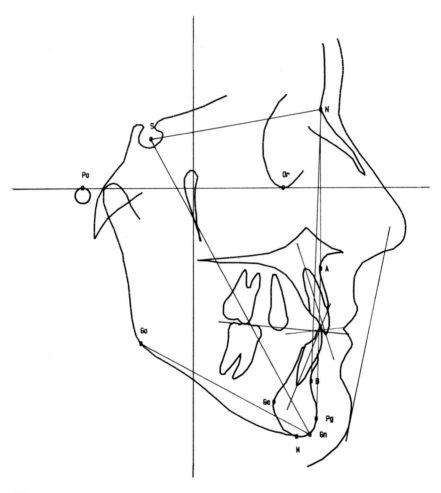

(B)

MODIFIED STEINER ANALYSIS

SKELETAL

MEASUREMENT	NORM	ACTUAL	COMMENT
SNA	80.0° to 84.0°	80.4°	
SNB	78.0° to 82.0°	78.4°	
ANB	0.0° to 4.0°	2.0°	SKELETAL CLASS I
WITS	-2.0mm to 2.0mm	-0.3mm	SKELETAL CLASS I
UPPER FACIAL HEIGHT	45.0%	43.6%	
LOWER FACIAL HEIGHT	55.0%	56.4%	
Go-Gn to SN	28.0° to 36.0°	37.2°	SKELETALLY OPEN
Y-Axis to SN	63.0° to 69.0°	70.5°	CLOCKWISE GROWER
			Open bite tendencies.
OCCL to SN	14.0° to 15.0°	15.0°	
Pg to NB	1.5mm to 3.5mm	2.6mm	

DENTAL

MEASUREMENT	NORM	ACTUAL	COMMENT
UP1 to NA DIST	4.0mm	3.4mm	
UP1 to NA ANG	20.0° to 24.0°	18.0°	LINGUOVERSION
LOW1 to NB DIST	4.0mm	3.7mm	
LOW1 to NB ANG	23.0° to 27.0°	20.7°	LINGUOVERSION
LOW1 TO UP1	120.0° to 140.0°	139.3°	
A-Pg to LOW1	-2.0mm to 3.0mm	1.3mm	
6+6 to PTV	19.0mm	12.4mm	BE SURE ENOUGH TUBEROSITY EXISTS TO DISTALLIZE MOLARS IF NECESSARY

SOFT TISSUE

MEASUREMENT	NORM	ACTUAL	COMMENT
UPPER LIP	0.0mm to 2.0mm	6.1mm	
LOWER LIP	0.0mm to 2.0mm	5.3mm	

used. The ability to direct individual attention for example to a lingually blocked-in bicuspid by adjustments to a lingual arm makes the Crozat the appliance of choice for such circumstances. Crozats are also superior if the case is more narrow anteriorly than posteriorly. If wide enough in the molar region but still narrow in the bicuspids due to anterior tapering of the upper arch in Leghorn Analyzer fashion, the Fan-type appliance may also be used. Since a certain degree of relapse always accompanies efforts at lateral development, compensation traditionally takes the form of overcorrection past Schwarz or Pont limits laterally in the posterior area. The Wilson 3-D series may also be used instead of Crozats.

Once lateral development is complete and lateral limits have been reached (remembering to overexpand), the remaining crowding may be relieved by distalizing slightly with a Sagittal I if needed or going directly to the Straight Wire appliance to perfect arch form. Either way will be greatly facilitated by the removal of the second molars, even before the case is developed laterally. For, as stated in previous chapters, after lateral development without second molar extraction the case relapses with the molars drifting *mesio*lingually. However, after lateral development with second molar extractions performed first, the anticipated relapse that might occur causes the first molar to drift *disto*lingually, which in these circumstances is desirable.

Division 1 flaring of maxillary central incisors in Class I cases may be retracted in Straight Wire with power chain, which is the particular technique of choice if the arch is *asymmetrical*. The upper four anteriors may also be retracted by means of elastics running from the hooks on the molar bands to the soldered hooks on a round .18 or .20 arch wire distal to the cuspids, but only if the outline of the arch is symmetrical. The forces needed to retract the anteriors are not great. An elastic tension of 50−150 grams per side (as measured with a Dontrix tension gauge) is the usual fare popular with most clinicians. The elastic force may be supplied by a variety of sources: elastics, Pletcher springs, and even Saif springs on occasion. However, the 5/16-inch or 5/8-inch 2-ounce elastics are some of the most commonly used in these situations, depending on the amount of force desired and the linear distance between the hook on the molar bracket and the hook on the arch wire (which is usually soldered distally to the lateral).

The bicuspids are retracted first if need be; the second bicuspids are first retracted to the molar, and ligated to it with wire ligature to form a sort of "orthodontic double abutment" which serves as anchorage. Next, the first bicuspid is retracted back up against the "double-abutted" second bicuspid (and first molar). Next, these three posterior teeth are ligated together with a common steel ligature wire to "triple abut" them together for maximum anchorage. Then, and only then, may the cuspids be retracted against them. The cuspid root is long and offers considerable resistance to displacement by means of orthodontic forces in *any* direction. Note: Cuspids are considered as posterior teeth here.

Once retracted and ligated to the rest, the whole four-tooth span serves as anchorage against which the four remaining anteriors may be retracted en masse with elastic forces to the whole arch wire. The afore-mentioned 5/16, 5/8, etc, elastics are hooked up from the respective molars to the soldered hooks (or crimpable hooks) on the arch wire distal to the laterals. As previously discussed, cephalometrics determines whether round or rectangular wires are used.

Of course, rectangular wire usage implies somewhat heavier forces in the 150 g per side range due to (1) the friction of a rectangular arch wire in a rectangular bracket slot, and (2) the fact that *translation*, and not mere tipping, is being attempted. Root angulation and position is the determining factor in wire selection: tipping calling for round wire, translation calling for rectangular wire. Sometimes the amount of retraction required is so slight that, in all honesty, this becomes a moot point. Again, this method of running elastics to hooks on the arch wires distal to the laterals is for *symmetrical* retraction of the anterior arch when all the spaces between the centrals and laterals are of roughly equal size. However, if these spaces vary in size, the gaining of anchorage by ligating the four teeth posterior to the laterals together with wire ligatures is employed similar to the technique used for symmetrical retraction; but for asymmetrical arch condensation, power chain is stretched across from cuspid to cuspid so that the forces may be exerted unevenly through the elasticity of the chains needed to get all the teeth individually retracted proportional to their needs. Little, if any, anchorage will be lost posteriorly in either type of retraction method, since only the upper centrals and laterals have to be retracted.

Power chain is reserved more for simpler space condensation or for the aforementioned anterior arch retraction asymmetrically. It is not usually used for major anterior arch retractions in a molar-to-molar fashion. Without the employment of the anchorage systems described above, in major arch condensation and anterior arch retraction situations, the power chain elastic systems used will have a tendency to pull the first molars, to which the elastic system is attached by hooks on the buccal tubes, forward slightly along with the other teeth in front of them. Mesiorotation of the first molars will also occur, especially if lighter wires or coaxial wires are used. This may be prevented by the proper use of compensating lingual elastic forces, such as "K" modules or power thread running from lingual buttons on the molar brackets to "acid-etched" lingual buttons on the lingual surfaces of first bicuspids or cuspids. Some may even resort to the old Oliver-type internal Class II labial bow in conjunction with Class II elastics. But the ligation method is easiest.

Open-ended molar tubes on molar brackets are required so that the retracting arch wire may express its excess out the back of the molar brackets as the wire is pulled distally by the elastics. However, this method of round wire usage is viable only if excessive angulation (labial crown torque) is present prior to treatment. Round wire usage will merely tip the teeth back at the clinical crown while the point of rotation is the apex. This in effect uprights the whole tooth bodily as well as causes the crowns to be pulled in lingually. If the angulation of the long axes of the four anteriors (especially the centrals) is already upright enough, the round wire may "overupright" them too much due to its purely tipping action. In this case a rectangular wire of the .16 × .16 or the hefty .18 × .25 variety is substituted to effect more of a bodily movement of the teeth (which also takes longer than mere tipping) to keep root angulation constant. But beware of the big mandibular arc of closure.

Common methods of evaluating angulation of the upper and lower incisors are the Steiner, Downs, Ricketts, Sassouni, McNamara, and Bowbeer. The plethora of analyses that allow for this type of evaluation result from the assumption that the case is indeed skeletal Class I. Were the case to be a skeletal Class II only, the Sassouni and parts of the Steiner may be justifiably used (of the analyses discussed in this text). The Sassouni relates the angulation and position of the upper and lower incisors to base reference lines that are not affected by the position of the mandible either before treatment, in its Class II retruded state, or after treatment, in its advanced and lowered state.

All the other analyses relate their upper and lower incisors either partially or entirely to base reference lines running from some landmark or another in the maxilla to some sort of landmark in the mandible, which automatically negates their validity in skeletal Class II mandibular retrusive situations, since the mandible is not going to remain retrusive for long once an FJO-oriented treatment plan is initiated. Once mandibular advancement takes place, the angulation of the base reference line of the particular system swings forward, automatically changing the angulation of the long axes of the upper and lower incisors to that reference line, which renders the significance of their pretreatment angulations meaningless. On the other hand, for our discussion here of Class I situations, all these aforementioned reference lines for evaluating incisor angulation that are constructed to run from the maxilla to the mandible *are* valid. Some, however, need even further qualifications.

An example of an analysis that requires such qualifications is the Steiner. The *angulation* of the maxillary central is 22 degrees to the NA line, with *position* in turn determined by the ideal of a 4-mm distance between the tip of the maxillary central incisor's incisal edge and the NA line. However, this assumes that the maxilla is in the right place with respect to the cranial base. To verify proper maxillary location when using only the Steiner, one might be tempted to merely check the SNA,

Steiner's method of determining maxilla location, with the ideal being 82 degrees. Yet this may be suspect due to possible variance of S or N. Thus the NA line, used as the base reference line for evaluating incisor angulation and position, has no way of being proven properly angulated to begin with when using the Steiner. If the SN line is at or very near 7 degrees to FH and the SNA does approach 82 degrees, it may safely be assumed that the maxilla is in the proper location. This is due to the fact that Bimler determined, after much research and clinical observation, that SN is on the average angulated 7 degrees to Frankfort. If such is the case, the angulations of the Steiner may hold up as valid.

The evaluation of the lower incisors is also predicated upon these same conditions, since their ideal location of 25 degrees of the long axis of the lower central incisor to NB, and incisal tip to NB of 4 mm, is predicated on the proper location of N. In a Class I case it is assumed that the mandible (and therefore B-point) is located adequately forward at proper vertical. Therefore, for this reference system to be valid, N must be correctly positioned (again a product of the angulation of SN line to FH and a correspondingly proper SNB angle of 80 degrees). Obviously, a Class II skeletal mandibular retrusion may not affect the referencing system of the upper incisor, but the referencing system of the lower incisor, with its biased and incorrect NB line, is negated.

Thus it may be seen that an important series of qualifications must be present to permit the Steiner to be used in evaluation of the proper position and angulation of anterior incisors, and only in "surefire" skeletal Class I situations. Class II mandibular retrusions automatically invalidate the NB referencing values. A system such as the Ricketts, Downs, Tweed, etc, that references its incisor angulation and positioning against base reference lines running from the maxilla to the mandible becomes suspect in skeletal Class II retrusive conditions.

The problem with methods of incisor evaluation like the Downs, Ricketts, McNamara, and Bowbeer analyses in evaluation of lower incisor angulations, interincisal angulations, or upper incisor positioning is that none of them evaluate both *position and angulation* at the same time, nor do they use separate reference lines (that are specific for each tooth, upper and lower) that are not constructed from one jaw to the other. Here again, the Sassouni shines.

The Sassouni allows the evaluation of both maxillary and mandibular skeletal positioning by means of the location of ANS, the tip of the maxillary central incisor, and Pog on the Anterior Arc, A-point and B-point on the Basal Arc, and Go on the Posterior Arc (at age 12—the beginnings of the stage of the permanent dentition). With the upper incisor *positioned* (even if it is only relatively positioned to the maxillary apical base once any necessary qualifying corrections are made according to the indications of PNS and the cribriform vertical), there remains only the evaluation of the incisor's long axis *angulation*. From Beistle's

Sassouni Plus, we see that the angulation between the long axis of the upper incisor and the palatal plane (ANS-PNS) is 110 to 113 degrees. This may also indicate the amount of flexure between the premaxilla and the main body of the palate, but either way it serves as a good guide to proper relative incisor angulation. The angulation of the lower incisors is 95 degrees plus or minus 5 degrees to the Sassouni version of the mandibular plane, ie, a line drawn from Me to the lowest point on the ramus just posterior to the Antegonial Notch (if present) at the posterior corner of the angle of the jaw.

Now in all fairness to the other systems, maxillary anteriors that are flared forward are almost invariably *tipped* forward and thus require not bodily retraction but the importation of lingual crown torque to tip them back in lingually to proper angulations once again. In such circumstances the other methods of evaluating incisor positioning will prove adequate, especially the McNamara, since it uses the A-point perpendicular as its reference line for positioning the maxillary central (labial surface of maxillary central 4 to 5 mm anterior to A-point perpendicular).

The same may be said of the similar method of location used in the Bowbeer analysis (incisal edge of maxillary central 3 to 5 mm anterior to the A-point perpendicular). Therefore, if one suspects that the incisors are positionally flared forward, but are already fairly upright, angulation-wise, detailed cephalometric analysis will determine if rectangular arch wires firmly ligated to the anterior brackets will be necessary to effect actual bodily translation of the anteriors lingually during retraction in order to prevent too steep an interincisal angle from being effected and to prevent excessively vertically angulated posttreatment upper anteriors in the overall attempt to obtain coupling. However, such differentiations are seldom needed. But when they are, cephalometrics provides the "tip-off." (No pun intended.)

With respect to treatment, Division 1 flaring of the anteriors is also easily retracted by the action of the labial bow of the Schwarz plate if that appliance is used first to obtain proper arch form when the case is more than 5.0 mm short of proper cross arch width. Even if the case is within the 5-mm limit for Straight Wire, the Schwarz is a nice appliance to easily gain that extra little bit of arch form and width necessary to retract Division 1 proclined anteriors, and its removable aspect makes it very popular with patients.

Division 2 problems in the adult dentition again offer one of the rare exceptions to the "develop laterally first" concept. The Division 2 retroclined incisors may be compromising the TMJs due to the *NRDM/ SPDC* phenomenon (superior posterior displacement of the condyle due to the inclined plane action of the lower anteriors against the lingual surface of the upper anteriors, resulting in neuromuscular reflexive displacement of the mandible). This means leaving the second molars intact and advancing the maxillary anteriors to their proper interincisal angle with the Sagittal II. Again, a modicum of overcorrection in the form of extra labial crown torque is always indicated (as are concerted periods of retention) in the correction of Division 2 retroclined upper incisors because they have a *strong propensity* to relapse lingually once again after treatment. Once they are properly proclined, one may follow up the case with the previously discussed crowded or Division 1 treatment process if needed. This is what is meant when Division 2 cases are "untreatable"; ie, they have to figuratively be "made into Division 1's first," then treated from there.

When Division 2 situations exist in Class I skeletal and dental categories, the bite is often closed, and once the anteriors are moved forward, retained adequately, and stabilized, the case may need to have its vertical increased by use of the Bionator (remember to keep the lingual retention wire of that appliance snug against the lingual surfaces of the upper anteriors to prevent their incessant desire to relapse lingually). The construction bite of the Bionator in the skeletal Class I deep overbite case must also be taken in the neutral position or actually only slightly advanced to compensate for the distal autorotational effect on the mandible of the bite opening during wax bite registration. The amount of bite opening required in such cases is not great, and the Bionator phase of treatment to open the bite a little may only take 9 months or so. There is a great deal of acceptable tolerance for vertical in the ANS-Me LFH area, and as a result the amount of incisal overbite (about 2 mm ideal) is often the best guide when the case is already skeletally within the normal range of orthopedic limits for vertical.

The severe case of Class I anterior flaring with an interincisal angle of less than 120 degrees presents problems similar to the anterior open bite, which it very nearly is. Some clinicians advocate expanding the case over Schwarz's, or Pont's individually corrected limits with a Crozat or similar appliance to gain sufficient room into which to retract the anteriors; they believe that the increased arch length gained in such a manner will allow room for the desired lingual directed crown movement of the protruding anterior teeth. But this, combined with retaining the second molars, is a scenario for failure, since overexpansion laterally is an unfavorable and extremely unstable state in nature. It must be remembered that when laterally developed cases relapse with second molars in place, the relapse is always mesiolingual, something not needed in this type of case.

Two alternatives offer better chances of success. One may seek to secure adequate arch width, extract second molars, and distalize upper and lower posterior quadrants with the Sagittal I, finally retracting the anteriors with a Bionator II, as in anterior open bite cases. If retracting these teeth would create excessive anterior overbite as the interincisal angle increases, the case may have to be finished in a Bionator I, provided the case can stand the increase in vertical cephalometrically.

If not, the second alternative comes into play. As previously discussed in the chapter "The Great Second Molar Debate," there are a few
rare exceptions when four-bicuspid-extraction treatment may be performed with impunity. If the vertical is already excessive, distalizing
posterior quadrants will only open it more. And if those same posterior
quadrants have drifted anteriorly enough to cause severe anterior protrusion in the classic bimaxillary protrusion situation, and adequate arch
width also already exists, extracting the four bicuspids and closing down
both the bimaxillary protrusion and excessive vertical by conventional
Straight Wire extraction appliances with brackets designed specifically
for bicuspid extraction cases may be entirely indicated. Paramount attention must be paid to the face and TMJs so as not to compromise their
integrity. However, cases with this unique list of qualifications that
require such forms of treatment are extremely rare.

CHAPTER 8

Class II Malocclusions

If ever there were a type of condition in which the full prowess of the FJO system of treatment might extend itself to its maximal and most dramatic capabilities, it is surely in the Class II malocclusion. Designed for this type of malocclusion from the very beginning, functional appliances such as the Bionator work hand in hand with Nature to help with the downward and forward growth of the maxillofacial complex in its proper directions out from under the relatively stable anterior and posterior cranial bases and calvarium. It is the deficiency and lack of fulfillment of this growth and development in either the vertical plane, horizontal plane, or both that is responsible for the Class II skeletal and dental conditions.[26-28]

Unlike the bone-growth-retarding effects of four-bicuspid-extraction treatment in conjunction with headgear, an often-used method of therapy in the past for Class II conditions, the FJO system's thrust of energy lies in the entirely opposite direction. Functional appliances are very poor bone "shrinkers," but they are superb bone "stretchers." And that is exactly what is orthopedically needed to correct skeletal Class II mandibular deficiencies. Functional appliances merely effect the result Nature was trying to accomplish in the first place. The Class II malocclusion in

479

both the mixed and permanent dentitions is by far the most commonly seen type of malocclusion and the one that has the greatest effect on the appearance of the face (with the possible exception of the severe deformity of the Class III mandibular prognathism as the result of a condition such as acromegaly).

Surveys have proved that people will be far more tolerant and accepting of a slightly protrusive profile of the lower face and jaw than a structurally retrusive profile.[29, 30] The weak and unassuming chin, sunken corners of the mouth, and lack of lower lip support are extremely uncomplimentary to facial appearance. The two growth and development discrepancies that stand out as responsible above all others for this condition are both orthopedic in nature, the lack of forward mandibular development and the lack of vertical. Both must be increased to their normally balanced orthopedic relationships before proper correction of this type of condition may even begin to be seriously addressed. Ignoring these two important needs negates even the most heroic of orthodontic efforts to the level of a compromised result. The needs of Class II deep overbite cases are conceptually simple, straightforward, and basic—mandibular advancement and vertical, and that means Bionators!

Just because a Class II situation exists does not mean that the first thing the clinician does is reach for the Bionator. The status of the arches must again be considered individually since the Bionator is defined as an "arch-aligning appliance." If the arches are improperly shaped, shortened, narrowed, or crowded, they must first be prepared by one of the arch-preparing appliances and techniques previously described, before the final arch alignment of the Bionator may be called upon. A certain percentage of cases treated with the Bionator may be followed by the arch-perfecting treatment of the Straight Wire appliances, as needed. Again the question to answer is, "What are the patient's needs?" Where are we starting from, and where do we want to go? Clinical examination, two-dimensional cephalometric analysis, and three-dimensional model analysis provide the answers. After enumerating the needs, we choose the most efficient combination of appliances that will address those needs and utilize them in a treatment plan designed to take advantage of the particular attributes of the appliances selected in the most expedient and logical sequence.

But upon sufficient experience in the field, one will soon realize that the central figure in the Class II case is still the Bionator. There are an almost endless variety of arch-preparing methods and devices available to the practitioner to accomplish the preliminary work of getting the individual arches ready for proper alignment. After the Bionator's use, individual perfection of tooth position may be desired and easily accomplished with Straight Wire appliances. But the treatment techniques used before or after treatment with the Bionator cannot detract from its prominent position as the leading component of Class II treatment. In classic Class II cases it may easily be seen that orthopedic mandibular advancement and procurement of adequate vertical are the chief concerns. All else before or after, though also very important, is secondary. It is just that, for the Bionator to be able to express its full effects in correcting skeletal Class II problems, all other problems are necessarily corrected by implication.

CLASS II MIXED DENTITION

The very early Class II mixed dentition case, where the first permanent molars have just erupted and the upper and lower permanent anteriors are just starting to appear, offers a situation that, due to the very young age of the patient, is not considered critical. At about age 6 or 7 the full force of the growth of the mandible may not as yet have manifested itself. In addition, the extremely young age of the patient may possibly be an obstacle to consider relative to cooperation in appliance wear. Combating the latter is entirely justified in the "urgency" type of case, for those are situations in which the early interception of the malocclusion is extremely important and beneficial to the patient. But in the Class II condition in the 6- to 7-year-old, interception is not quite as critical, especially if the case is only a marginal Class II.

As the first permanent molars continue erupting, opening the vertical as they do, the mandibular growth may accelerate sufficiently to regain Class I status, especially if the Class II status was only marginal to begin with. Even if it does not, and in a majority of severe skeletal Class II mandibular retrusive situations it will not catch up completely, waiting for the child to mature a little more to the preferred 9- to 11-year age bracket will not usually complicate the case but allow the doctor to work with a much more manageable patient from a psychological point of view, and a more predictable situation relative to the actual amount of bone growth latent in the mandible from an orthopedic point of view. Should there be any hidden tendencies to excessive growth of a pseudo-Class III nature, premature advancement of what at first may appear to be a straggling Class II mandible at age 5–6 to Class I may result in a full-fledged structural Class III once the full genetic potential has had time to be realized relative to the proportional differences in bone growth by age 10–11, especially in males. By age 9–10 a child should give a quite accurate impression of his growth patterns as divulged by appropriate cephalometric analysis. The Y-axis of the Bjork, Steiner, or Ricketts analysis or the Suborbital Facial Index of the Bimler should be able by that time to reveal the direction of the main component of growth. (This will be discussed later.)

But if by age 9, 10, or 11, the classic signs of a structural Class II deep bite condition become steadily more prevalent with large overjets starting to appear in the 7–10 mm range accompanied by near 100% overbites (the complete disappearance of the lower incisors up behind the upper incisors upon closure), interceptive orthopedic and orthodontic treatment should be considered. If instituted at that time, the treatment during that phase of development will always be complete long before the patient exfoliates all the deciduous teeth and reaches the full adult dentition. Hence, the practitioner must make the patient and parents aware of the concept of ongoing treatment and remind them that some further treatment may be necessary once the entire adult dentition arrives. However, with correct orthopedic balance already having been obtained by the earlier Bionator treatment, the chances are the treatment that might be needed once the full dentition finally arrives will be minimal and usually only orthodontic in nature. Without the benefits of obtaining proper skeletal Class I balance at the earlier age, at the later adolescent age when the full set of adult dentition arrives on the scene, both orthodontic *and* orthopedic correction will be needed. With early treatment, interception and correction may turn out to also be prevention. Given a "normal" and orthopedically correct posttreatment starting position as the child enters the teenage years, the child may then at least have the potential to develop the rest of the way "normally," without complication. Without the benefits at an orthopedically balanced starting position, ie, a position in which structural imbalances already have a foothold, the child simply hasn't got a chance.

One thing that can always be said about such circumstances to inquiring parents and plaintive children is that left untreated the condition will most likely worsen. But starting Class II treatment in the mixed dentition is sort of like buying life insurance; the time to do it is when you have the need and the means. The need is determined diagnostically. The means are threefold: the technique, the parents' approval, and the patient's volition.

Dentally, the Angle Class II is defined as that interdigitation of teeth whereby the mesiobuccal cusp of the upper first permanent molar is anterior to the buccal groove of the lower first permanent molar and the maxillary permanent cuspid is anterior to its customary place in the embrasure between the mandibular permanent cuspid and first bicuspid. Thus, it may be seen that we may actually have a case where we could hypothetically have a Class II molar situation posteriorly and a Class I cuspid situation anteriorly (but not without some jumbling and crowding of the bicuspids between the upper cuspid and molar along the way). Conversely, the molars could hypothetically be in a Class I relationship posteriorly with the upper and lower cuspids Class II anteriorly, but this would imply excessive anterior flaring of the maxillary incisors or blocked-in lower bicuspids. Thus, we see that even the Angle dental classification of teeth for the Class II is not as simple as it might appear, for on top of this there are the separations of the Class II dental designations into the three divisions according to interincisal angulation as well as the skeletal or structural designations to deal with, which may or may not correspond. The structural Class is determined cephalometrically.

The cephalometric varification of the skeletal aspects of the Class II type of malocclusion are also somewhat more involved due to the factor of "multiple variability." In the Class I case, both the maxilla and the mandible must equally contribute to the defined orthopedically balanced standards of proportion to qualify the arrangement as acceptable skeletal Class I. But in the Class II situation, the skeletal components of the jaw-to-jaw relationship may be such that, due to the factor of multiple variability, the maxilla as a whole may be solely at fault by being too protrusive, although in modern times this is thought to be quite rare. The mandible may be solely at fault by being too retrusive, or both may contribute in varying degrees simultaneously to the Class II structural circumstance. What is needed from the cephalometric analysis, as far as the clinician is concerned, is not only the knowledge of whether or not the case is in fact a structural Class II but also which member of the jaw-to-jaw relationship is errant and to what extent. For it is this knowledge that is the key to which appliances and techniques he selects for the correction and treatment of the problem. Being in possession of such important diagnostic information prior to the beginning of therapy allows for the most efficient and orderly clinical management of the appliances to be used in the most expedient, purposeful, and well-directed treatment plan possible. Also, the key aspects of a particular case that would require modifications of standardized appliance designs or treatment techniques may be elucidated, allowing the practitioner to implement such modifications as the case may dictate to obtain the maximum therapeutic benefit from the appliances he has chosen for his treatment plan. Proverbially, forewarned is truly forearmed.

The aforementioned Wits analysis is ideal for a simple and expedient determination of the structural class of the case cephalometrically. The BO perpendicular will fall distally to the AO perpendicular by considerably more than the 2-mm defined limit, even in the mixed dentition. But here is where the usefulness of the Wits ends. For although this system does clearly denote the skeletal Class II discrepancy, it in no way gives any hints as to exactly where the source of the problem is. Is the difference between AO and BO due to a flared forward and protrusive premaxilla carrying its A-point landmark anteriorly with it as it goes, or is it due to a deficient mandible's inability to bring B-point far enough forward in its arc of closure, or is it a combination of both?

Being able to determine cephalometrically to what extent the maxilla and mandible are involved in creating the structural Class II relationship is sort of a diagnostic proving grounds for cephalometric analysis systems. Such orthopedically oriented cephalometric analysis systems that rise to such an occasion and help provide the clinician with such information vital to a correct diagnosis are the McNamara, the Sassouni, and the Bimler.

Though older systems, such as the Steiner, use angular relationships such the SNA and SNB to describe the relative cephalometric relationships of the upper and lower jaws, their criteria are based on the relative stability of the location of the landmarks S and N, which may not always be taken for granted as being immutable. But the primary problem which makes reliance on such methods suspect is that it fails to take into consideration the important and mitigating effects of the degree of ANS-Me LFH which McNamara has shown unequivocally to have a direct relation on the relative horizontal locations of A-point and B-point.

From the McNamara analysis we know that in the average 9-year-old with a well-balanced face the effective lengths of the maxilla and mandible should be 85 mm and 105 to 108 mm, respectively. But such a normally balanced case will also exhibit (and this is what is important here) a maxillomandibular linear differential of 20 to 23 mm. This is all predicated, however, on an ANS-Me LFH of around 60 to 62 mm. It must be remembered that for every millimeter the ANS-Me measurement *closes* it has the effect of *advancing* Pog (and therefore neighboring B-point) about 1 mm, and for every millimeter ANS-Me is *extended* beyond that point it in effect rotates Pog *posteriorly* about 1 mm relative to the horizontal plane. This relationship greatly aids in the determination of exactly what is happening between the maxilla and mandible. Correlating this information with the determination of A-point relative to the N-perpendicular (A-point on the N-perpendicular, the normal 9-year-old maxillary skeletal status) and the location of Pog relative to the N-perpendicular (−8 to −6 mm, the normal 9-year-old mandibular skeletal status), the diagnostician may determine how much the maxilla and mandible contribute to the Class II structural relationship and whether the status of the mandibular skeletal component is being masked by an unconventional ANS-Me LFH linear measurement into appearing either more or less Class II structurally than it really is.

Since the determination of both size and position of the maxilla and mandible, as well as the relative degree of existing vertical dimension, are critical to diagnosis of the skeletal Class II deep bite condition, it may be seen why the Sassouni offers valuable diagnostic assistance in determining these matters. As previously stated, it is not only important to evaluate the maxilla relative to the mandible, but it is also important to evaluate the maxilla relative to the cranial base. This is done in an effort to detect whether a retruded maxilla might not be disguising an equally retruded mandible into only appearing Class I with respect to the maxilla, when it might in fact be skeletally Class II with respect to the cranial base. The maxilla size and position in the younger 9- to 11-year-old mixed dentition patient are evaluated with respect to the locations of ANS and PNS to the Anterior Arc and cribriform perpendicular, respectively, according to conventional Sassouni technique. The vertical dimension is evaluated as a proportion of UFH versus LFH. It must be remembered that the first Inferior Arc is constructed by placing the point of a compass at ANS and opening it until the pencil tip touches supra-orbitale (SOr). This distance is then transferred by rotating the compass to strike a small arc in the area of the symphysis which intersects the Anterior Arc. Opening the compass 10 mm, a second small arc is scribed. These two lower or inferior arcs delineate the individualized range of normality for Me. Vertically, the UFH should equal the LFH at age 4. At age 8, LFH = UFH + 3 mm. At age 10, LFH = UFH + 4.5 mm. And at age 12, LFH = UFH + 6 mm. Thus by measuring the location of Me to the uppermost of the two Inferior Arcs and comparing that to the age of the patient, an evaluation of the vertical dimension of occlusion may be made. This then is correlated to the size and location of the mandible. At age 8 to 10 the Basal Arc relationship should show A-point and B-point aligning with it, while the Anterior Arc should be *slightly anterior to ANS and Pog* (which both should be on the separate ANS Arc). By age 12 the ANS, tip of maxillary central incisor, and Pog should all fall on the Anterior Arc. A-point and B-point should be on the Basal (A-point) Arc. Gonion should fall on the Posterior Arc. Variation of Pog either in front of or behind the Anterior Arc is *not* the determinant of skeletal position (Class I, II, or III) of the mandible but rather that determination is made by evaluating the location of A-point and B-point with respect to the Basal Arc. With A-point and B-point on the Basal Arc, variance in Pog location with respect to the Anterior Arc is a product of simple variation in chin-button size. This is usually no problem in the mixed dentition stage since it has not had time to manifest itself to a great extent as yet. However, if B-point is posterior to the Basal Arc, and the vertical dis-crepancy is *not* a major contributing factor (although it may in fact be masking the retrusion in a deep bite case), then the case is a skeletal Class II. A protruded maxilla, or Pog and Go being displaced posteriorly from their respective arcs, only intensifies the skeletal Class II retrusion. Any combination of maxillary protrusion or mandibular retrusion of 3 mm or more which is confirmed by the relationship of B-point to the A-point arc is a true skeletal Class II.

From the Bimler we see that in a Class II malocclusion in the mixed dentition the Anterior Profile Angle would be a positive 10 degrees and up. The Factor 6 Stress Axis may not be applicable here as the full complement of adult dentition may or may not yet have completely replaced the deciduous dentition (ie, the maxillary first bicuspid may not have fully erupted or even have completed apexification yet). Also, the Factor 8 ramal line may be in any one of its three possible positions as a mere reflection of the amount of vertical present in the case. The com-parison of the AT, T-TM and DLM linear measurements should reveal the status of the skeletal proportions of the maxilla and mandible.

Class II mixed dentition treatment goals   The treatment goals in the true skeletal Class II mixed dentition case will vary slightly from that of the adult for the simple reason that the entire adult dentition has not arrived on the scene yet. Though orthodontic considerations are important at this stage of the child's development to be sure, the primary thrust of the clinician's concern at this important time of the patient's development should be for orthopedic relationships. In what manner the rest of the adult dentition will finally arrive is intimately related to the size, shape, and orthopedic relationships of the jaws into which the adult teeth are going to erupt. Providing a correct and balanced set of arches in which this process may proceed as normally as possible gives Nature every chance to correctly carry out the transition from deciduous to adult dentitions with only minimal assistance from the doctor at the end, if any is needed at all. This is the basic premise of the concept of ongoing treatment. Thus it is with a certain casualness and tolerance for slight orthodontic imperfections that one initiates treatment in the mixed dentition stage. One goes about the business of forming, preparing, and aligning the arches with the knowledge that should various individual teeth persist in orthodontic misalignment during treatment they may always be corrected by arch-perfecting appliances such as SWA once the adult dentition is fully erupted. If major orthodontic movement of individual adult teeth is needed, the Brehm Utility Arch system may be called on also, which of itself in certain instances may be all that is needed to correct the needed orthopedic charges.

For the Class II mixed dentition case the entire treatment plan will revolve around what ancillary techniques must be employed in conjunction with the *main* goal in Skeletal Class II mixed dentition treatment, which is proper vertical and horizontal arch to arch alignment with the Bionator.

Class II mixed dentition "urgency" cases   Since the Class II condition implies at least some degree of excessive overjet, the anterior crossbite cannot exist, but the other two conditions of posterior crossbite and anterior or lateral open bite from a tongue-thrust or thumb/finger-sucking habit may certainly exist, and if so they should receive the most expeditious attention. Posterior crossbites are treated identically to Class I mixed dentition cases, with a maxillary Schwarz plate. The labial bow may or may not be added depending on the degree of flare or rotation to the permanent maxillary anteriors. The acrylic occlusal coverings, which would convert the Schwarz into a Transverse appliance, may be used if no crowding exists in the lower arch or if some TMJ symptoms are present. Once the proper arch form and width are attained, the case is placed in a Bionator to advance the mandible and open the vertical to correct the Class II problems.

When the anterior open bite is complicated by Class II mandibular deficiency, it is treated in the conventional manner as described for Class I mixed dentition anterior open bite treatment with the Bionator II. But under these circumstances of Class II the construction bite is taken in the mandible in the advanced position. This causes the appliance to take on the multiple functions of both closing down the anterior open bite while at the same time advancing the mandible from Class II to Class I. With activation of the midline expansion screw minor crowding in the lower anterior area may also be relieved when necessary. With the lingual wire cut and adjusted as previously described, along with the swallowing exercises, also previously described, the tongue receives the needed stimuli and myofunctional training to help it return to its proper nonthrusting-type swallowing and resting posture patterns. The labial bow of the Bionator II is kept in its proper position contacting the maxillary anteriors at the appropriate places on the facial surfaces of the procumbent teeth.

In the event both conditions of posterior crossbite and anterior open bite exist in a Class II mandibular deficiency, the old rule of thumb still applies; correct posterior crossbites first (which is the same as developing laterally first), followed by routine Bionator II treatment. The lateral development of the upper arch will open the bite even more and if the case is already excessively protrusive in the maxilla (a rare finding), it may well qualify for four-bicuspid-extraction treatment, but extreme care must be exercised here to be sure this is truly the indicated treatment of choice.

Class II mixed dentition conventional treatment One should be cautious not to institute Class II treatment too early with functional appliances in the mixed dentition stage. By the age of 9–10 the child will usually correctly manifest its growth tendencies, and the patient is greatly helped in his growth and development of the maxillofacial complex if glaring discrepancies in the relation of the mandible to the maxilla are corrected. Though less willing to admit openly to concern, children of that age are going through psychological growth periods of self-awareness at that time and are often very sensitive about their appearance, especially if that appearance is a seemingly protruding set of upper anterior teeth jutting out over a retruded chin. This self-consciousness and personal sensitivity can sometimes cause great vulnerability in an insensitive world.

We must have the teeth in the right place before we may concern ourselves with determining whether or not the arches are ready for the Bionator. If moderate crowding exists with narrow or pointed arch form the case is developed laterally first with a maxillary Schwarz or Fan and mandibular Jackson appliances. Once proper arch form is attained the case is finished in the Bionator in the usual manner. If, however, the arch form is reasonably good and the anterior open bite exists in a Class II mandibular deficiency, and mandibular advancement and bite closing would result in the production of a bilateral posterior crossbite due to the narrowness of the upper arch prior to mandibular advancement, the old rule of thumb still applies: Correct posterior crossbites first (which is the same as developing laterally first), followed by routine Bionator II treatment for both advancing the mandible and closing down the anterior open bite, retraining the tongue and perioral musculature along the way.

Class II, Division 1 treatment: mixed dentition   With all the concern over the proper orthopedic alignment of the jaws in a skeletal Class II mixed dentition situation, one must not forget to pay close attention to the Angle Dental Class II relationships also. For here we may be possibly fooled a little by a trick of Nature. As previously described in the chapter on Sagittal appliances, if decay or other reasons have brought about the premature loss of any of the deciduous second molars, there may result the phenomenon of what we have previously referred to as lost "E" space. If once the upper deciduous second molar is prematurely lost, either unilaterally or bilaterally, and proper space maintainence procedures have not been implemented, the first permanent molars, which should normally by aligned directly on top of one another with their mesial surfaces on that imaginary vertical line known as the flush terminal plane, have the capability to drift mesially into the now empty space vacated by the missing "E" and cause a dental Class II situation to appear. This should be corrected *not* by advancing the entire mandible forward to make the molars a dental Class I again, but by distalizing the upper first molars unilaterally or bilaterally as needed with Sagittal I technique until the upper "E" space is regained.

A similar technique may be used in the mandible with a lower Sagittal to correct what may appear to be a super-Class I molar relationship back once again to the flush terminal plane. So one merely distalizes enough to make room for what the missing "E" would have occupied had it not been lost. Then one may proceed to conventional mandibular advancement. The first permanent molars may distalize quite easily in the early mixed dentition if the second molars are so far down in the alveolar process and so far from erupting that they offer little or no resistance to the movement of the distalizing first molars. However, if routine radiographic survey reveals the second molars in proximity to the first and reasonably close to the surface so as to offer a resistance to distalization, and third molars are present, the removal of the seconds is indicated. This, however, assumes distalization is required as a result of mesial migration of posterior quadrants (in this specific example; however it is only the first molars) and that the anterior incisors are *not* in need of labial crown torque. If the anterior incisors are in need of such labial movement, they are corrected *first* with the aid of leaving the "distalization-obstructing" second molars in place for the purposes of providing the needed anchorage to permit moving the anteriors forward.

Once accomplished, if arch lengthening is still needed, the second molars may be removed to permit the forward-drifted first molars to be properly distalized back to their proper locations (a location not impinging over the path of the second bicuspid that will be erupting in the future). This allows adequate room for the developing permanent second bicuspids to erupt. This space can be held by filling it in with acrylic once the Bionator is constructed. The acrylic is then adjusted clear of the area once the second bicuspid begins to erupt.

Another "trick" that Nature may attempt to get by with is the disguising of true Class I skeletal and dental relationships in the form of half-Class II dental relationships due to the mesiorotation of the upper first permanent molars. As a result of being mesially rotated, the huge mesiolingual cusps of the upper first molars force the mandible to close in a more retruded arc of closure in order to permit the most stable and complete interdigitation of the large upper cusp tips with the fossae of the lower first molars. This will cause some slight retrusion of even a true skeletal Class I mandible and make the upper and lower first molars appear half-Class II dentally, especially in the mixed dentition. Simple distal rotation and expansion with either custom or preformed Brehm Utility Arches will not only easily correct the rotational problems associated with the upper first molars and allow the mandible to naturally advance to Class I skeletally, but will also retract the Division 1 procumbency of the upper anteriors in doing so if need be due to the natural action on the anterior part of the arch wire expressed by the toe in bends. However, this phenomenon is predicated on the case honestly being skeletally Class I to begin with, since true skeletal Class II deficiencies that would still exist after molar correction, anterior retraction, and bite opening with Utility Arches must still be corrected with functional appliance therapy such as a Bionator not only for the good of the bones but also for the sake of the muscles and joints.

We must make every attempt to make sure we have the teeth in the right place sagittally and laterally before we concern ourselves with determining whether the arches are ready for the Bionator. Minor molar class discrepancies, arch width, and mandibular alignment problems may be corrected with Brehm Utility Arches and conventional Straight Wire technique in the usual manner. If moderate crowding exists with narrow or pointed arch form, deficiencies greater than the 5-mm limit for Straight Wire Utility Arches only, the case is developed laterally first with maxillary Schwarz and mandibular Jackson appliances. Once proper arch form is attained, the case is finished in the Bionator in the usual manner. If, however, the arch form is reasonably good and the crowding is slight and confined to the lower anterior area, one may proceed directly to the Bionator and relieve the crowding in the lower anterior area by expansion of the midline screw. The appropriate adjustments are made to the inside of the acrylic bite plate cap to ensure smooth lateral movement of the teeth and the desired angulation of the long axes of the teeth. Proper and timely adjustment of the labial bow controls the degree of retraction of the Division 1 maxillary anteriors. Concern for the inter-

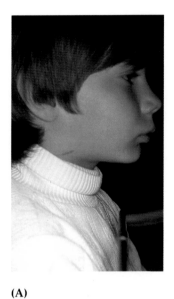

(A)

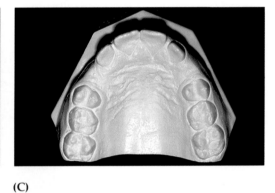

(B)   **(C)**

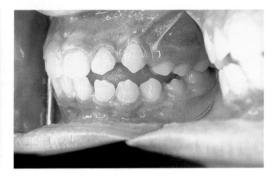

(D)   **(E)**

Figure 8–1   Class II, Division 1 (mixed dentition). A 10-year-old boy exhibited a classic Class II, Division 1 malocclusion in the mixed dentition. Note the skeletal deep bite and full skeletal Class II mandibular retrusion as evidenced by the profile, various cephalometric analyses, and study models **(A)**, **(B)**. The ANB angle is 8.6 degrees, and the Wits analysis reads 5.8 mm. Also note the Division 1

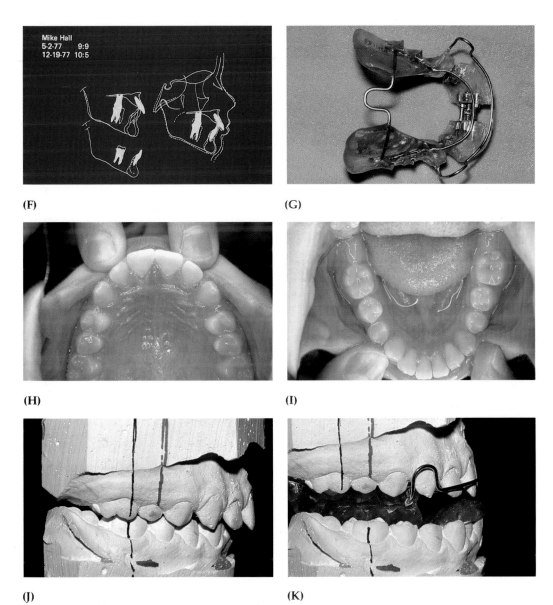

Mike Hall
5-2-77   9:9
12-19-77 10:5

(F)

(G)

(H)

(I)

(J)

(K)

flaring of the maxillary anteriors (C) and the crowding of the lower anterior area (D). Treatment began with insertion of a Bionator (not pictured) to advance the mandible and increase the vertical. The midline jackscrew and Coffin spring were serially activated to develop the arches laterally. After 7 months of treatment, with the mandible in the "as if" position, note the relief of crowding and the characteristic appearance of the occlusion with the posterior molars most near full occlusal contact and the bite progressively opening forward to the bicuspid area (E), although the actual biting occlusion shows only partial correction from Class II to Class I (F). Expansion of Bionator midline screw and Coffin spring eventually produces fairly good arch form, albeit slightly pointed with some open contacts (G)–(I). Second Bionator is constructed to bring mandible to final state of

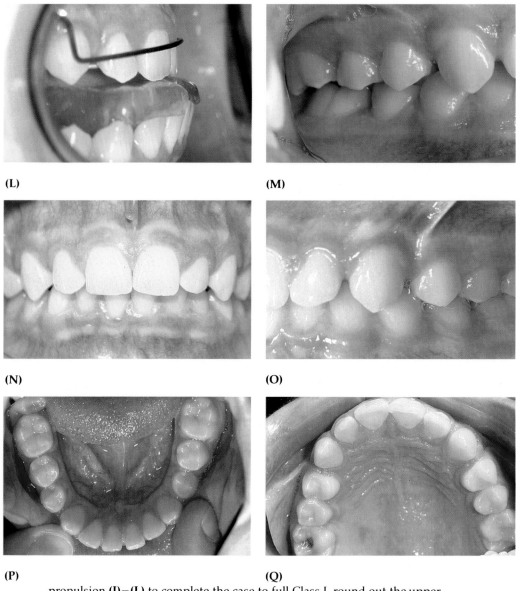

(L)

(M)

(N)

(O)

(P)

(Q)

propulsion **(J)**−**(L)** to complete the case to full Class I, round out the upper
and lower arches, and close contacts (labial bow effect of Bionator) **(M)**−**(Q)**.
Continued use during second Bionator phase of treatment of the midline
screw/Coffin spring combination to further develop arches laterally also aids
in obtaining final, fully rounded arch form. Various cephalometric analyses
reveal full skeletal correction from mandibular retrusive Class II state to Class I
(R), as does clinical observance of the face **(S)**, **(T)**.

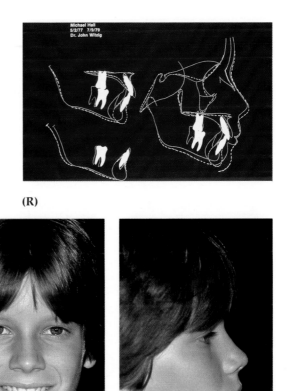

(R)

(S)   (T)

incisal angle and placing the facial surface of the maxillary anteriors within 4 to 5 mm of the A-perpendicular and the facial surface of the lower anteriors within 2 to 3 mm of the A-Pog line, according to McNamara, will produce the desired anterior coupling in about the 130-degree interincisal angle range.

Once Class I skeletal and dental status is attained and the anteriors have been properly coupled the case may be monitored throughout the rest of its growth and development with any additional treatments implemented as necessary. Once given such a proper start the potential reasonably exists for mixed dentition patients to make it the rest of the way on their own.

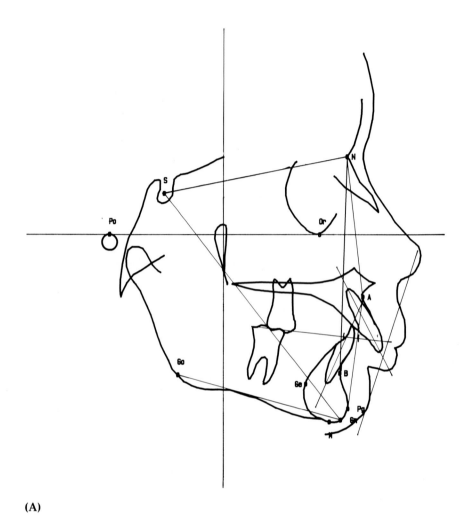

(A)

MODIFIED STEINER ANALYSIS

SKELETAL

MEASUREMENT	NORM	ACTUAL	COMMENT
SNA	80.0° to 84.0°	85.5°	PROGNATHIC MAXILLA
SNB	78.0° to 82.0°	77.0°	RETROGNATHIC MANDIBLE
ANB	0.0° to 4.0°	8.6°	SKELETAL CLASS II
WITS	-3.0mm to 1.0mm	5.8mm	SKELETAL CLASS II
UPPER FACIAL HEIGHT	50.0%	46.6%	
LOWER FACIAL HEIGHT	50.0%	53.4%	
Go-Gn to SN	28.0° to 36.0°	26.2°	TENDENCY FOR INSUFFICIENT VERTICAL DEVELOPMENT
Y-Axis to SN	63.0° to 69.0°	62.4°	COUNTERCLOCKWISE GROWER
			Closed bite tendencies.
OCCL to SN	14.0° to 15.0°	17.2°	ANY CHANGE IN POSTERIOR VERTICAL SUPPORT WILL HAVE A THREE-FOLD PROPORTIONAL CHANGE IN ANTERIOR VERTICAL
Pg to NB	1.5mm to 3.5mm	3.7mm	PLENTY OF BONE STRUCTURE FOR MOVING MANDIBULAR TEETH ANTERIORLY

DENTAL

MEASUREMENT	NORM	ACTUAL	COMMENT
UP1 to NA DIST	4.0mm	5.6mm	
UP1 to NA ANG	20.0° to 24.0°	21.4°	
LOW1 to NB DIST	4.0mm	5.3mm	
LOW1 to NB ANG	23.0° to 27.0°	22.7°	LINGUOVERSION
LOW1 TO UP1	120.0° to140.0°	127.3°	
A-Pg to LOW1	-2.0mm to 3.0mm	-1.3mm	
*6+6 to PTV	13.0mm	17.4mm	

SOFT TISSUE

MEASUREMENT	NORM	ACTUAL	COMMENT
UPPER LIP	0.0mm to 2.0mm	5.8mm	
LOWER LIP	0.0mm to 2.0mm	5.3mm	

Figure 8-2 Pretreatment **(A)** and posttreatment **(B)** Steiner cephalometric analysis of patient in Figure 8-1. Note change in Wits analysis from pretreatment 5.8 mm to posttreatment -2.1 mm and the change in the ANB angle of the Steiner from a pretreatment 8.6 degrees to a posttreatment 3.7 degrees.

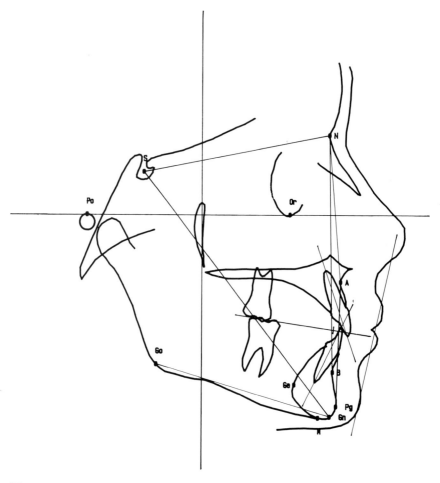

(B)

MODIFIED STEINER ANALYSIS

SKELETAL

MEASUREMENT	NORM	ACTUAL	COMMENT
SNA	80.0° to 84.0°	83.7°	
SNB	78.0° to 82.0°	80.0°	
ANB	0.0° to 4.0°	3.7°	SKELETAL CLASS I
WITS	-3.0mm to 1.0mm	-2.1mm	SKELETAL CLASS I
UPPER FACIAL HEIGHT	50.0%	46.7%	
LOWER FACIAL HEIGHT	50.0%	53.3%	
Go-Gn to SN	28.0° to 36.0°	27.3°	TENDENCY FOR INSUFFICIENT VERTICAL DEVELOPMENT
Y-Axis to SN	63.0° to 69.0°	62.9°	COUNTERCLOCKWISE GROWER Closed bite tendencies.
OCCL to SN	14.0° to 15.0°	19.6°	ANY CHANGE IN POSTERIOR VERTICAL SUPPORT WILL HAVE A THREE-FOLD PROPORTIONAL CHANGE IN ANTERIOR VERTICAL
Pg to NB	1.5mm to 3.5mm	1.2mm	NOT MUCH BONE STRUCTURE FOR MOVING MANDIBULAR TEETH ANTERIORLY

DENTAL

MEASUREMENT	NORM	ACTUAL	COMMENT
UP1 to NA DIST	4.0mm	2.6mm	
UP1 to NA ANG	20.0° to 24.0°	14.4°	LINGUOVERSION
LOW1 to NB DIST	4.0mm	4.0mm	
LOW1 to NB ANG	23.0° to 27.0°	27.7°	BUCCOVERSION
LOW1 TO UP1	120.0° to140.0°	134.2°	
A-Pg to LOW1	-2.0mm to 3.0mm	1.4mm	
6+6 to PTV	15.0mm	17.0mm	

SOFT TISSUE

MEASUREMENT	NORM	ACTUAL	COMMENT
UPPER LIP	0.0mm to 2.0mm	1.1mm	
LOWER LIP	0.0mm to 2.0mm	1.4mm	

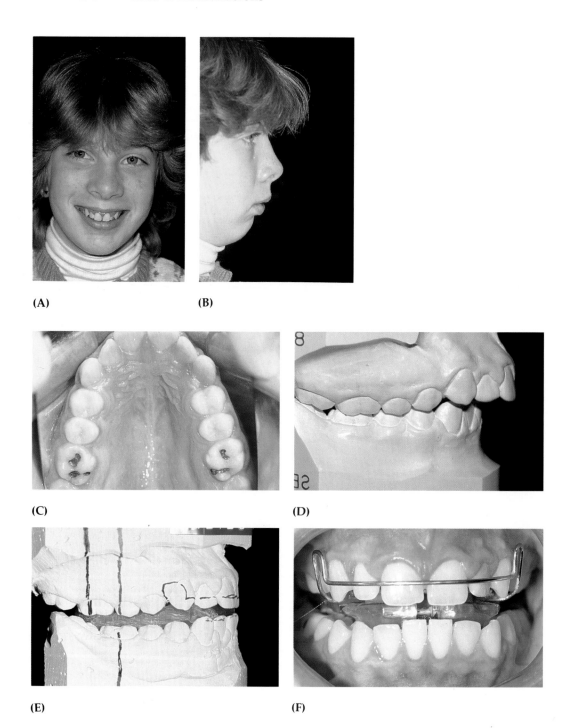

(A)

(B)

(C)

(D)

(E)

(F)

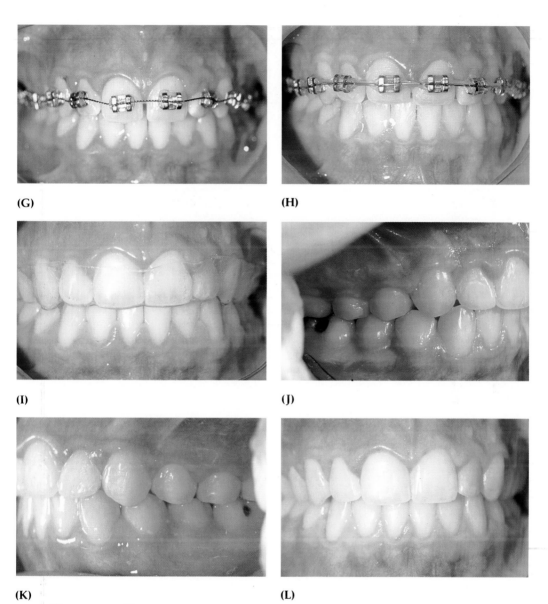

(G)

(H)

(I)

(J)

(K)

(L)

Figure 8–3 Class II, Division 1 (early adult dentition). A girl, aged 12 years, 7 months presented to Dr Witzig's office with a severe skeletal Class II malocclusion and reciprocal clicking in both TMJs. The mandible also locked occasionally. Consultation at another office resulted in an opinion to extract four bicuspids and treat the case using traditional fixed-appliance technique. The mother of the patient refused to submit her child to this treatment because it involved extracting the four bicuspids. Proper treatment for this case involved use of the more advanced philosophical approaches of FJO methodology. Because

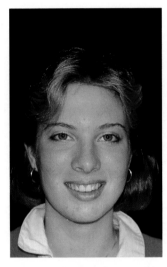 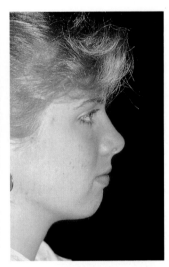

(M)   **(N)**

this was a "high angle" case due to the steep mandibular plane, and the arch form, though symmetrical, was nevertheless still narrow and gothic in shape in the anterior region, the principle of directional decrowding was employed. To expand the arches to traditional arch widths invites relapse, because high-angle cases are usually associated with leptoprosopic facial patterns and narrower overall arch forms. There was also a slight tendency to an open bite in spite of the severe mandibular retrusion. High-angle cases tend to open the bite very quickly when traditional Bionator I or Orthopedic Corrector I technique is used. Therefore, since the arch was not crowded, albeit narrow, and adequate vertical was already present, the first appliance used in this case was the Orthopedic Corrector II. The acrylic pads of this appliance hold the already substantial vertical constant while advancing the mandible. The narrow arches are widened only slightly by expansion of the midline screw and Coffin spring of the appliance so as to avoid any chance of relapse due to overdevelopment laterally (directional decrowding). Note typical Class II retruded facial appearance **(A)**, **(B)**, narrow arch form **(C)**, and severity of overjet, 8.2 mm **(D)**. Construction bite for OC II **(E)**, and insertion of appliance **(F)** is per standard OC II technique. After 12 months of wear, the mandible was fully advanced and final bite closure was effected by extraction of all four second molars, which also aided in preserving slight increases in arch width gained by midline screw and Coffin spring adjustment of the OC II. Straight Wire appliances on uppers only for 9 months **(G)**, **(H)**, followed by Tru-tain retainers **(I)** finishes the case nicely **(J)**−**(L)**. Note full face and improved facial profile **(M)**, **(N)**.

Class II, Division 2 treatment: mixed dentition   Class II, Division 2 treatment in the mixed dentition could almost qualify as the type of malocclusion that should be listed under the "urgency" treatment category. This type of malocclusion is usually accompanied by deep overbite and concomitant orthopedic loss of vertical denoted by the proportionally short ANS-Me LFH. The characteristic high interincisal angle of the upper and lower anteriors along with the crowded out and flared forward upper lateral incisors is a condition that does not usually manifest itself until later in the mixed dentition stage of development. But once it has the chance to fully express itself, the results, especially over the long term, may be potentially devastating to the proper stability, comfort, and function of the TMJs. In the Class II structural relationship the effect of neuromuscular reflexive displacement of the mandible (NRDM) has occurred to such an extent that a full skeletal Class II deficient mandible has resulted. There may even be classic symptoms of TMJ malarthrosis, such as recurrent headaches, facial pain, or facial muscular fatigue upon prolonged chewing (as children of that age are prone to do, especially on things like bubble gum). Pain may also be reported in the cervical area.

Though the face may suffer more in appearance, the joint would probably suffer less in Class II, Division 2, deep bite situations if the mandible were somehow to remain structurally deficient and undersized in its skeletally Class II status. This would at least temporarily allow the lower jaw to be housed within and under the upper dental arch without exerting an excessive strain on the TMJ. However, when the mandible strains to express its full genetic potential for forward growth and attempts to attain full normal structural Class I size, as a surprising number will prove to do, it becomes locked in its arc of closure behind the interfering retroclined upper anteriors, and the extra length must express itself the only way it can, out the back. The longer mandible causes the lower anteriors to strike the lingually locking surfaces of the retroclined Division 2 upper anteriors such that the full arc of closure to maximum interdigitation during occlusion jams the condyle up and back in the TMJ.

Joint problems may often already be present in the mixed dentition stages if mandibular retrusion and loss of vertical are great enough. And the prospects for the patients getting steadily worse as they progress into the full adult dentition are exceedingly great. As with Class 1, Division 2 conditions (which would merely be an earlier variety of the Class II, Division 2 condition that has not had time to come to fruition yet), the case must be "unlocked" first by restoring the interincisal angle of the anterior teeth to its more correct 130-degree range or better before *any* other type of treatment may be initiated, even lateral development. This is why one will occasionally hear such a malocclusion referred to (some-what tongue-in-cheek) as "untreatable," stressing the concept that no

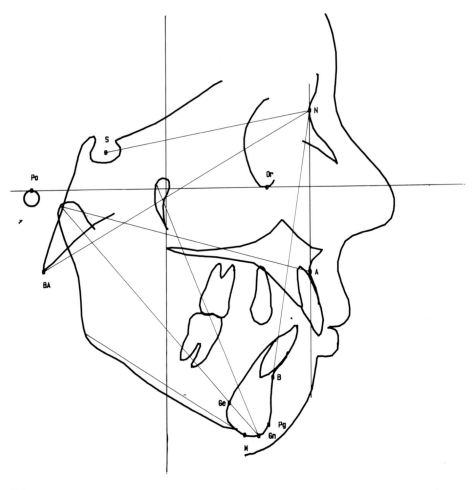

(A)

FUNCTIONAL ORTHOPEDIC ANALYSIS

MEASUREMENT	NORM	:ACTUAL	COMMENT
A. RELATING THE MAXILLA TO THE CRANIAL BASE			
A Pt to N Perp	-1.0mm to 3.0mm	-0.2mm	
B. RELATING THE MANDIBLE TO THE MAXILLA			
Eff. MAXILLA Lgth	***	101.0mm	
Eff. MANDIBLE Lgth	130.5mm to135.5mm	117.4mm	SHORT MANDIBLE
Diff=MAX-MAND Lgth	***	16.4mm	
Lower Facial Ht[Vert Dim]	71.1mm to 76.7mm	76.4mm	
C. RELATING THE UPPER INCISOR TO THE MAXILLA			
Up1 to A Perp	4.0mm to 6.0mm	5.0mm	
D. RELATING THE LOWER INCISOR TO THE MANDIBLE			
Low1 to A-Pg Line	1.0mm to 3.0mm	1.2mm	
E. MANDIBULAR POSITION			
Pg to N Perp	-4.6mm to -0.4mm	-16.5mm	POSSIBLE RETRUSION
F. OTHER USEFUL CEPHALOMETRIC MEASUREMENTS			
SNA	80.0° to 84.0°	79.2°	RETROGNATHIC MAXILLA
SNB	78.0° to 82.0°	71.0°	RETROGNATHIC MANDIBLE
ANB	0.0° to 4.0°	8.2°	SKELETAL CLASS II
Interincisal Angle	120.0° to140.0°	127.7°	
Mandibular Plane Angle	20.0° to 30.0°	30.3°	HIGH VERTICAL DIMENSION
Facial Axis (Ricketts)	86.5° to 93.5°	97.3°	OPEN BITE TENDENCIES
WITS	-2.0mm to 2.0mm	8.0mm	SKELETAL II

Figure 8–4   Pretreatment Functional Orthopedic **(A)** and Bimler **(B)** and posttreatment Functional Orthopedic **(C)** and Bimler **(D)** cephalometric analysis of patient in Figure 8–3. In the pretreatment state this "high-angle" case exhibits a slightly retruded maxilla and a short "effective mandibular length" shown by the Functional Orthopedic analysis. There is also a pre-existing abundance of lower face height, a severe mandibular retrusion, and steep mandibular plane. The SNA and SNB angles are biased by the steep N-S Factor 7 line making the case appear more retruded in the maxilla and mandible than it may be, although the mandible is, in fact, quite retruded. The abundant pretreatment vertical uncovers the A-B difference in the Steiner ANB angle as an excessive bony overjet due to mandibular retrusion. This is especially clear in the pretreatment A-B distance of 14.7 mm in the Bimler. Note also the exceptionally long T-TM distance. The high gonial angle inspite of the hyperflexion of Factor 8 of the Bimler contributes to the steep Factor 3 in this "high-angle" case.

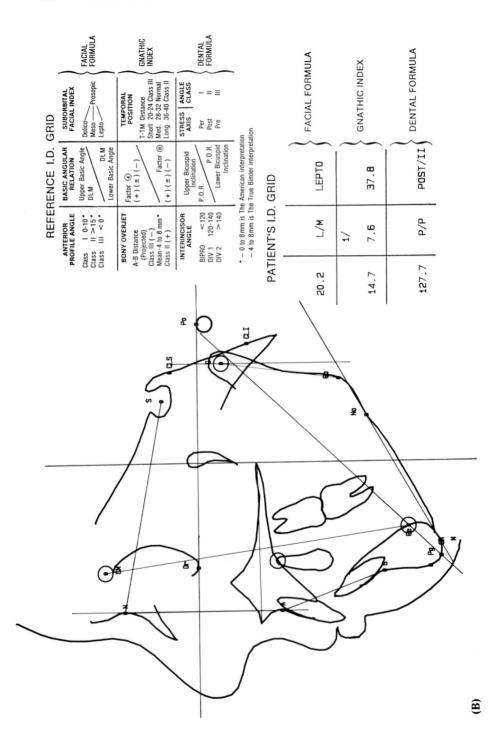

REFERENCE I.D. GRID

ANTERIOR PROFILE ANGLE	BASIC ANGULAR RELATION	SUBORBITAL FACIAL INDEX	FACIAL FORMULA
Class I 0-10°	Upper Basic Angle DLM	Dolico ———	
Class II >15°		Meso ——— Prosopic	
Class III < 0°	DLM Lower Basic Angle	Lepto ———	

BONY OVERJET		TEMPORAL POSITION	GNATHIC INDEX
A-B Distance (Projected)	Factor Ⓐ (+) (±) (−)	Factor Ⓑ (+) (±) (−)	T-TM Distance Short 20-24 Class III Med. 28-32 Normal Long 36-40 Class II
Class III (−)			
Mean-4 to 8 mm •			
Class II (+)			

INTERINCISOR ANGLE			STRESS AXIS	ANGLE CLASS	DENTAL FORMULA
BIPRO <120	Upper Bicuspid Inclination	P.O.R.	Per	I	
DIV 1 120-140	P.O.R.	Lower Bicuspid Inclination	Post	II	
DIV 2 >140			Pre	III	

* − 0 to 8 mm is The American interpretation
− 4 to 8mm is The True Bimler interpretation

PATIENT'S I.D. GRID

FACIAL FORMULA		
20.2	L/M	LEPTO

GNATHIC INDEX		
	1/	
14.7	7.6	37.8

DENTAL FORMULA		
127.7	P/P	POST/II

(B)

MODIFIED BIMLER ANALYSIS

MEASUREMENT	NORM	ACTUAL	COMMENT
FACTOR 1:			
UPPER PROFILE ANGLE N TO A	-1.0° to 1.0°	-0.2°	ORTHOGNATHIC
FACTOR 2:			
LOWER PROFILE ANGLE AB TO VERT		20.2°	
ANTERIOR PROFILE ANGLE (F1+F2)	0.0° to 10.0°	20.0°	SKELETAL CLASS II ()16 MAY INDICATE SURGERY)
FACTOR 3:			
MANDIBULAR INCLINATION		30.5°	
FACTOR 4:			
MAXILLARY INCLINATION ANS-PNS	-3.0° to 3.0°	1.0°	
LOWER BASIC ANGLE (F3-F4)	15.0° to 30.0°	29.5°	BALANCED GROWTH (MESO)
ALVEOLAR HEIGHT		6.5mm	
FACTOR 5:			
CLIVUS INCLINATION	60.0° to 70.0°	70.3°	STEEP POSTERIOR CRANIAL BASE
UPPER BASIC ANGLE (F5+F4)	60.0° to 70.0°	71.4°	LEPTO PROSOPIC
FACIAL HARMONY		L/M	CLOSED VERTICAL: L/D
SUBORBITAL FACIAL INDEX (A1M/AC)	1.00 to 1.05	1.04	MEDIUM
FACTOR 6:			
STRESS AXIS		119.8mm	CLASS II (POST)
FACTOR 7:			
N-S INCLINATION		10.6°	
FACTOR 8:			
MANDIBULAR FLEXION	-5.0° to 5.0°	7.6°	HYPERFLEXION - UNDER-DEVELOPMENT OF MIDDLE FACE; FAVORABLE IN CLASS III CASES; IT WILL BE REDUCED IN BITE OPENING IN TREATMENT

LINEAR MEASUREMENTS

MAXILLA LENGTH (AT)		56.3mm	
TEMPORAL POSITION (T-TM)	23.0mm to 32.0mm	37.8mm	EXTREMELY LONG (CLASS II)
OVERJET OF BONY BASES (A1-B1)		14.7mm	
MANDIBULAR LENGTH (B1-TM)		79.4mm	
MANDIBULAR DIAGONAL		116.3mm	
MANDIBULAR HEIGHT		94.1mm	
HORIZONTAL TOTAL		94.1mm	

ANGLES

UPPER INCISAL ANGLE		105.6°	
LOWER INCISAL ANGLE		126.7°	
INTERINCISAL ANGLE	120.0° to 140.0°	127.7°	
GONIAL ANGLE	105.0° to 120.0°	128.1°	LEPTOGNATHIC
IMPA		96.2°	

The posttreatment tracings reveal a slight retrusion of A-point which could be due to the changes in the location of nasion due to forward growth and/or the headgear effect of OC2. The slight increase in Factor 7 angulation, if accurate, would tend to support a change in nasion upward and forward. However, note how the Bimler Facial Angle reduction, advancement of the Stress Axis Factor 6 line to near apicale, reduction of the A-B distance, and increase in the maxillomandibular differential, all indicate a full-scale mandibular advancement and correction of the case from skeletal Class II to Class I. The advancement of

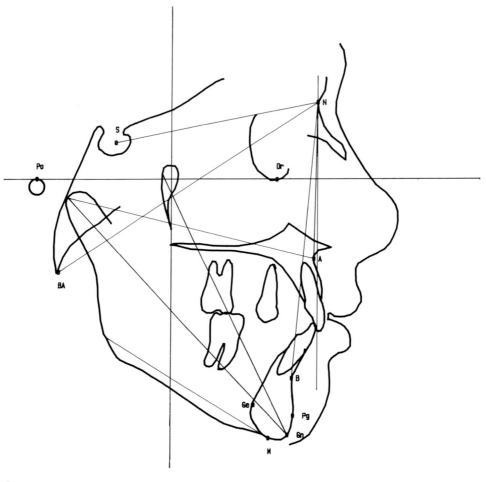

(C)

FUNCTIONAL ORTHOPEDIC ANALYSIS

MEASUREMENT	NORM	ACTUAL	COMMENT
A. RELATING THE MAXILLA TO THE CRANIAL BASE			
A Pt to N Perp	-1.0mm to 3.0mm	-1.5mm	UNDERDEVELOPED PRE-MAXILLA
B. RELATING THE MANDIBLE TO THE MAXILLA			
Eff. MAXILLA Lgth	***	99.0mm	
Eff. MANDIBLE Lgth	127.2mm to 132.2mm	124.7mm	SHORT MANDIBLE
Diff=MAX-MAND Lgth	***	24.2mm	
Lower Facial Ht[Vert Dim]	69.7mm to 75.0mm	76.9mm	LONG VERTICAL DIMENSION
C. RELATING THE UPPER INCISOR TO THE MAXILLA			
Up1 to A Perp	4.0mm to 6.0mm	4.4mm	
D. RELATING THE LOWER INCISOR TO THE MANDIBLE			
Low1 to A-Pg Line	1.0mm to 3.0mm	4.4mm	
E. MANDIBULAR POSITION			
Pg to N Perp	-3.9mm to 0.9mm	-9.4mm	POSSIBLE RETRUSION
F. OTHER USEFUL CEPHALOMETRIC MEASUREMENTS			
SNA	80.0° to 84.0°	77.5°	RETROGNATHIC MAXILLA
SNB	78.0° to 82.0°	73.5°	RETROGNATHIC MANDIBLE
ANB	0.0° to 4.0°	4.0°	SKELETAL CLASS I
Interincisal Angle	120.0° to 140.0°	132.3°	
Mandibular Plane Angle	20.0° to 30.0°	27.5°	
Facial Axis (Ricketts)	86.5° to 93.5°	96.2°	OPEN BITE TENDENCIES
WITS	-2.0mm to 2.0mm	1.6mm	SKELETAL CLASS I

pogonion as shown in the Functional Orthopedic analysis as well as a reduction in the "Wits" value also corroborate this despite other parameters that numerically indicate the case could still be a borderline Class II. The long T-TM distance no doubt had some effect on this.

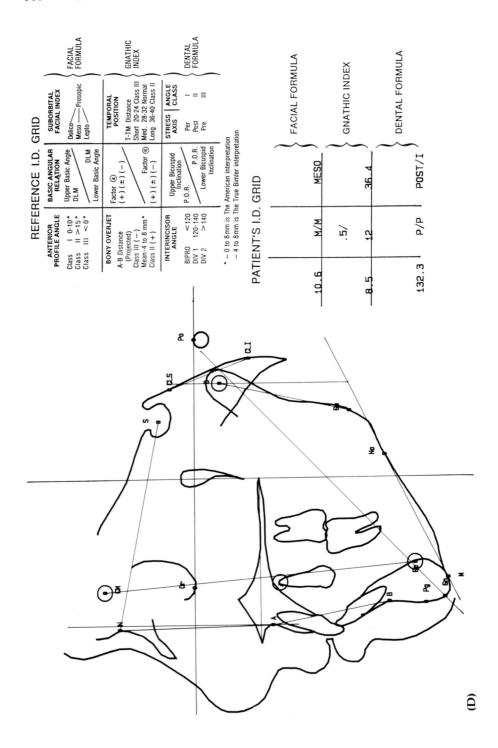

(D)

MODIFIED   BIMLER   ANALYSIS

MEASUREMENT	NORM	ACTUAL	COMMENT

FACTOR 1:
UPPER PROFILE ANGLE N TO A   -1.0° to 1.0°   -1.4° RETROGNATHIC

FACTOR 2:
LOWER PROFILE ANGLE AB TO VERT   10.6°

ANTERIOR PROFILE ANGLE (F1+F2)   0.0° to 10.0°   9.1° SKELETAL CLASS I

FACTOR 3:
MANDIBULAR INCLINATION   27.5°

FACTOR 4:
MAXILLARY INCLINATION ANS-PNS   -3.0° to 3.0°   0.5°

LOWER BASIC ANGLE (F3-F4)   15.0° to 30.0°   27.1° BALANCED GROWTH (MESO)

ALVEOLAR HEIGHT   5.8mm

FACTOR 5:
CLIVUS INCLINATION   60.0° to 70.0°   68.9° MEDIUM POSTERIOR CRANIAL
                                                             BASE

UPPER BASIC ANGLE (F5+F4)   60.0° to 70.0°   69.4° MESO PROSOPIC

FACIAL HARMONY   M/M   NEUTRAL (L/L, M/M, D/D)

SUBORBITAL FACIAL INDEX (A1M/AC) 1.00 to 1.05   1.09   LONG FACE

FACTOR 6:
STRESS AXIS   121.6mm CLASS II (POST)

FACTOR 7:
N-S INCLINATION   11.1°

FACTOR 8:
MANDIBULAR FLEXION   -5.0° to 5.0°   12.0° HYPERFLEXION - UNDER-
                                                             DEVELOPMENT OF MIDDLE FACE;
                                                             FAVORABLE IN CLASS III
                                                             CASES; IT WILL BE REDUCED
                                                             IN BITE OPENING IN TREATMENT

LINEAR MEASUREMENTS
MAXILLA LENGTH (AT)   55.6mm
TEMPORAL POSITION (T-TM)   23.0mm to 32.0mm   36.4mm EXTREMELY LONG (CLASS II)
OVERJET OF BONY BASES (A1-B1)   8.5mm
MANDIBULAR LENGTH (B1-TM)   83.5mm
MANDIBULAR DIAGONAL   123.5mm
MANDIBULAR HEIGHT   98.5mm
HORIZONTAL TOTAL   92.0mm

ANGLES
UPPER INCISAL ANGLE   102.9°
LOWER INCISAL ANGLE   124.8°
INTERINCISAL ANGLE   120.0° to 140.0°   132.3°
GONIAL ANGLE   105.0° to 120.0°   129.6° LEPTOGNATHIC
IMPA   97.3°

other form of treatment should be started until the Division 2 status of the anterior teeth has been corrected. Bicuspid extraction in these cases is universally and totally contraindicated, because the results to both the face and joint, regardless of the type of treatment employed, would be disastrous. Enlargement of the arches, not constriction, is needed. This again implies the use of the Sagittal II, or, if conditions warrant, the Brehm Utility Arches may also be used.

The Sagittal II is employed leaving the upper second molars intact to serve as anchorage. The appliance can be used to both develop the premaxilla forward orthopedically if needed or, by means of appropriate adjustments to the appliance, as discussed previously, advance offending teeth to their proper proclination by imparting labial crown torque to them. Once attained, the proper interincisal angle relationship is retained by use of upper and lower Sagittals if need be for a period of several months before further treatment is begun. This allows for much needed time for the teeth to stabilize and let the muscle environment adapt to the teeth in their new position.

Premature withdrawal of the appliance without the benefit of alternative forms of retention leaves the teeth too "green" in their sockets, which consequently invites relapse in a lingual direction once the appliance is removed in favor of some other device such as a Bionator. Another reason overcorrection is favored is that Bionators have a natural tendency to bring the upper anteriors down and in lingually. Once the Division 2 is converted to an overcorrected Division 1, if the arches need lateral development, which is rare, it may be instituted by the maxillary Schwarz, which also acts as a retainer during treatment to hold the recently advanced upper centrals forward during the lateral development of the arch.

Upper Transverse appliances may be used in a similar manner if TMJ symptoms are still present. Not much concern is given to slight-to-moderate crowding in the mandibular area, since this may be corrected with the activation of the midline screw of the Bionator or again the lower Brehm Utility Arch prior to institution of Bionator therapy. Only if the Pont "W" index is grossly deficient need the lower arch be prepared also with the Jackson. Once the arches have been properly prepared in this manner, and the case does not "spontaneously" correct, indicating true vertical and mandibular deficiences, the Bionator may be inserted to attain Class I dental and skeletal status and open the vertical to the required amount. (However, since the case is in the mixed dentition, this may not necessarily mean treating to traditional Angle Class I molar interdigitation, since the "E's" may still be present. Using cephalometrics to check structure and the concepts of the flush terminal plane to aid in dental alignment, the case may not need quite the amount of mandibular skeletal advancement as the traditional alignment of the molars in Angle Class I relationship might indicate. Although a slight excess of protrusion of the uppers is *well tolerated* by both the face and the TMJs, the difference would only be the leeway space, ie, not much.) Also, it must be remembered that relative to lateral development, the case may often be directly advanced from the Sagittal II appliance (after adequate overcorrection or retention) to the Bionator, since Class II, Division 2 upper arches are by their very nature seldom if ever collapsed in laterally. The Division 2 aspect of the upper arch form seems to act in some way as an inhibitor to excessive narrowness of the upper arch. Conversely, if the upper arch is quite narrow, it more often than not seems to force the anteriors labially rather than lingually, resulting in a Division 1 rather than a Division 2 situation.

The tongue in both resting and swallowing posture is often the culprit in the production of the narrow arch with its flared forward anterior teeth in Division 1 angulation. Other factors may contribute also. But there is no doubt as to what is happening muscularly in the Division 2 case. The power of the perioral musculature is far greater than the counteracting intraoral forces of the tongue, and the shortening of the arch and retroclination of the anteriors result as a product of the hypertonic external musculature having its way. The forces pushing in from the front are greater than the forces pushing out from behind. The teeth show the effect. This hypertonic perioral muscle activity may still attempt to exert itself even after the maxillary anteriors have been corrected to the proper interincisal angle, since the muscles may not have had time to accommodate to nor be retrained by the new dental environment. And since the Bionator is often the second appliance in line in the treatment plan of severe Class II, Division 2 cases, the clinician must make sure that the lingual retention wire is constructed properly so as to contact the *lingual* surfaces of the crowns of the upper anterior teeth, which have just been torqued labially, so as to adequately retain them in their advanced or even slightly overcorrected position.

If there is any doubt that the contact is complete, the wire may be cut in the middle and bent slightly forward to ensure proper contact. The labial guide bow of the Bionator is kept off the upper anterior teeth for the first 3 months of wear to take advantage of the distal drive effect on the maxillary first molars by muscle tension on the appliance. This necessitates periodically adjusting the lingual retention wire in such a manner described, since the appliance drifts distally slightly during the first 3 months, pulling the lingual retention wire with it as it goes. Left unadjusted during these changes so as to be in full contact with the recently proclined upper anteriors, these teeth have an even more intensified tendency to relapse lingually without adequate tension being placed on them by the lingual wire. In anticipation of such circumstances, one may wish to substitute lap springs in place of the individual heavier lingual wire. These may be adjusted individually to contact the anterior teeth in the cingulum area. Remember, active forces are not required, merely firm but passive contact. This is one of the reasons a period of retention, wearing the Sagittal II as its own retainer without turning the screws, serves to prepare the upper arch better to absorb the effects of the Bionator and allows more time for muscular readaptation and tooth/socket stabilization.

Special cases   There may occur a combination of circumstances in the Class II mixed dentition stage, or for that matter in any stage of development, that offer peculiar problems to the clinician attempting to devise a treatment plan. One example would be the case where, due to a variety of factors, the first permanent molars are in a reasonably normal Class II distocclusion, but where the premaxilla is *so* protrusive orthopedically that anterior coupling with Bionator technique translating the mandible forward would result in an iatrogenic bimaxillary protrusion and dental Class III molars. In other words, simple advancement of the mandible to its cephalometrically correct orthopedic position would still leave the overjet so great that upper and lower anterior coupling would still be impossible.

Applying an improperly anchored Straight Wire appliance to the upper arch and attempting to consolidate it with elastics will only pull the upper first molars forward incorrectly, "burning anchorage" as it does and generating a pseudo-dental Class II all over again. This then requires the aforementioned arch retraction methods with ligated molars, bicuspids, and cuspids for either symmetrical arch retraction (arch wire with hooks distal to laterals) or asymmetrical arch retraction (power chain cuspid-to-cuspid) retraction, or maybe even the possibility of external or extraoral force in the form of headgear to properly anchor the upper first molars if the retraction distances are inordinately large. This may also be accomplished by the use of the old Oliver or newer Truitt-style internal Class II labial bow, but this again is predicated upon totally adult dentition so that Class II mechanics may be employed.

It may also be determined that for a special case interceptive treatment may be by far the best choice, as waiting for the full adult dentition to erupt would only make the task of correction more difficult. Such conditions backed up with sound diagnostic data derived from clinical, cephalometric, and model analyses might indicate the need for services that are not within the spectrum of what the FJO series of appliances and techniques are capable of delivering. The FJO system is not all-inclusive as far as the number of malocclusions that it is capable of treating; no system is. But one of the ways to manage this system best is to know its limits and avoid forcing it to attempt correct completion of treatments for which none of its components were originally designed. When the diagnosis clearly indicates a technique is needed for the case which is outside the domain of the FJO system as we have discussed it, the clinician should be prepared to either provide that extraneous technique or refer the patient to another practitioner whose talents and training qualify him to deliver it. Special cases require specialized techniques and should receive special attention to ensure that the patients receive what is best for them. The patient should not be made to fit the demands and the needs of the available techniques. The techniques should be selected and made available, one way or another, to fit the demands and needs of the patient. Fortunately, the number of malocclusions or maxillofacial developmental aberrations that fall outside the rather broad treatment limits of the FJO family of therapeutic methods are rare. But they do exist, and when periodically discovered by the clinician they should be recognized for what they are, and given the appropriate consideration that is their due and should not be relegated to the servitude of an intentionally myopic diagnostic eye and prejudiced treatment-planning heart.

Class II, Division 3: excessive maxillomandibular dental protrusion   Occasionally, one will be confronted with a case in the Class II mixed dentition that is so protrusive as far as upper and lower anterior labial crown torque is concerned that substitution of a lower Schwarz plate for the conventional lower Jackson are made. When the interincisal angle is in the 120-degree range or less, both upper and lower anterior teeth are tipped labially too far. Such conditions have only recently been dubbed "Division 3" designations. The distortion of the dental arch in this case usually brings with it a narrowing of the arch posteriorly. Hence, upper Schwarz plate treatment to widen the maxillary dental arch and retract the maxillary anteriors by means of the labial bow is indicated. But on the lower arch the mandibular incisors are also tipped too far labially and need to be retracted and uprighted. Since the lower Jackson cannot work at all with a labial bow, the lower Schwarz is substituted in its place. As the midline expansion screw is activated, the tension in the labial bow may be taken advantage of to apply constant pressure to the lower anteriors tipping them back lingually to their normal posture. The acrylic lingual to the cingula of the teeth must be removed so that the teeth may be properly retracted. The retraction of these upper and lower teeth to a more vertical inclination automatically deepens the bite anteriorly. As the upper and lower incisors move (tip) lingually to the proper interincisal angle relationship, the vertical overbite will become greater and greater as the uppers overlap farther and farther down the facial surface of the lowers as the interincisal angle is increased. Once retracted, the case may be completed to proper vertical, through posterior tooth eruption, with the Bionator. During the Bionator phase of treatment, one must not only advance the mandible from Class II to Class I and open the vertical, but also express concern for the activity of the tongue.

Cases of this degree of anterior protrusion of anterior teeth in the Division 3 category must obviously have some etiological agent responsible for the very low interincisal angle. It is often the tongue. Even if one does not suspect such, it would do well to assume so and treat the case similar to those of anterior open bite associated with tongue thrust, not in the selection of the Bionator II necessarily, but rather in the way the type of Bionator selected to finish the case is adjusted. Cutting the lingual retention wire at its midpoint and bending it posteriorly at the end of its cut tips and instituting swallowing exercises nightly with the appliance in place should be given serious consideration in Class II, Division 3 cases. The Bionator I is used in the conventional manner if both mandibular advancement *and* vertical are needed, or the Bionator III may be used if only the mandibular advancement is needed and the vertical is already satisfactory. But this is quite rare, since the anterior overbite almost always seems to be excessive once the protruded upper and lower incisors are retracted by either active plates or fixed appliances to their more correct upright position.

In Class II, Division 3 situations in the mixed dentition, arch length and crowding are never the problem. Arch width, arch-to-arch alignment, and extremely low or acute anterior interincisal angle problems dominate. One must also always remember to keep an eye out for improper muscle function, ie, the tongue.

CLASS II PERMANENT DENTITION

It is the Class II malocclusion in the permanent dentition that allows the practitioner the fullest variety of choices of appliances and techniques for correction and treatment of the problem. Not only are the Crozat and full-arch Straight Wire appliances now available, as they are seldom used in the mixed dentition, but also the techniques of Class II mechanics and the use of the Class II internal labial bow as additional adjuncts to adult dentition fixed appliance therapy are available. But one thing that treatment for the adult dentition stage of Class II malocclusions has in common with its mixed dentition counterpart is that when the orthopedic aspects of the case are indeed actually in a full structural Class II situation, the mandible must be likewise translated with the Bionator to its correct skeletal Class I relationship in the conventional manner. The old nemesis of both bone and musculature deficiences must still be directly addressed. The preliminary treatments of arch preparation and the final phases of arch perfecting follow similar patterns of appliance selection and sequencing. There may be some slight variance in the order in which they may be performed in certain instances as opposed to mixed dentition treatment, but other than that, the philosophies behind the orthopedic and orthodontic development of the case are the same. Address the patient's needs. Balance and align the bones and teeth in a coordinated effort that gives the patient the best possible function and esthetics.

Using cephalometric proportional balance as a guide for the orthopedics and Andrews' six keys to occlusion as a guide to the orthodontics, we have a clear guide to lofty treatment goals. We also know that seldom will we ever attain perfection. But we are encouraged by the fact that we now have the treatment methods available to come closer to perfection than we ever have. Our standards may be justifiably high because of the capabilities of our appliances and the power of our knowledge.

The inculcation of these methods in this review may verge at this point on the tedious, but the importance of developing a balanced, esthetic, and functional occlusion in a balanced, orthopedically proportional set of jaws governed by healthy, unstrained, uncompressed TMJs is a total treatment goal, the importance of which cannot be overstressed. The patients must be assured of our desire and determination to attain these goals while under our care. For if not, and it were within our powers to deliver such, they will have been deprived of the total patient care that is rightfully theirs. By failing to deliver such a standard of care, we incur the responsibility of having possibly produced a compromised or less than complete case. But taking the total aspects of the patient's condition—the face, teeth, jaws, and TMJ—into consideration, and addressing each of them according to its requisites with the appropriate techniques in our treatment plan, we ensure that our patients will receive all that is best for them under the prevailing conditions.

The FJO system of therapeutics has the power to treat each of these aspects in a total patient care fashion, especially in the Class II permanent dentition type of malocclusion where the treatment system potential may be executed to its fullest. By employing such a system, the clinician exhibits his concern and awareness of these factors and his desire for a more comprehensive approach to what the Class II malocclusion represents in the patient. For assuming this posture, regardless of the methods by which he came to it, he is to be commended. For as the English poet Edward Young so aptly wrote nearly 300 years ago, "who does the best his circumstance allows, does well, acts nobly, angels could do no more."

From clinical examination and model analysis we may determine if the molars and cuspids are both in dental Class II relationships or if one or the other may be still in Class I due to crowding, etc. Generally, all four reference teeth will be in dental Class II. Only rarely will lower bicuspids be so crowded out that a lower molar has drifted forward enough to be in Class I while the cuspids are still Class II. This could be a tip-off that molar distalization is needed, ie, a pseudo-Class I.

The cephalometric indications of the Class II malocclusion in the permanent dentition are similar to those for the younger patient still in the mixed dentition Class II stage, and vary only in degree. The Wits will show the usual separation of AO and BO perpendiculars. As far as the Steiner goes, if the S-N line is near 7 degrees to FH, and if the vertical is not at either of the two extremes of being too open or too closed, the ANB angle will be larger than the ideal 2 degrees. But again neither of these analyses divulges which component, maxilla or mandible, is errant. However, Sassouni, Bowbeer, Lynn, McNamara, and Bimler become quite definitive here, each in his own way.

From the McNamara we may analyze the position of A-point relative to the N-perpendicular to judge the degree of protrusion of the maxilla. A true maxillary protrusion on a structural basis of any great extent will be found to be relatively rare. We also may see from the analysis of Pog relative to the N-perpendicular the degree of the mandibular deficiency. In the mixed dentition Pog may often be seen quite far back from the N-perpendicular due to the mandible's natural tendency to lag slightly in growth behind that of the maxilla. Its normal range in the average 9-year-old is −8 to −4 mm from N-perpendicular. However, in the adult female or medium-sized person, it should lie only −4 to 0 mm from the line. The adult male or large-sized person has Pog in a range from −2 to +2 mm to the N-perpendicular. Thus a teenage boy of average stature with a Pog to N-perpendicular linear distance of −4 mm might not be as pronounced a Class II skeletally as the reading might lead one to believe, simply because (1) a young teenage boy of average stature can be considered as a medium-sized person, and (2) the prominence (or lack thereof) of the bony chin button may have some bearing on the interpretation of the case. Since all growth might not be complete yet and since the patient is male, it would be hoped that mandibular growth would cause the mandible to "catch up" to the −2 to +2 mm range in this case by fully mature adulthood.

At present, in this example more information would be useful in deciding the skeletal status of the case. We also have the effective lengths of the maxilla and mandible to compare. In the true Class II skeletal case, the effective length of the mandible will by necessity always be *proportionally* less than that of the maxilla. The maxillomandibular differential in the average 9-year-old is 20 to 23 mm (effective length of maxilla 85 mm, effective length of mandible 105 to 108 mm). However, in the adult female, the maxillomandibular differential is 26 to 29 mm (effective length of maxilla 94 mm, effective length of mandible 120 to 123 mm). This norm also serves for what McNamara calls a middle-sized person, which just as easily could be a mid-teenage male. For the fully adult male, the differential is 30 to 33 mm (effective length of maxilla 100 mm, effective length of mandible 130 to 133 mm). The advantage of using the maxillomandibular differential is that it represents a proportional difference between the two jaws, regardless of what their specific actual size may be. And with an effective mandibular length sporting a 3-mm range, the differential is limited enough to be fairly useful. But it must be remembered that the maxillomandibular differential alone still does not divulge which of the two jaws is errant. Other components of the analysis must be considered for this information, for the maxillomandibular differential of the McNamara, like the AO-BO relationship of the Wits, and the A-point/B-point relationship of the Basal Arc of the Sassouni, merely expresses the horizontal discrepancy in the alignment of the upper and lower jaws to each other.

To continue our example of a young teenage male with Pog −4 mm to N-perpendicular, the further corroborative evidence of a maxillo-mandibular differential of, say, 26 mm, which is on the low side for a medium-sized person, wouldn't do anything to help make the case appear Class I. But then it wouldn't be all that conclusive for skeletal Class II either, because although the patient in our example is male, and adult males should be 30 to 33 mm, the adolescent status of the patient mitigates this norm somewhat. Yet we still have another parameter left to consult. The consideration of the ANS-Me LFH is also critical to determining the degree of relative mandibular insufficiency. Quite often there is a diminished LFH linearly in structural Class II cases, which is usually observed clinically as deep overbite. This disguises the mandible into appearing less structurally Class II than it really might be because as the mandible rotates to an overclosed position, B-point, Pog, Me, and the entire mandibular symphysis are brought by the act of rotation more forward relative to the horizontal.

To return to our example of a young teenage male with a maxillo-mandibular differential of 26 mm and a Pog to N-perpendicular distance of −4 mm, if we give him an ANS-Me LFH of, say, 60 mm, we have the clue that will give the answer to how to classify just such a case. As previously stated in the discussion of the McNamara analysis, a general rule of thumb assumes that for every millimeter of vertical distance that the bite is *closed*, the mandibular symphysis (and all its landmarks) moves *forward* approximately the same distance due to the path of arc of rotation of the mandible. Conversely, for every millimeter that the bite is *opened*, the mandibular symphysis "autorotates" approximately 1 mm *backward*. Thus our classification puzzle of the above example is solved. With a 60-mm ANS-Me LFH, the case is obviously overclosed in a deep bite situation. If the bite is opened to even the 66-mm level, which only represents the low-end range for vertical for females and medium-sized persons (something our young teenage male patient of this example won't be for long), the autorotational effect of the symphysis moving posteriorly 6 mm, due to the arc of rotation of the mandible, puts Pog −10 mm from the N-perpendicular, an indisputable skeletal Class II for any type of individual!

From the Sassouni, the first thing that will be noticed is that B-point falls posterior to the Basal Arc in the adult skeletal Class II mandibular retrusion and usually by more than just a millimeter or two. A 3-mm differential is the accepted limit to differentiate between Class I and Class II. This will also be corroborated by the location of Pog, which will be found to be posterior to the Anterior Arc. However, a wealth of detailed analytical information is available relative to the skeletal status from the Sassouni. The location of B-point may deceivingly fall on or very near the Basal (A-point) Arc; yet the case can still be a full skeletal Class II. This situation occurs when A-point itself is retruded. This would result in ANS falling posterior to the Anterior Arc, thus by default generating its own ANS Arc. In such circumstances, Pog could very well be on or near the ANS Arc, and B-point could be on or near the Basal Arc, indicating the mandible is in a seemingly skeletal Class I relationship to the maxilla but only a skeletal Class II relationship to the cranial base, as evidenced by the appearance of the ANS Arc in the first place. The distance from the ANS Arc to the Anterior Arc indicates the degree of retrusion of the maxilla. Stretching terminology a bit, it is as if the maxilla itself is "skeletally Class II" to the cranial base. This is why seeming skeletal Class I cases can in fact be TMJ cases with retruded mandibles and posteriorly displaced condyles. The retruded maxilla deceptively camouflages the case into merely appearing Class I to the naked eye.

The eye of cephalometrics sees deeper. The location of Go with respect to the Posterior Arc is also important. Gonion in the Sassouni is "constructed" or "cephalometric gonion," ie, the intersection of the mandibular plane with the ramal line; therefore, it is a space mark. It should fall on or very near the Posterior Arc at age 12. If the maxilla is properly positioned with ANS on the Anterior Arc, and the mandible is proper in size but merely bodily retruded, cephalometric Go will be displaced posteriorly past the Posterior Arc by the same distance that Pog is displaced posteriorly to the Anterior Arc, and also by the amount B-point is displaced past the Basal Arc. However, this is for the 12-year-old. Gonion moves posteriorly as the individual grows older. In 12-year-olds Go and sella posterior (Sp) should fall on the Posterior Arc, and N and Pog should fall on the Anterior Arc. Therefore at age 12, the corpus length of the mandible equals the cranial base. At age 16, Go should be found 4 mm posterior to the Posterior Arc in males. At adulthood it should be 6 mm behind the Posterior Arc in males but only 4 mm behind the Posterior Arc in females. If the distances that Pog and Go are displaced posteriorly from their respective reference arcs are uneven and the Pog/Anterior Arc distance is the greater of the two, it indicates that the mandible is not only displaced posteriorly but it is also underdeveloped anteriorly. Should Go fall in its relatively age-related correct place but Pog be posterior to the Anterior Arc, the mandible is more likely to be underdeveloped anteriorly. However, it could also be a bodily small mandible that is displaced posteriorly.

The Sassouni is also very helpful with respect to therapeutic correction of the above situations. Obviously, if the maxilla is in the correct location (ANS on the Anterior Arc), and the mandible is a retruded skeletal Class II (B-point more than 3 mm posterior to the Basal (A-point) Arc), and both Pog and Go are posterior to their respective arcs by the same amount (or if different amounts, Go the larger of the two discrepancies), then simple Bionator-effected advancement of the mandible is indicated after proper *dental* arch preparation. However, if the maxilla is also retruded (ANS posterior to Anterior Arc), it is quite likely a certain amount of *orthopedic* arch preparation will be required prior to Bionator therapy to advance the mandible.

The key to determining which therapeutic approaches will serve best to correct the retruded maxilla (thus exposing the true severity of the skeletal Class II mandibular retrusion for what it is) is in the evaluation of not only ANS relative to the Anterior Arc, but also PNS relative to the cribriform vertical. Should the PNS fall on the cribriform vertical, as it should ideally, and ANS fall short of the Anterior Arc, the maxilla is short anteriorly. Now, if the distance is not far (in the neighborhood of 1 to 2 mm), *and* if the angulation of the maxillary incisor is less than the 110- to 113-degree norm (ie, more acute), Sagittal II technique may be used to impart the necessary labial crown torque to the upper centrals and laterals in an effort to attain the alignment of the incisal edges of the centrals on the Anterior Arc.

Depending on the adjustment process used on the appliance, the age of the patient, and the level of cooperation in appliance wear, efforts may even be made at orthopedically advancing the entire premaxillary area somewhat by opening the premaxillary sutures with the expanding appliance. However, if the angulation of the upper central is beyond the 110- to 113-degree norm, and ANS and the central's incisal edge is still short of the Anterior Arc, which would indicate a small maxilla posteriorly displaced, the previously described technique could torque the upper anteriors too far labially to an unfavorable angulation to the apical base. Therefore, forward-pulling headgear (FPHG) may be needed for a brief period to bring the entire maxilla and upper arch forward en masse.

Another indication for this is if PNS falls posterior to the cribriform vertical. The molars will usually be in conventional Angle Class II dental relationship, and the mesial surface of the maxillary first molar will be distal to a noncorrected Midfacial Arc. Such circumstances are usually indicative of a normal-sized maxilla that is posteriorly displaced. These factors in conjunction with a maxillary central incisor angulation in the 110- to 113-degree range or greater all but mandates FPHG usage prior to Bionator advancement of the mandible. One of the hallmarks of the Sassouni is that alterations of the vertical *do not* affect the relationship of any of the mandibular landmarks with respect to their respective arcs, since the mandible itself rotates on an arc as it opens, keeping approximately the same linear relationship of its parts to the reference arcs of the analysis.

Analyzing the gonial angle by means of the split-gonial-angle method of the Sassouni is also helpful once the maxillary arch and apical base have been both orthodontically and orthopedically prepared for the

Bionator advancement of the mandible out of its skeletal Class II retrusive state. As previously stated, the Sassouni gonial angle is split into upper and lower angle components. The normal range for the upper angle is 52 to 55 degrees, while the normal range for the lower angle is 70 to 75 degrees. The upper angle identifies the slant of the ramus. If it is large, the main component of growth will be forward. If it is small, growth tends to be downward and backward. The lower angle identifies the slant of the corpus of the mandible. If the lower angle is large, the main component of growth tends to be downward. If it is small growth tends to be forward.

This is pertinent to Bionator construction bite registration. Vertical growers usually do better if the construction bite favors the protrusive, since vertical changes come easily enough (or at least relatively easily enough, since increasing vertical is always somewhat difficult, especially compared with mandibular advancement). Conversely, horizontal growers seem to do better if the construction bite favors the greater interocclusal distance (ie, thicker cap on the finished appliance), since horizontal advancement of the mandible is somewhat enhanced by the growth pattern.

Still another factor to consider that comes to us from the Sassouni in diagnosing and planning treatment for the adult Class II case is the position of the lower incisor(s) relative to the functional occlusal plane. If the mandible is Class II and the vertical is diminished relative to the location of Me above the uppermost of the two lower arcs, and the incisal edge of the lower incisor is slightly above the occlusal plane (as it should be), conventional Bionator therapy is employed to advance the mandible and to increase vertical. However, if the vertical is adequate, Me will be between, or maybe even below, the two lower arcs, and if the incisal tip is *on* the occlusal plane, mere Class II advancement with a Bionator II or III is indicated (depending on the location and angulation of the upper incisors). A third possibility exists in which the vertical is already adequate *skeletally* according to the location of Me between the two lower arcs, but the incisal edge of the lower incisors is decidedly above the occlusal plane. This indicates extruded lower incisors and a deep curve of Spee, and serious consideration should be given to sequential lower incisor retrusive mechanics to help lessen the severe *dental* overbite. Once Bionator therapy is instituted to advance the mandible in such a case as this, the vertical should be maintained with the interocclusal acrylic pads of the Bionator II or III.

One of the handy things about Sassouni is its relative ease of determining that a case is only *dentally* Class II while structurally it is *skeletally* Class I. In this instance the maxilla is seen to be correctly positioned with ANS, perhaps even the incisal edge of the maxillary central on the Anterior Arc. The mandible is also seen to be correctly positioned in such a case as Pog and Go are on (or relatively positioned as per age) the Anterior and Posterior Arcs, respectively, while B-point also is on the Basal (A-point) Arc. However, dentally, the first molars are full Angle Class II with the mesial of the maxillary first molar well forward of the Midfacial Arc (and by necessity cuspids are usually blocked out labially). This is due to the forward migration of the maxillary posterior *dental* segments and *does not* require orthopedic realignments of the jaws to correct. The skeletal relationships are truly Class I. This is merely an orthodontic problem. Treatment consists of first acquiring proper maxillary incisor position and angulation, then extracting second molars, and relieving remaining crowding by distalization techniques.

From the Bimler, in addition to the analysis of Anterior Profile Angle and the NS-AT-TTM-DLM Bimler ratios, the Factor 6 Stress Axis may also be considered in diagnosis of skeletal Class II cases now that we have the full complement of adult dentition present. The Stress Axis line will fall posterior to apicale in the POST designation, indicating a mandibular retrusion. The Posterior Profile Angle may also shed some light on the degree of vertical present in the lower face. We know that Bimler defines balanced faces as those where the Upper Basic Angle (UBA) and Lower Basic Angle (LBA) coincide, such as D/D, M/M, or L/L. If a loss of a vertical is present, the discrepancy will be reflected in the lower angle, such as M/D or L/D relationship, or any other combination where the UBA is greater than the LBA. This shows that the volume of lower facial development is deficient relative to the volume represented by the upper angle. An increase in vertical (McNamara's ANS-Me LFH) should bring the face back into properly balanced proportions orthopedically. Analysis of the DLM versus the critical T-TM linear measurements also reveals the degree of success that may be projected during Bionator therapy. (This will be discussed in further detail later.)

Even the soft tissue profile oriented systems like the Bowbeer or Lynn analyses can be used to diagnose the more pronounced skeletal Class II malocclusions. Both use the soft tissue profile of the upper lip as a gauge to the proper position of the maxillary central incisors and apical base. This is important in the evaluation of any Class II condition, since advancement of the mandible out of its Class II retrusive state depends on the maxilla and its dental arch being properly positioned with respect to the cranial base so that the amount of mandibular advancement may be properly gauged.

The Bowbeer analysis specifies that A-point should fall on, or within 3 mm ahead of, the N vertical. However, since there is a possibility of variance in N location, the ultimate criterion is the location of the profile of the upper lip. In the Bowbeer, esthetics takes precedence over orthopedics. Although the criteria for proper upper lip position (hence, indirectly A-point and maxillary incisor position) is for one third to one half the upper lip to be beyond the BNV, this may at times be difficult to decipher from the radiograph. The upper lip angle (ULA) is easier to discern, but its range of 20 to 30 degrees is a bit broad, and hence less specific. The range of the maxillary central incisor tip of 3 to 5 mm ahead of A-point vertical is more specific. The hallmarks of the Class II condition, however, are the mentalis crease (MC) and the location of B-point. In the full skeletal Class II, MC will be clearly seen to fall posterior to the BNV by more than the −2 mm inner limit of the range of ±2 mm from the BNV. B-point will also be seen to be more than its −6 mm limit behind the A-point perpendicular.

From the Lynn analysis it may be seen that the actual pretreatment profile generally falls posterior to the matrix-constructed ideal profile, especially in the lower lip, MC, and soft tissue Pog areas. As with all analysis systems, lack of adequate vertical masks the location of the mandibular symphysis as well as all of its hard and soft tissue landmarks into appearing slightly further forward (and hence less Class II) than they actually are. This would be revealed should the mandible be merely opened to its proper level of cephalometrically balanced vertical without the benefit of also being correspondingly advanced.

An often overlooked, but simple, way of analyzing the degree of loss of vertical in a Class II case is by observing the amount of overbite in the anterior area. Ideally, the upper centrals normally overlap the lowers vertically by no more than about 1−2 mm. Any more overbite at a corrected interincisal angle than this requires the elevation of the occlusal plane posteriorly to obtain correct overbite anteriorly, assuming the anteriors have not supererupted.

Class II, Division 1 Permanent Dentition Treatment

The concept of an "urgency" case in the mixed dentition, especially of posterior crossbite and anterior open bite, stresses the interceptive value of treatment at that time so that patients may avoid worsening the situation as they make the transition to full adult dentition. Treatment, though not necessarily exceptionally difficult in the adolescent dentition, is nevertheless more involved and usually lasts longer once the level of full permanent dentition is achieved (especially for the case suffering from open bite). Hence, once these conditions pass untreated from the extremely bioplastic growth and development stage of the mixed dentition to the more complete adult counterpart, the chance at interceptive orthodontics has been lost. At that point the philosophy of treatment lapses into what may be described as purely corrective. The notion of describing the condition of a malocclusion such as a crossbite or an open bite as an "urgency" case becomes a moot point. Now that the full adult dentition has arrived, the specific aspects of the malocclusion must be enumerated and dealt with by a treatment plan based on current needs. It may be easy to use hindsight and infer what should have been done in an earlier stage of the patient's development, but the task at hand is not concerned with hindsight but with foresight and with what must be done under the present circumstances to correct the conditions for the future.

The most innocuous-appearing Class II, Division 1 malocclusion may be the one where both upper and lower arches are already in fairly good arch form with no posterior crossbites, no major rotations, or otherwise orthodontically compromised teeth, but just a well inter-digitated set of arches in a full skeletal and dental Class II relationship, with possibly some slight degree of crowding in the lower anterior area. Upon first inspection, the clinician may be tempted to conclude that he has one of the Haupl-Andresen "miracle cases," and that treatment will entail nothing more than the sole use of a Bionator. Not so. One must remember to not only determine the status of the arches in relation to one another while the patient occludes in his present situation, but also observe what the jaw relationship will be in the future once the mandible is advanced by the Bionator. This may be easily viewed clinically by having the patient assume the "as if" position, ie, have him advance his own lower jaw to the position that it would occupy after treatment with the molars reasonably aligned in a vertical relationship over one another approximating a dental Class I and the lower incisors near 0 mm overbite. Asking the patient to bite not quite far enough forward to hit end to end in the anteriors usually suffices to accomplish the desired observational alignment.

Once this "as if" position is attained, instruct the patient not to move his teeth at all while you are parting his lips to observe the posterior quadrants. Sometimes it will be observed in this "preview" position that the upper molars are situated too far lingually to allow proper overjet and interdigitation in the desired normal cusp fossa relationship, once their vertical position is enhanced by Bionator treat-ment. This occurs because the maxillary arch in such cases is too narrow. It must be remembered that both arches widen as they go posteriorly, and, when the mandible is advanced, the given portion of cross-sectional width at a specific spot on the mandibular arch is advanced to a position beneath a more anterior, hence, narrower, portion of the upper arch. If this more anterior part of the upper arch is not wide enough to accom-modate the wider and newly advanced more posterior part of the lower arch, it must be corrected prior to Bionator placement by lateral develop-ment techniques. If not, the teeth of the upper arch will be in a posterior crossbite or buccal cusp end-to-end relationship relative to the lower posteriors once they erupt to contact after mandibular advancement with the Bionator.

A Schwarz or Pont analysis of the maxillary arch in such cases should also reveal that arch-widening procedures will be necessary prior to Bionator placement. This assumes the patient to be 13 or 14 years of age when naturally occurring arch width growth generally ceases. The 9-,

10-, or 11-year-old is usually not in the full adult dentition yet, and therefore a somewhat "prorated" value of the Schwarz or Pont indices should be considered. For the 12-year-old, or equivalent to near completion of lateral bone growth, adult values may be used, since by the time the treatment and retention are complete, the age of completion of lateral bone growth will have been reached anyway. The somewhat jocular mental image of the Leghorn Analyzer may also be of some use as a warning of this complication, since the more pointed or gothic the arches are in outline prior to treatment, the more prone they are to exhibit this phenomenon, especially if the mandible is to be translated a considerable distance.

If it is determined that arch widening is needed in either one or both arches of the Class II, Division 1 case, the practitioner has a variety of appliances for such at his disposal. If the case is slightly crowded and the anterior teeth are in reasonable proximity to the 130-degree interincisal angle, the arches may be developed with a Straight Wire appliance (SWA) starting out with either straight twisted wire blanks, Nitinol, or arch-formed twisted arch wires that are *flared to the buccal* posteriorly. The option of starting with SWA as opposed to more conventional archwidening appliances is governed by the degree of arch width deficiency present. If the case is within 3 to 5 mm of Pont's or Schwarz's facial type corrected indices, the SWA may be used, running from the smallest to the largest twisted, round, then final finishing rectangular arch wires. (However, the 5-mm limit is considered by some as still too much for SWA only.) Some only take the case to the largest round wire (say a .020) and proceed directly to the Bionator, since the teeth will shift once again while the vertical is being increased anyway. Once the Bionator phase is complete and the case is back to skeletal and dental Class I, the SWA may be reapplied if necessary to level, align, and rotate for the final perfection as desired. But certainly if it is anticipated that SWA will be used at the completion of treatment for final leveling, alignment, and rotation, the mere efficiency of the treatment plan would dictate that the earlier efforts at the minimal arch width gain be obtained with a more easily initiated removable appliance of some sort. To be quite frank, lateral development was never considered as one of the goals SWA was originally designed to correct and as a result it is not exactly its forte. It will be found in clinical practice that the Bionator is truly the star of Class II orthopedic treatment. But surely as it is, it is also true that indeed the SWA is its leading lady.

However, if the case is narrower than the 5-mm limit, the clinician may choose from a variety of appliances, depending on the symmetry of the arches. If the arches are deficient in width symmetrically across both the bicuspids and the molars they may be developed laterally by either the upper and lower Schwarz appliances or the combination of an upper Transverse and lower Schwarz if TMJ symptoms are present. Upper and

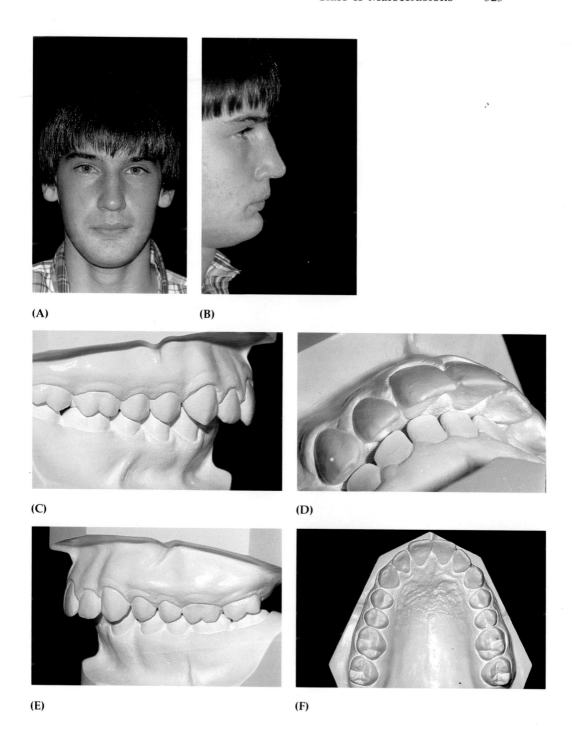

(A)

(B)

(C)

(D)

(E)

(F)

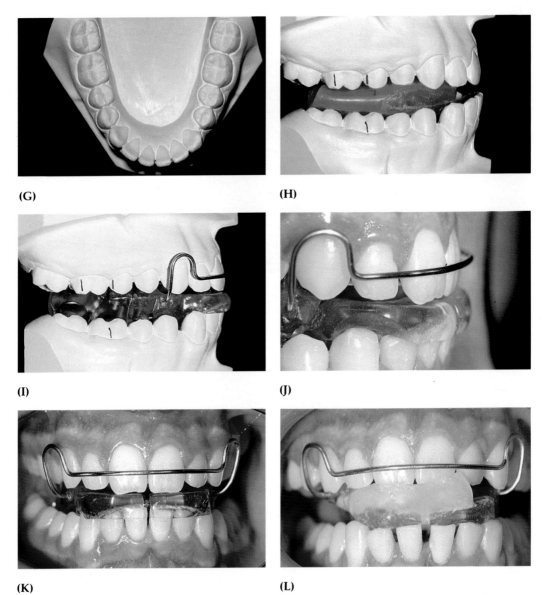

(G)   **(H)**

(I)   **(J)**

(K)   **(L)**

Figure 8—5   Class II, Division 1 (permanent dentition). This patient was treated for approximately 2 years with conventional fixed appliances in another orthodontic office. He was told he needed surgery to advance his mandible to eliminate the remaining deep overbite, skeletal Class II mandibular retrusion problems. He and his parents were also told that no other treatment would be successful at his age of 17 years, 4 months. A second opinion was obtained at Dr Witzig's office and he treated the patient for 1 year with an Orthopedic Corrector I appliance. Observe the results. Note the Class II retrusion of the lower face **(A)**, **(B)**. Also note that the previous 2 years of fixed appliances obtained good arch

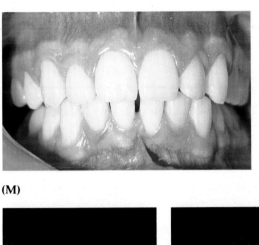

(M)

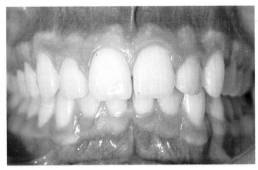

(N)

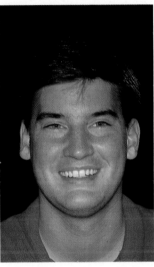

(O)   **(P)**

form but not good arch *alignment* **(C)**−**(G)**. Construction bite was registered in end-to-end position **(H)**, and an Orthopedic Corrector I was constructed that could progressively advance the mandible due to side screw activation **(I)**−**(K)**. Removal of the cap to aid in overjet correction (tipping the lower incisors forward somewhat) and increasing cap thickness to speed posterior eruption, combined with midline screw activation (also to "rock posteriors loose" to speed eruption), are steps carried out in the later stages of treatment **(L)**. Note how slight overcorrection laterally settles in nicely after appliance withdrawal **(M)**, **(N)**. Final facial appearance **(O)**, **(P)** shows improvement of lower facial profile. Final photographs **(N)**−**(P)** were taken 3 years after appliance withdrawal, and clinically it is impossible to manipulate the mandible back to its former skeletal Class II retrusive position!

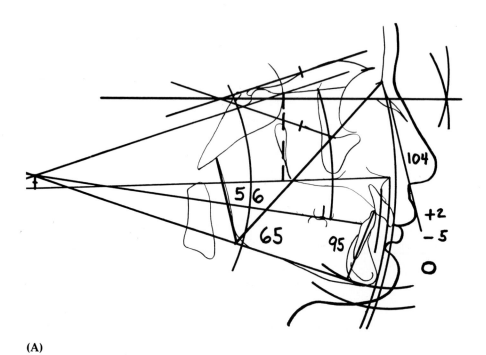

(A)

THE CEPHALOMETRIC "BOTTOM LINE"

CIRCLE THE PROPER RESPONSE

SKELETAL AP: I (II) III IIT IIIT

SKELETAL VERTICAL: N OB (DB) OBT DBT

UPPER INCISOR: (N) P R

LOWER INCISOR: (N) P R

GROWTH DIRECTION: N CW (CCW) CWT CCWT

MAXILLA LENGTH: N L (S) -- (P) A

MAXILLA POSITION: N (P) A

UPPER 6 POSITION: N P (A)

MANDIBLE LENGTH: N L (S) -- (P) A

MANDIBLE POSITION: N (P) A

UPPER LIP ANGLE: (N) P F R

Figure 8–6 Pretreatment Sassouni **(A)** and Steiner **(B)** and posttreatment Sassouni **(C)** and Steiner **(D)** cephalometric analysis of patient in Figure 8–5. Note how in this particular case the change in the Steiner ANB angle from a pretreatment 4.3 degrees to a posttreatment 3.2 degrees is deceptive and *does not* reflect the true amount of mandibular advancement that has taken place. The Wits analysis reflects a change from 7.6 to 0.1 mm. Also note retraction of maxillary incisors due to action of labial bow adjustment and proclination of lower incisors due to trimming of cap of appliance. Patient cooperation in appliance wear was excellent.

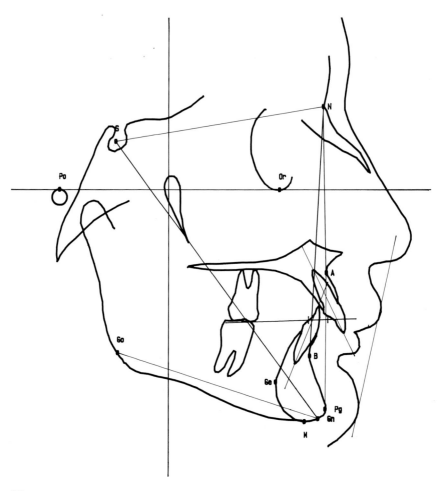

(B)

MODIFIED STEINER ANALYSIS

SKELETAL

MEASUREMENT	NORM	ACTUAL	COMMENT
SNA	80.0° to 84.0°	81.7°	
SNB	78.0° to 82.0°	77.4°	RETROGNATHIC MANDIBLE
ANB	0.0° to 4.0°	4.3°	SKELETAL CLASS II
WITS	-3.0mm to 1.0mm	7.6mm	SKELETAL CLASS II
UPPER FACIAL HEIGHT	45.0%	46.0%	
LOWER FACIAL HEIGHT	55.0%	54.0%	
Go-Gn to SN	28.0° to 36.0°	27.1°	TENDENCY FOR INSUFFICIENT VERTICAL DEVELOPMENT
Y-Axis to SN	63.0° to 69.0°	62.5°	COUNTERCLOCKWISE GROWER
			Closed bite tendencies.
OCCL to SN	14.0° to 15.0°	7.4°	
Pg to NB	1.5mm to 3.5mm	7.3mm	PLENTY OF BONE STRUCTURE FOR MOVING MANDIBULAR TEETH ANTERIORLY

DENTAL

MEASUREMENT	NORM	ACTUAL	COMMENT
UP1 to NA DIST	4.0mm	7.1mm	
UP1 to NA ANG	20.0° to 24.0°	25.3°	BUCCOVERSION
LOW1 to NB DIST	4.0mm	3.2mm	
LOW1 to NB ANG	23.0° to 27.0°	19.5°	LINGUOVERSION
LOW1 TO UP1	120.0° to 140.0°	130.9°	
A-Pg to LOW1	-2.0mm to 3.0mm	-2.4mm	
6+6 to PTV	19.0mm	23.5mm	

SOFT TISSUE

MEASUREMENT	NORM	ACTUAL	COMMENT
UPPER LIP	0.0mm to 2.0mm	0.3mm	
LOWER LIP	0.0mm to 2.0mm	5.1mm	

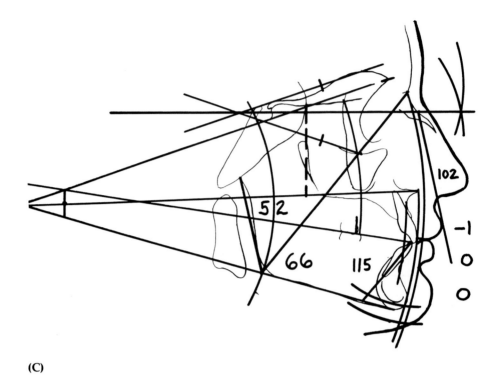

(C)

THE CEPHALOMETRIC "BOTTOM LINE"

CIRCLE THE PROPER RESPONSE

SKELETAL AP:	(I) II III IIT IIIT
SKELETAL VERTICAL:	(N) OB DB OBT DBT
UPPER INCISOR:	N P (R)
LOWER INCISOR:	N (P) R
GROWTH DIRECTION:	N CW (CCW) CWT CCWT
MAXILLA LENGTH:	N L (S) -- (P) A
MAXILLA POSITION:	N (P) A
UPPER 6 POSITION:	(N) P A
MANDIBLE LENGTH:	N L (S) -- (P) A
MANDIBLE POSITION:	N (P) A
UPPER LIP ANGLE:	(N) P F R

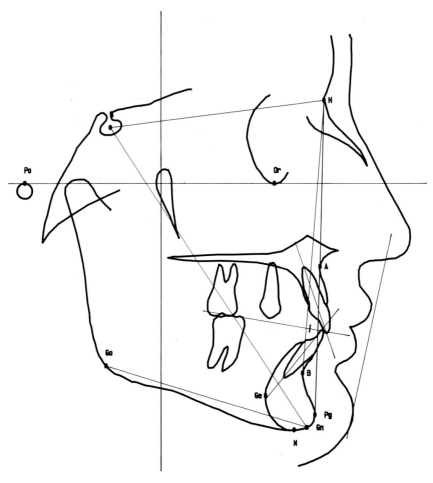

(D)

MODIFIED STEINER ANALYSIS

SKELETAL

MEASUREMENT	NORM	ACTUAL	COMMENT
SNA	80.0° to 84.0°	81.5°	
SNB	78.0° to 82.0°	78.3°	
ANB	0.0° to 4.0°	3.2°	SKELETAL CLASS I
WITS	-3.0mm to 1.0mm	0.1mm	SKELETAL CLASS I
UPPER FACIAL HEIGHT	45.0%	44.9%	
LOWER FACIAL HEIGHT	55.0%	55.1%	
Go-Gn to SN	28.0° to 36.0°	23.7°	TENDENCY FOR INSUFFICIENT VERTICAL DEVELOPMENT
Y-Axis to SN	63.0° to 69.0°	63.1°	
			Normal skeletal bite.
OCCL to SN	14.0° to 15.0°	16.4°	ANY CHANGE IN POSTERIOR VERTICAL SUPPORT WILL HAVE A THREE-FOLD PROPORTIONAL CHANGE IN ANTERIOR VERTICAL
Pg to NB	1.5mm to 3.5mm	6.2mm	PLENTY OF BONE STRUCTURE FOR MOVING MANDIBULAR TEETH ANTERIORLY

DENTAL

MEASUREMENT	NORM	ACTUAL	COMMENT
UP1 to NA DIST	4.0mm	4.5mm	
UP1 to NA ANG	20.0° to 24.0°	21.0°	
LOW1 to NB DIST	4.0mm	6.9mm	
LOW1 to NB ANG	23.0° to 27.0°	35.1°	BUCCOVERSION
LOW1 TO UP1	120.0° to140.0°	120.7°	
A-Pg to LOW1	-2.0mm to 3.0mm	2.3mm	
6+6 to PTV	21.0mm	18.2mm	BE SURE ENOUGH TUBEROSITY EXISTS TO DISTALLIZE MOLARS IF NECESSARY

SOFT TISSUE

MEASUREMENT	NORM	ACTUAL	COMMENT
UPPER LIP	0.0mm to 2.0mm	1.7mm	
LOWER LIP	0.0mm to 2.0mm	4.6mm	

lower Crozats may also be used if more individualized control of the arch form is desired. If the arches are anteroposteriorly asymmetrical, which means more deficient across the bicuspids than the molars (ie, gothic-arch-shaped), the clinician may choose between the Crozats or a combination of first the Schwarz plates followed by Fan-type appliances. The double-appliance therapy of the Schwarz and Fan appliances would be necessary, for example, in the maxilla to correct the difference in bicuspid and molar widths that such eccentric arch width loss demands. If only a Schwarz were used on such a case where the arch was short of individualized Schwarz or Pont limits by 8 mm in the bicuspid area and only 4 mm in the molar area, for instance, once the Schwarz were to obtain the increase of width by 4 mm apiece at each expansion screw site, its symmetrical expansion would not allow the remaining 4 mm to be gained at the bicuspids without overwidening the molars. Hence at that point the Fan appliance would have to be used to gain the other 4 mm asymmetrically across the bicuspids. 3-D Wilsons are also handy here.

A different approach to this problem may be taken in the mandible. If the lower arch needs similar eccentric development laterally, the lower Schwarz may be used at first and the molar area developed followed by picking up the asymmetrical difference in the mandibular cuspid and bicuspid region with the activation of the midline screw of the Bionator. Such minor complications as these bring to the forefront the beauty of the Crozat appliance. By using only one set of appliances, the clinician may develop the arches to their proper arch form either symmetrically or eccentrically with equal ease. However, both methods described work well, and the practitioner will usually select the methods that work best in his own hands and those with which he is most comfortable.

But the Division 1-type of malocclusion also has another aspect to it that favors the Schwarz or Fan appliance in turn, that of the interincisal angle. In the Division 1 category the lower incisors are usually very near the 90-degree range or slightly above in the old IMPA of the Tweed or in an angulation in the 115-degree range of the Bimler Lower Incisal Angle as measured against FH. Since the interincisal angle range of variance for Division 1 designation is between 120 and 130 degrees, and the lower incisors often are near normal, the 10-degree variance usually appears to be expressed in the amount of labial flaring of the maxillary anteriors. This puts their angulation in the 115−125 degree range of the Bimler Upper Incisal Angle. The McNamara would also show this as having the facial surface of the maxillary incisor beyond the 4−5 mm limit relative to N-perpendicular, which denotes maxillary dental protrusion. With this much labial crown torque present the advantages of retraction with the labial bow of the Schwarz during the lateral development of the arch offers an ideal situation. Further retraction may also be accomplished with proper Bionator technique once that appliance is inserted.

One note with regard to the angulation of the lower incisors: If it is determined that they are angulated back too far lingually such as to preclude proper coupling with the uppers once the mandible is advanced, they may be given the extra needed labial crown torque (1) with a lower Sagittal II, (2) by removing the lip of the cap of the bite plate on the Bionator upon its insertion, or (3) by Wilson Lingual Arch technique with or without SWA. Regardless of technique, the status of these teeth should always receive the closest scrutiny so that their eventual position in the arch may be ensured that it is correct. Anterior incisal guidance of lateral and protrusive movements of the mandible is a must once the case is complete.

In the event a posterior crossbite exists in conjunction with the Class II, Division 1 malocclusion, the crossbite is to receive attention prior to the placement of any other appliance. Again, as with Class I adult dentition crossbites, the use of the Crozat appliance is contra-indicated. This leaves the clinician the choices of the Schwarz , Transverse (if TMJ symptoms exist), Nord (for the few rare cases that actually are unilateral), or, if the patient is not too old, the Rapid Palatal Expander. If the case is severely narrow in the posterior areas such that both maxillary posterior quadrants are in full crossbite during occlusion and the patient is an *early* adolescent, the use of the Rapid Palatal Expander should receive serious consideration. It must also be remembered that in all forms of lateral development, the usual precautions are taken at the appropriate times during and at the end of treatment to ensure that any balancing side interferences during lateral excursive movements are eliminated.

But the discrepancy in arch shape may not always be in its width; it could be in its length. In some Class II, Division 1 cases not only are the anteriors flared forward, but there is also crowding. In the instance of an arch shortened anteroposteriorly the cuspids are usually blocked out labially, with the posterior quadrants drifted forward (although the entire anterior set may be *positioned back* albeit *angulated forward*) and some degree of crowding to the anterior teeth. The laterals may or may not be blocked in lingually, depending on the intensity of the crowding anteriorly. When arches with this type of loss of arch length are on or close to Pont's or Schwarz's corrected indices as far as arch width is concerned, it is obvious that no amount of lateral development would relieve the crowding. It would be near physiologically impossible to move the posterior teeth apart laterally far enough to allow for the anterior crowding to be relieved and the arches to subsequently be rounded out. And even if they were overexpanded to such an exaggerated degree, the relapse would collapse them back quicker than the appliances had pushed them out. The reason for the nearly 100% guaranteed chances of relapse being that, what is needed in the above example is not lateral arch width but AP arch *length*. Such circumstances call for an arch-lengthening appliance, and that means Sagittals.

Now this is not to say that lateral development prior to Sagittal lengthening is not important, nor is it to be discarded if it has been determined that a Sagittal appliance will eventually be used. The case should still be analyzed by Schwarz's or Pont's facially corrected methods, and if deficient the arches should still be developed to their indexed width with the appropriate techniques prior to Sagittal appliance treatment.

But once the properly indexed width is gained and arch crowding still exists, the question that immediately presents itself is, should the arch be lengthened anteriorly or posteriorly? Should second molars be extracted and posterior quadrants be distalized, or should the second molars be retained to act as anchorage and allow for the development of the arch anteriorly? The answer lies in both clinical examination and the old diagnostic standby—cephalometric analysis!

To determine which of the two Sagittal appliance techniques to employ in the maxilla, first observe the degree of protrusion of the anterior teeth. If they are flared forward too far, one would obviously not wish to increase their degree of angular protrusion by the use of Sagittal II technique, but would most likely wish to reduce their protrusion to a more proper angulation. This obviously indicates the use of the Sagittal I in conjunction with second molar extraction, to relieve the crowding and bring the cuspids into proper position. But if the maxillary anteriors are not protrusive to a great extent, the determinations clinically are more

---

Figure 8—7 Class II, Division 1 (permanent dentition). This patient presented with a dental and skeletal Class II, Division 1 malocclusion with severe crowding and all four permanent cuspids blocked out labially **(A)—(G)**. Overbite and overjet were also profound, and the maxillary arch was only slightly short of width at the first bicuspids according to the Schwarz index. Treatment consisted of removal of all four second molars (since cephalometric evaluation indicated the need for distalization with Sagittal I technique to relieve AP crowding, not forward movement of the anteriors), followed by 6 months of upper and lower Sagittal I appliance treatment **(H)—(K)**. This was followed by 6 more months of Sagittal I treatment with a second set of appliances **(L)—(P)**. Note the diastemata present in upper and lower arches **(Q)—(R)**, indicative of slight overcorrection, which is favorable. Although arches become "decrowded" **(S)**, **(T)**, the Class II status remains. Thus an Orthopedic Corrector I is constructed and inserted **(U)** and after 9 months of treatment the mandible is advanced nicely **(V)—(X)**. This is followed by 5 months of Straight Wire technique for the maxillary arch to level, align, and rotate teeth **(Y)**. Tru-tains are used in conventional manner. Cephalometric comparison of before and after treatment shows the degree of mandibular advancement and increase in vertical effected by the functional appliance phase of treatment. Final occlusion and facial appearance **(Z)—(CC)**: Note full broad smile and straight lower facial profile with full lips well supported at the corners of the mouth.

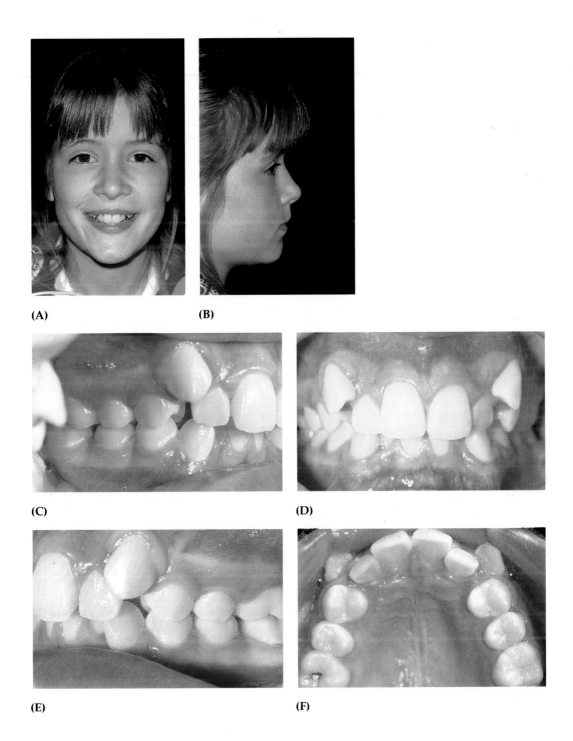

(A)   (B)

(C)   (D)

(E)   (F)

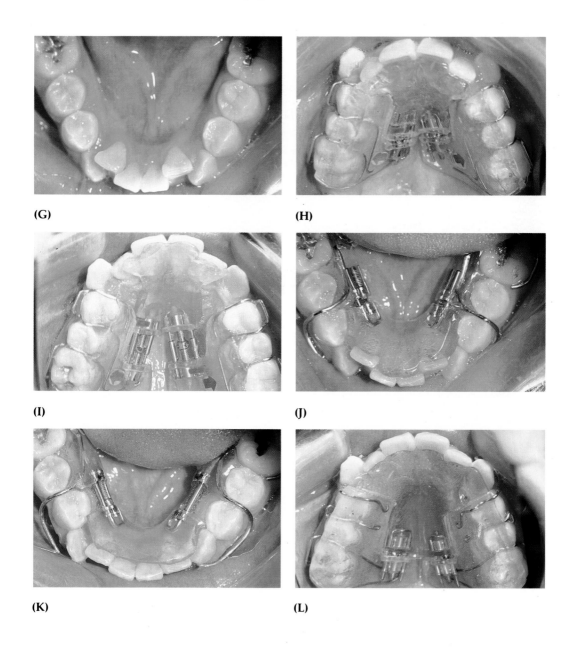

(G)

(H)

(I)

(J)

(K)

(L)

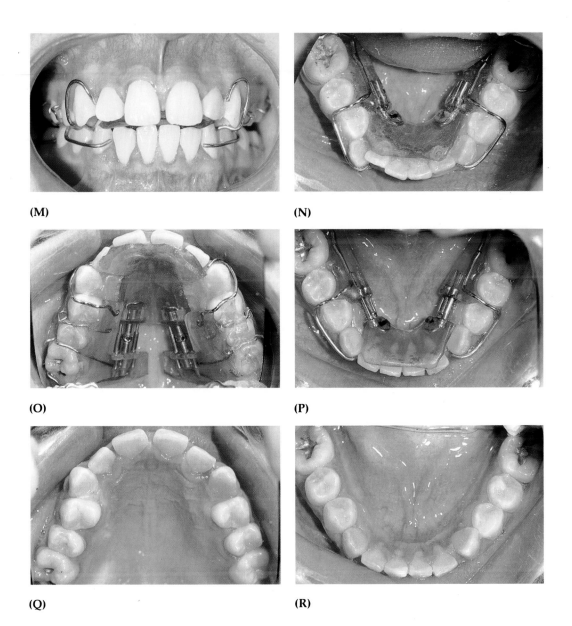

(M)

(N)

(O)

(P)

(Q)

(R)

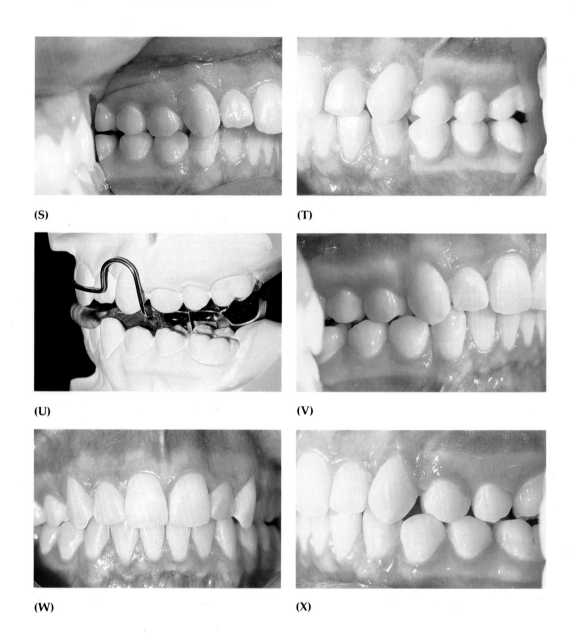

(S)

(T)

(U)

(V)

(W)

(X)

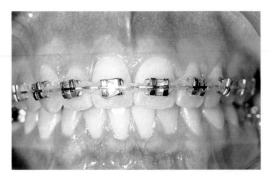

(Y)

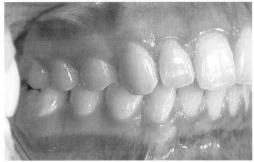

(Z)

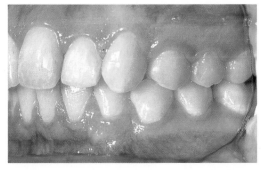

(AA)

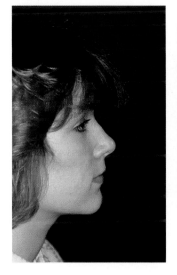

(BB)

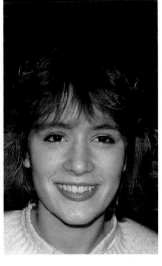

(CC)

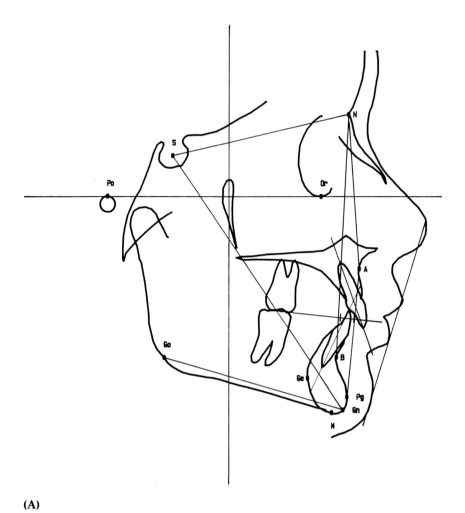

(A)

MODIFIED STEINER ANALYSIS

SKELETAL

MEASUREMENT	NORM	ACTUAL	COMMENT
SNA	80.0° to 84.0°	81.1°	
SNB	78.0° to 82.0°	74.1°	RETROGNATHIC MANDIBLE
ANB	0.0° to 4.0°	7.0°	SKELETAL CLASS II
WITS	-2.0mm to 2.0mm	5.3mm	SKELETAL CLASS II
UPPER FACIAL HEIGHT	50.0%	44.7%	
LOWER FACIAL HEIGHT	50.0%	55.3%	
Go-Gn to SN	28.0° to 36.0°	28.8°	
Y-Axis to SN	63.0° to 69.0°	68.3°	
			Normal skeletal bite.
OCCL to SN	14.0° to 15.0°	18.9°	ANY CHANGE IN POSTERIOR VERTICAL SUPPORT WILL HAVE A THREE-FOLD PROPORTIONAL CHANGE IN ANTERIOR VERTICAL
Pg to NB	1.5mm to 3.5mm	5.0mm	PLENTY OF BONE STRUCTURE FOR MOVING MANDIBULAR TEETH ANTERIORLY

DENTAL

MEASUREMENT	NORM	ACTUAL	COMMENT
UP1 to NA DIST	4.0mm	1.5mm	
UP1 to NA ANG	20.0° to 24.0°	16.1°	LINGUOVERSION
LOW1 to NB DIST	4.0mm	4.9mm	
LOW1 to NB ANG	23.0° to 27.0°	23.0°	
LOW1 TO UP1	120.0° to140.0°	133.9°	
A-Pg to LOW1	-2.0mm to 3.0mm	-1.4mm	
6+6 to PTV	14.0mm	14.6mm	

SOFT TISSUE

MEASUREMENT	NORM	ACTUAL	COMMENT
UPPER LIP	0.0mm to 2.0mm	0.4mm	
LOWER LIP	0.0mm to 2.0mm	0.3mm	

Figure 8−8   Pretreatment Steiner **(A)** and Functional Orthopedic **(B)** and posttreatment Steiner **(C)** and Functional Orthopedic **(D)** cephalometric analysis of patient in Figure 8−7. Observe how in this case two major cephalometric analysis systems dramatically disagree with not only each other as to the pretreatment and posttreatment status of the case but also with what may be clearly observed clinically. By modified McNamara standards in the pretreatment condition, the premaxilla is overdeveloped, the mandible is at the outer limits of the acceptable range for length, and the ANS-Me LFH is excessive. This is the opposite of what the Steiner shows. It says the mandible is retruded and the maxilla is on the more retruded end of the acceptable range. The real discrepancy

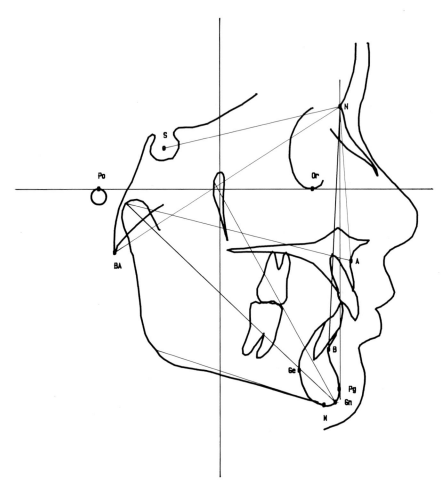

(B)

```
F U N C T I O N A L   O R T H O P E D I C   A N A L Y S I S

    MEASUREMENT                    NORM          ACTUAL     COMMENT

A. RELATING THE MAXILLA TO THE CRANIAL BASE
   A Pt to N Perp            -2.0mm to  2.0mm     4.2mm   OVERDEVELOPED PRE-MAXILLA


B. RELATING THE MANDIBLE TO THE MAXILLA
   Eff. MAXILLA Lgth             ****N,48,$   90.4mm      EFFECTIVE MAXILLA LENGTH
                                                          AFTER ADJUSTMENT FOR 'A'
                                                          PT. LOCATION: 86.2

   Eff. MANDIBLE Lgth       106.2mm to111.2mm    111.0mm

   Diff=MAX-MAND Lgth            ***              24.8mm

   Lower Facial Ht[Vert Dim] 60.5mm to 64.2mm    64.7mm   LONG VERTICAL DIMENSION


C. RELATING THE UPPER INCISOR TO THE MAXILLA
   Up1 to A Perp             4.0mm to  6.0mm      2.9mm


D. RELATING THE LOWER INCISOR TO THE MANDIBLE
   Low1 to A-Pg Line         1.0mm to  3.0mm     -1.4mm


E. MANDIBULAR POSITION
   Pg to N Perp             -5.4mm to -1.6mm     -0.5mm   POSSIBLE PROTRUSION


F. OTHER USEFUL CEPHALOMETRIC MEASUREMENTS
   SNA                       80.0° to 84.0°       81.1°

   SNB                       78.0° to 82.0°       74.1°   RETROGNATHIC MANDIBLE

   ANB                        0.0° to  4.0°        7.0°   SKELETAL CLASS II

   Interincisal Angle       120.0° to140.0°      133.9°

   Mandibular Plane Angle    20.0° to 30.0°       15.8°   LOW VERTICAL DIMENSION

   Facial Axis (Ricketts)    86.5° to 93.5°       92.8°

   WITS                      -2.0mm to  2.0mm      5.3mm  SKELETAL II

***See Instructions RE: Reliability of analysis with uncertain Porion location.
```

appears in comparison of posttreatment evaluations. Functional Orthopedic analysis standards show the case to be "right on" in almost every category while the Steiner shows the finished case to be short in the maxilla, retruded in the mandible, and low in vertical dimension (mandibular plane angle), while at the same time the Ricketts Facial Axis indicates slight open bite tendencies! Lesson: In cephalometrics what you see is not always what you get! Observing identical pretreatment and posttreatment cephalometric locations of "stable" landmarks is almost impossible due to changes by growth, altered head position during exposure, tracing error, etc. Observe beautiful final face and occlusion.

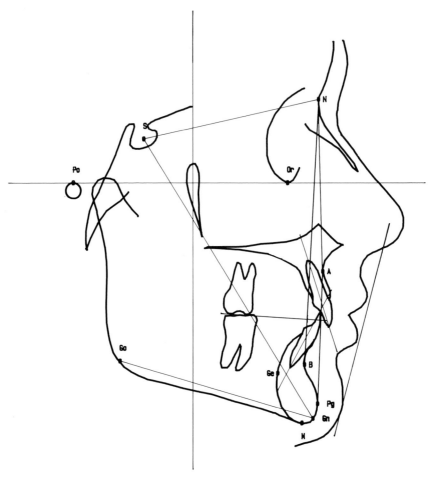

(C)

MODIFIED STEINER ANALYSIS

SKELETAL

MEASUREMENT	NORM	ACTUAL	COMMENT
SNA	80.0° to 84.0°	78.9°	RETROGNATHIC MAXILLA
SNB	78.0° to 82.0°	74.3°	RETROGNATHIC MANDIBLE
ANB	0.0° to 4.0°	4.6°	SKELETAL CLASS II
WITS	-2.0mm to 2.0mm	4.9mm	SKELETAL CLASS II
UPPER FACIAL HEIGHT	45.0%	44.7%	
LOWER FACIAL HEIGHT	55.0%	55.3%	
Go-Gn to SN	28.0° to 36.0°	28.6°	
Y-Axis to SN	63.0° to 69.0°	70.7°	CLOCKWISE GROWER
			Normal skeletal bite.
OCCL to SN	14.0° to 15.0°	16.2°	ANY CHANGE IN POSTERIOR VERTICAL SUPPORT WILL HAVE A THREE-FOLD PROPORTIONAL CHANGE IN ANTERIOR VERTICAL
Pg to NB	1.5mm to 3.5mm	6.0mm	PLENTY OF BONE STRUCTURE FOR MOVING MANDIBULAR TEETH ANTERIORLY

DENTAL

MEASUREMENT	NORM	ACTUAL	COMMENT
UP1 to NA DIST	4.0mm	3.3mm	
UP1 to NA ANG	20.0° to 24.0°	16.8°	LINGUOVERSION
LOW1 to NB DIST	4.0mm	5.5mm	
LOW1 to NB ANG	23.0° to 27.0°	25.9°	
LOW1 TO UP1	120.0° to140.0°	132.7°	
A-Pg to LOW1	-2.0mm to 3.0mm	-0.1mm	
6+6 to PTV	19.0mm	12.1mm	BE SURE ENOUGH TUBEROSITY EXISTS TO DISTALLIZE MOLARS IF NECESSARY

SOFT TISSUE

MEASUREMENT	NORM	ACTUAL	COMMENT
UPPER LIP	0.0mm to 2.0mm	1.3mm	
LOWER LIP	0.0mm to 2.0mm	1.0mm	

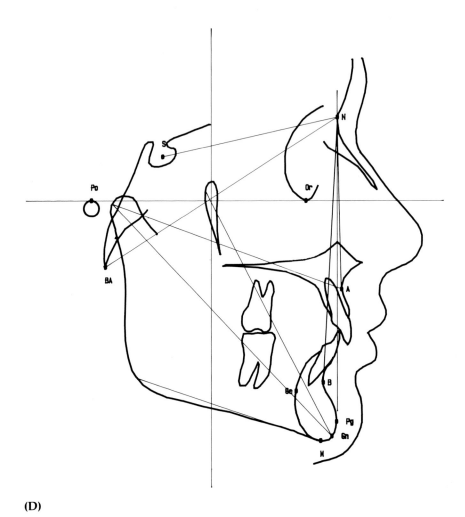

(D)

FUNCTIONAL ORTHOPEDIC ANALYSIS

MEASUREMENT	NORM	ACTUAL	COMMENT
A. RELATING THE MAXILLA TO THE CRANIAL BASE			
A Pt to N Perp	-1.0mm to 3.0mm	1.6mm	
B. RELATING THE MANDIBLE TO THE MAXILLA			
Eff. MAXILLA Lgth	***	95.2mm	
Eff. MANDIBLE Lgth	120.8mm to125.8mm	122.9mm	
Diff=MAX-MAND Lgth	***	29.4mm	
Lower Facial Ht[Vert Dim]	66.9mm to 71.7mm	69.6mm	
C. RELATING THE UPPER INCISOR TO THE MAXILLA			
Up1 to A Perp	4.0mm to 6.0mm	3.7mm	
D. RELATING THE LOWER INCISOR TO THE MANDIBLE			
Low1 to A-Pg Line	1.0mm to 3.0mm	-0.1mm	
E. MANDIBULAR POSITION			
Pg to N Perp	-3.5mm to 1.5mm	-0.4mm	
F. OTHER USEFUL CEPHALOMETRIC MEASUREMENTS			
SNA	80.0° to 84.0°	78.9°	RETROGNATHIC MAXILLA
SNB	78.0° to 82.0°	74.3°	RETROGNATHIC MANDIBLE
ANB	0.0° to 4.0°	4.6°	SKELETAL CLASS II
Interincisal Angle	120.0° to140.0°	132.7°	
Mandibular Plane Angle	20.0° to 30.0°	16.1°	LOW VERTICAL DIMENSION
Facial Axis (Ricketts)	86.5° to 93.5°	94.3°	OPEN BITE TENDENCIES
WITS	-2.0mm to 2.0mm	4.9mm	SKELETAL II

subtle and the use of cephalometrics becomes increasingly valuable. In using the Sassouni analysis to analyze Class II, Division 1 malocclusions with blocked out cuspids, if one observes that the mesial surface of the upper first molar falls anterior to the Midfacial Arc, distalization is indicated. From the McNamara we know the position of the facial surface of the maxillary central should be 4−5 mm from N-perpendicular. As a result of this, combined with the fact that the Division 1 category, by definition, implies a range of interincisal angles from 120 to 130 degrees, and also fortified by the fact that a truly orthopedically protrusive premaxilla is rare, the decision in such circumstances is soon weighed in favor of the Sagittal I in combination with second molar extraction.

For the Sagittal of choice in the mandible the decision is a knotty one. Since the mandible is Class II, its advancement changes cephalometric landmark baseline relationships. Observance clinically often only leaves the clinician guessing whether (1) the tilted forward lower cuspids should be distalized along with the rest of the teeth in the posterior quadrants (which really consists of uprighting the lower cuspids) or whether (2) the four lower anteriors be "dumped" forward labially with a lower Sagittal II or SWA technique. If considerable mandibular advancement is to follow, one could use the tracing cutout method of McNamara to advance the mandible to its predicted position on paper and analyze the angulation of the lower incisors relative to the AP line from there. But this is tedious. We could also use his technique of estimating the number of millimeters the mandible will advance after Bionator treatment and "retrude" A-point distally by the same amount and evaluate the position of the lower incisor to the new hypothetical AP line. But this again leaves the clinician guessing a little. One could just as easily have the patient advance the mandible to the "as if" position and observe the degree of overjet still present. By again estimating how much the maxillary anteriors will be retracted during treatment, the doctor might be able to judge if the position of the lower incisors is presently adequate. If so, or if it is clearly obvious that the incisors are tipped forward enough to couple with the upper anteriors once these teeth are retracted, the Sagittal I is indicated to distalize posterior quadrants and upright the tipped forward lower cuspids by means of the cuspid clasps in conjunction with lower second molar extraction. But if in this "as if" position the lower incisors are obviously retroclined in appearance, the lower Sagittal II is indicated.

Another "guesstimate" method of determining preadvancement lower incisor relative procumbancy is comparing its facial surface to the old N-B line in millimeters, being anterior to the line by +4 mm as ideal. This method, though still tenuous since it is predicated upon an estimate of the amount of mandibular advancement necessary to effect an ideal A-B difference, is less affected geometrically by translation of the mandible since the facial surface of the lower incisor and B-point would move less differentially upon advancement relative to the longer N-B radius. The only danger here is that it is assumed N is in its correct place and not retruded, an assumption that may not always be valid. We also have the Lower Incisal Angle of the Bimler analysis to consult for some help. With an interincisal angle of 130 degrees, the ideal Upper and Lower Incisal Angles as both measured against the FH plane hover around 115 degrees. If the angular departure of the lower central incisor in one direction or another is great, it can serve as a guide to appliance selection, especially if the lower incisors are retroclined making the Lower Incisal Angle lower than 115 degrees.

From the Sassouni we know the angulation of the long axis of the lower incisor to the mandibular plane is defined as having a range of ±5 degrees either side of a 95-degree mean (measured internally at the intersection of the two lines). As previously stated, this is a rather wide range that reflects a bit more favor of the protrusive as compared to more traditional norms and reflects concern for coupling with slightly more protrusive uppers, which is a current trend reflecting concern over lip support and protecting the all-important mandibular arc of final closure from anterior incisal interference and the NRDM/SPDC phenomenon. The treatment-planning output sections of the Smith computerized diagnostic programs are also extremely helpful in determining proper angulation and position of both upper and lower anterior incisors as well as final net movements necessary to effect correct molar position, and even the final position of maxillary and mandibular osseous segments.

If it is too difficult to tell from all of the above, one can always resort to simple direct observation of a study cast or the patient's actual lower arch. After looking at teeth every day of one's life, one can usually tell if lower incisors are, relative to the alveolar ridge, retroclined too much. The combination of clinically observing the patient and the amount of overjet in the "as if" position, along with the analysis of the Bimler Lower Incisal Angle, should be able to guide the clinician in the right direction as to which way to lengthen the lower arch. It must be remembered that if the upper molar is being distalized, its final position must ultimately be Class I dentally with the lower. So if the lower is only half-Class II or not very far into the dental Class II retruded position, by the time the mandible is in turn advanced, it could develop a Class III if the Sagittal discrepancy on the lower is not relieved first. Until the lower arch is uncrowded, it probably shouldn't be put in a Bionator, barring slight lower anterior crowding that may be relieved with the Bionator's midline expansion screw.

Another important consideration to keep in mind that greatly simplifies the decision as to which way to lengthen moderately crowded mandibular arches with lower incisors already within a reasonably acceptable range of angulation in skeletally Class II mandibles is the concern for the safety of the TMJs. For the sake of discussion, adequate arch width is assumed to exist either naturally or as a result of prior lateral development. If the lower incisors are well within the acceptable range of angulation, they may be considered "protrusive enough," and the mandibular arch may be subsequently decrowded by means of second molar extraction and Sagittal I distalization techniques. This places the entire dental arch safely far enough back on the mandibular apical base to allow enough mandibular advancement in subsequent Bionator treatment to make sure the condyles do not become (or remain) compressed due to a combination of excessive mandibular bodily length (DLM, Bilmer; effective mandibular length, McNamara) and insufficient bodily mandibular advancement. Lower anteriors flippantly "dumped" forward to the outer limits of cephalometrically acceptable angulations could possibly provide just enough anterior incisal interference during full occlusion by virtue of striking what may be just a bit too retracted a set of maxillary anteriors, in conjunction with a slightly bigger than anticipated mandible to add up to an NRDM/SPDC phenomenon and resultant TMJ trouble.

Sometimes a combination of treatment techniques is required. A case might be considered for Sagittal II treatment first to give just a bit more protrusion to anteriors that are on the high (steep) end interincisal angle-wise of the Division 1 category before extracting the second molars and converting the appliances to a Sagittal I for distalization purposes. (This might also serve well as a possible solution to the problem of which way to go with the lower arch that needs arch length due to possibly retroclined incisors.)

Once the maxillary arch has been relieved of its crowding with either of the Sagittal techniques, the case is retained for 3—4 months with the appliance acting as its own retainer. This is a critical period during the arch preparation phase of treatment with the Sagittal appliances. If the treatment has been with the Sagittal II, the important retentive phase allows time for the teeth to stabilize prior to the insertion of the Bionator. If the treatment has been with Sagittal I, the movement of teeth in the sagittal direction distally is relatively stable. Since the teeth are often distalized rather quickly, due to a combination of heavy function on the appliance, faithful patient cooperation in wearing it, and two turns of the expansion screws per week, this may result in the tipping of the crowns of the teeth posteriorly ahead of the roots. The marginal ridges may even become stepped like edges of a row of dominoes, all tilted together at an angle. Once the active phase of distalization is complete, the patient must continue to wear the appliance for 2—3 months to allow the functional stimuli of the forces of occlusion of the lower teeth against the bite blocks of the plate to bring about the leveling of the teeth. This brings the marginal ridges back into line and parallels the roots. The more function the better, so stress constant wearing of the appliance during this time with special emphasis on trying to wear it during the ultimate of all functional stimuli—eating!

Having completed the task of shaping and securing the arches, the Class II, Division 1 adult dentition is ready to be advanced to the second phase of treatment, which is usually the Bionator.

Before constructing the Bionator, there are several factors the practitioner may wish to consider relative to the cephalometric data he has on hand that might alter the way he manages the use of the Bionator during treatment.

We know that the purpose of the Bionator in Class II treatment is to translate the mandible down and forward to bring the lower jaw with its "passenger teeth" back to a skeletal and dental Class I at proper vertical dimension of occlusion. This net movement, viewed from the lateral aspect, as in a cephalogram, is in a relatively straight line at approximately a 45-degree angle down from the Frankfort plane. But, as with all net movements, it may be divided into horizontal and vertical vectors. We can take advantage of these vectors in the way we construct the Bionator to accentuate either one component or the other of the net movement, depending on which is most deficient in the patient. Since not every patient's maxillofacial complex grows in the exact same net direction down and out from under the cranial base, each patient's particular dominant vector of growth, either horizontal, neutral, or vertical, may be analyzed and, if found to be dominantly horizontal or vertical, may be compensated for in the contruction bite of the Bionator used to treat the skeletal Class II problem of that individual.

Some individuals' horizontal and vertical components of growth are about equal, hence the usual technique for construction bite registration will suffice.

However, certain patients have a dominance of the horizontal growth vector and are referred to as horizontal growers. This would allow the clinician to take a construction bite for a Bionator to be used on such a patient, with a more accentuated consideration for the "vertical-addressing" properties of the appliance. The construction bite could be made thicker vertically, and the distance between the incisal edges of the upper and lower anterior teeth could be left at, say, 4 mm, instead of having the patient close to within the usual 2 mm. This, in conjunction with taking the bite at the usual horizontal level of protrusion of the lower incisors past the uppers, produces a Bionator which has more effect on stimulating the teeth in the posterior quadrants to "supraerupt" than it would in an appliance constructed on a conventional wax bite.

For a patient who is predominantly a horizontal grower (a "brachycephalic facial type" if using American terminology or a "dolichoprosopic facial type" if using Bimler terminology—we won't go into this clockwise or counterclockwise business here because it's simply too confusing!), this vertical accentuation appliance is favored, since not much stimuli will be needed to advance the mandible forward because the patient's main component, or vector of growth, is primarily in that direction anyway. Since the vertical forces of growth are less dominant in this type of individual, we would want to accentuate those types of stimuli the appliance delivers to help erupt the posterior teeth as much as possible to more quickly open the diminished vertical dimension of occlusion. This is the main purpose of constructing the Bionator on a slightly thicker construction bite. Once processed on such a bite, the acrylic bite cap over the lower anteriors is correspondingly thicker, and this holds the teeth in the posterior quadrants farther apart in the finished appliance, which in turn increases the functional stimuli to this area and aids in counteracting a diminutive vertical growth tendency. This is exactly what the doctor ordered for advancing the mandible and opening the vertical in a horizontal grower.

Conversely, if an individual shows that the vertical component of growth is dominant, the opposite would be true. Individuals whose vertical vector of growth is greater than their horizontal vector are referred to as vertical growers. Such individuals in Class II treatment with a Bionator would be best managed if the appliance were constructed from a construction bite that gave the finished appliance a more accentuated consideration for the "horizontal-addressing" properties of the device. The construction bite could be made with the mandible in a slightly more protruded position of, say, 3—4 mm past end to end in the incisor area. This, coupled with keeping the bite at the usual level of thickness vertically, produces a Bionator which has more effect on stimulating bodily mandibular translation horizontally to correct orthopedic balance than on increasing vertical through supraeruption of teeth in the posterior quadrants.

For a patient who is predominantly a vertical grower (a "dolichocephalic facial type" if using the American terminology or a "leptoprosopic facial type" if using Bimler terminology—and if that's not confusing enough, we can still bring back this clockwise, counterclockwise business, but don't worry, we won't!) this is favored, since the patient's main component or vector of growth is in the vertical direction anyway, and added vertical growth will come easily enough. What is needed in a mandibular retrusion case such as this is to stimulate as much as possible the advancement of the mandible. We would also want to stimulate to an increased degree its concomitant muscle reattachment and condylar growth to compensate for the straggling horizontal development.

In some cases this vertical component of development may be already so great that the case merely needs mandibular advancement with no increase in vertical at all. This is an indication for the Bionator III. The percentage of incisor overbite, the ANS-Me LFH, and the general appearance of the face in the "as if" position may all be analyzed to verify this point.

The value of our discussion on facial types is now apparent. When the clinician realizes the type of growth patterns and facial type that the patient represents (horizontal grower, vertical grower, or balanced or neutral grower) he or she may then best decide how to make the subtle changes in the appliance construction so as to seek that extra bit of performance out of them. Many patients will not be at the clearly observable extremes of the two accentuated growth vector categories, but will merely exhibit "tendencies." Such tendencies have a certain amount of light shed on them by use of the Sassouni split-gonial-angle evaluation. Careful observation of these tendencies to either the vertical or horizontal type of dominance will offer practitioners the option to take advantage of the appropriate appliance modifications of the Bionator (by means of the modified construction bite) if they so desire. Consideration of such factors will not only lead to better chances for a satisfactory result, but also will most likely contribute to shortened treatment times.

Two other methods of determining if the patient has anything other than a balanced or neutral component of growth are (1) the various members of the Y-axis family of determinations of either the Downs, Bjork, or Ricketts analyses, or (2) by consulting the Suborbital Facial Index of the Bimler. If the patient is developing normally (other than being skeletally Class II) the mesocephalic, mesofacial, or mesoprosopic designation (no confusion here!) indicates that the construction bite for the Bionator may also be normal. (Note: Special plastic Truitt bite positioners are now available that greatly facilitate the taking of normal and modified construction bites. These little plastic sticks are of two types: a blue bite positioner that is notched with both 2-mm and 4-mm vertical opening thicknesses in conjunction with either end-to-end or 2-mm advanced situations; yellow bite positioner notched with 2-mm and 4-mm vertical opening thickness in conjunction with either end-to-end or 4-mm advanced relationships.)

Another concept that we will insert here is that of arch perfecting with SWAs after Sagittal appliance (or lateral development) therapy but *before* insertion of the Bionator. This has the advantage of aligning the teeth in the arch, consolidating spaces, eliminating rotations, etc, so that once the Bionator is inserted it will have an easier time of coupling the entire upper and lower arches to each other and obtaining proper tooth-to-tooth interdigitation. Or once the Bionator is removed the SWA may then be placed also. Which to do first can only be decided on an individual case-by-case basis. There is a certain degree of tolerance for the particular sequence in which the SWA is used as far as perfecting individual tooth positions. The determining factor might be the observation of the arches in the "as if" position. If it appears that the arches simply aren't arch shaped enough due to improper orthodontic positioning of various teeth, use of the SWA first may be advantageous. The degree of mesiorotation of the molars is also an important factor to consider, since more correct and balanced arch form is obtainable once the mesiorotated molars are distally rotated to a proper state with SWA. As stated previously, this distal rotation of upper first molars that are incorrectly mesially rotated may also help with the advancement of the mandible out of Class II back into Class I. Actually what is happening in the multi-appliance-requiring malocclusions is that the case is being brought out of a deep hole orthodontically by the various arch preparation appliances such as Sagittals, Schwarz types, Crozats, Fan types, etc prior to arch alignment.

Once the arches start assuming reasonably acceptable form as a result of treatment with the arch lengtheners and arch wideners, the case is judged by the same standards as the *simple* Class II malocclusion in the adult dentition, which, as previously stated, if within 3 to 5 mm of Pont's or Schwarz' facialy corrected indices of width, may first be "touched up" if desired with the SWA *prior* to the insertion of the Bionator. However, there are those whose experience and skills are such that they can perform a modicum amount of individual tooth movement with the Bionator itself by means of the use of lap springs instead of a lingual retaining wire; others may also use the acrylic drop method, etc, and as a result these practitioners will tolerate more individual tooth misalignment or arch imperfection prior to Bionator insertion than others might be willing to accept.

But, on the other hand, once the case is fully Class I in both the dental as well as orthopedic relationships, the clinician then is more capable of judging just where he or she wants to place a given tooth relative to another. This allows for the most precise degrees of arch perfection to be achieved with the SWA—hence the rationale of the alternative route of placement of the SWA appliance *after* the Bionator phase of treatment!

So what finally resolves the issue is the idea of doing whatever must be done to first get good arch form, then good interarch alignment, followed by arch perfection, after having once attained that state of correct jaw alignment. How particular practitioners obtain each of these stages of correction is not measured by the methods they use, but merely by the results they produce. The active plate/functional appliance/Straight Wire combination of treatment modalities gives them the power to produce these results on a predictable, respectable, profitable basis to extremely high standards of excellence.

It must also be noted here that some cases of Class II, Division 1 malocclusions may be treated on a nonextraction basis with SWAs only in conjunction with Class II mechanics. Serious concern must be given to the analysis of the cephalometrics in such cases so as not to leave the orthopedics wanting. Another very important factor to consider is the musculature. As a major etiological agent in the production of the Class II malocclusion, the musculature must be given serious consideration in both the diagnosis and treatment planning of the Class II case. Functional appliances such as the Bionator have Class II musculature correction already built into their fundamental design. Class II fixed appliance mechanics do not.

The fixed appliance and Class II elastic route is primarily a technique for Class II *dental* situations already in near Class I orthopedic relationship. But the main subject matter of this text is the management of the *orthopedically* oriented removable appliances. Advanced Class II fixed appliance mechanics here are relegated to the level of an alternative but not necessarily superior method. Those who ardently espouse the theories of orthopedic treatment of Class II skeletal conditions with functional appliances feel strongly that Class II fixed appliance mechanics are contraindicated when true structural and muscular Class II deficiencies exist. They feel, and correctly so, that once the case has been both orthopedically and "muscularly" corrected by functional appliances out of its pretreatment skeletally retrusive mandibular position to structural Class I, the need for extensive Class II fixed mechanics no longer exists. In addition, their advocation of second molar extraction principles enabling upper posterior quadrants to be moved nearly anywhere desired just about "cements their case."

Class II, Division 2 Permanent Dentition Treatment

There was never a stronger case by which the arch preparation removable appliances such as the Sagittal may prove their worth than in that of the correction of Class II, Division 2 malocclusions. These types of malocclusion not only cause the orthodontic malposition and malocclusion of teeth, but are also extremely dangerous situations relative to a more distant component of the maxillofacial complex, the TMJ. When combined with deep overbite, as they almost always are, the Class II, Division 2 malocclusion is capable of not only restraining the forward development of the mandible but also, because of the inclined plane action of the lower incisors against the retroclined upper incisors, can result in the mandible being forced rearward and upward during the path of closure to full posterior molar occlusion. This neuromuscular reflexive displacement of the mandible and its associated rearward and upward displacement of the condyle due to the incisal interferences anteriorly is a combination of events that universally leads to compressed TMJs, forward displaced intraarticular discs, fatigued muscle and ligament tissues, stretched posterior attachment ligaments in the bilaminar zone, and a whole raft of various forms of chronic headache, neck, and myofacial pain and discomfort symptoms. Even young children suffering from Class II, Division 2 deep bite malocclusions are not immune to these symptoms and the observant clinician will often find that adolescents with this type of malocclusion routinely have a history of somewhat more frequent than normal headache or muscle soreness in the facial or temporal area, especially in the more severe examples of the malocclusion.

In the path of growth and development of the maxillofacial complex down and out from under the cranial base, the mandible is straining to free itself from the trapping influences of the Division 2 retroclined upper anteriors. But every time the teeth occlude (1500—2000 times per day just for swallowing), due to the incisal interference anteriorly, the mandible is forced up and back in its full arc of final closure, the complete opposite direction in which it is trying to grow. Under such circumstances compression of the TMJ cannot help but occur. Extracting four bicuspids in such a case and making the upper arch even smaller, which correspondingly forces the lower arch to be also smaller, will only compound the problem and cause the mandible to be retained even further posteriorly and just about guarantee serious TMJ complications after treatment. The only way to "liberate" the mandible, and consequently its attending TMJ, is to convert the Class II, Division 2 into a Division 1 and proceed from there as if it were a routine case with the remainder of treatment.

The Class II, Division 2 appearance of the maxillary arch is of a truly classic appearance and may be of two varieties. The purest (most prime) example of a Division 2 anterior tooth arrangement is one of *severely* retroclined maxillary central incisors accompanied by crowded and flared forward adjacent laterals. Care must be taken to remember this configuration when tracing the cephalogram so as not to mistakenly trace the protruded lateral in place of the more vertical central, thus giving a false impression of greater labial crown angulation than actually exists for these teeth. Extremely steep interincisal angles are noted often in such arrangements that register well beyond the somewhat arbitrary 140-degree limit for Division 2 designation. The tip of the upper central in such circumstances will be found to fall short of the ANS Arc (or the Anterior Arc if ANS is on the Anterior Arc) of the Sassouni, while it will also be seen to be short of the innermost limit of 4 mm to the A-point perpendicular of the McNamara. The Upper Incisal Angle (UI) of the Bimler will be seen to be less than 105 degrees with respect to FH. But empirically the upper arch as a whole in these cases seldom if ever seems to be "crowded in" with the centrals rotated or overlapped. What one does see only occasionally, however, is that the arch may be a little more gothic in shape, requiring slight fanlike widening anteriorly with either an appliance like the Fan plate or a Crozat. However, this is rare.

The second general type of Class II, Division 2 upper anterior incisor arrangement often seen is a bit more tenuous in appearance than the more dramatically obvious variety described above, but nevertheless, may still pose an equal level of potential danger to the long-term health of the TMJ in the untreated state due to the same old anterior incisal interference problem of inducement of the NRDM/SPDC. This type of arrangement shows all four of the upper anteriors in reasonably good arch form and fairly free of rotations, yet it still exhibits a rather vertical appearance to the long axis of the upper centrals and laterals. This, in conjunction with deep overbite or a crowded forward lower anterior, acts in the same manner as the previously described more intense version of the Division 2 arrangement in causing incisal interference during occlusion. This again produces a reflexive muscular inhibition of proper natural advancement of the mandible during growth and development. These types of upper arches are not usually too pointed or gothic in outline but display the more conventional Roman arch shape. Some may be so normal in appearance that if it were not for the history of symptoms the diagnostician may be tempted to pass the entire occlusal relationship off as being merely a little short of vertical. This is most likely to happen in the Class I dentition where the interincisal angle may be close to the Division 2 interincisal angular boundary of 140 degrees.

When a severe Class II mandibular retrusion accompanies a Division 2 arrangement anteriorly, the improper muscle function may have had such an effect in inhibiting the growth and development of the mandible that the mandibular insufficiency is great enough to prevent anterior coupling during occlusion. In such cases the lower incisors "dig in" to the palatal tissues above, which as a result may even exhibit lingual stripping of the gingivae from the necks of the lingual surfaces of the upper anteriors, usually the centrals. This is a case that exhibits three glaring needs: an increase in vertical, an advancement of the interfering Division 2 incisors out of the way anteriorly, and mandibular advancement.

There is usually so much mandibular retrusion in a structural Class II situation of this type that if it is accompanied by only mild Division 2 tendencies in the upper anteriors there is correspondingly sufficient overjet by default (due to the severe mandibular insufficiency) so as to preclude incisal interference from remaining as the prime initiator of the NRDM-SPDC phenomenon. But there may be no doubt that at one time early in the development of the case it played an important part in the etiology of the Class II, Division 2 malocclusion. The *improper muscle function* has now replaced incisal interference in such cases as the prime factor in holding the mandible back. As the whole skull and maxilla mature, they gain slightly in size, possibly accounting for the anterior coupling to be lost as the premaxilla "pulls away" slightly while the powerful, albeit improper, muscle function below holds the mandible back, thus producing a slight overjet that puts the lower incisors just onto the palatal tissues in spite of the Division 2 high interincisal angle. This type of case exhibits the greatest need for active plate/functional appliance correction. One would never want to extract bicuspids to obtain anterior coupling, ie, bringing the premaxilla back in these cases, since this would perpetually lock the mandible in a compressed TMJ situation.

But even when the Division 2 tendency is only slight in the upper anteriors and coupling also exists with the lowers, and the molars only appear as a marginal dental Class I or half-Class II, the net effect on the TMJ may still be eventually the same as the full-fledged Class II, Division 2 situation. One must not be fooled by the innocuous appearances of such "mild" cases, which may actually be serious TMJ-involving malocclusions in orthodontic disguise. The joints never lie.

The clinician must take a careful and detailed history when such marginal Division 2 conditions are observed. If symptoms crop up indicating a myofacial-TMJ involvement of some sort, the joint may be assumed to be compromised, and *regardless* of how well the teeth appear to align the case should be considered the same as a full "TMJ-compromising" structural Class II, Division 2 malocclusion. This is especially so when the occlusion is accompanied by deep overbite (and by "deep" is meant 50% or greater overlap of the incisal edges of the upper anteriors down over the crowns of the lower incisors). The upper incisor angle of the Bimler and the comparison of the facial surface of the upper central to the A-perpendicular of the McNamara may also be called upon to shed some light on the subject, since sometimes one may receive a false impression of what is seen clinically about the degree the upper anteriors are retroclined or the extent the crowns are torqued lingually.

For the sake of the joints, it is imperative to not only consider upper incisor *angulation* but also *position*, and that means maxillary location. A maxilla short anteriorly or even underdeveloped on a wholesale basis coupled with a relatively longer mandible and even the most innocent-appearing angulation of the upper anteriors can easily add up to a net effect of anterior incisal interference and a resultant NRDM/SPDC-induced TMJ problem. The retrusion of the entire maxillary arch, as represented by the location of A-point, is a vital element in the determination of the actual Class II, Division 2 malocclusion or the "Division 2 effect," which as far as the joints are concerned amounts to the same thing. The previously discussed methods of the Sassouni for determining maxillary position, along with the Factor 1 of the Bimler (being a negative angle), as well as the location of A-point less than −2 mm to McNamara's N-perpendicular, and the effective maxillomandibular differential are helpful here too.

Of course, the ultimate proof of a dental or orthopedically induced NRDM/SPDC TMJ-type mandibular retrusion is the reduced posterior joint space seen in the common transcranial radiograph! The point is that more than just the angulation of the upper anteriors must be considered in the Division 2 effect as far as the joints are concerned. In this vein, full scale maxillary arch retropositioning has the same effect as steep anterior incisor angulation. One must always consider the net effect of the maxillary arch (A-point) position, upper anterior incisor retraction, steepness of the upper anteriors, proclination of the lowers, and degree of overbite in the overall evaluation of what actually constitutes Division 2 category versus Division 2 effect, especially with respect to the all-important mandibular arc of final closure, and the TMJs.

Sometimes we are surprised to see how "straight up and down" some reasonably normal-appearing upper incisors can actually be when examined under the unbiased scrutiny of a cephalometric x-ray analysis system mitigated by considerations of a mandibular arc of closure evaluation, and the resultant final location of the condyles during full occlusion. The joints are blind and cannot see what is up front causing their problems, nor do they care what the source is; they only know what they *feel*!

Cephalometrics is not needed for the diagnosis of the more profound or classic Class II, Division 2 cases, since the "towed in" upper centrals, flared and crowded upper laterals, and the deep overbite are conditions the receptionist could diagnose from across the room. But in the more innocent-appearing cases where the bite is not too deep, the posterior quadrants only half-Class II, and the upper anteriors appear fairly normal, a little more careful scrutiny of the cephalogram will be required along with thorough analysis of the occlusion and history. The consideration of the TMJ must remain paramount. Even if the upper anteriors appear near normal on the cephalogram but symptoms and other orthopedic data off the radiograph or transcranial x-ray indicate a need for mandibular advancement and increased vertical by means of the Bionator to decompress the joint and recapture a forward displaced intraarticular disc, the mandible must indeed be relocated down and forward to a position acceptable to the joint. The mandible, however, cannot be prematurely advanced without having the lower anteriors collide with the Division 2 retroclined upper anteriors. These upper anteriors must be cleared out of the way by pushing them forward, by imparting labial crown torque to them so the next phase of treatment with the Bionator may be properly employed without reservations. Hence the almost universal use of the Sagittal II as a first appliance prior to Bionator usage in such cases is due to the need to clear away anterior incisal interferences from the proposed future, Bionator-effected, more advanced posttreatment mandibular arc of closure.

Cephalometrically, when the interincisal angle approaches the 140-degree range or beyond in the Division 2 category, the Upper Incisal and Lower Incisal Angles of the Bimler approach the 100–90 degree range as opposed to their more normal 115-degree value. Remember, the interincisal angle, and Upper and Lower Incisal Angles of the Bimler analysis all add up to 360 degrees. This is a helpful cross-reference for checking the "uprightness" of the centrals as opposed to the method of analyzing their position in the McNamara (which has the facial surface of the upper central 4–5 mm from the A-perpendicular). If A-point is slightly retruded due to an underdeveloped premaxilla, it could give a false impression

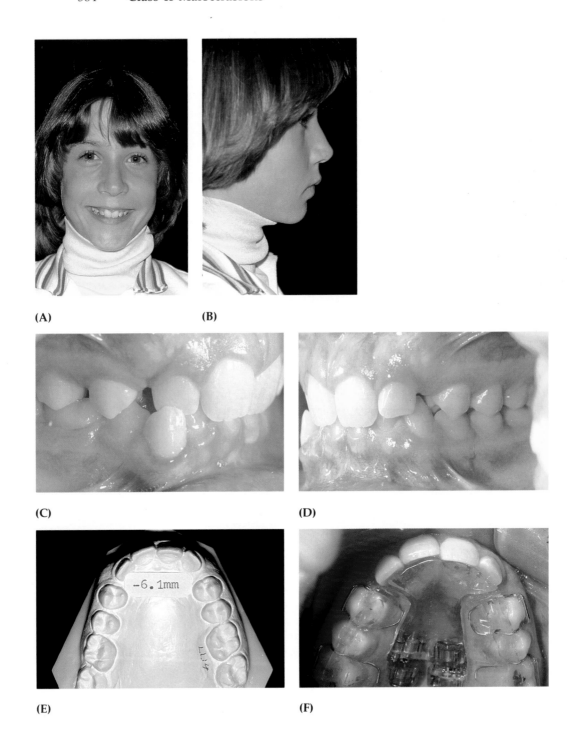

(A)

(B)

(C)

(D)

(E)

(F)

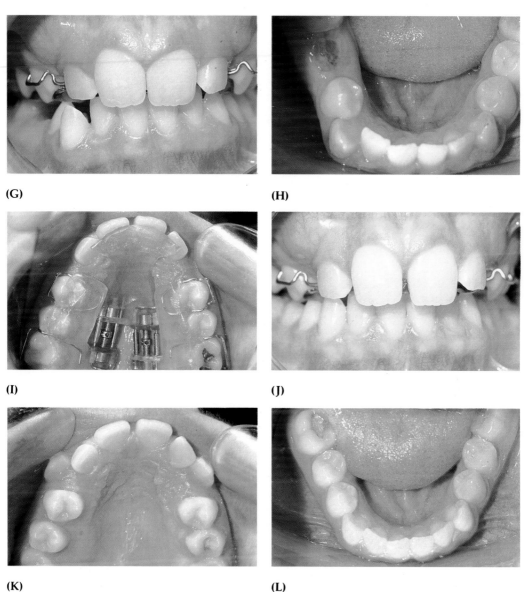

(G)   **(H)**

(I)   **(J)**

(K)   **(L)**

Figure 8−9   Class II, division 2 (permanent dentition). This patient exhibited a
Class II, Division 2 malocclusion with blocked-out upper cuspids and a lower
cuspid in crossbite **(A)−(D)**. Because of the Division 2 nature of the anterior
incisors **(E)**, an upper Sagittal II appliance was inserted to develop the anterior
premaxillary area forward **(F)**, **(G)**. With lower second molars removed and the
natural exfoliation of the lower right deciduous second molar **(H)**, no appliances
were needed to correct crowded mandibular right cuspid, which self-corrected
spontaneously. After 10 months note the development of the maxillary anteriors
forward and self-correction of lower arch **(I)−(L)**. With erupting cuspids still

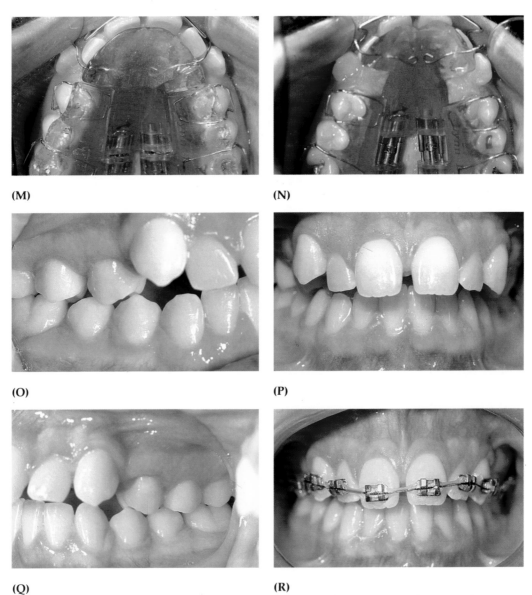

(M)   (N)

(O)   (P)

(Q)   (R)

slightly short of space, a second Sagittal II was used for 6 more months **(M)**–**(N)**. Note again the extent of overcorrection. As cuspids erupt **(O)**–**(Q)**, they do not assume ideal position, and upper right lateral still acts as a source of deflection of the mandibular arc of closure, thus "trapping" the mandible in a Class II retrusion; therefore, Straight Wire appliance technique is used for 6 months to perfect the arch form **(R)**, **(S)**. A Hawley retainer was used during sleep only **(T)**. With the unlocking of the occlusion, the mandible spontaneously advanced itself **(U)**. Final pictures were taken 3 ½ years after completion of treatment **(V)**, **(W)**.

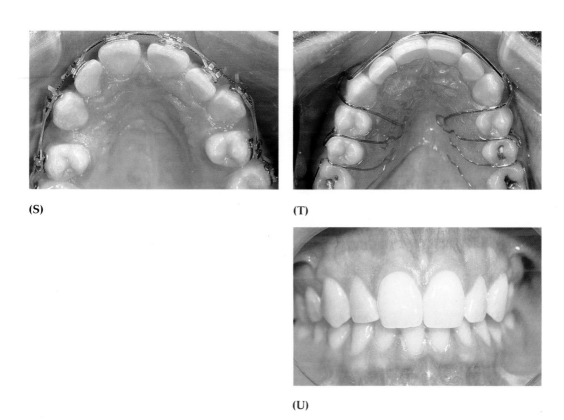

(S)

(T)

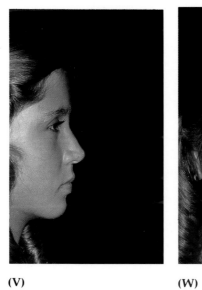

(U)

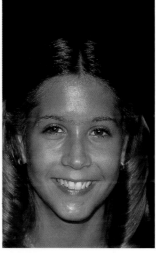

(V)

(W)

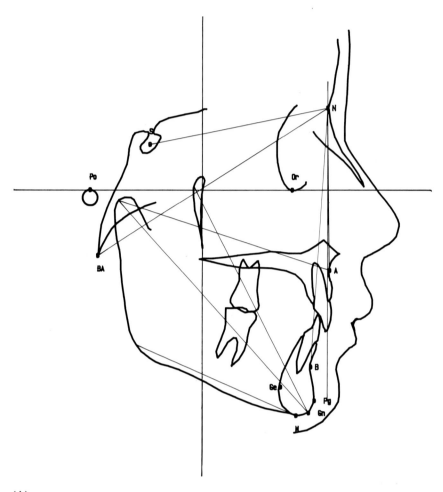

(A)

FUNCTIONAL ORTHOPEDIC ANALYSIS

MEASUREMENT	NORM	ACTUAL	COMMENT
A. RELATING THE MAXILLA TO THE CRANIAL BASE			
A Pt to N Perp	-1.0mm to 3.0mm	0.8mm	
B. RELATING THE MANDIBLE TO THE MAXILLA			
Eff. MAXILLA Lgth	***	86.7mm	
Eff. MANDIBLE Lgth	106.9mm to 111.9mm	109.7mm	
Diff=MAX-MAND Lgth	***	23.0mm	
Lower Facial Ht[Vert Dim]	60.8mm to 64.6mm	64.0mm	
C. RELATING THE UPPER INCISOR TO THE MAXILLA			
Up1 to A Perp	4.0mm to 6.0mm	0.8mm	
D. RELATING THE LOWER INCISOR TO THE MANDIBLE			
Low1 to A-Pg Line	1.0mm to 3.0mm	-1.3mm	
E. MANDIBULAR POSITION			
Pg to N Perp	-4.3mm to 0.3mm	-5.1mm	POSSIBLE RETRUSION
F. OTHER USEFUL CEPHALOMETRIC MEASUREMENTS			
SNA	80.0° to 84.0°	79.3°	RETROGNATHIC MAXILLA
SNB	78.0° to 82.0°	74.8°	RETROGNATHIC MANDIBLE
ANB	0.0° to 4.0°	4.6°	SKELETAL CLASS II
Interincisal Angle	120.0° to 140.0°	149.5°	
Mandibular Plane Angle	20.0° to 30.0°	21.0°	
Facial Axis (Ricketts)	86.5° to 93.5°	94.4°	OPEN BITE TENDENCIES
WITS	-2.0mm to 2.0mm	1.5mm	SKELETAL CLASS I

Figure 8−10 Pretreatment **(A)** and posttreatment **(B)** Functional Orthopedic cephalometric analysis of patient in Figure 8−9. Note the advancement of A-point (Downs) from a pretreatment location of 0.8 mm to the N-perpendicular to a posttreatment location of 2.0 mm from N-perpendicular. Also note the advancement of the maxillary centrals from 0.8 mm to A-point perpendicular to 3.9 mm to A-point perpendicular. Correction of the Division 2 upper anterior incisor angulation caused the "untrapped mandible" to spontaneously advance to its correct and physiologically balanced anatomical location. Pogonion advanced from −5.1 to −1.0 mm to N-perpendicular. Change in Wits was due to action of Sagittal II on premaxilla in spite of slight leveling of cant of occlusal plane.

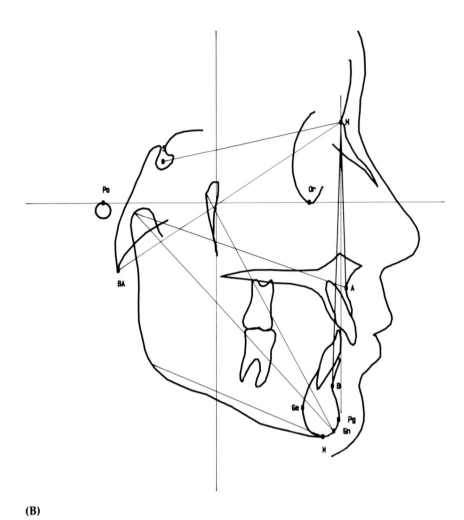

(B)

FUNCTIONAL ORTHOPEDIC ANALYSIS

MEASUREMENT	NORM	ACTUAL	COMMENT
A. RELATING THE MAXILLA TO THE CRANIAL BASE			
A Pt to N Perp	-1.0mm to 3.0mm	2.0mm	
B. RELATING THE MANDIBLE TO THE MAXILLA			
Eff. MAXILLA Lgth	***	87.3mm	EFFECTIVE MAXILLA LENGTH AFTER ADJUSTMENT FOR 'A' PT. LOCATION: 85.3
Eff. MANDIBLE Lgth	104.7mm to109.7mm	113.6mm	LONG MANDIBLE
Diff=MAX-MAND Lgth	***	28.2mm	
Lower Facial Ht[Vert Dim]	59.8mm to 63.5mm	66.6mm	LONG VERTICAL DIMENSION
C. RELATING THE UPPER INCISOR TO THE MAXILLA			
Up1 to A Perp	4.0mm to 6.0mm	3.9mm	
D. RELATING THE LOWER INCISOR TO THE MANDIBLE			
Low1 to A-Pg Line	1.0mm to 3.0mm	-0.8mm	
E. MANDIBULAR POSITION			
Pg to N Perp	-3.5mm to 1.5mm	-1.0mm	
F. OTHER USEFUL CEPHALOMETRIC MEASUREMENTS			
SNA	80.0° to 84.0°	79.8°	RETROGNATHIC MAXILLA
SNB	78.0° to 82.0°	76.0°	RETROGNATHIC MANDIBLE
ANB	0.0° to 4.0°	3.8°	SKELETAL CLASS I
Interincisal Angle	120.0° to140.0°	138.9°	
Mandibular Plane Angle	20.0° to 30.0°	19.8°	LOW VERTICAL DIMENSION
Facial Axis (Ricketts)	86.5° to 93.5°	93.9°	OPEN BITE TENDENCIES
WITS	-2.0mm to 2.0mm	2.3mm	SKELETAL II

that the upper centrals are torqued far enough forward when they may not be. Low Upper and Lower Incisal Angles in the 110-degree range or less may be a tip-off that a marginal Class II, Division 2 case is in fact exhibiting the incisal interference NRDM-SPDC phenomenon if TMJ symptoms are present. Even if TMJ symptoms are not yet present, the potential for their appearance in the mild or marginal half-Class II, Division 2 malocclusion still exists (especially in females) and may arise at any time later in the patient's adult life when orthodontic and ortho-pedic treatments are more difficult, impractical, last longer, and after the time when natural growth and development have ceased and can no longer be taken advantage of by the treating clinician. And, from a purely idealistic viewpoint, a marginal Class II, Division 2 is not a correct occlusion. It is not the Class I normal condition exhibiting the Andrews six keys that structurally and functionally well-balanced patients should have. Thus, treatment of such cases is always justified by more than just the desire for improved appearance.

Some cases that are teetering on the verge of NRDM-SPDC TMJ conditions may actually look pretty good to the untrained and unsuspect-ing eye of the clinician as well as the layman. But the TMJs could care less about deceptive appearances anteriorly. Their only concern is normal healthy balance and function posteriorly. And when they are deprived of this by joint compression they speak out the only way they can in the form of audible clicking or pain. And when they do in fact speak, they never deceive! Even if treatment of such a case would cause the opening up of anterior contacts with the creation of slight spacing between the anterior teeth as a means to the ultimate end of being able to tolerate the mandibular advancement (which sometimes may only have to be mini-mal), it is still justified as opposed to the complications of allowing the compromised TMJ area to slowly worsen (which it will, especially in menopausal females).

It is quite possible once the case is complete that the forward thrust of the retained second molars, which would be left intact in the mouth in such cases, may be enough over the years to gradually push everything forward enough to "reclose" the artifically created diastemata. Once deter-mined that the need for treatment actually exists, it would be far better to have the slight spacing between the interproximals of the upper anterior teeth and have a sound healthy TMJ with a balanced, stable occlusion than to have the teeth remain tight and have the space in the retrocon-dylar or bilaminar zone of the TMJ subsequently narrowed. It is easier to close anterior interproximal spaces with modern orthodontic or even operative methods if need be than to close the space of a 5-inch incision required to permit removal of a mangled intraarticular disc!

Using FJO methods to treat the Class II, Division 2 malocclusion, whether active TMJ symptoms have already appeared or not, is always the same. First the case is treated with a maxillary Sagittal II to regain the lost upper anterior labial crown torque. This requires that the upper second molars be left intact as anchorage. The occlusal coverings of the plate over the posterior teeth act as a TMJ splint to open the vertical and decompress the joint slightly, which is often enough to give relief of some of the TMJ symptoms almost immediately, especially in the younger adult patients.

At this point it would seem appropriate to expound upon and clarify some of the issues concerning the addressing of Division 2 problems with Sagittal appliances. There are two major delineations of Sagittal appliance technique: Sagittal I, in which second molars are extracted and posterior quadrants are distalized, and Sagittal II, in which second molars are left intact to serve as anchorage to develop the anterior segments forward. However, there is another delineation of the Sagittal II technique itself that must be borne in mind, that of *orthodontic* Sagittal II technique *v orthopedic* technique. Both have application to Division 2 problems (and even Division 2 effect problems, which as far as the joints are concerned are the same thing).

In the orthodontic Sagittal II technique the middle portion of the appliance is constructed and adjusted so that only the lingual surfaces of the upper anteriors are contacted by the acrylic of the appliance. This results in the teeth being tipped forward (labial crown torque) as the appliance is opened, and little else. The premaxilla orthopedically is pretty much left alone. In the orthopedic Sagittal II technique, however, the middle portion of the appliance is left in full contact with the palatal gingivae in the nasopalatine and rugae areas. This results in more bodily movement of the teeth forward (although some labial crown torque is imparted also) as well as a generalized forward development of the premaxillary alveolar crest and even portions of the apical base (if the patient is faithful in wearing the appliance all day and night and during eating). The younger (and more faithful) the patient is, the better this technique works.

On the heels of this discussion follows the notion of treating the retruded maxilla. A retruded A-point leaves the treating clinician in a quandary as to when to use orthopedic Sagittal II technique and when to resort to more drastic measures such as FPHG. No hard-and-fast rule exists on this issue other than common sense—when the distance is short and the amount of A-point retrusion is quite minimal, orthopedic Sagittal II technique will suffice. When the amount of A-point retrusion is great, FPHG is indicated. The question is then, what constitutes the boundary between the two? Many factors come into play here. The noted authority on this technique, Dr Merle Bean of Des Moines, Iowa, feels that the angulation of the maxillary central in such situations offers a clue as to treatment choice. He states that if the angulation of the upper central is greater than 108 degrees to S-N and the patient suffers from a retruded A-point, FPHG is indicated. The use of even the orthopedic

Sagittal II technique in such instances would result in too much labial crown torque being ultimately imparted to the upper anteriors, leaving them too proclined (and therefore unstable) with respect to the maxillary apical base. This evaluation of the long axis of the upper centrals to S-N is predicated upon S-N being the standard 7 degrees with respect to FH. Should S, N, or both landmarks vary in location to cause a different angulation, either plus or minus, to FH, the amount of correction is simply transferred to the 108-degree limiting value. An even easier way is to relate the central to FH. Figuring that S-N to FH should be 7 degrees, add 7 degrees to the 108-degree value for a new standard of reference of central angulation to FH of 115 degrees, which would be safely independent of S-N variance.

Dr Richard Beistle of "Sassouni Plus" analysis fame uses a similar approach to diagnosis of this issue. He relates the long axis of the upper central incisor to the *palatal plane* with the range of normality at 110 to 113 degrees. If A-point is more than 1.5 to 2.0 mm retruded and the patient has any sort of TMJ situation whatsoever, he employs FPHG, using 1 gm per side per year of age of the patient, feeling also that any extra form of labial crown torque imparted by even orthopedic Sagittal II technique would leave the upper anteriors too proclined if they are already beyond the 113 degrees at the start. The general consensus among most practicing clinicians concerning the movement of A-point forward with orthopedic Sagittal II technique seems to be limited to about 2 mm with some variance for age, cooperation, length of wear, and vault depth (shallower vaults offer less for the acrylic of the appliance to push against).

Another thing to keep in mind is that FPHG hooked up to either a Sagittal appliance with elastic hooks or SWA is predicated upon proper arch form and well-aligned molars with respect to the upper arch form. If the arch is not properly shaped (continuous), the forward-pulling forces will only serve to increase the degree of collapse. Thus it may be necessary to distalize, "mesialize," or develop laterally to obtain correct arch forms prior to hooking up the FPHG. Thus it may be seen that molar position is important when considering such treatment.

Another valuable tip in Sagittal II technique concerning the adjustment of the occlusal bite surfaces of the Sagittal II, or any other active plate with occlusal acrylic when having it double as a TMJ splint, is to "forward grind" the occlusal markings. By this technique the indentations on the occlusal surface of the acrylic against which the opposing lower posterior teeth articulate are ground with acrylic burs such that the acrylic mesial to the indentations is reduced in a graduated fashion so that the distal slopes of the indentations remain untouched but the mesial slopes of the indentations make a gradual or feathered angulation to the surface. This aids in sliding the mandible forward slightly during occlusion with the plate. The steep unreduced distal slopes of the indentations act to "kick" the cusps of the lower teeth forward upon occlusion. With the mesial slopes of the indentations reduced and out of the way, the mandible may not only slide forward, but is encouraged by inclined plane action with the acrylic to do so. This helps relieve some of the constriction of the condyle in the joint area, in an attempt to hasten symptomatic relief before the full decompressing effects of the Bionator may be instituted.

As with most forms of arch modification with removable active plates, when developing either laterally or anteroposteriorly, *overcorrect a little*. Once the arch has been first rounded out anteroposteriorly with the Sagittal, it may then be reevaluated for any arch width deficiencies. If upper Schwarz or Fan appliances are subsequently required, the anterior acrylic portion of these "follow-up" plates will act as a retentive force for the newly forward repositioned upper anteriors while the rest of the arch is being developed laterally. If Crozat appliances are used for this secondary lateral development, the lingual crossover retention wires must be carefully and regularly observed and adjusted so as to provide sufficient anterior force to the lingual surfaces of the upper central and laterals to prevent their relapse. This can be difficult.

If after the initial Sagittal arch lengthening, further lateral development is *not* needed, one must not be too hasty to go right to the Bionator phase of treatment. It would serve the case better to retain the anteriors in their new position for 3–4 months or so to allow for better stabilization to take place in order to help resist relapse in case the patient is less than completely faithful in his Bionator wear. Once the arches have been shaped and retained sufficiently to permit the insertion of the Bionator, the lingual retention wire of that appliance should be properly constructed to provide similar retentive lingual contact.

Prior to construction of the Bionator, the patient's main component of growth should be analyzed by either the Bimler Suborbital Facial Index, Sassouni split gonial angle, or any of the various Y-axis determinants, since Class II, Division 2 malocclusions are often seen in either horizontal or neutral growers. Since they are also often associated with a severe loss of vertical, these two factors may be considered and taken advantage of when construction bites are registered to construct an appliance that produces a greater stimulation to increased vertical.

Since we are discussing adult Class II, Division 2 cases here, it may also be noted that often this implies some of the patients being treated may be old enough or in such a working or social environment where they find wearing the Bionator during the day somewhat impractical, yet are able to handle keeping the Sagittal in place until home from school or work where the phonetic impracticability or social intolerance of the Bionator is nonexistent. When patients are in a program of wearing the Sagittal II during the day and the Bionator in the late afternoon, evening, and night, after 3–5 months it may appear that the mandible has repositioned itself enough, at least on a muscular level, so that the forces of occlusion of the newly advanced lower anteriors against the lingual surfaces of the upper anteriors appear to be able to hold the upper anteriors out labially at the correct interincisal angle on their own. But this is no reason to entertain a cavalier attitude concerning the regularity of continued wear of the Sagittal appliance. Sometimes only 3—4 months are needed to push the upper anteriors forward to the desired angulation in the first phase of treatment prior to the second phase with the Bionator. And after 3 months (or 4—5 if worn only during the evening and night) of Bionator wear when the mandible appears to be fairly stable in the new position, the total time the upper centrals may have been in their own new position may be only 6—8 months. The muscle function in the upper lip that brought about the anterior deformation of the arch is a powerful force, as evidenced by the original pretreatment position of the upper anterior teeth. And in that short of a treatment time the muscle's functional habits may have not yet been completely altered or become accustomed to the new dental environment and therefore may still have enough of a "memory component" of their "old ways" remaining to cause some lingual relapse difficulties if neither the Sagittal II nor the Bionator are worn during the day.

Sagittal I development in a posterior direction is very stable. Sagittal II development in an anterior direction has the nagging potential to be very *unstable* until the case has truly had sufficient time for the alveolar osseous reorganization to take place around the roots of the teeth and for hypertonic muscle function to be retrained. If sufficient attention is not given to retraining the musculature through wear of both the Sagittal and Bionator in the day/night combination as previously described, or by the more clinically desirable and effective means of Bionator wear exclusively, a sort of biological or muscular duel begins between the forces of retention and muscular retraining offered by the appliance while it is being worn, on the one hand, *v* the improper forces of the perioral musculature against the premaxilla and upper anterior teeth due to "memory" while the appliances are not being worn. This can lead to patients presenting with appliances that no longer fit quite right, which in turn contributes to a vicious cycle of poor patient cooperation in appliance wear, and only complicates and prolongs treatment time. The basic principles of treatment cannot be ignored: Patients must wear the appliances as instructed; they must activate them properly as instructed; and they must keep the appliances in place as instructed until treatment is complete. One should not be fooled into permissiveness in appliance wear simply because results appear to the eye to have occurred quickly. It is perfectly normal for both patient and doctor to anxiously await the resolution of the case and to try to expedite the treatment as quickly as possible. But if one does not have the time or commitment to do it right, how will one find the time and commitment to do it over?

Counter-condensation   As with all cases completed with Bionators, final arch perfection of individual teeth may be easily accomplished with the SWAs if needed. However, there may be times when the SWA is called upon *prior* to insertion of the Bionator. This brings us to the consideration of a very important concept, that of "counter-condensation" of the maxillary dental arch. In some Class II, Division 2 cases of the adult dentition, correction of Division 2 reclined upper anteriors often leads to sizable multiple diastema formation between the anterior incisors, and in some instances even distal to the cuspids, especially if the maxilla itself is somewhat orthopedically retruded. In younger adolescent adult dentition patients of this type, the forward thrust of the second molars is sometimes enough to eventually close up the spaces once the case is complete and natural "settling in" has occurred. However, if the spaces are large and the anteriors have been torqued labially a considerable degree, and if the patient is well into adulthood, the spaces may be very slow to close, thus allowing for the possibilities of the problems of lingual relapse to manifest themselves. This possibility is heightened by the use of the Bionator, which has a modicum of distal drive effect on the upper arch. If the labial bow is left *on* the teeth when the appliance is inserted, it can cause some unwanted lingual relapse of the upper anteriors in a lingual direction as the mandible advances. If it is kept *off* the upper anteriors during the mandibular advancement phase of treatment, it applies all of its distal driving effect (the result of the "stretch" forces of the musculature) to the bicuspids and first molars, which may add to the spacing problem posteriorly. Even if this was not a problem, an upper arch expanded out anteroposteriorly in an effort to protect TMJs from the NRDM-SPDC phenomenon and sporting diastemata between all the teeth makes proper cusp/fossa alignment of the arches during subsequent Bionator advancement of the mandibular arch difficult at times, due to the uneven positioning of recently moved upper teeth. This occurs because, after the Sagittal II phase of treatment, even though the upper anteriors are now properly positioned forward enough, the posterior quadrants might still remain back too far. This is especially true with respect to the future position of the mandibular arch that is still waiting to be advanced as a whole by the Bionator phase of treatment yet to come. Overcorrection might be thought of as a solution, but this leaves the clinician guessing as to final position of the maxillary anterior teeth; ie, how much relapse will occur? Although some overcorrection is always advisable in Division 2 correction situations, other methods prove more controllable. One is to put small wires distal to the cuspids (or distal to the laterals in the younger patient if the cuspids have not arrived yet) to keep the anterior contacts closed between the six front teeth as the middle section of the Sagittal II appliance moves them forward. This only leaves a space distal to the cuspids, which is more acceptable esthetically. A more comprehensive method, however, is the process of maxillary arch "counter-condensation" with the SWA. First, the diastema between the upper centrals is closed with elastic power chain, a process that takes about 2 weeks or so, depending on the size of the space to be closed.

Next, the upper laterals are condensed to the fixed centrals. Then the two cuspids are condensed, either simultaneously if spaces are small or unilaterally if larger, forward with power chain to the four fixed centrals and laterals. Sequentially, the first bicuspids are condensed (as a pair) against the six fixed anteriors followed by the condensation of the second bicuspids forward against the front eight using sequentially longer and longer sections of power chain as more and more teeth are engaged. Finally, the molars are condensed against the front ten teeth, which when ligated together as a single unit form enough anchorage to easily pull molars forward instead of vice versa. This results in a tight, fully advanced, fully condensed, forward positioned arch against which Bionator advancement of the mandible may be more easily effected with better cusp/fossa alignment of the individual teeth arch to arch. This must of course be done against the reinforcement of the old Sagittal II appliance that has been appropriately trimmed of any acrylic or wires that would interfere with the sequential forward condensation of the teeth. This process is also usually confined to the six anteriors.

Class II, Division 3 Bimaxillary Protrusion

A rarely occurring type of malocclusions is the Class II, Division 3 bimaxillary protrusion. (The term "Division 3" is a recently invented designation for a malocclusion with severely proclined anteriors such that the interincisal angle is less than 120 degrees.) As previously stated in the section on Class I, Division 3 protrusive cases, the Class II "bipro" is one of the few instances in which four-bicuspid-extraction treatment may be seriously and legitimately considered, albeit even under more restrictive conditions than the Class I counterpart. In the presence of initially adequate vertical, or maybe even *excessive* pretreatment vertical, a *leptoprosopic* face, severe forward drift of the posterior segments, intense protrusion, and proclination of the anteriors and no third molars in a post-teen young adult, the extraction of the bicuspids will allow the retraction of the remaining teeth into the extraction site which will reduce the amount of protrusion in both upper and lower arches anteriorly. By virtue of the reciprocal forces of this action, molars will move forward slightly (unless full anchorage is retained with some sort of headgear) and the vertical will also be reduced. However, extreme care must be exercised to ensure that this process will not result in an excessive reduction of the anterior lip support so as to result in a sunken-in perioral facial appearance. Likewise, the orthopedic status of the mandible must receive the most scrutinizing attention so as to be fully translated forward to its cephalometrically correct position prior to such consolidation so as to ensure that after treatment the patient has a balanced face and uncompromised TMJ. When the anteriors are retracted, they should be done so with great caution so as to avoid undoing all that the Bionator will be attempting to do orthopedically. By being retrieved to cephalometrically correct overjet and overbite relationships their effect on the mandibular arc of final closure must constantly be monitored so as to avoid initiation of the NRDM-SPDC phenomenon.

If the degree of skeletal Class II mandibular insufficiency is not great but the amount of upper anterior protrusion and overjet is enormous (above the 10-mm level), some authorities advocate extracting only the upper bicuspids and retracting the anterior teeth with headgear anchorage of the first molars and making the upper arch fit the lower arch while leaving the case in *dental* Class II molar relationships. Being able to advance the entire mandibular skeletal Class II lower arch greatly aids such circumstances, since it reduces the degree of retraction necessary to bring the upper anteriors to coupling as well as ensures that no retropositioned condyles and compromised TMJs will remain after treatment. Although the true "firebrand" FJO enthusiasts cringe at the thought of extracting bicuspids under any circumstances, we must be honest and admit that under the right circumstances of a rarely (and I do mean *rarely*) occurring and long list of definitive qualifications, bicuspids may be extracted and the case delivered satisfactorily: face, smile, occlusion, TMJ, and all. To deny such is to become close-minded and subservient to a dogma, and those who insist on such in all circumstances may wind up painting themselves into a methodological corner when special cases arise.

But therein lies the key to understanding the rationale of this or any other form of treatment: special cases require special measures, and extraordinary cases require extraordinary measures. One must always remember to treat to the *needs* of a given individual, not to the mindless dictates of a treatment-planning paradigm. Mandibular advancement with a Bionator may be necessary prior to initiation of this bimaxillary protrusion reduction technique to ensure a balanced profile and a decompressed joint prior to anterior retraction. These are special circumstances that occur infrequently, and their correction via the route of bicuspid extraction by no means is a violation of the FJO philosophy. It is in complete adherence to what the philosophy dictates—to give the patient what he needs: balanced, stable, functional occlusions in a balanced face while ensuring healthy, sound TMJs.

In these unusual malocclusion circumstances of the biprotrusion variety, the clinician can only work with what cards Nature has dealt him. The FJO system of appliances, as previously stated, are great bone "stretchers" but poor bone "shrinkers." And if the patient presents with bones that are already grossly "overstretched" prior to treatment, modifications in therapeutic approach must obviously be made to accommodate the existing dysplasias. But the long list of special and rarely occurring indications must be truly present for such radical forms of treatment to be instituted, and the diagnosis and treatment plan must be verified by sound and thorough levels of justifying diagnostic information.

Another method of approaching such a case advocated by others considers that if the biprotrusion is not too severe, the second molars may be extracted and the case developed to Pont's or Schwarz's corrected indexed widths if needed followed by distalizing the posterior quadrants with upper and lower Sagittal I therapy to give the upper and lower anteriors room in which to be retracted. Often the Class II mandible is advanced into Class I skeletal relationship, taking advantage as much as possible of the retracting powers of the Bionator's labial bow action along the way. Final retraction of the upper anteriors may then be completed by use of a Hawley-type upper palatal appliance, anchored by clasps and posterior interproximal projections of acrylic and with a labial bow (and elastic hooks) to retract the upper anteriors (keeping the lingual acrylic behind them out of the way to prevent it from interfering). The labial bow wire of such an appliance is activated to pull the bow labially against the upper anteriors, which, as they retract, work against the overly protruded lowers to help upright them and increase the extremely low (120 degrees or less) biprotrusion type of interincisal angle.

Lower arch condensation procedures with SWA and power chain also aid in retracting overly tipped and protruded lower incisors. However, an *increase in vertical* will result from the distalizing of both upper and lower posterior quadrants; hence an already adequate or excessive vertical obviates this type of treatment. Due to the infrequency of either Class I or Class II true bimaxillary protrusion cases, each patient must be assessed on an individual basis to determine which treatment techniques may be best tolerated and most effective in addressing that patient's needs.

Special Considerations in Class II Treatment: Skeletal *v* Dental Resolution

There are occasions when the clinician may be confronted with the problem of deciding which way to go on a marginal Class II or half-Class II situation with little or no lower arch crowding. After proper arch width is secured, the clinician knows he may round out the crowded upper arch and develop it anteriorly with fixed Straight Wire mechanics, Sagittal II technique anchoring against retained second molars, followed by advancing the lower arch to Class I with a Bionator. However, he also sees the opportunity for an alternative and completely opposite approach, that of extracting the upper second molars and distal driving the upper first molars, thus regaining the lost maxillary arch form by relieving the crowding by means of posterior quadrant distalization and, coincidentally, acquiring the dental Class I status in the process.

Both treatments are readily feasible, but which will be best for the face, stability of the occlusion, and the joints? The answer again lies in cephalometrics. For assistance in this decision the clinician may wish to consider the Factor 6 Stress Axis of the Bimler. If it is of a POST designation, the case obviously needs mandibular advancement so that the long axes of the teeth may have their best architectural advantage in absorbing the stresses of occlusion. Hence, the treatment of choice would utilize a Sagittal II to develop the upper arch anteriorly followed by conventional Bionator treatment to bring the mandible forward, genion with it, and hence bring the Stress Axis forward into proper location through apicale. Upon careful analysis of the Factor 6, he may otherwise possibly see that the Stress Axis line does fall through apicale, which would be designated as PER, indicating a *skeletal Class I* in spite of the molars actually being in a *dental Class II*. With a Stress Axis in a PER configuration, other aspects of the Bimler will also lend support to the skeletal Class I aspect of such a marginal case.

Which should the clinician accept as being the most accurate representation of the case, the tooth-to-tooth half-Class II, or maybe even full-Class II dental relationship of the occlusion, or the bone-to-bone PER designation of the Factor 6 Stress Axis relationship? If the Stress Axis is the diagnostic criteria that is correct (which it almost always is) in this seemingly orthodontic/orthopedic contradiction, it would indicate that the upper and lower jaws are horizontally aligned correctly with respect to one another but the maxillary posterior teeth and cuspids are by default tipped forward in the alveolar trough of the maxilla, thereby producing the Class II dental relationship while the orthopedic relationship actually remains as a Class I. Such a case appears to be a Class II (because of the relationship of the cusps of the teeth), but it is actually a Class I. Treating it as a true Class II would entail developing the lower anteriors forward, tipping of the bicuspids, and might leave the Upper Incisal Angle of the Bimler a little high. And when the Class II molar relationship is then subsequently corrected with the Bionator the mandible will be drawn past its normal orthopedic Class I starting position, pulling genion and, as a result, the Factor 6 Stress Axis line with it anteriorly. This results in a PER designation, which is an indication of Class III tendencies and might tend to leave the lower face too full.

To ensure better orthopedic balance and increase the chances for better posttreatment long-term stability, one would most likely wish to preserve the PER Stress Axis designation when selecting which way to develop the arches anteroposteriorly. Once the Stress Axis is on PER or orthopedic Class I, mandibular advancement procedures in dental Class II/skeletal Class I cases described above tend to bring on the loss of orthopedic Class I status and might easily lead to slight anterior overdevelopment. This is why certain cases of this nature, due to the anterior drifting or tipping of the posterior segments, when treated as if they were actually skeletal Class II, tend to look a little protrusive. This is why it helps to understand how to coordinate direct, clinically observed orthodontic cusp-to-cusp anatomical relationships with cephalometrically analyzed orthopedic bone-to-bone relationships to better understand the full significance of each in the malocclusions at hand. If the maxillary teeth are at fault by having tipped forward resulting in a crowded anterior cuspid and half-Class II or near full-Class II molars, the deciding factor could well be the fidelity of the Factor 6 Stress Axis line. It will remain in true orthopedic Class I relationship in the PER category. Hence, the indication is to distal drive.

Further considerations of the location of the mesial surface of the upper first molar with respect to the Midfacial Arc (or corrected Midfacial Arc if ANS is not on the Anterior Arc) from the Sassouni analysis is also helpful in this decision. Sagittal I technique would be indicated if crowding exists anteriorly (crowded out cuspids) and the mesial surface of the maxillary first molars are anterior to the Midfacial Arc. The location of B-point on the Basal Arc would also corroborate the Sagittal I choice and obviate the use of a Bionator; ie, the case is purely orthodontic. However, with a maxillary first molar mesial surface on (tangent) the Midfacial Arc in the same situation and a B-point location slightly distal to the Basal Arc, the combination would then alternatively cause the clinician to opt for the Sagittal II technique of leaving the upper molars essentially where they are and relieving the crowding by developing the arch anteriorly. Yet this method would also result in increasing overjet in the process. But this is no problem, since B-point is going to be retruded somewhat from the Basal Arc (cause for the retrusion of the passenger mandibular dental arch distally enough to qualify the case as Class II) and will be corrected with Bionator advancement anyway. This corrects the temporary Sagittal-appliance-induced overjet.

The reason for the dental Class II situation in the example described above comes from the fact that due to one reason or another, during the transition from the deciduous dentition to the adult dentition, the space-holding aspects of the transitional dentition in the maxillary arch were somehow lost which allowed the crowns of the teeth in the upper posterior quadrants to *tip* forward even though their apicies remained in their original and orthodontically correct location high up in the basal bone. This forced the eruption of the straggling upper cuspids to follow a path more mesofacially oriented in a "blocked out" fashion. Hence the Class II molar relationship ensues, not because of a lower molar that is too far back but because of an upper molar that is too far forward. What the needs are in this type of case are for the reverse actions to take place—the artificial undoing of what has already naturally occurred. The offending teeth, namely the upper posteriors, simply need to be driven back distally, or maybe only tipped distally to their more original upright position, which would not only restore Class I dental status to the arches and relieve crowding anteriorly but also allow the Factor 6 Stress Axis line to remain unadvanced and continue to correctly pass through the nearly stationary apicale. This would keep the stresses of occlusion more favorably and biomechanically aligned with the long axes of the roots of the posterior teeth aiding in securing long-term orthodontic functional balance and retention. Hence, treatment would involve second molar extraction followed by Sagittal I technique so as to restore the upper teeth that have drifted or tipped forward back to their originally correct and more distal locations in the maxilla.

Corroboration of the above will also be possible with additional analysis of maxillary anterior positioning by means of the McNamara. This system of determining how much anterior protrusion is acceptable is excellent for deciding where to place anterior teeth, but the degree of variance of analysis of mandibular positioning (-8 to $+2$ mm) makes that particular cephalometric analysis point worthless in marginal or border line "disguised" Class II cases of the nature described above. The extremely wide range of acceptability of the mandible's position would not help one decide whether to develop anteriorly and translate a little, or to leave the mandible alone and distal drive upper posterior quadrants. Obvious discrepancies indicate obvious treatments, but slight discrepancies only hint at a number of treatment possibilities. Some may feel that since the discrepancy is slight, any of a number of choices of varying treatments will be acceptable. Maybe so. But it is comforting to be able to determine which of the choices is the exact best. In its grand design of the human form Nature never guesses. Who are we to tolerate lesser standards when we intervene?

Individual Teeth and the Bionator

Although we have consistently referred to the Bionator's ability to align the arches as separate whole units, it may also be modified or adjusted to place specialized attention to specific areas.

The first area is arch-to-arch midline horizontal alignment. It may occur that a lower Class II arch is symmetrical in shape but more retruded or deficient in growth on one side than another. The right side, for instance, may be a full Class II while the left side is only half-Class II. When this is accompanied by good lower arch form and symmetry, unilateral distalization of the less retruded Class II molars is totally contraindicated. Rather than correcting the half-Class II segment with a lower Sagittal I to "even up" the degree of retrusion of the first molars prior to Bionator advancement of the entire lower arch back to Class I again, the problem is solved by simply taking the construction bite with the mandible not only advanced but also shifted to the correct side such that the upper and lower orthopedic midlines coincide. This also assumes that the soft tissue (frenum) and toothy midlines will then coincide in their respective arches. This will allow the shorter side of the mandible (in the above example the right side) to be advanced more than the longer left side. Overcorrection in such cases is entirely contraindicated.

Mandibular advancement is an adaptive response unlike that of moving an individual tooth where the transeptal fibers that have a protracted elastic memory try to return the tooth to its original position. During the "muscle slippage" that occurs in the first 3 to 4 months of Bionator wear, only that muscular repositioning which is needed to adapt to the mandible's new position will occur. When it does occur and is once complete, there is no equivalent of the elastic memory of the tooth-moving situation.

CHAPTER 9
Class III Adult Dentition Treatment

Describing effective removable appliance treatment for the true Class III malocclusion isn't easy: It's impossible. The best the clinician may hope for is that the case initially presents itself, and will remain, as a marginal or near pseudo-Class III throughout the entire adolescent and young adult growth period. But the true skeletal Class III or malocclusions simulating leptoid dysplasia and/or mandibular prognathisms with anterior open bites are truly candidates for surgery.

For the marginal case where the bite is end to end in the anteriors and there is hopefully a little anterior crowding in the maxillary incisors, the Sagittal II may be employed to advance the premaxilla and its teeth in an effort to restore the anterior overjet to the incisors, relieve the crowding in the upper anterior area, and round out the maxillary arch. Once the upper anteriors have cleared the lowers, a Bionator II fabricated from a wax bite taken in neutral occlusion, but merely open 2 mm, may be inserted in an effort to increase the anterior overbite a little to try and "house" the lower anteriors. Sagittal II treatment may create spacing distal to the cuspids. Some practitioners advocate finishing the case in

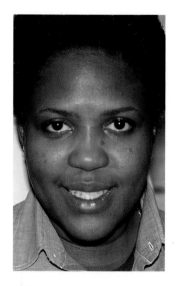

(A)

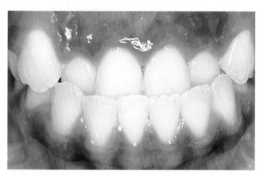

(B)

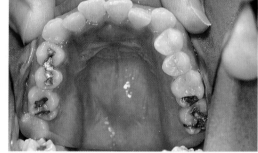

(C)

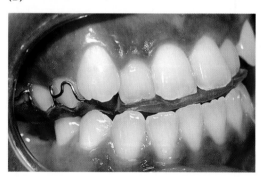

(D)

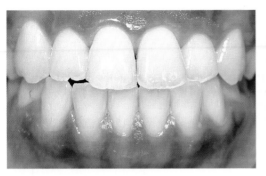

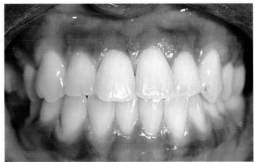

(E)   **(F)**

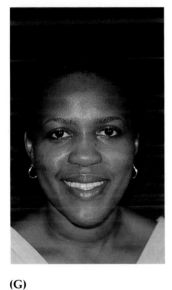

(G)

Figure 9–1   Class III (permanent dentition). This patient presented at 30 years of age with a Class III-type malocclusion that is very similar to an anterior crossbite **(A), (B)**. Note the foreshortened appearance of the anterior maxillary arch form **(C)**. Treatment consisted of 4 months with the first Sagittal II appliance, 8 months with a second Sagittal II, and 6 more months with a third Sagittal II to effect slight overcorrection, which subsequently settled in nicely to a well-finished case **(D–G)**.

fixed appliances, of a standard Straight Wire setup on the upper against a fixed labial arch on the lower and the use of Class III elastics (elastics running from a hook on the cuspid area of the lower fixed appliance to the Class II hook on the buccal tube of the upper molar band). If such is employed, the space that may occur distal to the upper cuspids (after Sagittal II development forward has advanced the anterior teeth) will most likely close.

But two precautions must be noted when initiating such treatment. First, concern must be shown for the TMJ, since the forces of Class III elastic mechanics will force the mandible to its most retruded position which, as far as the TMJ is concerned, is tenuous at best. Should TMJ symptoms appear, the use of the elastics may have to be discontinued. The second point to remember in attempting to use fixed appliances in any Class III situation, is to never under any circumstances finish the case in the lower arch with a rectangular wire. The rectangular arch wire is designed to impart labial crown torque to the lower anteriors, a normally desired circumstance especially in Class II situations.

But labial crown torque is the last thing one needs in a Class III situation. If anything, a little lingual crown inclination may be desirable if possible to allow the upper anteriors the chance to obtain proper overbite and overjet relative to the lowers. The labial crown torque provided by the rectangular finishing arch wires would only undo this situation. Therefore, only finish in a *round* wire!

A third consideration to make in Class III treatment is whether the patient could stand the protrusion that such Sagittal III treatment as discussed above may impart to the face. If the mandibular arch is already protruded and one does successfully thrust the premaxilla far enough forward to house it, what will be the effects in the patient's face? Unfortunately, there is no way to assume an "as if" position by advancing the maxilla to ponder such an effect. But one can easily imagine what would happen if a premaxilla were to be advanced improperly beyond the esthetically acceptable limits of the face in an effort to house the lower Class III arch. Although man has much in common with the ape, parents are not particularly fond of having their children look like one.

This is where the Lynn analysis serves as a most valuable aid. The Bio-Facial Matrix acts as an ideal medium to enable the clinician to get a reasonably accurate idea of the differences between the pretreatment and posttreatment states of the facial profile. It also gives an estimate of the feasibility of the treatment considered to correct the problem. The use of the matrix value (MV) serves to individualize the Matrix, hence the constructed posttreatment profile, to the individual patient's own proportionalized specifications. A freehand sketch of where the upper teeth and bony lip support, and if the clinician is creative enough even an outline of the profile of the upper lip itself, can be drawn over the cephalometric tracing with the lower incisors acting as a guide to show the minimum distance required to house the case. A simple human assessment of the esthetics of the projected posttreatment profile along with an analysis of the cephalometric readings such a profile would generate are usually all that is needed to determine if the results would be acceptable. Even if the premaxilla could be moved that far forward and assuming it would remain there with no tendency to relapse, an overly protrusive lower facial profile would obviously preclude satisfactory orthodontic treatment. Cephalometric considerations of present and projected anatomic relationships as divulged by the Lynn analysis may act as a guide here.

Another approach advocated by some is the use of the Class III Frankel appliance or Functional Regulator III (abbreviated FR III). Dr Rolf Frankel of East Germany developed a whole series of removable functional appliances during the 1960s to treat various types of malocclusions. He developed four basic types of "functionsregler" or Functional Regulator appliances: the FR I for Class I, and Class II, Division 1 malocclusions; the FR II for Class II, Division 2 malocclusions; the FR III for Class IIIs; and an FR IV for anterior open bites and bimaxillary protrusions. Their use was first promoted on a large scale in America by Dr J. McNamara of cephalometric analysis fame. These appliances operate on an entirely different principle than the Bionators and active plates we have discussed so far. The Bionator, Sagittal, Schwarz, and Transverse appliances are all tooth-borne devices, whereas the Frankel series of appliances are tissue-borne. The basic premise behind the Frankel is that if tension can be placed on the periosteum over the bone or alveolar process of a jaw, it will stimulate bone movement, through adaptive growth, in the vectored direction of that particular artificially produced stimulating tension. But the impression procedures, construction, adjustment, and general management of this series of appliances is so different than that of the appliances we have already discussed that time and space do not permit their discussion in this text. The only reason that these appliances are mentioned here at all is that of the entire series of Functional Regulators the FR III might *just be the simplest, easiest, and most efficient to use.* For this reason, it is advocated by some who normally do not favor the use of such appliances as an alternative form of treatment for marginal Class III cases. Hence, the reader may wish to pursue this independently.

CHAPTER 10
The Final Steps

The final steps in any treatment plan should always include at least a consideration of two things: retention and the posttreatment conference. Both are very important to the completion of a well-planned and correctly treated case, and either one may take on a variety of forms. Both may take on the structure of being active and formal or more passive and casual, depending on the circumstances of the case involved. The one is a product of concern for the biological principles that were utilized in the correction of the case, while the other is a product of concern for the courtesy due to the individuals responsible for the patient's account!

RETENTION

There are numerous forms of retention that have been indulged in since orthodontics began over 100 years ago. It has been a nagging problem since dentists first started moving teeth. We only have time to discuss some of the simplest and most effective principles of retention here. One may or may not be in a position on a given case to use an actual retentive appliance constructed specifically for that purpose, but whenever any form of orthodontic or orthopedic procedure is performed in the oral cavity, the clinician will always have to deal with the retention of his effort either directly or indirectly. The case may have been treated in such a way that an actual retainer is not needed once the final appliance in the treatment plan has been removed. But that is because, due to the circumstances of that particular case, the last appliance used has most likely been doubled over to serve as its own retainer. But in many other instances the retainer *is* the last appliance in the sequence.

When single-appliance treatment plans are indicated, such as those requiring only a Schwarz plate, Sagittal, anterior single-tooth crossbite appliance, etc, the active plate may serve as its own retainer once active treatment is complete. Sagittal I distalization techniques are the most stable of all active plate procedures. But, as previously stated, a 2−4 month posttreatment wearing of the Sagittal is required for functional leveling of the crowns of the teeth moved. Lateral development should be retained also by either the active plated used to attain it or, if too bulky or unhygienic, a simple more streamlined Hawley-type palatal retainer. Active retention with these devices (wearing the appliance 24 hrs a day) may take the form of 3−5 months in the mixed dentition to 4−6 months in the adult dentition, depending on the degree of expansion and the time in which it was accomplished. Having moved something a long way in a short time would obviously require longer periods of active retention than for something moved a short distance at a more leisurely pace. At the point when the clinician considers the case stable enough to diminish retainer wear to the passive stage (night) the first week of such will tell him if the patient is ready. If the retainer becomes progressively tighter or ill fitting over the first days of passive retention, the return to active wear is obviously indicated. Function is a terrific helper in retaining orthodontic and/or orthopedic movements. Anteriorly or posteriorly, good cusp/fossa interdigitation (or incisal overjet and overbite in the anterior area) serves the patient well in helping keep things put.

Other than the first 3−4 months of wear, retention with the Bionator is automatically built into the treatment plan. Whatever is accomplished in the later stages of a Bionator phase of treatment is a simple matter of "what you have, you have" if the incisal overbite is only 50%. If you move up to only 25% it will not revert back down to 50%. Posterior teeth do not "retreat" back down into their sockets! The one consideration that should be made retentivewise in the use of the Bionator is in the treatment of tongue-thrust patients. Once the case is resolved orthopedically and orthodontically, there is no reason to assume it is also resolved myofunctionally. Extended periods of nighttime wear are indicated if the least suspicion at all exists that there may be residual thrusting reflexes remaining. Also, once the appliance phase of Bionator II treatment is complete, the appliance may have to be converted to a Bionator III to prevent an unwanted surplus of overbite.

Even in conventional Bionator treatment, once posterior molar support is attained there is no harm in a period of nighttime wear after the case is near complete to "tighten every thing up" and seek that last little bit of performance out of the appliance, especially in the permanent dentition.

The most glaring example of where active retention is acutely important is in cases that are finished in fixed appliances. The leveling and aligning effects of the SWA are relatively stable but relative to retention, rotations are "murder." Whenever a tooth is rotated more than 20 degrees about its own long axis, three things should be seriously considered: (1) overrotation to a slight extent with rotation wedges, (2) a modified Edwards technique, (3) active retention after fixed appliance removal with spring retainers used for the anterior teeth. The worse the rotation, the more precautions of this nature should be employed to retain the tooth once it has been corrected. As far as leveling and alignment of teeth are concerned, the removal of second molars will all but ensure these types of positionings of individual teeth will remain acceptably unchanged (although there is always some degree of "posttreatment change"). But the transeptal fiber is the true culprit as far as rotations are concerned.

Spring Retainers

The spring retainer is a great advancement over the more traditional Hawley-type retainers that preceded it in that it imparts an exacting, albeit suboptimal, tooth-positioning force on the teeth.

The upper spring retainer may be of two types, either with or without the added acrylic Hawley-type palatal coverage. The method by which these simple yet highly effective retainers obtain their active forces is a product of the ingenious way in which they are constructed. A plaster cast of the posttreatment arch is made and the anterior teeth on the model are carefully sliced interproximally and removed from the model. They are then repositioned back on the model in the most anatomically ideal positions, free of all minor rotations or in-and-out discrepancies that they might have exhibited on the original model. A wire loop is then fabricated to actively contact both facial and lingual surfaces of the six anterior teeth encircling the teeth in a loop cuspid to cuspid. Next a thin bead of clear acrylic is processed on to the wire loop making detailed and positive contact to all the facial and lingual surfaces of the anterior teeth as well as the interproximal contact areas. When this setup is transferred to the mouth, the taut wire loop anticipates an ideal arrangement of the natural teeth similar to that on which it was processed. But, the natural teeth may have minor in-and-out or rotational imperfections still remaining. When snapped into place down over the natural teeth, their deviation from the ideal setup anticipated by the retainer distorts it by prying the wire loop with its acrylic bead apart slightly in a facial-lingual direction. The tension created in the bare wire at its ends, where it crosses over from facial to lingual distal to the cuspids, causes the two facial and lingual halves of the retainer to try and return to their original position, and this in turn puts pressure on the offending teeth by means of the flat surfaces of acrylic bead that are processed over the facial and lingual sections of the wire. Tension may be added to the appliance by crimping the bare hoop of wire slightly with a pair of three-pronged pliers at its exposed parts where it passes distal to the cuspids. This entire process actively moves the individual teeth to the ideal locations they would occupy if they were free of rotations (minor) and in-and-outs (minor), as was the man-made setup upon which the retainer was processed. A small isthmus of exposed wire connects the Hawley palate to the upper spring retainer. The lower spring retainer is processed just to cover the lower six anterior teeth. Though these retainers are highly efficient and have the power to actively move teeth, they "can't move 'em a mile." Only *minor* rotations and in-and-out movements may be accomplished, and this is only possible if space for the movement to be affected already exists for the tooth. As the teeth move closer and closer to the ideal setup of the processing model, the tension will lessen in the wire and may be increased as described above, but too much of an increase will cause the retainer to "pop up" off the teeth and prevent its complete and proper seating.

Tru-tains

Another excellent form of retention device is the full-surface-contact, vacuum-molded, clear plastic retainers developed by Dr Lloyd Truax of Rochester, Minnesota—ie, "shrink wrapped teeth"! The resiliency of the special plastic sheets used in the process of vacuum forming a retainer over a model of the completed case allows ideal retentive devices to be formed, which are easy to trim with common scissors and easy to wear because of the proximity of fit between the clear plastic and the teeth and gingivae. They are extremely esthetic and possess superior retentive capabilities because of the enormous surface area of contact they exert between the plastic of the retainer and the teeth. Therefore, patient compliance with wearing the retainers is almost never a problem. They usually are not used for slight tooth movements like the spring retainers but are limited to use only when the teeth are in their final position. The plastic sheets and vacuum formers are commercially available under the registered trademark Tru-tain. Truax instructs his patients to wear them 24 hr per day for the first 3 days after placement, then 12 hr per day thereafter for 1 year. However, many clinicians take advantage of the extreme comfort and esthetics of these retainers to convince their patients to wear them in a fashion similar to the older-style Hawley retainers, ie, 24 hr per day for the first 6 months, then 12 hr per day for 6 more months. Truax also keeps a model of the finished case (or "one may be given to the patient") in case a retainer is lost or becomes completely worn out, since new ones can be made on the original model in less than 5 minutes.

> *"God and the doctor we like adore*
> *But only in danger and not before,*
> *The danger or'e both alike are requited,*
> *God is forgotten and the doctor slighted"*
> *John Owen—Welsh poet 1560–1622*

THE POSTTREATMENT CONFERENCE

The posttreatment conference is the natural end product of the evolution of the case from the point in the very beginning at which it all began, the pretreatment conference. Before briefly discussing the post-treatment conference, and for the sake of continuity, the pretreatment conference will be discussed first.

We know that for the sake of a proper diagnosis we should acquire a good set of study casts, a panoramic or full mouth set of x-rays, a cephalogram, a thorough health history, and a direct clinical examination. In addition, the chief concerns of the patients and parents should be written down. To be able to adequately explain the patient's problems to both the patient and parents, we must first thoroughly understand them and all their ramifications. By preparing a written outline of our treatment plan and a listing of the patient's individual needs that this treatment plan is designed to correct, we can make the problems which will be encountered during that treatment clear not only to ourselves, but also to the patient and parents, so that when complications arise during treatment all parties concerned will be prepared. At the pretreatment conference the goals of the treatment may be spelled out along with the prognosis for the attainment of those goals. One must always be totally frank and honest as to what is possible to achieve. Never promise what cannot be delivered and never make the case seem easier or less involved than it is. In predicting treatment duration it is better to err on the long side than on the short. Take careful note to address the patient's or parents' particular wants as to whether they are attainable, and, if so, to what degree.

Show the parties involved the recorded data, Pont's or Schwarz's deficiencies, skeletal and dental class, etc; simple and concise explanation of their meaning is all that is needed. The quantification of these conditions helps put the patient's condition into a perspective that they can easily understand. Where the TMJ is of concern, a simple explanation of how the FJO system addresses it is also in order. Using an ideal set of models of teeth as an example, compare the patient's condition against what would be normal. Also, due to the fact that many of the appliances are removable, explain that should patient cooperation become a problem (late teenage boys being the worst offenders), the treatment (and payments) may be stopped upon request. By the maximum application of the "inform before you perform" principle at the pretreatment conference, the concerned parties will be highly understanding of the problems facing the treating clinician and are less likely to generate unrealistic expectations. Explain also that optional extras (like a little Straight Wire perfection at the end) and legitimate complications (like lost appliances, recurrent myofunctional problems, etc) always cost extra. By laying the groundwork clearly and thoroughly at the pretreatment conference, the posttreatment conference takes on the aspect of a treatment progress "report card" and, if the results are good, such conferences act as an excellent practice-building opportunity.

At the posttreatment conference, the parties responsible for the case receive the formal attention of the treating clinician telling them that the case has gone well, the patient has definitely benefited from the treatment, and most or all of the pretreatment goals have been realized. This sounds at first redundant. The improved appearance of a successfully treated case acts as satisfaction enough for most lay people. However, we as doctors realize the ramifications of treatment of a far deeper level, and the significance of things that the layman, though informed of at the beginning of treatment, may have since become confused about or may have entirely forgotten. The posttreatment conference also allows the parents or patient to offer their opinions as to their satisfaction with the progress and present condition of the case and whether additional (and originally noted as optional) treatment should be considered.

Comparing the pretreatment models to the current status of the case is also a valuable practice-building procedure, because parents and patients (and even the treating clinician as well) sometimes forget just how far the case has come since the beginning of treatment. It is easy to be lulled, over a long period of treatment time, into a feeling that "well, the teeth weren't really that bad to begin with, were they?" Such revelations of original conditions prior to treatment tend to remind the parents of how worried they might have originally been for the sake of their child before treatment relieved them of their anxiety, which only acts to raise the level of esteem they have for the treating practitioner. It also tends to make them less critical of any persistent minor imperfections. It must also be frankly stated that in this world of space and time, true, ideal, and pristine perfection is only a fantasy!

For mixed dentition cases that are being treated on an ongoing basis, the posttreatment conference also provides an opportunity for the practitioner to remind the parents that although treatment is presently complete and the case is currently at the normal level of development for a child that age, there is no guarantee that further problems will not appear in the future and require additional treatment. However, this is also a time to ensure them that the child now has just as good a chance as any other to successfully make the transition to the full adult dentition without being sidetracked by the development of further malocclusion. Also, note that even if further work is required, it will be less severe than if the interceptive mixed dentition treatment had not been instituted at all.

The posttreatment conference usually lacks the formality of the pretreatment conference, since a much more casual and relaxed mood permeates the air. It may be only a brief few minutes of the doctor and parents/patient mutually agreeing that things have turned out pretty well. Some may feel it is only a ruse to seek psychological "stroking" from the parents and/or patient for the doctor. But, such an accusation is only immature and venial. It is a celebration! Considering all that modern orthopedic and orthodontic techniques are capable of, and considering how unfortunate the patient's life would be without the benefit of this treatment that we as practitioners now seem to take for granted, once the case is brought to successful completion there is certainly more than enough cause for celebration. And should this turn out to be an occasion where the parties concerned express their gratitude and delight with the efforts the practitioner has produced, all the better. He or she deserves it! Smiles look just as good on the doctor as they do on the patient.

SEQUENCING FOR SUCCESS!

After a careful consideration of this review of generalized treatment methods, we see that it reveals that not only is the sequencing of the appliances we use to correct malocclusions important, but the implementation of that sequence is really nothing more than the reversal of the step-by-step process by which the arches collapsed, failed to develop, and became maloccluded in the first place. We also have seen that the methods employed have a great affinity for simplicity, practicality, and efficiency, the lifeblood of the daily workings of a private practice. We have also seen that the thorough delineation of the patient's individual problems or needs, by means of perceptive and accurate diagnosis, just about points the way by itself to the selection of the appliances and procedures needed for correction of the case.

But what we have not yet seen at the completion stage of treatment is how the results of this process shall endure, for that requires an ongoing observation over a period of many years. But one thing that may be safely predicted is that in every case there will always be some degree of posttreatment change. If a case is treated by means of properly sequenced appliance therapy based on sound diagnosis, that posttreatment change will most likely be imperceptible to the human eye, but it will nevertheless be there. If for no other reason than the long-term interproximal wear and occlusal attrition, the case will no doubt change slightly in time. This posttreatment change may, on the other hand, be clearly perceptible to the eye, in which case it will be of two types: a favorable change, as when a case completes its "settling in" after withdrawal of the appliance, or an unfavorable change. If unfavorable, the question then becomes at what point does it become unacceptable? Only the parties involved may make that individual value judgment. But, posttreatment change is a factor that the patient and parents must always be made aware of prior to treatment. It is a reality that must always be confronted.

However, over the many years of clinical experience techniques have evolved, as we have attested to, that deal quite well with these as well as other important issues. But being able to call upon the full benefits of these techniques requires that maximum effort be directed toward obtaining as proper and complete a diagnosis as possible. Gathering as much information as possible prior to the treatment of the case best prepares clinicians for the treatment problems that lie ahead and helps them make the best choices of appliances and techniques to bring their cases to the highest level of success.

But even after once being successfully completed, it may be discerned through hindsight that a slight modification here or a brief change in sequencing there might have produced an even better case. The fear of such circumstances of hindsight always crosses the mind of the practitioner contemplating the treatment plan of a case prior to initiation of therapy. Though this is the product of a truly concerned and conscientious mind and is to be commended, it should not act as an impediment to what has been determined to be obviously needed treatment. The FJO system is generally forgiving and tolerant enough in many of its aspects to allow the practitioner the liberty to modify or amend a given treatment plan en route as new or heretofore unnoticed circumstances arise and manifest themselves.

The best the treating clinicians may do beforehand is to thoroughly prepare themselves by means of a proper and comprehensive diagnosis and to be fully aware of the treatment capabilities of the appliances and techniques at their disposal. Given the fact that if the patient cooperates in the prescribed wearing and activation of the appliances, and if the clinician correctly adjusts them as required and properly sequences their use, they will impart the full powers inherent in their design to the case and as a result they will work every time. In the light of these undeniable facts, and governed by the knowledge that the effects of a series of appliance selections and sequencing in a given treatment plan are merely a direct issuance of the dictates of the diagnosis, the clinician soon readily surmises that once that particular diagnosis has been verifiably secured, all that remains is to do it!

"Success is never final
failure is never fatal,
it's courage that counts."
Winston Churchill 1874−1965
English Prime Minister

"There's a skirmish of wit between them."
Much Ado about Nothing
William Shakespeare

CHAPTER 11
Interlude

As we look back on this brief review of the coordination of appliance selection and sequencing with the representative diagnostic and cephalometric findings of a particular case, a wide variety of generalizations could readily be made. A proper and reasonably comprehensive diagnosis implies a thorough clinical examination of the patient by the treating practitioner. Yet, two extremely critical components of effecting a diagnosis are the accompanying disciplines of model analysis and cephalometric analysis. Three-dimensional model analysis has been adequately covered in Volume I. The emphasis of this text (Volume II) with respect to diagnostics has been placed on the expansive science of cephalometrics. With respect to each of these components, several things must be kept in mind, things which prove critical to the level of understanding the clinician will possess and the level of success the final case will ultimately achieve.

First, concerning model analysis, it is true that it is important to understand the detailed workings of the Schwarz analysis with its facial corrections, the Pont analysis and its Linder-Harth corrections, the mixed dentition analysis, and the Carey analysis. The concept of directional decrowding is an important mode of thinking to employ in the augmentation of these various arch form analysis systems. But there is also another concept that follows directly on the heels of the notion of directional decrowding that is even more difficult to verbalize in precise quantitative terms. It is a notion that is easily demonstrable through clinical observation, and the understanding of its principles greatly aids in the successful correction of various types of arch form problems. It is a notion that, for want of a better set of terms, might best be described as the concept of correction *v* development. The temptation is strong, for the sake of more rapid assimilation of the overall idea, to refer to it as correction *v* expansion. But the term "expansion" has been associated with various untoward definitions in orthodontics over the years, and as a result would bring with it too many unwanted overtones that might lead to confusion. Hence the term "development" will have to suffice.

By the term "correction" is meant the movement of teeth to their correct original location, ie, a location where they might have originally developed and resided but because of the various numbers of factors acting on them have been subsequently forced somewhere else. The prime example of such is the forward movement of posterior quadrants mesially as a result of the tremendous thrust of the second molars. Such forward drift can easily block out the cuspids labially. Treatment in the form of removal of the second molars and distalization of the posterior quadrants with a Sagittal I appliance or similar technique is an example of correction. It is extremely stable. The teeth are moved back to their original locations in the alveolus, the places where they erupted. The disrupting force moving them improperly forward is eliminated almost instantly via the extraction forceps. Distalization (correction) of the teeth of the posterior quadrants along their own alveolar trough is always very stable.

Development, on the other hand, implies the movement of a group of teeth to an entirely new location, a location which, although the teeth might actually and ideally belong there, they nevertheless have not yet achieved. Moving retroclined upper anteriors forward in Division 2 cases and moving posterior quadrants laterally in reduced arch width cases are examples of development. Development is an extremely unstable situation that requires long and intense periods of retention. Teeth can erupt correctly and then be shoved somewhere else (usually forward), hence the concept of correction. But in cases where development is needed, the teeth are usually residing right where they erupt. The entire alveolar process in which they develop and erupt is slightly misplaced itself due to improper muscle function that surrounds the area and perpetually acts upon it, albeit in an unbalanced manner. Obtaining proper arch form consists of not only moving the teeth to a more desirable location but also in retraining and rehabilitating the surrounding musculature. Functional appliances can do this in certain instances and so can prolonged periods of retention, but, oddly, only to a point! This is why it will be observed that moving retroclined Division 2 upper anteriors forward to more proper interincisal angles in order to free a locked mandible and retruded mandibular arc of closure is a procedure fraught with relapse problems. If such a forward development procedure is performed too quickly and not retained long enough, the surrounding oral muscle environment, which has not had time to get used to the new dental environment, persists in its old imbalanced ways and endeavors to push the anteriors back in again. The older the patient, the more likely this will occur such that Division 2 development (or even division 2 effect development) forward in adult patients to eliminate NRDM/SPDC TMJ problems is often attended by the use of lifetime, night-only retainers. Sometimes you really *can't* teach old muscles new tricks. The source of the problem cannot be eliminated instantly by the surgeon as in the case of the forward crowding of the correction example (second molars), but it must be dealt with on a long-term basis. The longer the muscles have had their way, generally the more difficult it is *in development problems* to retrain them. Somehow, almost miraculously, this dictum *does not* pertain to retraining muscles to move the whole mandible forward all at once with functional appliances such as the Bionator. But then in such cases as this, the mandible is merely being taken to the orthopedically balanced position to which *it* had always belonged per the dictates of the joint.

Moving posterior quadrants laterally has always been an endeavor that has met with a great deal of controversy. "You can't expand arches laterally." "The intercanine distance in the mandible is one of the most immutable in Nature." Such statements have long echoed through the chambers of orthodontic therapeutics. The reason statements of this nature appeared in the first place is that excessive lateral expansion has always been proven highly unstable and highly subject to relapse. Yet every clinician who treats malocclusion is sooner or later forced to develop a certain number of very narrow arches laterally to obtain acceptable arch form. In many of these cases excellent and quite stable results are obtained on a regular basis.

What is happening? Well, no one really knows for sure; but there are some pretty good ideas currently in circulation. A general consensus of forward-thinking individuals seems to center around the idea of uprighting lingually tipped lower teeth to obtain proper mandibular arch form. Barring AP crowding problems for the moment for the sake of our discussion, development of the mandibular arch laterally consists of the uprighting of lingually tipped lower teeth and even the tipping of them as far buccally as possible to obtain reasonable mandibular arch form according to the dictates of the mandibular deep apical base.

Attempts at bodily moving the entire tooth, apex, alveolar envelope, and all, in a lateral direction might meet with considerable resistance; hence it might also be expected to exhibit serious relapse. It is common knowledge that mandibular expansion past a certain point, individual to each case, simply will not hold. Not only will the muscle environment not tolerate it, the bony environment will not tolerate it. Yet severely lingually collapsed mandibular arches can be developed to a more acceptable wider arch form that, if not taken past certain physiological limits will in fact demonstrate stability. This happens when lowers are uprighted over their apical bases. This would appear as lateral movement of the teeth, but in actuality is movement of crowns only. The tooth is not translated, apex and all, laterally over the apical base. Some retention is needed for lateral development (uprighting), because parts of the teeth (the upper parts) are being moved to a new, never-before-experienced, bony location. It must be remembered that the age of the patient is a factor here too, ie, the younger the better. It appears that retention past 6 months for lateral and even anterior development in the late mixed dentition and *early* adult dentition seems generally unnecessary. But in the late adolescent and early adult patient, more caution is advised because longer periods of retention will often prove necessary.

With the concept of correction *v* development in mind, we may now make sense out of the debate between two of the major schools of thought in orthodontics, the fixed appliance viewpoint *v* the functional appliance philosophy. For years the traditional fixed-appliance-oriented orthodontic community built their cases orthodontically around the mandibular arch. True, they obtained some degree of arch widening, but it was due to uprighting lingually tipped crowns of the posterior quadrants back out buccally. Barring extraction of bicuspids, which is a separate issue, such a fixed-appliance-produced (widened) arch was rock solid, since teeth were not translated beyond their apical base. Then believing the mandible with its new and now very stable mandibular arch form could not be moved bodily forward in any way, practitioners "solved" Class II large overjet problems by treating the maxillary arch back to the mandibular arch. That was their mistake. It was good orthodontics for the mandibular arch form, but bad orthopedics for the maxilla and joint.

The functional camp tried the opposite. They generally were thought of as preferring to develop the ideal maxillary arch with anteriors far enough forward to permit an "unlocked" mandibular arc of closure with respect to the dictates of the joint and posterior quadrants wide enough apart to permit the formation of ideal arch form according to precalculated tables of values, such as Pont's or Schwarz's. Then, with the arch-aligning capabilities of functional appliances such as the Bionator, they would bring the mandible forward and make it and its mandibular dental arch meet the maxilla and its idealized maxillary dental arch. However, this often led to unnecessary widening of the arches. Overexpansion then became their mistake. That was good orthopedics for the mandibular jawbone, but may prove out in some instances to be bad orthodontics for the maxillary teeth. Both schools of thought believed that certain basic therapeutic precepts of the other were dead wrong. In actuality, both were only partially wrong, which more euphemistically means that both were actually only partially right. Hence, the notion of directional decrowding enhanced by the concepts of correction *v* development becomes the obvious compromise in the search for stable arch form.

The beauty of the traditional fixed appliance school is that it produced, by default sometimes merely because they uprighted posteriors, nicely shaped, widened mandibular dental arches that were very stable, especially with respect to lateral development. Although they were incorrect in leaving the mandible in skeletal Class II orthopedic retrusion, they did have the key to proper orthodontic mandibular arch width stability. Therein lies the true orthodontic dental arch width measuring rod. It is individualized patient to patient and is closely related to frontal facial form and facial type. Using this as the key, the upper arch need only be widened enough so as to be able to adequately house the lower arch's very stable width. After arch width development laterally by means of uprighting lingually tilted lower posteriors, any further crowding in the arch must be relieved by posterior distalization (correction), anterior development, or varying combinations of both. It is imperative that the maxillary arch be able to *house the mandible far enough forward* so as to keep the TMJs properly articulated—condyle on disc—and allow for plenty of posterior joint space. So the traditional school was right in that the mandibular arch form, one that is properly developed and not overly expanded laterally, is the key to maxillary arch form, but only from an orthodontic (ie, arch width) standpoint. The key to the *orthopedic* correctness of the mandibular location is the TMJ, and its proper articulation and functional balance is predicated on the all-important mandibular arc of closure, which is predicated on the maxillary arch being far enough forward to allow decompressed, free mandibular operation. So if everybody would philosophically get together, the hybrid approach incorporating the best of both worlds would give the best results to the patient. Egos can wait.

As previously stated, along with model analysis, cephalometric analysis is also critical for obtaining a comprehensive diagnosis, especially with respect to the skeletal aspects of the case. We have seen some of the trailmarks of the path cephalometric analysis has followed from its inception to the present day. Our attention has focused almost exclusively on the clinical significance of the science and its role in helping the practitioner determine the best combined orthodontic *and* orthopedic treatment plan. We have seen how various experts set varying norms to use as standards of judgment for certain measurements and anatomical relationships. The sheer number of standards derived and the variability of their values indicates that no single set of numbers can serve as an ideal for all individuals. The clinical use of cephalometrics (and even model analysis) resolves itself down to a matter of relativity. One must not "treat to the numbers" but to the patient's needs. And the overriding need of all patients receiving orthodontic treatment, the one major issue that makes all cephalometric criteria truly relative, is the need for fully functioning, properly articulated, and adequately decompressed post-treatment TMJs. This must be obtained above all else. Where they are present, all other cephalometric criteria may be evaluated as to what is right and proper relative to where the mandible, maxilla, and dental arches subsequently align and as to what constitutes an acceptable case. When they are not present, ie, when they are imbalanced with condyles riding off the discs in both function and rest positions, all other cephalometric measurements, no matter how closely they comply with the most exacting ideal series of norms, are for all intents and purposes meaningless. Without proper joints a finished case can never be considered acceptable, regardless of how perfect the numbers are. Cephalometrics, like model analysis, can act as a very important guide in treatment planning. Both methodologies should be used in a fashion which reflects concern for the joint, the face, the total patient, and not just the dental occlusion.

However, the consideration of the significance of cephalometric criteria and its augmented interpretation relative to the dictates of the TMJ is subject matter that should be relegated to yet again an entirely different discussion. Hence it has been. But for now it is fitting that we first explore "classical" cephalometrics in an attempt to better understand what is "normal" before we attempt to consider what actually constitutes "abnormal." This is why we have emphatically stressed, both at the beginning and at the end of our discussion of this subject, that the theories and standards discussed in these pages are predicated upon a case already exhibiting properly articulated joints in the pretreatment state. The absence of obvious and direct relationships between various criteria of the cephalometric analyses discussed with the needs of the TMJs in no way negates their value as diagnostic tools. It must simply be remembered that their meaning must be interpreted in light of the needs of the joint, not in spite of them. It may take a bit more practice and insight to correlate one with the other, but to fail to do so is placing the success of the treatment plan and the well-being of the patient at serious risk. When the two are correlated, the patient receives the best chance for a truly successful outcome, and the clinician is producing the finest of standards of proper treatment, standards patients have trustingly come to expect.

As stated at the outset, cephalometrics is a language. We have looked at the meaning of some of its words. But putting the words together, as in a poem, requires more than mere reading. It requires interpretation, the seeking of deeper meanings. Incorporating the factors of the face, the joints, the arch form, and the occlusion into the language of cephalometrics helps the diagnostician interpret the meaning of the entire diagnostic process in a manner in which it is most apt to reveal the true needs and significance of the pretreatment status of a case. Again, it becomes not only a matter of determining "what is" but more properly "what is significant." This represents the finest efforts at diagnosis and treatment planning. But with the importance of proper facial appearance, proper occlusal function, and proper joint function being what they are, truly it can be no other way.

"In Nature's infinite book of secrecy, a
little I can read."
Antony and Cleopatra I, vi
William Shakespeare

SECTION II
References

1. Witzig JW, Spahl TJ: *The Clinical Management of Basic Maxillofacial Orthopedic Appliances*. Littleton, MA, PSG Publishing Company, 1987, pp 264–266.
2. Rogers JH: Swallowing patterns of a normal population sample compared to those of patients from an orthodontic practice. *Am J Orthod* 1961;47:674–689.
3. Rosenblum RE: Orofacial muscle activity during deglutition as revealed by physiologic cinematography. *Angle Orthod* 1963;33:162–176.
4. Cleall, JF: Deglutition: A study of form and function. *Am J Orthod* 1965;51: 566–594.
5. Subtleny JD: Oral habits—Studies in form, function, and therapy. *Angle Orthod* 1973;43:347–383.
6. Ardan GM, Kemp AG: A radiographic study of movements of the tongue in swallowing. *Dent Pract* 1955;5:252–261.
7. Kydd WL, Neff CW: Frequency of deglutition of tongue thrusters compared to a sample population of normal swallowers. *J Dent Res* 1964;43:363–369.
8. Profitt WR: Equilibrium theory revisited: Factors influencing position of the teeth. *Angle Orthod* 1978;48:175–186.
9. Kydd WL: Maximum forces on the dentition by the perioral and lingual musculature. *J Am Dent Assoc* 1957;55:646–651.
10. Weinstein S, Haack DC, Morris LY, et al: An equilibrium theory of tooth position. *Angle Orthod* 1963;33:1–26.
11. Rogers AP: Exercises for developing the muscles of the face with a view to increasing their functional activity. *Dent Cosmos* 1918;60:857–876.
12. Rogers AP: Muscle training and its relation to orthodontia. *Int J Orthod* 1918;4:555–577.
13. Rogers AP: Making facial muscles our allies in treatment and retention. *Dent Cosmos* 1922;64:711–730.
14. Rogers AP: Living orthodontic appliances. *Int J Orthod* 1929;15:1–14.
15. Lear CSC, Flanagan JB, Moorrees CFA: The frequency of deglutition in man. *Arch Oral Biol* 1965;10:83–99.
16. Straub WJ: Malfunction of the tongue. Pt I. The abnormal swallowing habit: Its causes, effects, and results in relation to orthodontic treatment and speech therapy. *Angle Orthod* 1960;46:404–424.
17. Graber TM: The "Three M's": Muscle, malformation, and malocclusion. *Am J Orthod* 1963;49:418–450.
18. Kydd WL, Adamine JS, Mendel RA, et al: Tongue and lip forces exerted during deglutition in subjects with and without an anterior open bite. *J Dent Res* 1963;42:858–866.

19. Wildman AJ: Analysis of tongue, soft palate, and pharyngeal wall movement. *Am J Orthod* 1961;47:439–461.

20. Swindler DR, Sassouni V: Open bite and thumb sucking in rhesus monkeys. *Angle Orthod* 1962;32:27–37.

21. Graber TM: *Orthodontics: Principles and Practice*. Philadelphia, WB Saunders Co, 1961, pp 235–257.

22. Hitchcock HP: Preventative orthodontics. *Oral Health* 1977;6:19–28.

23. Baum L: Physiological tooth migration and its significance for the development of occlusion. *J Dent Res* 1950;29:123–132.

24. Brauer JC, et al: *Dentistry for Children*, ed 5. New York, McGraw-Hill Co, 1946, p 486.

25. Graber TM: *Orthodontics: Principles and Practice*. Philadelphia, WB Saunders Co, 1960, pp 77–79.

26. Luzi, V: The CV value in analysis of sagittal malocclusions. *Am J Orthod* 1982;81:478.

27. Moyers RE, et al: Differential diagnosis of Class II malocclusion. *Am J Orthod* 1980;78:477–494.

28. Gottlieb EL: A new look at Class II malocclusion. *J Clin Orthod* 1982;16: 571–572.

29. Riedel RA: An analysis of dentofacial relationships. *Am J Orthod* 1957;43: 103–119.

30. Peck H, Peck S: A concept of facial esthetics. *Angle Orthod* 1970;40:284–317.

INDEX

AB distance, 270–271, 284
A-B line, 144
Ac. *See* Acanthion
Acanthion, 5
Adams, Philip, 45
Adult dentition. *See* Permanent dentition
Adult skull, 6–7
AFH. *See* Anterior face height
Airway constriction, 228
AT, AT' length, 282
Al.P. *See* Prosthion
Alveolar bone stimulation, 55
Alveolar height, 271–272
Alveolar point (prosthion), 18
Alveolar process
  maxilla and, 71–72
  thrusting-type swallowing reflex and, 415
Alveolar surface of mandible, 77–78
Anatomical landmarks, 4–25
Anatomical P, 216
ANB angle
  Steiner analysis and, 153–157, 161
  Wits analysis and, 135–137
Andresen, Viggo, 272–273
Andrews, Larry, 315
Angle
  ANB
    Steiner analysis and, 153–157, 161
    Wits analysis and, 135–137
  anterior profile, 240
  basic; *See* Basic angle
  Bimler analysis and, 238–239
  of convexity, 143–144, 145
  cranial base, 318
  facial, 317
    Downs analysis and, 143
    Rickett's analysis and, 317
  incidental, 264–267
  interincisal, 159–160

lower
  basic. *See* Basic angle, lower
  incisal, 265, 267
  profile, 240–242
  mandibular plane, 79–80
    Downs analysis and, 144
    Frankfort's, 166
    Ricketts analysis and, 320
  maxillary incisor–palatal plane, 205
  N-S-Ar, 104
  profile, 242–244
    posterior, 123, 128, 244–251
  saddle, 104
  SNA, 306–307
  SND, 158–159
  upper
    basic. *See* Basic angle, upper
    profile, 240–242
  upper lip
    Bowbeer analysis and, 309–310
    Class II permanent dentition and, 522
    Sassouni plus and, 203
Angle, Edward, 131–133, 134
  cuspid classification of, 341
  dental definition of, 93
ANS. *See* Anterior nasal spine
ANS-Me
  Class II mixed dentition and, 484
  Sassouni analysis and, 178
ANS-Me LHF, 221–222
ANS-PNS, 175, 177
Antegonial notch, 5
Anterior arc, 177, 182
Anterior cranial base, 258–260
Anterior crossbite, 383–386
Anterior face height, 295
  Sassouni plus and, 188
Anterior incisor
  computer and, 344

Anterior incisor *(contd)*
  facial profile and, 295–296
Anterior nasal spine. *See also* ANS *entries*
  anterior arc and, 177, 182
  arc and, 177, 209
  Class II malocclusion and, 184
  definition of, 8
  maxilla size and, 178
  Sassouni plus and, 189, 190
  stability of, 88–89
Anterior open bite
  Class II mixed dentition urgency and,
    486–487
  myofunctional therapy and, 414
  timing of treatment and, 393–412
Anterior profile angle, 240
Anterior protrusion, 513–514
Anterior vertical dimension, 177
Anteroposterior dysplasia, 151, 152
Ap. *See* Apicale
Apicale, 8
  Bimler analysis and, 232
A-point, 8, 12
  stability of, 88–89
A-point retrusion, 573–574
Ar. *See* Articulare
Arc
  anterior, 177, 182
  anterior nasal spine, 177, 209
  basal, 177, 182
  midfacial, 177, 182
  posterior, 177, 183
Arch
  Bowbeer analysis and, 303
  computer preparation and positioning
    and, 343–344
  ideal versus actual, 346–347
  mesoprosopic facial type and, 120
  Sassouni analysis and, 173–186. *See also*
    Sassouni analysis
Arch length analysis, computerized,
  337–348
Arch perfecting, 557–558
Arch plot, 341
Arch-to-arch midline horizontal alignment,
  583–584
Articulare, 12–13
Auditory meatus, 216–217
Auxiliary esthetic plane, 360–361
Axis

facial, 317–318
stress, 252–258, 286–288

Backward growth, 80
Ba. *See* Basion
Basal arc, 177, 182
Base reference line, 92–93
Basic angle
  lower, 123, 125
    Bimler analysis and, 248
    dolichoprosopic facial type and, 128
  upper, 123–126
    Bimler analysis and, 246, 248
    dolichoprosopic facial type and, 128
Basion, 13
Bean, Merle, 299
Beistle, Richard, 186–213
Bicuspid
  Class I permanent dentition and, 472–473
  extracting of, 579
  longitudinal axis inclination and, 253–254
Bilateral posterior crossbite, 80
Bimaxillary protrusion, 578–580
Bimler, Hans Peter, 51–52
Bimler analysis, 230–293
  Class II mixed dentition and, 485
  Class II permanent dentition and, 521
  color code and, 235–239
  computer and, 328
  diagnostic interpretation and, 290–293
  factor analysis and, 240–262
  incidental angle and, 264–267
  linear measurement and, 268–272
  nomenclature and, 231–232
  orthogonal reference coordinate and,
    232–234
  ratio and, 272–273
  reference factor line and, 235
  Suborbital Facial Index and, 121, 123
  timing of treatment and, 407, 411
  tracing sheet and, 262–264
Bimler index, 122
Bio-facial matrix, 348–364
  Class III and, 588–589
Bionator
  anterior open bite and, 419
  Class II malocclusion and, 480–481
    division 2, 575–576
  individual teeth and, 583–584
  McNamara analysis and, 221–222

as retention, 591–592
timing of treatment and, 395–396
Bionator II, 520
Biprotrusion, 579–580
Bite, open. *See* Open bite
Bjork, Arne, 51
Bjork analysis, 170
    growth tendencies and, 557
Blumenbach's plane, 20
BNV. *See* Bowbeer Nasion Vertical
Bolton, Charles Bingham, 353
Bolton plane
    Broadbent registration point R and,
        98–99
    S-N resurgent and, 99–100
Bolton point, 13
Bone, 52–85
    formation of, 53–54
    maxillofacial complex and, 64–80
Bony overjet, 270–271, 284
Bony suture, 87–88
Bowbeer, Grant, 299
Bowbeer analysis, 299–316
    Class II permanent dentition and,
        521–522
Bowbeer Nasion Vertical, 307
BP. *See* Bolton point
B-point, 13
Brachycephalic facial type, 127, 128, 130
    Class II, division 1, permanent dentition
        and, 555–556
Brash, J. C., 74
Brehm utility arch
    Class I mixed dentition and, 429, 454
    Class II mixed dentition and, 489
Broadbent, B. Holly, 13
    sella nasion and, 86, 95
Broadbent registration point, 13,
    98–99
Broadbent serial growth study, 91
Broadbent-Bolton cephalometer, 35, 36
Broadbent-Bolton line, 20
Broca's line, 20
Brodie, Allen G., 38–39, 45
    constant facial pattern and, 92
    normative concept and, 108–109
    S-N resurgent and, 99–100
B-TM distance, 271
Buccal cortical plate, 58
Burstone, Charles, 298

C. *See* Capitulare
Calvarium, 55–56
Camper's line, 20
Campion, G., 35
Cant of occlusal plane, 144, 146
Capitulare, 13
    Bimler analysis and, 232
Capsular functional matrix, 83, 84
Capsule, orofacial, 84
Carey analysis, computerized, 337–338
Cartilage, formation of, 53–54
Cartilage-membrane bone, 56–64
CC point. *See* Center of cranium
CCC. *See* Color–coding
Cd. *See* Condylion
Center of cranium, 105
Centro-Masticale, 254
Centro-Masticale CM, 252, 288–289
Chaconas, S. J., 354
Chain, power, 473
Charles, S. W., 74
Chevron, 161
Chin button, 396, 415
Chin tissue plane, 360
Circle, Sassouni's, 164–167
Class I malocclusion, 422–478
    definition of, 131–132
    mesoprosopic facial type and, 120
    mixed dentition and, 423–455
    permanent dentition and, 455–478
Class II malocclusion, 479–584
    Bowbeer analysis and, 314
    definition of, 132
    division 1, 522–559
    mixed dentition, 481–514
        conventional treatment of, 487–514
        treatment goals, 485–486
    permanent dentition and, 514–584
        treatment and, 522–559
    Saussoni analysis and, 184
Class III malocclusion
    adult dentition and, 585–589
    Centro-Masticale CM and, 288
    definition of, 133
    Saussoni analysis and, 184
Clivion inferior, 232
Clivion superior, 232
Clivus, 14, 250
Closed bite
    Class I mixed dentition and, 454–455

Closed bite *(contd)*
  Saussoni analysis and, 184
Coben, S. E., 103
Coben's two-bone concept, 106–107
Color-coding, 235–239, 278–281, 283,
    285–286, 289–290
Computerized cephalometric analysis,
    316–348
  history of, 49–50
  R. Ricketts and, 105
Co. *See* Condylion
Concave profile, 245
Condyle
  cephalometrics and, 366
  condylion and, 14
  mandibular
    functional matrix theory and, 84–85
    growth and, 75–76
  Ricketts analysis and, 318, 320
Condylion, 14
Constancy of facial pattern, 109–110
Convexity, 245, 295–296
  Downs analysis and, 143–144, 145
  Ricketts analysis and, 318, 319
Coronoid process, 83
Correction versus development, 600–602
Correlative classification, 256
Correlometer, 238–239
Cortical bone of mandible, 58
Countenance, 294–299
Counter-condensation, 576–578
Cranial base
  anterior, 258–260
  bone growth and, 64–68
  flexure of, 110–111
  functional matrix theory and, 82
  Ricketts analysis and, 318
Cranial base to mandible relationship,
    227–229
Cranial base to maxilla relationship,
    216–219
Cranial component, functional, 83–84
Craniomaxillary bone, 103–105
Craniometrics, 33
Cranium, center of, 105
Cribriform plane, 101
Crossbite
  anterior, 383–386
  posterior

bilateral, 80
Class I mixed dentition and, 451–454
Class I permanent dentition and,
    463–466
Class II mixed dentition urgency and,
    487
Class II permanent dentition and, 537
timing of treatment and, 388–393
tongue thrust and, 418–421
Crowding
  Class I mixed dentition and, 426–428,
    431–454
  posterior crossbite and, 463–466
  Sassouni plus and, 211
  tongue and, 72–73
Crozat appliance
  Class I posterior crossbite and, 420–421
  Class I permanent dentition and, 467, 472
  Class II permanent dentition and, 536
  posterior crossbite and, 537
Curve of Spee, 253, 286
Cuspid, 472–473

DeCoster's line, 20
Dental arch. *See* Arch
Dental formula, Bimler's, 277–278
Dental midline deviation, 340
Dental versus skeletal resolution 580–583
Denture, 133
Depository bone, 58–59
Development
  correction versus, 600–602
  growth versus, 53
  McNamara analysis and, 229
Dewey, M. N., 34
Diagonal length of mandible, 271
Displacement
  primary, 59, 61
  secondary, 61
  superior posterior, of condyle, 137
    neuromuscular reflexive mandibular
    and, 501. *See also* Neuromuscular
    reflexive displacement of mandible
Distocclusion. *See* Class II malocclusion
Divine proportion, 171, 172–173
Dolichocephalic facial type, 129–130
  Class II permanent dentition and, 556
Dolichocran facial type, 125, 126, 127
Dolichoprosopic facial type, 130

Bimler analysis and, 267
Class II permanent dentition and, 555–556
Dorsum sellae, 14
Downs, William B., 41
Downs analysis, 41, 43, 44, 143–149
growth tendencies and, 557
Drift, 58
alveolar process and, 71–72
Ds. *See* Dorsum sellae
Dysplasia
anteroposterior, 151, 152
jaw, 130
leptoid, 292–293
microrhinic, 290–292
microtic, 292

Early adult dentition, Class II, 500
Early treatment, 381–383
Endosteal bone, 59
Enhancer, computer, 330–331
Enlow, D. H., 299–300
E-plane, 318
Esthetic line, 24
Esthetic plane
Bio-Facial Matrix and, 358–359
Ricketts analysis and, 318
Esthetics, facial, 294–299
Exercise
lip, 416
swallowing, 417
External auditory meatus, 216
Extraction
bicuspid, 579
second molar
Bowbeer analysis and, 299
Class I permanent dentition and, 467

Face height
anterior, 295
lower, 271
posterior, 177
Sassouni plus and, 188
Facial angle
Downs analysis and, 143
Ricketts analysis and, 317
Facial axis, 317
Facial esthetics, 294–299
Facial formula, Bimler's, 273–274
Facial index, suborbital, 283

Facial pattern constancy, 90–93
critics of, 109–110
Facial type, 118–131
Bimler tracing sheet and, 264
Class II permanent dentition and, 555–557
Factor analysis, Bimler, 240–262
Fan appliance
Class II permanent dentition and, 536
thumb-sucking and, 418
FH plane. *See* Frankfort horizontal plane
FH-P. *See* Frankfort horizontal plane,
porion and
Fibonacci sequence, 171
First molar, maxillary
Angle's classification and, 131–132
Sassouni plus and, 194–195
Fissure, pterygomaxillary, 18
Fixed appliance
retention and, 592
functional appliance versus, 602–606
FJO. *See* Functional jaw orthopedics
Flexure of cranial base, 66–67, 110–111
Forward–pulling headgear, 519, 573–574
Fossa, 318
Ricketts analysis and, 318
FPHG. *See* Forward-pulling headgear
Frankel appliance, 589
Frankfort horizontal plane, 20, 105–106
McNamara analysis and, 217
porion and, 93–94
Frankfort mandibular plane angle, 166
Frontal bone, 66
Functional versus fixed appliance, 602–606
Functional cranial component, 83–84
Functional jaw orthopedics
computer and, 328
history of, 26–52
Functional matrix, 81–85
Functional regulator III, 589

Garson index, 122
Gl. *See* Glabella
Glabella, 14
Gn. *See* Gnathion
Gnathic index, 274–277, 284–286
Gnathion, 14
Gnathostatics, 29
Go. *See* Gonion
Golden section, 169–170

Gonion, 14–15
  Bimler analysis and, 232, 266, 267
  Sassouni plus and, 200
Graber, T. M., 109
Gregory, W. K., 35
Grid for Bimler analysis
  facial typing, 264
  summation, 273–290
Growth
  backward, 80
  Broadbent serial study of, 91
  development versus, 53
  horizontal, 80, 111
    Class II permanent dentition and, 555
  McNamara analysis and, 228, 229
  prediction of, 111
  vertical, 80, 111
    Class II permanent dentition and,
      556
Growth center, 56–57
Growth direction indicator, 200
Growth proportionate template, 111–115
Growth site, 56
Gummy smile, 310–311

Half-Class II dental relationship, 489, 580
Harmony line, Holdaway, 23, 296–297
Hawley-type palatal retainer, 591
Head gear
  reverse, 207
  forward-pulling, 519, 573–574
Height, anterior face, 295
  Sassouni plus and, 188
Hellman, Milo, 31–32, 33, 294
Herron, 298
Higley, L. B., 39, 45
His' plane, 22
Hixon, E. H., 109
Hofrath, Herbert, 35
Holdaway harmony line, 23, 296–297
Horizontal grower, 80, 111
  Class II permanent dentition and, 555
Horizontal length
  maxillary, 269
  mandibular, 271
Horizontal plane, Frankfort, 20–22, 105–106
  with porion, 93–94
Horizontal total length, 271
Humphrey, G., 74

Hunter, John, 74
Huxley's line, 23–24
Hyperflexion, 276
Hypoflexion, 276

Ideal profile, 361
Identification grid, 264, 273–290
Identification line, 263
Image tracing landmark, 10
Incidental angle, 264–267
Incisal angle
  lower, 265, 267
  upper, 264–265
Incision inferius, 15
Incision superius, 15
Incisor
  anterior
    computer and, 344
    facial profile and, 295–296
  anterior lingual crossbite and, 383–386
  Class I permanent dentition and, 474
  mandibular
    McNamara analysis and, 224–227
    Sassouni plus and, 198
  maxillary
    Downs analysis and, 144–145
    McNamara analysis and, 223–224
    Sassouni plus and, 192–193
    Ricketts analysis and, 318
    Tweed's triangle and, 165
Incisor-palatal plane angle, 205
Infantile thrusting–type swallowing reflex,
  394
II. *See* Incision inferius
Integumental bone, 54–56
Interincisal angle
  Bimler analysis and, 267
  Steiner analysis and, 159–160
Internal auditory meatus, 216
IS. *See* Incision superius

Jacobson, Alex, 135, 142
Jaw dysplasia, 130
Joint, temporomandibular. *See* Temporo-
  mandibular joint

Kieth, A., 35
Kollmann index, 122
Krogman, W. M., 35, 45

Landmark
anatomical, 4–25
stability of, 85–101
Lateral cephalogram
golden section and, 172
relationships in, 117–118
Leptoid dysplasia, 292–293
Leptoprosopic facial type, 128, 130
Bimler analysis and, 267
Class II, division 1 and, 556
Class II, division 3 and, 578
LFH, McNamara analysis and, 220
Liddle, David, 299
Linder-Harth correction, 341
Line
Broadbent's 20
Broca's, 20
Camper's, 20
DeCoster's, 20
Huxley's, 23
Margolis, 24
Ramus, 24
reference factor, 235
Ricketts', 296–297
Steiner's, 296–297
Von Baer's, 24
Von Ihring's, 25
Linear measurement in Bimler analysis,
268–272, 282–286
Lingual cortical plate, 58
Lingual crossbite, 383–386
Lingual wire, 396
Lip
Bowbeer analysis and, 309
exercise for, 416
swallowing and, 415
Lip angle, upper
Bowbeer's analysis and, 307, 309–310
Class II permanent dentition and, 522
Sassouni plus and, 203
Lip puncture plane, 359–360
Locus O, 175, 176
Longitudinal axis inclination, 253–254
Lost E space, 488
Lower basic angle, 123, 125
Bimler analysis and, 248
dolichoprosopic facial type and, 128
Lower face height, 271
Lower incisal angle, 265, 267

Lower incisor, 318
Lower profile angle, 242–244
Luzi, V., 43
Lynn, Jack, 348–364
Lynn analysis
Class II permanent dentition and, 521,
522
Class III and, 588–589

Malocclusion. *See* Class I
malocclusion; Class II malocclusion;
Class III malocclusion
Mandible. *See also* Mandibular *entries*
advancement of
Class II, division 3 and, 579
computer and, 344
A-P position and, 303–305
bone growth and, 74–80
Bowbeer analysis and, 308
Coben's theory and, 103–105
condyle and, 84–85
cortical bone of, 58
development of, 56–64
diagonal length of, 271
landmark stability and, 89
length of
Bimler analysis and, 271
Wylie analysis and, 150
neuromuscular reflexive displacement of,
501
retrusion and. *See* Mandibular retrusion
Steiner analysis and, 155
Mandible to cranial base relationship,
227–229
Mandible to maxilla relationship, 219–223
Mandibular arch, 314
Mandibular incisor
McNamara analysis and, 224–227
Sassouni plus and, 198
Mandibular flexion, 260–262
Mandibular plane, 24
Bimler analysis and, 232, 246, 267
Downs analysis and, 144
mandibular incisor angle to, 144 144
Ricketts analysis and, 320
Sassouni analysis and, 175
Tweed's triangle and, 166
Mandibular retrusion
anterior open bite and, 419–420

Mandibular retrusion *(contd)*
  Class I versus Class II, 481
  Class II permanent dentition and, 561
  Sassouni plus and, 191
Margolis, H. I., 39
Margolis line, 24
Martin, Rudolph, 119
Matrix, functional, 81–85
Matrix value, 358
Maxilla. *See also* Maxillary *entries*
  bone growth and, 68–73
  Bowbeer analysis and, 306–307, 308
    A-P position and, 302–303
  correctness of, 43
  length of
    horizontal, 269
    projected, 282
  protrusion and
    McNamara analysis and, 217
    Sassouni plus and, 191
  retrusion of, 217
  Sassouni analysis and, 178
Maxilla to cranial base relationship, 216–219
Maxilla to mandible relationship, 219–223
Maxillary arch
  Bowbeer analysis and, 303
  ideal, 342
Maxillary incisor-palatal plane angle, 205
Maxillary plane
  anterior, 132
  Bimler analysis and, 246–251
  Sassouni analysis and, 174, 175
Maxillary tooth
  first molar and, 131–132
  incisor and, 223–224
  Downs analysis and, 144–145
  Sassouni plus and, 192–193
Maxillofacial complex, 64–80
Maxillofacial triangle analysis, 40–41
Maxillomandibular dental protrusion, 513–514
Maxillomandibular differential, 516–517
MC. *See* Mentalis crease
McNamara, James A., 50–51, 106
McNamara analysis, 214–230
  Class II mixed dentition and, 484
  Class II permanent dentition and, 516
    division 1, 536
  computer and, 328

growth and development and, 229–230
mandible to cranial base relationship and, 227–229
mandibular central incisor to mandible relationship, 224–227
maxilla to cranial base relationship and, 216–219
maxilla to mandible relationship and, 219–223
maxillary central incisor to maxilla relationship, 223–224
Membrane bone, 54–56
Mentalis crease, 303, 305, 307
Mentalis muscle, 396, 415
Mesethmoidal-frontal, 66
Mesial drift, 71–72
Mesioclusion. *See* Class III malocclusion
Mesofacial type, 130
Mesognathic, 148–149
Mesoprosopic facial type, 119, 130
  Bimler analysis and, 267
Microrhinic dysplasia, 290–292
Microskeletal unit, 81–82
Microtic dysplasia, 292
Midfacial arc, 177, 182
Mixed dentition
  Class I malocclusion and, 423–455
  Class II malocclusion and, 481–514
  computerized analysis and, 338–340
Molar
  computer analysis and, 341, 344
  mandibular growth and, 80
  maxillary first
    Angle's classification and, 131–132
    Sassouni plus and, 194–195
  posterior crossbite of, 388–393
  second. *See* Second molar
Molar tube, 473–474
Moore, A. W., 101–103
Morphogenesis, 53–54
Moss, Melvin, 81
Myofunctional therapy, 412–421
  timing of treatment and, 393–394
Myth of protruded maxilla, 43

N. *See* Nasion
Nasal airway, 84
Nasal dorsum/skeletal class relationship, 354
Nasal growth, 353–355

Nasal plane, 356
Nasal spine
  anterior. *See* Anterior nasal spine
  posterior
    definition of, 17
    Sassouni analysis and, 178
Nasal tip superior, 356
Nasion
  definition of, 15
  Bio-Facial Matrix and, 356
Nasion vertical, 299
Nasion-porion on Frankfort, 95
Nasion-sella–articulare, 306–307
Nasolabial point, 356
Neuromuscular reflexive displacement of
    mandible, 501
  NRDM/SPDC phenomenon, 553, 554
    Class II permanent dentition and, 561
    temporomandibular joint and, 562, 572
Neutroclusion, 131
No. *See* Antegonial notch
Nomenclature, 231–232
Norma lateralis
  anatomical landmarks of, 5–19
  lines and planes of, 20–25
Normative standard, 108
Nose, growth changes and, 353–355
NRDM. *See* Neuromuscular reflexive
    displacement of mandible
NRDM/SPDC phenomenon, 553, 554
  Class II permanent dentition and, 561
  temporomandibular joint and, 562, 572
N-S linear length, 271
N-S-Ar angle, 104
NV. *See* Nasion vertical

Obturated airway, 228
Occlusal plane, 24
  Downs analysis and, 144, 146
  Sassouni analysis and, 175
Op. *See* Opisthion
Open bite
  anterior
    Class II mixed dentition urgency and,
        486–487
    myofunctional therapy and, 414
    timing of treatment and, 393–412
  Sassouni analysis and, 183–184
Opisthion, 15

Optic plane, 178, 180
Or. *See* Orbitale
Orbital plane, 24
Orbital-canine law, 29, 32
Orioitale, 15
Orofacial capsule, 84
Orthognathic, 149
Orthogonal reference system, 232–234, 281,
    286
Overbite
  Class II malocclusion and, 132
  computer analysis and, 341
Overjet
  Bimler analysis and, 270–271, 284
  Class II mixed dentition and, 486
  computer analysis and, 341

P. *See* Pogonion; Porion
Pacini, A. J., 33–34
Palatal plane, 22
  Bimler analysis and, 246–251
  Sassouni analysis and, 175
Palatal retainer, 591
Palate, 69–70
Parallel plane, 174, 175
Pattern, facial, 90–93
Periosteal bone, 59
Periosteal functional matrix, 83
Permanent dentition
  Class I malocclusion and, 455–478
  Class II malocclusion and, 514–584
    division 1, 522–559
    division 2, 559–578
    early, 500
  Class III malocclusion and, 585–589
  crowded, 463–466
Pharyngeal airway, 84
Pharynx, 228
Pg. *See* Pogonion
Plane
  Blumenbach's, 20
  Downs analysis and, 144, 146
  Frankfort horizontal, 20–22
    McNamara analysis and, 217
    with porion, 93–94
  His', 22
  lip puncture, 359–360
  mandibular. *See* Mandibular plane
  occlusal

Plane (contd)
  definition of, 24
    Downs analysis and, 144, 146
    Sassouni analysis and, 175
  orbital, 24
  Sassouni analysis and, 174, 175
Plane angle, mandibular, 79–80
  Downs analysis and, 144
  Tweed's triangle and, 166
Plane inclination, palatal maxillary, 246–251
PNS. See Posterior nasal spine
Po. See Pogonion
Pog. See Pogonion
Pogonion
  definition of, 15
  Sassouni plus and, 189, 190
Pont's analysis
  Class II permanent dentition and, 523–524
  computer analysis and, 341
Porion, 15–16, 89–90
  Frankfort horizontal with, 94
Porion-nasion on Frankfort parallel, 94
Positional analysis, 29–30
Posterior arc, 177, 183
Posterior crossbite
  bilateral, 80
  Class I mixed dentition and, 451–454
  Class I permanent dentition and, 463–466
  Class II mixed dentition and, 487
  Class II permanent dentition and, 537
  timing of treatment and, 388–393
  tongue thrust and, 418–421
Posterior face height ratio, 188
Posterior nasal spine
  definition of, 17
  Sassouni analysis and, 178
Posterior profile angle, 123
  Bimler analysis and, 244–251
  dolichoprosopic facial type and, 128
Posterior vertical dimension, 178
Posttreatment conference, 594–596
Power chain, 473
Premaxilla
  bone growth and, 70
  Class II mixed dentition and, 512
  mesial drift and, 72
Primary displacement, 59, 61
Profile
  Lynn analysis and, 361

types of, 245
Profile angle, posterior
  Bimler analysis and, 244–251
  dolichoprosopic facial type and, 128
Prognathic, 149
Projected length of maxilla, 282
Prosthion, 18
Protrusion
  anterior, 513–514
  bimaxillary, 578–580
  maxillary
    myth of, 43
    Sassouni plus and, 191
  maxillomandibular dental, 513–514
  premaxillary, 512
Pterygomaxillary fissure, 18
Puncture plane, lip, 359–360
Pupil of eye, 356

Ramus
  bone growth and, 76–77
  growth and development of, 59
  stress and, 56
Ramus line, 24
Rapid palatal expander, 537
Ratio
  Bimler's, 272–273
  golden section and, 169–170
  posterior face height, 188
Rectangular wire
  Class I permanent dentition and, 473
  Class III, 588
Reference factor line, 235
Reflex, swallow, 394
Reflexive displacement, neuromuscular
    mandibular, 501
Registration point R, Broadbent, 98–99
Reidel, Richard A., 42–43
Relocation versus displacement, 61, 63
Remodeling, 69
Removable acrylic plate, 383–386
Resorption, bone, 57–58
Resorptive field, 77
Retention, 590–594
Retrognathic, 149
Retrusion
  mandibular
    anterior open bite and, 419–420
    Class I versus Class II, 481

Class II permanent dentition and, 561
  Sassouni plus and, 191
maxillary skeletal, 217
Reverse head gear, 207
Ricketts, Robert M., 47–48, 48–49, 105,
    115, 168–169, 316–323
Ricketts analysis
  esthetic line and, 24
  golden section and, 172
  growth tendencies and, 557
Riesner, S., 34
RMDS. *See* Rocky Mountain Data Systems
Rocky Mountain Data Systems, 322
Roentgenocephalometrics, 4
  growth prediction and, 92–93
  history of, 33–52
  purpose of, 117
Rotation, mandibular, 78–80
Round wire, 588

Saddle angle, 104
Sagittal appliance
  Class II
    division 1, permanent dentition and,
      543, 552, 554
    division 2, 559
    permanent dentition and, 573, 576
  as retention, 591
  reversed head gear and, 207
Sagittal I appliance
  Class II, division 3, permanent dentition
    and, 582
  timing of treatment and, 401
Sagittal II appliance
  Class II mixed dentition and, 429
  timing of treatment and, 396
Saller, Karl, 119
Salzmann, J. A., 45, 47
Sassouni, Viken, 50–51
Sassouni analysis, 173–186
  Class II mixed dentition and, 484–485
  Class II permanent dentition and,
    517–518, 518–519, 520–521
    division 1, permanent dentition and,
      552
  interpretation of, 180–186
Sassouni plus, 186–213
  growth direction indicator, 200–203
  mandibular A-P length and, 195–196

mandibular A-P position and, 196–197
  mandibular incisor position and, 197
  maxillary A-P position and, 193–194
  maxillary first permanent molar position
    and, 194
  maxillary incisor position and, 192–193
  skeletal A-P alignment and, 189–191
  skeletal vertical dimension and, 191–192
  upper lip angle and, 203–213
Sassouni split-gonial-angle evaluation, 557
Sassouni's circles, 164–167
Schudy, F. F., 295
Schwartz, Rudolf, 27, 29
Schwartz computerized analysis, 333–337
  Class II permanent dentition and, 523–524
    division 1, 536
Schwartz plate
  maxillomandibular protrusion and, 513
  posterior crossbite and, 389
    adult Class I, 420–421
  tongue thrusting and, 417–418
Second molar
  extraction
    Bowbeer analysis and, 299
    Class I permanent dentition and, 467
  premature loss of, 488
Secondary displacement, 61
Sella, 18
  stability of, 86
Sella-nasion reference line, 95, 97
  Bimler analysis and, 258
  Brodie's, 99–100
  stability of, 86–88
  Steiner analysis and, 161
Serial growth study, Broadbent, 91
Simon, P., 29–33
Simpson, C. O., 34
Skeletal retrusion, 217
Skeletal unit, 81–82
Skeletal vertical dimension, 191
Skeletal versus dental resolution, 580–583
Skull shape, 126
  adult, 6–7
S-line, 296–297
  Steiner analysis and, 158
Smile, gummy, 310–311
Smith, D. D., 324–348
Smith, Norman, 324–348
S-N. *See* Sella-nasion reference line

SNA angle, 306–307
SND angle, 158–159
Soft tissue nasion, 356
Space, functioning, 83
Space maintenance, 345
Spee's curve, 253, 286
Sphenomesethmoidal synchondrosis, 66
Spheno-occipital synchondrosis, 19
  bone growth and, 66
  growth at, 104
Spine, nasal
  anterior. See Anterior nasal spine
  posterior
    definition of, 17
    Sassouni analysis and, 178
Split-gonial-angle evaluation, 557
Spring retainer, 592–593
Standard, normative, 108
Steiner, Cecil, 44
Steiner analysis, 44, 153–164
  color coding and, 236–237
  computer and, 328
  timing of treatment and, 405, 409
  Wits analysis versus, 139
Steiner line, 296–297
Straight profile, 245
Straight wire appliance
  Class II permanent dentition and, 524
  pseudo-dental Class II and, 512
Straight wire utility arch, 489
Stress axis, 252–258, 286–288
Subnasion, 19
Suborbital Facial Index, 121, 123
  Bimler analysis and, 281–282, 283
  determination of, 130–131
  growth tendencies and, 557
Subspinale, 8, 12
Subtleny, J. D., 353
Summation grid, 273–290
  Bimler tracing sheet and, 264
Superior posterior displacement of condyle,
    137
  NRDM/SPDC phenomenon and, 553, 554
    Class II permanent dentition and, 561
    temporomandibular joint and, 562, 572
Supramentale, 13
Supraorbital plane, 174, 175
Surgery, 345
Suture, bony, 87–88

SWA, Class II permanent dentition and
  division 1, 557–558
  division 2, 576–577
Swallowing
  myofunctional therapy and, 413–421
  thrusting-type, 394
Synchondrosis
  sphenomesethmoidal, 66
  spheno-occipital, 19
    growth at, 104

Template, growth proportionate, 111–115
Temporalis muscle, 83
Temporomandibular joint
  Bowbeer analysis and, 312
  cephalometrics and, 366
  Class II, division 2 and, 560, 562, 572
  Class II, division 3 and, 578
  Class II mixed dentition and, 501
  Class III, 588
  computer analysis and, 345
  fixed versus functional, 603–604
  growth of, 57
  neuromuscular reflexive mandibular
    displacement and, 562, 572
  posterior crossbite of, 388
  Ricketts analysis and, 323
  Sassouni plus and, 208–209, 210, 213
Thompson, J. R., 42
TMJ. See Temporomandibular joint
Todd, T. Wingate, 95
Tongue, 511
Tongue thrust, 393–412
Tooth bed development, 55
Topogenesis, 53
Trabecular structure, 54
Tracing sheet, Bimler, 262–264
Transformation, bone, 54
Transitional dentition analysis,
    computerized, 340
Translation, 59
Transverse appliance
  Class I mixed dentition and, 453
  posterior crossbite and, 389
Treatment-planning output, 342–348
Triangle, Tweed's, 39, 164–167
Triangle analysis, maxillofacial, 40–41
Truitt, J. W., 417, 323
Trutains, 593–594

T-TM measurement, 268–269, 270, 282–283
Tube, molar, 473–474
Tuberculum sellae, 19
Tweed, Charles, 39
Tweed's triangle, 39, 164–167
Two-bone concept, 103–104, 106–107
Typing grid, facial, 264

ULA. *See* Upper lip angle
Upper basic angle, 123–126
  Bimler analysis and, 246, 248
  dolichoprosopic facial type and, 128
Upper incisal angle, 264–265
Upper lip angle
  Bowbeer analysis and, 307, 309–310
  Class II permanent dentition and, 522
  Sassouni plus and, 203, 203–213
Upper profile angle, 240–242
Upper transverse appliance, 510–511
Urgent treatment, 381–383
  Class II mixed dentition, 486–487

Van Loon, J. A. W., 27
Vertical dimension
  Bowbeer analysis and, 305–306
  Sassouni analysis and, 178

anterior, 177
skeletal, 191
posterior, 178
Vertical grower, 80, 111
  Class II permanent dentition and, 556
Von Baer's line, 24
von Garson, Vorschlag, 119–120
Von Ihering's line, 25

Wigglegram, 185, 186
Wire
  rectangular
    Class I permanent dentition and, 473
    Class III, 588
  round, 588
  straight. *See* Straight wire *entries*
  tongue-restraining, 396
Wits analysis, 133–143, 483
Wylie, Wendell, 40
Wylie analysis, 149–152

XY-axis, 317–318

Y-axis, 25
  McNamara analysis and, 228
Yerkes, Ira, 299